INSTRUCTOR'S RESOURCE MANUAL FOR

OLDS' MATERNAL-NEWBORN NURSING & WOMEN'S HEALTH ACROSS THE LIFESPAN

EIGHTH EDITION

Anne M. Krouse
Pam Hamre

Instructor's Resource Manual for

Olds' Maternal-Newborn Nursing & Women's Health Across the Lifespan

Eighth Edition

Michele R. Davidson, PhD, CNM, CFN, RN
ASSOCIATE PROFESSOR OF NURSING AND WOMEN'S STUDIES,
GEORGE MASON UNIVERSITY, FAIRFAX, VIRGINIA, STAFF MIDWIFE WOMEN'S
HEALTHCARE ASSOCIATES, LANSDOWNE, VIRGINIA

Marcia L. London, RNC, MSN, APRN, CNS, NNP
SENIOR CLINICAL INSTRUCTOR AND DIRECTOR OF NEONATAL NURSE
PRACTITIONER PROGRAM, BETH-EL COLLEGE OF NURSING AND HEALTH
SCIENCES, UNIVERSITY OF COLORADO, COLORADO SPRINGS, COLORADO,
STAFF CLINICAL NURSE, URGENT CARE AND AFTER HOURS CLINIC, COLORADO
SPRINGS, COLORADO

Patricia A. Wieland Ladewig, PhD, RN
PROFESSOR AND ACADEMIC DEAN, RUECKERT-HARTMAN SCHOOL FOR HEALTH
PROFESSIONS, REGIS UNIVERSITY, DENVER, COLORADO

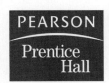

PEARSON
Prentice
Hall

Upper Saddle River, New Jersey 07458

Publisher: Julie Levin Alexander
Assistant to Publisher: Regina Bruno
Editor-in-Chief: Maura Connor
Executive Acquisitions Editor: Pamela Lappies
Associate Editor: Michael Giacobbe
Managing Editor, Development: Marilyn Meserve
Editorial Art Manager: Patrick Watson
Media Product Manager: John J. Jordon
Director of Marketing: Karen Allman
Senior Marketing Manager: Francisco del Castillo
Marketing Specialist: Michael Sirinides
Managing Editor, Production: Patrick Walsh
Production Editor: Heather Willison, Carlisle Publishing Services
Production Liaison: Anne Garcia
Media Project Manager: Stephen Hartner
Manufacturing Manager: Ilene Sanford
Manufacturing Buyer: Ilene Sanford
Senior Design Coordinator: Maria Guglielmo
Printer/Binder: Bind-Rite Graphics
Composition: Carlisle Publishing Services
Inteior Design: Rae Grant
Cover Design: Cheryl Asherman
Cover Illustration: *Kaleidoscopic VIII: The Sun, the Moon . . . and the Stars.* A quilt designed and made by Paula Nadelstern, copyright 1991
Cover Printer: Phoenix Color

Pearson Education Ltd.
Pearson Education Singapore, Pte. Ltd.
Pearson Education Canada, Ltd.
Pearson Education—Japan
Pearson Education Australia PTY, Limited

Pearson Education North Asia Ltd.
Pearson Educación de Mexico, S.A. de C.V.
Pearson Education Malaysia, Pte. Ltd.
Pearson Education Inc., Upper Saddle River, New Jersey

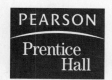

10 9 8 7 6 5 4 3 2 1
ISBN-13: 978-0-13-156799-3
ISBN: 0-13-156799-3

CONTENTS

PREFACE

Nurses play a central role in all aspects of the childbearing experience, from the earliest days of pregnancy, through the moments of birth, and during the early days of parenthood. ***Olds' Maternal-Newborn Nursing & Women's Health Across the Lifespan,*** Eighth Edition, was written to help students develop the skills and abilities they need now and in the future in an ever-changing healthcare environment. This accompanying **Instructor's Resource Manual** is designed to support your teaching in this stepped-up environment, and to reduce your preparation time for class. It will help you provide an optimal learning experience for your students and their many learning needs.

Each chapter in the **Instructor's Resource Manual** is thoroughly integrated with the corresponding chapter in the textbook ***Olds' Maternal-Newborn Nursing & Women's Health Across the Lifespan,*** Eighth Edition. Chapters are organized by objectives, and the teaching unit flows from these objectives. You will find the following features to support them:

- The **Concepts for Lecture** in this manual may be used in their entirety for class presentation or they may be merged with the classroom activities for a mixture of teaching styles that will meet the needs of students with various learning styles.

- The **Lecture Outlines** can be found on your Instructor's Resource DVD-ROM in PowerPoint. The number in the slide icon ▯ refers to the Concept for Lecture to which the slide correlates. Some lecture concepts have more than one slide, in which cases the slide icon will contain a letter after the Concept for Lecture number.

- **Suggestions for Classroom and Clinical Experiences** attempt to go beyond the traditional activities that have been the mainstay of nursing education for many years.

- The **Resource Library** identifies for you—the instructor—all the specific media resources and activities available for that chapter on the Prentice Hall Nursing MediaLink DVD-ROM, Companion Website, and Instructor's Resource DVD-ROM. Chapter by chapter, the Resource Library helps you decide what resources from the Prentice Hall Nursing MediaLink DVD-ROM, Companion Website, and Instructor's Resource DVD-ROM to use to enhance your course and your students' ability to apply concepts from the book into practice.

This **Instructor's Resource Manual** also contains a brand new "Strategies for Success" module written by Sandra DeYoung. Included within are Learning Theories,

Planning for Instruction, How to Use Effective Pedagogies, Assessing Learning, and more! There is also a guide on "Teaching Nursing to Students Who Speak English as a Nonnative Language." This tool is intended to guide you in reaching across cultural barriers to train nurses.

Finally, the following additional resources are also available to accompany this textbook. For more information or sample copies, please contact your Prentice Hall Sales Representative.

- **Prentice Hall Nursing MediaLink DVD-ROM—** This DVD-ROM is packaged with the textbook. It provides an interactive study program that allows students to practice answering NCLEX®-style questions with rationales for right and wrong answers. It also contains an audio glossary, animations and video tutorials, and a link to the Companion Website (an Internet connection is required). *Note: Prentice Hall Nursing MediaLink CD-ROM version is available for purchase on www.MyPearsonStore.com*

- **Companion Website** www.prenhall.com/Davidson— This on-line study guide is designed to help students apply the concepts presented in the book. Each chapter specific module features Objectives, NCLEX® Review Questions with rationales, Chapter Outlines for lecture notes, Case Studies, Critical Thinking Exercises, WebLinks, Audio Glossary, and more.

- **MyNursingLab to accompany** *Olds' Maternal-Newborn Nursing & Women's Health Across the Lifespan* (ISBN: 0-13-159647-0) is a user-friendly site that gives students the opportunity to test themselves on key concepts and skills. By using *MyNursingLab,* students can track their own progress through the course and use customized, media-rich, study plan activities to help them achieve success in the classroom, in clinical, and ultimately on the NCLEX-RN®. **MyNursingLab** can also help you, the instructor, monitor class progress as students move through the curriculum.

- **Workbook to Accompany** *Olds' Maternal-Newborn Nursing & Women's Health Across the Lifespan* (ISBN: 0-13-240149-5)—This workbook incorporates strategies for students to focus their study and increase comprehension of concepts of nursing care. It contains a variety of activities such as multiple choice, fill-in-the-blank, case studies, and more.

- **Clinical Handbook for Maternal-Newborn Nursing & Women's Health Across the Lifespan** (ISBN: 0-13-232441-5)—This pocket guide serves as a portable, quick-reference to maternal-newborn nursing care. Covering from pregnancy through the postpartum and newborn stages, this handbook allows students to take the information they learn in class into any clinical setting.

- **Instructor's Resource DVD-ROM** (ISBN: 0-13-225233-3)—This cross-platform DVD-ROM provides text slides and illustrations in PowerPoint for use in classroom lectures. It also contains an electronic test bank, animations, and video clips from the Prentice Hall Nursing MediaLink DVD-ROM, and question-and-answer slides for Classroom Response Systems. This supplement is available to faculty upon adoption of the textbook. *Note: Instructor's Resource CD-ROM also available upon request.*

It is our hope that the information provided in this manual will decrease the time it takes you to prepare for class and will optimize the learning experience for your students.

TEACHING NURSING TO STUDENTS WHO SPEAK ENGLISH AS A NONNATIVE LANGUAGE

We are fortunate to have so many multinational and multilingual nursing students in the United States in the 21st century. As our classrooms become more diverse, there are additional challenges to communication, but we in the nursing education community are ready. Our goal is to educate competent and caring nurses to serve the health needs of our diverse communities.

We know that English as a nonnative language (ENNL) students experience higher attrition rates than their native English-speaking counterparts. This is a complex problem. However, there are teaching strategies that have helped many students be successful.

The first step toward developing success strategies is understanding language proficiency. Language proficiency has four interdependent components. Each component is pertinent to nursing education. *Reading* is the first aspect of language. Any nursing student will tell you that there are volumes to read in nursing education. Even native speakers of English find the reading load heavy. People tend to read more slowly in their nonnative language. They also tend to recall less. Nonnative speakers often spend inordinate amounts of time on reading assignments. These students also tend to take longer to process exam questions.

Listening is the second component of language. Learning from lectures can be challenging. Some students are more proficient at reading English than at listening to it. It is not uncommon for ENNL students to understand medical terminology, but to become confused by social references, slang, or idiomatic expressions used in class. The spoken language of the teacher may be different in accent or even vocabulary from that experienced by immigrant students in their language education. ENNL students may not even hear certain sounds that are not present in their native languages. Words such as *amoxicillin* and *ampicillin* may sound the same. Asian languages do not have gender-specific personal pronouns (he, she, him, her, etc.). Asian students may become confused when the teacher is describing a case study involving people of different genders.

Speaking is the third component of language proficiency. People who speak with an accent are often self-conscious about it. They may hesitate to voice their questions or to engage in discussion. Vicious cycles of self-defeating behavior can occur in which a student hesitates to speak, resulting in decreased speaking skills, which results in more hesitation to speak. Students may develop sufficient anxiety about speaking that their academic outcomes are affected. Students tend to form study groups with others who have common first languages.

Opportunities to practice English are therefore reduced, and communication errors are perpetuated. When the teacher divides students into small groups for projects, ENNL students often do not participate as much as others. If these students are anxious about speaking, they may withdraw from classroom participation. ENNL students may feel rejected by other students in a small-group situation when their input is not sought or understood.

The fourth aspect of language is *writing*. Spelling and syntax errors are common when writing in a nonnative language. Teachers often respond to student writing assignments with feedback that is too vague to provide a basis for correction or improvement by ENNL students. When it comes to writing lecture notes, these students are at risk of missing important details because they may not pick up the teacher's cues about what is important. They might miss information when they spend extra time translating a word or concept to understand it, or they might just take more time to write what is being said.

Another major issue faced by ENNL nursing students is the culture of the learning environment. International students were often educated in settings where students took a passive role in the classroom. They may have learned that faculty are to be respected, not questioned. Memorization of facts may have been emphasized. It may be a shock to them when the nursing faculty expect assertive students who ask questions and think critically. These expectations cannot be achieved unless students understand them.

Finally, the European American culture, which forms the context for nursing practice, creates challenges. Because they are immersed in European American culture and the culture of nursing, faculty may not see the potential sources of misunderstanding. For example, if a teacher writes a test question about what foods are allowed on a soft diet, a student who understands therapeutic diets may miss the question if he or she does not recognize the names of the food choices. Nursing issues with especially high culture connection include food, behavior, law, ethics, parenting, games, or choosing the right thing to say. These topics are well represented in psychiatric nursing, which makes it a difficult subject for ENNL students.

MINIMIZING CULTURE BIAS ON NURSING EXAMS

Our goal is not to eliminate culture from nursing or from nursing education. Nursing exists in a culture-dependent context. Our goal is to practice transcultural nursing and to teach nursing without undue culture bias.

Sometimes our nursing exam questions will relate to culture-based expectations for nursing action. The way to make these questions fair is to teach transcultural nursing and to clarify the cultural expectations of a nursing student in the European-American-dominated healthcare system. Students must learn the cultural aspects of the profession before they can practice appropriately within it. Like other cultures, the professional culture of nursing has its own language (for example, medical terminology and nursing diagnoses). We have our own accepted way of dress and our own implements, skills, taboos, celebrations, and behavior. The values accepted by our culture are delineated in the American Nurses Association Code of Ethics, and are passed down to our students during nursing education.

It is usually clear to nursing educators that students are not initially aware of all the aspects of the professional culture, and that these must be taught. The social context of nursing seems more obvious to educators, and is often overlooked in nursing education. Some aspects of the social context of nursing were mentioned above (food, games, social activities, relationships, behavior, what to say in certain situations). Students must also learn these social behaviors and attitudes if they are to function fully in nursing. If they do not already know about American hospital foods, what to say when someone dies, how to communicate with an authority figure, or what game to play with a 5-year-old child, they must learn these things in nursing school.

Try for yourself the following test. It was written without teaching you the cultural expectations first.

CULTURE-BIASED TEST

1. Following radiation therapy, an African American client has been told to avoid using her usual hair care product due to its petroleum content. Which product should the nurse recommend that she use instead?
   A. Royal Crown hair treatment
   B. Dax Wave and Curl
   C. Long Aid Curl Activator Gel
   D. Wave Pomade

2. A Jewish client is hospitalized for pregnancy-induced hypertension during Yom Kippur. How should the nurse help this client meet her religious needs based on the tradition of this holy day?
   A. Order meals without meat-milk combinations.
   B. Ask a family member to bring a serving of *Marror* for the client.
   C. Encourage her to fast from sunrise to sunset.
   D. Remind her that she is exempt from fasting.

3. Based on the Puerto Rican concept of *compadrazco*, who is considered part of the immediate family and responsible for care of children?
   A. Parents, grandparents, aunts, uncles, cousins, and godparents
   B. Mother, father, and older siblings

C. Mother, father, and any blood relative
D. Parents and chosen friends (*compadres*) who are given the honor of child care responsibility

4. A 60-year-old Vietnamese immigrant client on a general diet is awake at 11 p.m. on a summer night. What is the best choice of food for the nurse to offer to this client?
   A. Warm milk
   B. Hot tea
   C. Ice cream
   D. Iced tea

5. Which of the following positions is contraindicated for a client recovering from a total hip replacement?
   A. Side-lying using an abductor pillow
   B. Standing
   C. Walking to the restroom using a walker
   D. Sitting in a low recliner

When you took this test, did it seem unfair? It was intended to test nursing behaviors that were based on culture-specific situations. Your immigrant and ENNL students are likely to face questions like these on every exam.

Question 1 is about hair care products for black hair. Option C is the only one that does not contain petroleum. Students could know this, if they were given the information before the exam. Otherwise the question is culture-biased.

Question 2 is about the Jewish holiday Yom Kippur. To celebrate this holiday, it is customary to fast from sunrise to sunset, but people who are sick, such as the client in the question, are exempted from fasting. This question is only unfair if students did not have access to the information.

Question 3 expects you to know about *compadrazco*, in which parents, grandparents, aunts, uncles, cousins, and godparents are all considered immediate family. This can be an important point if you are responsible for visiting policies in a pediatrics unit.

Question 4 tests knowledge about the preferred drink for an immigrant Vietnamese client. Many people in Asia feel comforted by hot drinks and find cold drinks to be unsettling.

Question 5 does not seem so biased. If you understand total hip precautions, it is a pretty simple question, unless you have never heard of a "low recliner." An ENNL student who missed this question said, "I saw the chairs in clinical called 'geri chairs' and I know that the client cannot bend more than 90 degrees, but 'low recliner' was confusing to me. I imagined someone lying down (reclining) and I think this would not dislocate the prosthesis."

The best way to avoid culture bias on exams is to know what you are testing. It is acceptable to test about hip precautions, but not really fair to test about the names of furniture. The same is true of foods. Test about therapeutic diets, but not about the recipes (an African immigrant student advised us to say "egg-based food" instead of "custard").

Behavior in social and professional situations is especially culture-bound. Behavior-based questions are common on nursing exams. Make behavior expectations explicit. Especially when a student is expected to act in a way that would be inappropriate in his or her social culture, these are very difficult questions. For example, we expect nurses to act assertively with physicians and clients. It is inappropriate for many Asian students to question their elders. When a client is their elder, these students will choose the option that preserves respect for the client over one that provides teaching. We must make our expectations very clear.

Finally, talk with your ENNL and immigrant students after your exams. They can provide a wealth of information about what confused them or what was ambiguous. Discuss your findings with your colleagues and improve your exams. Ultimately your exams will be clearer and more valid.

The following strategies were developed originally to help ENNL students. An interesting revelation is that they also help native English speakers who have learning styles that are not conducive to learning by lecture, who read slowly, or who have learning disabilities or other academic challenges.

STRATEGIES FOR PROMOTING ENNL STUDENT SUCCESS

1. You cannot decrease the reading assignment because some students read slowly, but you can help students prioritize the most important areas.
2. Allow adequate time for testing. The NCLEX is not a 1-minute-per-question test anymore. Usually 1.5 hours is adequate for a 50-item multiple-choice exam.
3. Allow students to tape lectures if they want to. You might have lectures audiotaped and put in the library for student access.
4. Speak clearly. Mumbling and rapid anxious speech are difficult to understand. If you have a problem with clarity, provide handouts containing the critical points. You want to teach and test nursing knowledge, not note-taking skills.
5. Avoid slang and idiomatic expressions. This is hard to do, but you can do it with practice. When you do use slang, explain it. This is especially important on exams. When in doubt about whether a word is confusing, think about what the dictionary definition would be. If there are two meanings, use another word.
6. Allow the use of translation dictionaries on exams. You can stipulate that students must tell you what they are looking up, so they cannot find medical terminology that is part of the test.
7. Be aware of cultural issues when you are writing exams. Of course you will test on culture-specific issues, but be sure you are testing what you want to test (e.g., the student's knowledge of diets, not of recipes).
8. Feel free to use medical terminology. After all, this is nursing school. However, when you use an important new term, write it on the board so students can spell it correctly in their notes.

9. In clinical, make the implied explicit. It seems obvious that safety is the priority. However, if a student thinks the priority is respecting her elders, there could be a disaster when a client with a new hip replacement demands to get out of bed.
10. Hire a student who takes clear and accurate lecture notes to post his or her notes for use by ENNL and other students. The students will still attend class and take their own notes, but will have this resource to fill in the details that they miss.
11. SOA (spell out abbreviations).
12. Many international students learned to speak English in the British style. If something would be confusing to a British person, they will find it confusing.
13. Provide opportunities for students to discuss what they are learning with other students and faculty. A faculty member might hold a weekly discussion group where students bring questions. It can be interesting to find a student having no trouble tracing the path of a red cell from the heart to the portal vein, but having difficulty understanding what cream of wheat is ("I thought it was a stalk of grain in a bowl with cream poured on it").
14. Make it clear that questions are encouraged. If you think a student who is not asking questions may not understand, ask the student after class if he or she has questions. Make it easier for students to approach you by being approachable. Learn their names, and learn to pronounce them correctly. Hearing you try to pronounce their names might be humorous for them, and it will validate how difficult it is to speak other languages.
15. Take another look at basing grades on class participation. You may be putting inordinate demands on the ENNL students. Of course nurses must learn to work with others, but the nurse who talks most is not necessarily the best.
16. Be a role model for communication skills. You might even say in class when you talk about communication that if you respect a person who is trying to communicate with you, you will persist until you understand the message. Say, "Please repeat that," or "I think you said to put a chicken on my head, is that correct?" or "You want me to do what with the textbook?" It may be considered socially rude to ask people to repeat themselves. Make it clear that this is not a social situation. In the professional role, we are responsible for effective communication. We cannot get away with smiling and nodding our heads.
17. In clinical, if a student has an accent that is difficult for the staff to understand, discuss clarification techniques (#16 above) with the student and staff member. Make it explicit that it is acceptable for the student to ask questions and for the staff to ask for clarification.
18. If your college has a writing center where students can receive feedback on grammar and style before submitting papers, have students use it. If you are not so fortunate, view papers as a rough draft instead of

a final product. Give specific feedback about what to correct and allow students to resubmit.

19. Make any services that are available to ENNL students available to all students (such as group discussions and notes). These services may meet the learning needs of many students while preventing the attitude that "they are different and they get something I don't."

20. Faculty attitudes are the most important determinant of a successful program to promote the success of ENNL nursing students. Talk with other faculty about the controversial issues. Create an organized program with a consistent approach among the faculty. The rewards will be well worth the work.

STRATEGIES FOR SUCCESS

Sandra DeYoung, EdD, RN
William Paterson University
Wayne, New Jersey

IMPROVING OUR TEACHING

Every faculty member wants to be a good teacher, and every teacher wants the students to learn. In particular, we want to achieve the student learning outcomes that our educational institutions say we must achieve. How can we best meet both goals? We cannot just teach as we were taught. We have to learn a variety of teaching methods and investigate best practices in pedagogy. We also have to learn how to measure student learning outcomes in practical and efficient ways. The next few pages will introduce you to principles of good teaching and ways to evaluate learning. Keep in mind that this is only an introduction. For a more extensive study of these principles and pedagogies, you might consult the resources listed at the end of this introduction.

LEARNING THEORY

In order to improve our teaching, we must have some familiarity with learning theory. Nurses who come into educational roles without psychology of learning courses in their background should read at least an introductory-level book on learning theories. You should, for example, know something about stages and types of learning, how information is stored in memory and how it is retrieved, and how knowledge is transferred from one situation to another.

BEHAVIORIST THEORIES

Behaviorist theories are not in as much favor today as they were 25 years ago, but they still help to explain simple learning. Conditioning and reinforcement are concepts with which most educators are familiar. Conditioning explains how we learn some simple movements and behaviors that result in desired outcomes, such as a nurse responding when an alarm sounds on a ventilator. Reinforcement refers to the fact that behavior which is rewarded or reinforced tends to reoccur. Therefore, reinforcement is a powerful tool in the hands of an educator.

COGNITIVE LEARNING THEORIES

Cognitive learning theories are much more sophisticated. They deal with how we process information by perceiving, remembering, and storing information. All of these processes are a part of learning. One of the most useful concepts in cognitive theory is that of mental schemata.

Schemata (plural) are units of knowledge that are stored in memory. For example, nurses must develop a schema related to aseptic technique. Once a schema is stored in memory, related information can be built on it. For instance, changing a dressing is easier to learn if the learner already has a schema for asepsis.

Metacognition is another concept identified in cognitive theories. This concept refers to thinking about one's thinking. To help learners who are having difficulty mastering certain material, you might ask them to think about how they learn best and help them evaluate whether they really understand the material.

Transfer of learning occurs when a learner takes information from the situation in which it is learned and applies it to a new situation. Transfer is most likely to occur if the information was learned well in the first place, if it can be retrieved from memory, and if the new situation is similar to the original learning situation. Educators can teach for transfer by pointing out to students how a concept is applied in several situations so that learners know the concept is not an isolated one, and the students begin to look for similar patterns in new situations.

ADULT LEARNING THEORIES

Adult learning theories help to explain how learning takes place differently for adults than for children. Adults usually need to know the practical applications for the information they are given. They also want to see how it fits with their life experiences. When teaching adults, nurse educators need to keep in mind adult motivation for learning.

LEARNING STYLE THEORIES

Learning style theories abound. Research has shown that some learners are visually oriented, some are more auditory or tactile learners, some are individualistic and learn best alone, others learn best by collaboration, some deal well with abstract concepts, and others learn better with concrete information. Measurement instruments that can determine preferred learning styles are readily available. Although not many educators actually measure their students' learning styles, they should keep learning styles in mind when they plan their instruction.

PLANNING FOR INSTRUCTION

With some background knowledge of how students learn, the nurse educator can begin to plan the learning experiences. Planning includes developing objectives, selecting content, choosing pedagogies, selecting assignments, and planning for assessment of learning. All nurse educators come to the teaching process already knowing how to write objectives. Objectives can be written in the cognitive, psychomotor, and affective domains of learning. In the cognitive domain, they can be written at the knowledge, comprehension, application, analysis, and synthesis levels of complexity. The critical aspect of objectives is to keep referring to them as you plan your lesson or course. They will help you focus on the "need to know" versus the "nice to know" material. They will help you decide which assignments will be most suitable, and they will guide your development of evaluation tools.

SELECTING ASSIGNMENTS

Selecting and developing out-of-class assignments calls for creativity. You may use instructor's manuals such as this for ideas for assignments or you may also develop your own. To encourage learning through writing, you can assign short analysis papers, position papers, or clinical journals, all of which promote critical thinking. Nursing care plans of various lengths and complexity may be assigned. You may create reading guides with questions to help students read their textbooks analytically. You might also ask students to interview or observe people to achieve various objectives.

USING EFFECTIVE PEDAGOGIES

Selecting teaching methods or pedagogies takes considerable time. You must consider what you are trying to achieve. To teach facts, you may choose to lecture or assign a computer tutorial. To change attitudes or motivate learners, you may use discussion, role-playing, or gaming. Developing critical thinking may be done effectively using critical-thinking exercises, concept maps, group projects, or problem-based learning. There are traditional pedagogies, activity-based pedagogies, and technology-based pedagogies.

TRADITIONAL PEDAGOGIES

Traditional pedagogies include lecture, discussion, and questioning. Lecturing is an efficient way to convey a great deal of information to large groups of people. However, the lecture creates passive learning. Learners just sit and listen (or not) and do not interact with the information or the lecturer. Research has shown that students learn more from active learning techniques (i.e., from being able to talk about, manipulate, deduce, or synthesize information). If you are going to lecture, it would be wise to intersperse lecture with discussion and questioning.

Discussion gives students an opportunity to analyze and think critically about information that they have read or were given in a lecture. By discussing key concepts and issues, they can learn the applicability of the concepts and see how they can transfer to varied situations. Discussions can be formal or informal, but they generally work best if they are planned. For a formal discussion, students must be held accountable for preparing for it. The teacher becomes a facilitator by giving an opening statement or question, guiding the discussion to keep it focused, giving everyone a chance to participate, and summarizing at the end.

Questioning is a skill that develops over time. The first principle to learn is that you have to give students time to answer. Most teachers wait only 1 second before either repeating the question or answering it themselves. You should wait at least 3 to 5 seconds before doing anything, to allow students time to think and prepare a thoughtful answer. Research has revealed that most instructor-posed questions are at a very low level (lower-order), eliciting recall of facts. But questioning can be used to develop critical thinking if it is planned. Higher-order questions are those that require students to interpret information, to apply it to different situations, to think about relationships between concepts, or to assess a situation. If you ask higher-order questions during your classes or clinical experiences, students will rise to the occasion and will be challenged to provide thoughtful answers.

ACTIVITY-BASED PEDAGOGIES

Activity-based teaching strategies include cooperative learning, simulations, games, problem-based learning, and self-learning modules, among others. Cooperative learning is an old pedagogy that has received more research support than any other method. This approach involves learners working together and being responsible for the learning of group members as well as their own learning. Cooperative learning groups can be informal, such as out-of-class study groups, or they can be formally structured in-class groups. The groups may serve to solve problems, develop projects, or discuss previously taught content.

Simulations are exercises that can help students to learn in an environment that is low risk or risk-free. Students can learn decision making, for example, in a setting where no one is hurt if the decision is the wrong one. Simulations in skill laboratories are frequently used to teach psychomotor skills. Simulations can be written (case studies), acted out (role-playing), computer-based (clinical decision-making scenarios), or complex technology-based (active simulation manikins).

Games can help motivate people to learn. Factual content that requires memorization (such as medical terminology) can be turned into word games such as crossword puzzles or word searches. More complex games can teach problem solving or can apply previously learned information. Board games or simulation games can be used for these purposes.

Problem-based learning (PBL) provides students with real-life problems that they must research and analyze and then develop possible solutions. PBL is a group activity. The instructor presents the students with a brief problem statement. The student group makes lists of what they know and don't know about the problem. They decide what information they must collect in order to further understand the problem. As they collect the information and analyze it, they further refine the problem and begin to investigate possible solutions. The educator serves as a facilitator and resource during the learning process and helps keep the group focused.

Self-learning modules are a means of self-paced learning. They can be used to teach segments of a course or an entire course or curriculum. Modules should be built around a single concept. For example, you might design a module for a skill lab based on aseptic technique, or you could develop a module for a classroom course around the concept of airway impairment. Each module contains components such as an introduction, instructions on how to use the module, objectives, a pretest, learning activities, and a posttest. Learning activities within a module should address various learning styles. For example, you should try to include activities that appeal to visual learners and tactile learners, conceptual learners and abstract learners, and individual learners and collaborative learners. Those activities could be readings, audiovisuals, computer programs, group discussion, or skills practice. The educator develops and tests the module and then acts as facilitator and evaluator as learners work through the module.

TECHNOLOGY-BASED PEDAGOGIES

Technology-based pedagogies include computer simulations and tutorials, Internet use, and distance learning applications. Computer simulations include decision-making software in which a clinical situation is enacted and students are asked to work through the nursing process to solve problems and achieve positive outcomes. They also include simulation games such as SimCity, which can be a useful tool in teaching community health principles. Computer tutorials are useful for individual remedial work such as medication calculations or practice in answering multiple-choice test questions.

The Internet is a rich resource for classroom use and for out-of-class assignments. There are hundreds of Web sites that can be accessed for health-related information. Students need to be taught how to evaluate the worth of these Web sites. The criteria they should apply to this evaluation include identifying the intended audience, the currency of the information, the author's credentials or the affiliated organization, and content accuracy. Students may not know how to identify online journal sources compared to other Web sites. It is worth spending time, therefore, teaching students how to use the Internet before giving them such assignments. If your classroom is Internet access enabled, you can visually demonstrate how to identify and use appropriate Web sites. For example, if you want students to find relevant information for diabetic teaching, you can show them the differing value of information from official diabetes associations versus pharmaceutical sites versus chat rooms or public forums.

You may be using this instructor's manual in a distance learning course. Distance learning takes the forms of interactive television classes, webcasting, or online courses. In any form of distance learning, students are learning via the technology, but they are also learning about technology and becoming familiar with several computer applications. Those applications may include synchronous and asynchronous applications, streaming video, and multimedia functions.

ASSESSING LEARNING

You can assess or evaluate learning in a number of ways. Your first decision is whether you are just trying to get informal, ungraded feedback on how well students are learning in your class, or whether you are evaluating the students for the purpose of assigning a grade. Following are a number of techniques that can be used for one or both purposes.

CLASSROOM ASSESSMENT TECHNIQUES

Classroom assessment techniques (CATs) are short, quick, ungraded, in-class assessments used to gauge students' learning during or at the end of class. Getting frequent feedback on students' understanding helps educators to know if they are on the right track and if students are benefiting from the planned instruction. If you wait until you give a formal quiz or examination, you may have waited too long to help some students who are struggling with the material. The most popular CAT is probably the *minute paper*. This technique involves asking students to write down, in 1 or 2 minutes, usually at the end of class, what was the most important thing they learned that day or what points remain unclear. A related technique is the *muddiest point*, in which you ask the class to write down what the "muddiest" part of the class was for them. In nursing, *application cards* can be especially useful. After teaching about a particular concept or body of knowledge, and before you talk about the applications of the information, ask the students to fill out an index card with one possible clinical application of the information. This technique fosters application and critical thinking. Always leave class time during the following session to give feedback on the CAT results.

Another means of doing a quick assessment of learning in the classroom is the use of a *classroom (or student) response system*, sometimes called *clicker* technology. By the use of radio frequency technology, a laptop computer, a projector, and student remote controls (the clickers), an instructor can pose a written question on the screen and ask students to use their clickers to select the correct answer. The answers are then tallied and can be projected as a graph of results on the screen. This technology permits quick assessment of student understanding of critical information and keeps students active during a lecture. Classroom response systems are often made available by publishers in conjunction with their textbooks.

TESTS AND EXAMINATIONS

Tests and examinations are also used to assess or evaluate learning. Tests should be planned carefully to measure whether learning objectives have been met. You should form a test plan in which you decide the number of test items to include for each objective as well as the complexity of the items. Just as objectives can be written at the knowledge through synthesis levels of knowing, test items can be written at each level, too. Some types of items lend themselves to the lower levels of knowing, such as true-false and matching items, while multiple-choice and essay questions can be used to test higher levels.

TRUE-FALSE QUESTIONS

True-false questions are used simply to determine if the student can identify the correctness of a fact or principle. This type of question should be used sparingly, because the student has a 50% chance of guessing the correct answer. Well-written true-false questions are clear and unambiguous. The entire statement should be totally true or totally false. An example of a question that is ambiguous is:

(T F) A routine urinalysis specimen must be collected with clean technique and contain at least 100 mL.

The answer to this question is false because the specimen does not require 100 mL of volume. However, the clean technique part of the question is true. Because part of the statement is true and part is false, the question is misleading. A better question is:

(T F) A routine urinalysis specimen must be collected with clean technique.

True-false questions can be made more difficult by requiring the student to explain why the statement is true or false.

MATCHING QUESTIONS

Matching questions also test a low level of learning—that of knowledge. They are most useful for determining if students have learned definitions or equivalents of some type. They should be formatted in two columns, with the premise words or statements on the left and the definitions or responses on the right. You should have more responses than premises so that matching cannot be done simply by process of elimination. Instructions should be given that indicate if responses can be used more than once or even not used at all. An example of a matching question is:

Match the definition on the right with the suffix on the left. Definitions can be used only once or not at all.

_____ 1. -itis   a. presence of

_____ 2. -stalsis   b. abnormal flow

_____ 3. -rrhage   c. inflammation

_____ 4. -iasis   d. discharge or flow

_____ 5. -ectomy   e. contraction

                           f. surgical removal of

MULTIPLE-CHOICE QUESTIONS

Multiple-choice questions can be written at the higher levels of knowing, from application through evaluation. At these higher levels they can test critical thinking. A multiple-choice question has two parts. The first part, the question, is also called the *stem*. The possible answers are called *options*. Among the options, the correct one is called the *answer*, while the incorrect options are termed *distractors*. You can word stems as questions or as incomplete statements that are completed by the options. For example, an item written as a question is:

WHAT IS A QUICK WAY TO ASSESS THE APPROXIMATE LITERACY LEVEL OF A PATIENT?

a. Pay attention to her vocabulary as she speaks.

b. Give her an instruction sheet to read.

c. Administer a literacy test.

d. Ask her whether she graduated from high school.

The same knowledge can be tested by a stem written as an incomplete statement:

A QUICK WAY TO ASSESS THE APPROXIMATE LITERACY LEVEL OF A PATIENT IS TO

a. pay attention to her vocabulary as she speaks.

b. give her an instruction sheet to read.

c. administer a literacy test.

d. ask her whether she graduated from high school.

Notice the differing formats of each item. When the stem is a question it is also a complete sentence, so each option should be capitalized because each is also a complete sentence and each ends with a period. When the stem is an incomplete statement, it does not end with a period, so the options that complete the statement do not begin with a capital letter but do end with a period. Stems should be kept as brief as possible to minimize reading time. Avoid negatively stated stems. For example, a poor stem would be:

WHICH OF THE FOLLOWING IS NOT A GOOD WAY TO ASSESS A PATIENT'S LITERACY LEVEL?

It is too easy for readers to miss the word *not* and therefore answer incorrectly. If you feel compelled to write negative stems occasionally, be sure to capitalize or underline the word *not*, or use the word *except* as in the following example:

ALL OF THE FOLLOWING ARE GOOD WAYS TO ASSESS A PATIENT'S LITERACY LEVEL EXCEPT

In this case, the reader is less likely to miss the negative word because of the sentence structure and also because the word *except* is capitalized.

Options usually vary from three to five in number. The more options you have, the more difficult the item. However, it is often difficult to write good distractors. Be sure that your options are grammatically consistent with the stem. Next is a test item in which all of the options do not fit grammatically with the stem:

The lecture method of teaching is best suited to

a. when the audience already knows a lot about the topic.

b. large audiences.

c. times when you are in a hurry to cover your material and don't want to be interrupted.

d. young children.

Not only are the options grammatically inconsistent, they are also of varied lengths. Attempt to keep the options about the same length. The following restatement of the item corrects the problems with grammar and with length:

The lecture method of teaching is best suited to

a. an audience that already knows the topic.

b. an audience that is very large.

c. times when you must cover your material quickly.

d. an audience of young children.

Distractors that make no sense should never be used. Instead, try to develop distractors that reflect incorrect ideas that some students might hold about a topic.

ESSAY QUESTIONS

Essay-type questions include short answer (restricted-response questions) and full essays (extended-response questions). These types of items can be used to test higher-order thinking. Extended-response essays are especially suited to testing analysis, synthesis, and evaluation levels of thinking. An example of an essay that might test these higher-order levels of thinking is:

Explain how exogenous cortisone products mimic a person's normal cortisol functions and why long-term cortisone administration leads to complications. Also explain how nursing assessment and intervention can help to reduce those complications.

The educator must plan how the essay is going to be graded before the test is given. An outline of required facts and concepts can be developed and points given to each. Then a decision must be made as to whether it is appropriate to give points for writing style, grammar, spelling, and so on.

TEST ITEM ANALYSIS

After a test is given, an analysis of objective items can be conducted. Two common analyses are *item difficulty* and *item discrimination*. Most instructors want to develop questions that are of moderate difficulty, with around half of the students selecting the correct answer. A mixture of fairly easy, moderate, and difficult questions can be used. The difficulty index can be calculated by dividing the number of students who answered the question correctly by the total number of students answering the question. The resulting fraction, converted to a percentage, gives an estimate of the difficulty, with lower percentages reflecting more difficult questions.

Item discrimination is an estimate of how well a particular item differentiates between students who generally know the material and those that don't. In other words, a discriminating item is one that most of the students who got high scores on the rest of the examination got right and most of the students who got low scores got wrong. The discrimination index can be calculated by computer software or by hand using a formula that can be found in tests and measurement textbooks.

HELPFUL RESOURCES

These few pages are but an introduction to teaching techniques. To be fully prepared for the educator role, you will need to enroll in formal courses on curriculum and teaching or do more self-learning on educational topics. For more information, you might consult the following print and Web-based resources:

DeYoung, S. (2003). *Teaching Strategies for Nurse Educators*. Upper Saddle River, NJ: Prentice Hall.

Websites:

www.crlt.umich.edu/tstrategies/teachings.html

www.gmu.edu/facstaff/part-time/strategy.html

www.ic.arizona.edu/ic/edtech/strategy.html

Instructor's Resource Manual for
Olds' Maternal-Newborn Nursing & Women's Health Across the Lifespan

Eighth Edition

CHAPTER 1
CURRENT ISSUES IN MATERNAL-NEWBORN NURSING

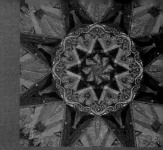

RESOURCE LIBRARY

PRENTICE HALL NURSING MEDIALINK DVD-ROM

Audio Glossary
NCLEX Review

COMPANION WEBSITE

Additional NCLEX Review
Case Study: *Cord Blood Banking*
Care Plan Activity: *Request for Second Trimester Abortion*
Applications: *Scope of Practice; Standards of Care*
Critical Thinking

📖 IMAGE LIBRARY

Figure 1.1 Individualized education for childbearing couples is one of the prime responsibilities of the maternal-newborn nurse.

Figure 1.2 No health insurance coverage among persons under 65 years of age by selected characteristics, United States, 2005.

Figure 1.3 The nation's health dollar, calendar year 2004.

Figure 1.4 A certified nurse-midwife confers with her client.

Figure 1.5 A collaborative relationship between nurse and physician contributes to excellent client care.

Figure 1.6 Leading causes of death for infants in the United States, 2003.

LEARNING OBJECTIVE 1

Relate the concept of the expert nurse to nurses caring for childbearing families.

CONCEPTS FOR LECTURE

1. Novice nurses become experts by drawing on their experiences and becoming more aware of client cues. They take on a more holistic approach, developing a clear perception of the possibilities of a given situation.

2. The holistic approach enables nurses to develop an inituitive approach to providing effective care. This intuition is an internalization of information. The "art of nursing" is an expression of this intuition, particularly in maternal-newborn nursing where rapid change occurs and nurses must become aware of client changes and needs.

POWERPOINT LECTURE SLIDES

(NOTE: The number on each PPT Lecture Slide directly corresponds with the Concepts for Lecture.)

1 Expert Nurses
- View situations holistically
- Are aware of subtle cues indicating change
- Have a clear vision of what is possible

2 Expert Nurses
- Knowledge and experience
- Intuition
- Internalization of information
- *Art of Nursing*

2a See Figure 1.1

SUGGESTIONS FOR CLINICAL ACTIVITIES

Have students shadow an expert and novice nurse in maternal-child health and have them discuss their observations in postconference, comparing and contrasting their observations.

Learning Objective 2

Discuss the impact of the self-care movement on contemporary childbirth.

Concepts for Lecture

1. Self-care took root in the late 1960s as health care consumers attempted to understand technology and took interest in caring for their own health. Practicing self-care requires that the consumer take an active role in acquiring information. Nurses play an integral role in fostering self-care by providing education and encouraging consumers to become actively involved in their own care.

PowerPoint Lecture Slides

(NOTE: The number on each PPT Lecture Slide directly corresponds with the Concepts for Lecture.)

 Self-care Movement
- Consumers seek to:
  - Understand technology
  - Take an interest in their own health
  - Take an interest in basic self-care skills

 Self-care Requires
- Assertiveness
- Taking an active role in seeking information

 Nurse's Role in Client Self-Care
- Provide information
- Encourage questions
- Encourage client to become actively involved in care

Suggestions for Clinical Activities

Have students interview women in a maternal-child clinic about their self-care activities.

Learning Objective 3

Compare the nursing roles available to the maternal-newborn nurse.

Concepts for Lecture

1. Maternal-newborn nurses function in many roles, both in the acute care setting and in the community. Their roles are defined by the level of education and specialization. Certified registered nurses have demonstrated expertise in a specific clinical area by taking a national certification exam. Nurse Practitioners (NP) and Clinical Nurse Specialists (CNS) have advanced education through a master's degree program and demonstrate expertise in a certain clinical area. A Certified Nurse Midwife (CNM) also receives advanced education through a master's degree program in nursing and midwifery. They independently manage the care of women at low risk for complications during pregnancy and birth and the care of normal newborns.

PowerPoint Lecture Slides

(NOTE: The number on each PPT Lecture Slide directly corresponds with the Concepts for Lecture.)

 Maternal-Newborn Nursing Roles
- Professional Nurse
- Certified Registered Nurse
- Nurse Practitioner
- Clinical Nurse Specialist
- Certified Nurse Midwife (Figure 1.4)

 See Figure 1.4

Suggestions for Classroom Activities

Invite maternal-child nurses with different roles to class to talk about their roles.

LEARNING OBJECTIVE 4

Identify specific factors that contribute to a family's value system.

CONCEPTS FOR LECTURE

1. Culture is based on socially learned beliefs, lifestyles, values, and integrated patterns of behavior that are characteristic of the family, cultural group, and community. Contributing elements of a family's value systems includes:
   - Religion and social beliefs
   - Presence and influence of the extended family, as well as socialization within the ethnic group
   - Communication patterns
   - Beliefs and understanding about the concepts of health and illness
   - Permissible physical contact with strangers
   - Education

POWERPOINT LECTURE SLIDES

(NOTE: The number on each PPT Lecture Slide directly corresponds with the Concepts for Lecture.)

1 Factors Contributing to Family Values
   - Religion and social beliefs
   - Presence and influence of the extended family
   - Socialization within the ethnic group
   - Communication patterns

1a Factors Contributing to Family Values
   - Beliefs and understanding about health and illness
   - Permissible physical contact with strangers
   - Education

SUGGESTIONS FOR CLASSROOM ACTIVITIES

Ask students to share their family values related to maternal-child health and the influences on their values.

LEARNING OBJECTIVE 5

Delineate significant legal and ethical issues that influence the practice of nursing for childbearing families.

CONCEPTS FOR LECTURE

1. Professional nurses must adhere to practice standards; institutional or agency policies; and local, state, and federal laws. Standards of care provide guidelines for the minimum level of competent delivery of nursing care. Nurses must also practice in an ethical manner. The focus of ethics is on duty, considering factors such as risks, benefits, other relationships, concerns, and the needs and abilities of persons affected by and affecting decisions. State nurse practice acts define the scope of practice by which every nurse must function.
2. Negligence is defined as omitting or committing an act that a reasonably prudent person would not omit or commit under the same or similar circumstances. Negligence consists of four elements:
   1. There was a duty to provide care.
   2. The duty was breached.
   3. Injury occurred.
   4. The breach of duty caused the injury (proximate cause).

POWERPOINT LECTURE SLIDES

(NOTE: The number on each PPT Lecture Slide directly corresponds with the Concepts for Lecture.)

1 Legal Issues
   - Standards of Care
     ○ Minimum criteria for competent, proficient delivery of nursing care
   - Institutional policies
   - Ethical Implications

1a Legal Issues
   - Scope of Practice
     ○ Defined by state's Nurse Practice Act
     ○ Identifies parameters within which nurses may practice
   - Laws

2 Negligence
   - There was a duty to provide care.
   - The duty was breached.
   - Injury occurred.
   - The breach of duty caused the injury (proximate cause).

SUGGESTIONS FOR CLASSROOM ACTIVITIES

Bring examples of professional standards of care, hospital policies, and laws to class for students to review.

Evaluate the potential impact of some of the special situations in contemporary maternity care.

CONCEPTS FOR LECTURE

1. Developments in technology have allowed for the treatment and monitoring of the fetus. The fetus is increasingly viewed as an individual client separate from the mother, although the mother is necessarily involved. The implication of this is that the interests of the mother and the fetus may be divergent. Most of the time, mothers protect their fetuses; however in some instances, women have refused interventions on behalf of the fetus and forced interventions have occurred. These include forced cesarean birth; coercion of mothers who practice high-risk behaviors, such as substance abuse, to enter treatment; and mandating experimental in utero therapy or surgery in an attempt to correct a specific birth defect. Non-therapeutic research requires that the risk to the fetus be minimal, that knowledge to be gained is important, and the information is unatainable by any other means. Therapeutic fetal research, which is aimed a treating a fetal condition, raises fewer ethical questions.

2. Intrauterine fetal surgery is a therapy for anatomic lesions that can be corrected surgically and are incompatible with life if not treated. Risks due to the surgery are significant and require subsequent delivery by cesarean birth because of the uterine incision. The ethical principle of autonomy arises from this surgery as it poses significant health risks to the woman.

3. Abortion, which has been legal in the United States since 1973, can be performed until the period of viability. After that, abortion can only be performed when the life or the health of the mother is threatened. Maternal rights supercede those of the fetus prior to viabiity and the reverse is true after viability. Nurses (and other caregivers) can refuse to assist with abortions if it conflicts with their moral and ethical beliefs; however, they run the risk of being dismissed for refusing. Therefore, nurses should carefully evaluate the philosophy and practices of the institution prior to accepting employment. Additionally, nurses must make sure that someone with adequate qualifications is available to provide care for that client.

4. Methods of resolving infertility may raise ethical questions including religious objections to artificial conception, financial and moral responsibility for a child born with a congenital defect, candidate selection and threats related to genetic engineering. Human stem cell research has demonstrated that these cells can be made to differentiate into other types of cells, which might then be used to treat problems such as diabetes, Parkinson's and Alzheimer's diseases, spinal cord injury, or metabolic disorders. The ethical issue that arises is the status of the embryo—as a person or a property and if a property, who is the owner. Cord blood may play a role in combating leukemia, certain other cancers, metabolic disorders, and other immune and blood

POWERPOINT LECTURE SLIDES

(NOTE: The number on each PPT Lecture Slide directly corresponds with the Concepts for Lecture.)

1 Maternal-Child Issues (Figure 1.5)
- Divergence between rights of mother and rights of fetus
  - Mother may refuse fetal intervention.
  - Fetal intervention may be forced on mother.
- Fetal research
  - Therapeutic vs. non-therapeutic

1a See Figure 1.5

2 Maternal-Child Issues
- Intrauterine fetal surgery
  - Therapy for anomalies incompatible with life
  - Health of the mother and fetus is at risk

3 Maternal-Child Issues
- Abortion
  - Can be performed until point of viability
  - After viability, if mother's health in jeopardy
- Nursing Role
  - Have right to refuse to assist
  - Responsible for ensuring a qualified replacement is available

4 Maternal-Child Issues
- Infertility
- Human stem cells
- Cord blood

system disorders. Ethical issues associated with cord blood banking include issues about ownership, informed consent, confidentiality, notification about testing results and the fair distribution of harvested blood.

SUGGESTIONS FOR CLASSROOM ACTIVITIES

Have students debate the various ethical/legal issues associated with the special situations noted above.

LEARNING OBJECTIVE 7

Contrast descriptive and inferential statistics.

CONCEPTS FOR LECTURE

1. The function of descriptive statistics is to describe or summarize a set of data.

   The function of inferential statistics is to draw conclusions or inferences about what is happening between two or more variables in a population and to examine causal relationships.

POWERPOINT LECTURE SLIDES

(NOTE: The number on each PPT Lecture Slide directly corresponds with the Concepts for Lecture.)

 Statistics
- Descriptive statistics
  - Describe or summarize a set of data
  - Report facts
- Inferential statistics
  - Draw conclusions about what is happening
  - Suggest or refute causal relationships

SUGGESTIONS FOR CLASSROOM ACTIVITIES

Bring research reports to class with examples of descriptive and inferential statistics. Have students discuss the implications of the findings based upon the types of statistics used.

LEARNING OBJECTIVE 8

Relate the availability of statistical data to the formulation of further research questions.

CONCEPTS FOR LECTURE

1. Research questions are formed from information retrieved from descriptive statistics. Inferential statistics answer specific questions and generate theories to explain relationships. Evidence-based practice is derived from the application of theory to practice.

POWERPOINT LECTURE SLIDES

(NOTE: The number on each PPT Lecture Slide directly corresponds with the Concepts for Lecture.)

1 Formulating Research Questions
- Descriptive statistics is starting point
- Inferential statistics
  - Answer specific questions
  - Generate theories to describe relationships

LEARNING OBJECTIVE 9

Delineate the benefits of evidence-based nursing practice to the client, the institution, and the profession of nursing.

CONCEPTS FOR LECTURE

1. Evidence-based practice is defined as nursing care in which interventions are supported by current research. It also considers other forms of evidence useful in making clinical practice decisions. Evidence-based practice improves efficiencies and provides better outcomes. Quality improvement is an essential part of evidence-based practice.

POWERPOINT LECTURE SLIDES

(NOTE: The number on each PPT Lecture Slide directly corresponds with the Concepts for Lecture.)

 Benefits of Evidence-Based Practice
   - Transforms research findings into clinical practice
     - Efficiency improvement
     - Better outcomes
     - Quality improvement

SUGGESTIONS FOR CLASSROOM ACTIVITIES

Have students find research reports related to maternal-child nursing interventions and discuss how they influence current evidence-based practice.

CHAPTER 2
CARE OF THE FAMILY IN A CULTURALLY DIVERSE SOCIETY

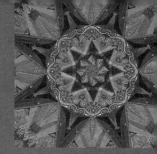

RESOURCE LIBRARY

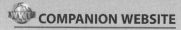 PRENTICE HALL NURSING MEDIALINK DVD-ROM

Audio Glossary
NCLEX Review

COMPANION WEBSITE

Additional NCLEX Review
Case Study: *Family Assessment*
Care Plan Activity: *Effects of Hispanic Culture on Infant Feeding Practices*
Applications: *Ethnocentrism and Health Care—Providing Culturally Sensitive Care; Examine Your Cultural Influences*
Critical Thinking

📖 IMAGE LIBRARY

Figure 2.1 Grandparents can offer nurturing and guidance to their grandchildren, not to mention lots of fun.

Figure 2.2 The traditional family of the mid-20th century consisted of a father who worked outside of the home, a mother who performed all homemaking and childrearing functions, and one or more children.

Figure 2.3 Today, 5% of married couples voluntarily choose to remain childless.

Figure 2.4 In an extended kin network family, two nuclear families live in close proximity to each other and share responsibilities and resources.

Figure 2.5 Single-parent families account for nearly one third of all US families.

Figure 2.6 Some gay and lesbian couples choose to adopt children in need of loving homes.

Figure 2.7 The Family Assessment tool.

Figure 2.8 Cultural assessment tool.

LEARNING OBJECTIVE 1

Explore factors that influence the values, decision making, and roles within the family unit.

CONCEPTS FOR LECTURE

1. The concept of family is defined in various ways including a legal definition of a family and a definition of family based on emotional bonds. Family is defined by a shared emotional closeness and a self-identified membership as part of a family. Legal definitions of a family include individuals joined together by marriage, blood, adoption and residence in the same household.
2. Family values guide interaction within the family unit and outside of it. These values are determined by the ideas, attitudes, and beliefs of the members of a family.
3. Influences on family values include cultural background; social norms; education; environmental influences; socioeconomic status, and beliefs held by peers, coworkers, political and community leaders, and other individuals outside of the family
4. An individual or group of individuals possess power to influence the others in the family unit. This individual will have the ability to influence the health behaviors and practices of the members of the family.

POWERPOINT LECTURE SLIDES

(NOTE: The number on each PPT Lecture Slide directly corresponds with the Concepts for Lecture.)

1 Defining Family
- Emotional closeness
- Defined membership
- Individuals joined together by marriage, blood, adoption, or residence in the same household

2 Family Values
- Ideas
- Attitudes
- Beliefs

3 Influences on Family Values
- Cultural background
- Social norms
- Education
- Environmental influences
- Socioeconomic status
- Beliefs held by peers, coworkers, political and community leaders, and other individuals outside of the family

CONCEPTS FOR LECTURE *continued*

5. Individual members of a family hold specific roles. These vary depending on age, position within the family, conflict within the family, stressors, cultural backgrounds, health status of family members, and demographic trends. Family roles are formed by normative behaviors based upon the expectations of a person in a certain position. Roles vary depending on age, position within the family, conflict within the family, stressors, cultural backgrounds, health status of family members, and demographic trends. Roles may be gender specific, may be assigned to the people who perform them, and individuals may have two or more roles in the family. Examples of roles may include th breadwinner, the homemaker, the nurturer, the social planner, and the peacemaker.

6. The role of the grandparent has become very important in US society. The role of the grandparent varies. Role functions may include being a witness who is simply present for the grandchildren, a protector who cares for and ensures safety, a peacemaker who helps to resolve conflict between parents and their children, and an active participant who maintains involvement in family life.

POWERPOINT LECTURE SLIDES *continued*

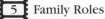 **4** Family Power and Decision Making
- Individual or group who possesses family power
  - Has potential or actual ability to change behavior of other family members
  - Influences family member response to health care

5 Family Roles
- Normative behaviors and expectations
- Roles vary depending on:
  - Age and position
  - Conflict and stressors
  - Cultural backgrounds
  - Health status and demographic trends

5a Family Roles
- Roles may be gender specific.
- Roles may be assigned to the people who perform them.
- Individuals may have two or more roles in the family.

5b Family Role Examples
- Breadwinner
- Homemaker
- Nurturer
- Social planner
- Peacemaker

 6 Grandparent Role Functions
- Acts as witness who is present for the grandchildren
- Provides care and ensures safety
- Helps resolve conflicts between parents and children
- Maintains involvement in family life

SUGGESTIONS FOR CLASSROOM ACTIVITIES

Have students interview each other about their own families and the roles within the family. Ask them to draw a family diagram. Discuss differences and similarities in family roles.

SUGGESTIONS FOR CLINICAL ACTIVITIES

Have students assess a client's family structure and the roles within the client's family.

LEARNING OBJECTIVE 2

Summarize employment, marital, and economic trends affecting the contemporary family.

CONCEPTS FOR LECTURE

1. The dual-earner family has become the norm in contemporary society.
2. Marriage rates are decreasing while there is an increase in the number of single-parent households, a later age for marriage and delayed childbearing, and a growing trend of childless families.
3. The household income of American families had steadily increased since 1973.

POWERPOINT LECTURE SLIDES

(NOTE: The number on each PPT Lecture Slide directly corresponds with the Concepts for Lecture.)

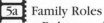 **1** Changes Affecting Contemporary Families
- Employment trends
- Marriage rates
- Growing trend to choose to remain childless
- Economic trends

LEARNING OBJECTIVE 3

Distinguish among several different types of families.

CONCEPTS FOR LECTURE

1. Nuclear families consist of a husband who works outside of the home, a wife who stays home, and children. This is no longer the most common type of family in the United States. Dual-career/dual-earner families are the most common type of family in the United States today. There is a growing trend for couples to remain childless due to infertility, delayed marriage, careers, the availability of contraception, and acceptance of the choice to remain childless. The extended family is one in which multiple generations share responsibilities within the family. This is more common in non-US cultures and working-class families. The extended kin network family is one in which two nuclear related families are sharing resources and living in close proximity to each other. The single-parent family makes up one third of all families in the United States. Families can be headed by a man or woman who has never been married or has been widowed, divorced, or abandoned. Stepparent families have become more common in the United States. These families have also been known as remarried, reconstituted, or blended families. Binuclear families have children who spend equal time between two nuclear families, the families of both the mother and the father. Nonmarital cohabitating families make up an increasing number of all families in the United States. The number of gay or lesbian families has also grown in the United States.

POWERPOINT LECTURE SLIDES

(NOTE: The number on each PPT Lecture Slide directly corresponds with the Concepts for Lecture.)

1 Types of Families
- Nuclear family
- Dual-career/dual-earner family
- Childless family
- Extended family
- Extended kin network family
- Stepparent family

1a Types of Families
- Binuclear family
- Nonmarital cohabitating heterosexual family
- Gay or lesbian family

LEARNING OBJECTIVE 4

Identify major developmental tasks to be completed by the childbearing family.

CONCEPTS FOR LECTURE

1. Family development refers to the dynamics or changes that families experience over time. The amount of time that the families spend in each stage and the duration between stages varies.
2. Duvall's eight-stage family life cycle is based on the nuclear family and describes the developmental process that each family encounters.

POWERPOINT LECTURE SLIDES

(NOTE: The number on each PPT Lecture Slide directly corresponds with the Concepts for Lecture.)

1 Family Development
- Changes that families experience over time, including:
  - Relationships
  - Communication patterns
  - Roles
  - Changes in interactions

2 Duvall Family Life Cycle 1979
- Stage 1: Beginning Families
- Stage 2: Childbearing Families

- Stage 3: Families with Preschool Children
- Stage 4: Families with School-age Children
- Stage 5: Families with Teenagers
- Stage 6: Families Launching Young Adults
- Stage 7: Middle-aged Parents
- Stage 8: Retirement and Old Age

SUGGESTIONS FOR CLASSROOM ACTIVITIES

Prepare case studies for student discussion of families in different stages of the life cycle. Have them discuss how the dynamics of the family change based upon the stages of the life cycle.

SUGGESTIONS FOR CLINICAL ACTIVITIES

Have students identify the stage of the family life cycle of their client based upon information obtained through the client interview. Interview the client about changes in his or her family dynamics.

LEARNING OBJECTIVE 5

Delineate the advantages of using a family assessment tool.

CONCEPTS FOR LECTURE

1. A family assessment should include the following:
   a. Name, age, sex, and family relationship of all family members residing in the household
   b. Cultural associations, including cultural norms and customs related to childbearing, childrearing, and infant feeding (discussed shortly)
   c. Religious affiliations, including specific religious beliefs and practices related to childbearing
   d. Support network, including extended family, friends, and religious and community associations
   e. Family type, structure, roles, and values
   f. Communication patterns, including verbal and written language barriers
2. A family health history should include the following:
   a. Current health practices
   b. Health promotion behaviors
   c. Nutritional assessment
   d. Exercise and activity patterns
   e. Sleep patterns
   f. Occupational exposures
   g. Use of prescription and nonprescription drugs and herbal remedies
   h. Use of alcohol and tobacco
   i. Use of illegal drugs
3. An assessment of environmental considerations should include the following:
   a. Availability of space for all family members
   b. Basic necessities for daily living
   c. Adequate cooking facilities
   d. Availability of a phone
   e. Resources needed for a new infant; for example, a safe place to sleep
   f. Potential hazards
   g. Neighborhood characteristics; for example, availability of resources, safety, transportation

POWERPOINT LECTURE SLIDES

(NOTE: The number on each PPT Lecture Slide directly corresponds with the Concepts for Lecture.)

1 Family Assessment
- Name, age, sex, and family relationship
- Cultural associations
- Religious affiliations
- Support network
- Family type, structure, roles, and values
- Communication patterns

2 Family Health History
- Current health practices and health promotion behaviors
- Nutritional assessment
- Exercise, activity, and sleep patterns
- Occupational exposures
- Use of prescription and nonprescription drugs and herbal remedies
- Use of alcohol and tobacco and illegal drugs

3 Environmental Considerations
- Availability of space and bare necessities
- Adequate cooking facilities
- Availability of a phone
- Resources needed for a new infant
- Potential hazards
- Neighborhood characteristics

LEARNING OBJECTIVE 6

Discuss the impact of culture in caring for the childbearing family.

CONCEPTS FOR LECTURE

1. Culture is defined as beliefs, values, attitudes, and practices that are accepted by a population, a community, or an individual. Ethnicity is a social identity that is associated with shared behaviors and patterns including family structure, religious affiliation, language, dress, eating habits, and health behaviors. Acculturation occurs when people from one culture adapt to the new cultural norms of the place in which they are living. Assimilation occurs when people from one culture completely assume the identity of the culture in which they are living. Ethnocentrism is the conviction that the values and beliefs of one's own cultural group are the best ones or the only acceptable ones. It is characterized by an inability or unwillingness to understand the beliefs or worldview of another group or culture. Culture has an impact on family structure, with many cultures outside of the United States having an extended family structure. Family beliefs about childbearing and childrearing greatly influence these life events. These include beliefs about the importance of children, beliefs and attitudes about pregnancy, health practices, and infant feeding behaviors.

POWERPOINT LECTURE SLIDES

(NOTE: The number on each PPT Lecture Slide directly corresponds with the Concepts for Lecture.)

 1 Definition of Terms
  • Culture
  • Ethnicity
  • Acculturation
  • Assimilation
  • Ethnocentrism

SUGGESTIONS FOR CLASSROOM ACTIVITIES

Have students discuss their individual cultural backgrounds in class.

LEARNING OBJECTIVE 7

Identify prevalent cultural norms related to childbearing and childrearing.

CONCEPTS FOR LECTURE

1. Family beliefs about childbearing and childrearing greatly influence these life events. These include beliefs about the importance of children, beliefs and attitudes about pregnancy, health practices, and infant feeding behaviors.

POWERPOINT LECTURE SLIDES

(NOTE: The number on each PPT Lecture Slide directly corresponds with the Concepts for Lecture.)

 1 Cultural Influences on Childbearing and Childrearing
  • Importance of children
  • Beliefs and attitudes about pregnancy
  • Health practices during pregnancy
  • Cultural norms regarding infant feeding practice

SUGGESTIONS FOR CLASSROOM ACTIVITIES

Have students present the practices of different cultures for childbearing and childrearing.

SUGGESTIONS FOR CLINICAL ACTIVITIES

Have students interview clients from different cultural backgrounds on their childbearing and childrearing customs.

LEARNING OBJECTIVE 8

Summarize the importance of cultural competency in providing nursing care.

CONCEPTS FOR LECTURE

1. Cultural competency is the skills and knowledge necessary to appreciate, understand, and work with individuals from different cultures. It requires self-awareness, awareness and understanding of cultural differences, and the ability to adapt clinical skills and practices as necessary.

POWERPOINT LECTURE SLIDES

(NOTE: The number on each PPT Lecture Slide directly corresponds with the Concepts for Lecture.)

 Cultural Competency
- The skills and knowledge necessary to appreciate, understand, and work with individuals from different cultures
- Requires self-awareness
- Requires an awareness and understanding of cultural differences
- Requires the ability to adapt clinical skills and practices as necessary

SUGGESTIONS FOR CLASSROOM ACTIVITIES

Have students present the practices of different cultures for childbearing and childrearing families.

SUGGESTIONS FOR CLINICAL ACTIVITIES

Have students interview clients from different cultural backgrounds on their childbearing and childrearing customs.

LEARNING OBJECTIVE 9

Discuss the use of a cultural assessment tool as a means of providing culturally sensitive nursing care.

CONCEPTS FOR LECTURE

1. A beginning development of cultural competency is through knowledge development about the culture. One way that nurses can begin to do this is by doing a cultural assessment. Giger and Davidhizar (2004) developed a transcultural assessment tool that identifies the cultural background, communication patterns, issues related to personal space, social organization, time, roles within the environment, biologic variations, and a nursing assessment.

POWERPOINT LECTURE SLIDES

(NOTE: The number on each PPT Lecture Slide directly corresponds with the Concepts for Lecture.)

 Transcultural Assessment Model (Giger & Davidhizar, 1995)
- Biological differences
- Communication patterns
- Nonverbal communication
- Touch
- Space
- Time orientation

SUGGESTIONS FOR CLASSROOM ACTIVITIES

Have students interview each other doing a transcultural assessment.

SUGGESTIONS FOR CLINICAL ACTIVITIES

Have students interview a client using the transcultural assessment model.

LEARNING OBJECTIVE 10

Identify the key considerations in providing spiritually sensitive nursing care.

CONCEPTS FOR LECTURE

1. It is vital for nurses to understand the influence of religion and spirituality on the care of their client. Religion and spirituality mean different things to different people. Religion is often defined as an institutionalized system that shares a common set of beliefs and practices, whereas others define it as a belief in a transcendent power. Spirituality is concerned with the spirit or soul. Nurses should make every attempt to accommodate religious rituals or practices in the care of their clients.

POWERPOINT LECTURE SLIDES

(NOTE: The number on each PPT Lecture Slide directly corresponds with the Concepts for Lecture.)

1 Impact of Religion and Spirituality
- Religion
  - Institutionalized system that shares a common set of beliefs and practices
  - Belief in a transcendent power
- Spirituality
  - Concerned with the spirit or soul

SUGGESTIONS FOR CLASSROOM ACTIVITIES

Ask students to define what religion and spirituality mean to them and to share any religious practices that they have that should be considered in a healthcare experience.

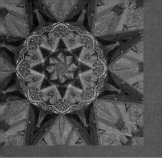

CHAPTER 3
COMPLEMENTARY AND ALTERNATIVE THERAPIES

RESOURCE LIBRARY

 PRENTICE HALL NURSING MEDIALINK DVD-ROM

Audio Glossary
NCLEX Review
Video: *Massage for Pregnancy*

COMPANION WEBSITE

Additional NCLEX Review
Case Study: *Complementary Therapies*
Care Plan Activity: *Use of CAM in High-Risk Adolescent Pregnancy*
Applications: *Complementary Therapies; Internet Information on Complementary Therapies*
Critical Thinking

IMAGE LIBRARY

Figure 3.1 Traditional Chinese symbol of the opposing forces of *yin* and *yang* in perfect balance, representing integration and wholeness.
Figure 3.2 Pregnant woman practices the movements of *Qigong*.
Figure 3.3 Meditation does not have to be practiced in a particular pose, but can be incorporated into each day.

Figure 3.4 Pregnant woman receiving massage.
Figure 3.5 Infant massage.
Figure 3.6 Foot reflexology points.
Figure 3.7 Pregnant woman doing a hatha yoga stretch.
Figure 3.8 During pregnancy, Therapeutic Touch is often helpful in easing pain and reducing anxiety.
Figure 3.9 Complementary and alternative medicine (CAM) use by race/ethnicity.

LEARNING OBJECTIVE 1

Distinguish between *complementary* and *alternative therapies*.

CONCEPTS FOR LECTURE

1. Complementary therapies are health products or procedures that are used in conjunction with conventional treatment. In contrast, alternative therapies are used in place of conventional treatment.

POWERPOINT LECTURE SLIDES

(NOTE: The number on each PPT Lecture Slide directly corresponds with the Concepts for Lecture.)

 Definitions
- Complementary therapy
  - Used with conventional treatment
- Alternative therapy
  - Used in place of conventional treatment

SUGGESTIONS FOR CLASSROOM ACTIVITIES

Have students do an Internet search for complementary and alternative medicine (CAM). Evaluate the Web sites for accurate and up-to-date information.

SUGGESTIONS FOR CLINICAL ACTIVITIES

Have students interview clients about their knowledge and use of CAM.

LEARNING OBJECTIVE 2

Identify several factors that have contributed to the rise in popularity of complementary and alternative therapies in the United States and Canada.

CONCEPTS FOR LECTURE

1. The rise in the poularity of complementary and alternative therapies over the past decade has resulted travel, increased media attention, and the increased from increased consumer awareness of the limitations of conventional medicine, increased internationaluse of the Internet. Factors that made consumers more aware of these limitations include increased health care costs, a decrease in the "human touch" of health care and the increase in technology.

POWERPOINT LECTURE SLIDES

(NOTE: The number on each PPT Lecture Slide directly corresponds with the Concepts for Lecture.)

1 Complementary/Alternative Medicine (CAM)
- Factors contributing to popularity
  ○ Increased awareness of limitations of conventional medicine
  ○ Increased international travel
  ○ Increased media attention
  ○ Advent of the Internet

SUGGESTIONS FOR CLASSROOM ACTIVITIES

Conduct a group discussion about the use of complementary and alternative therapies currently used by students and their families and discuss the reasons for their use.

LEARNING OBJECTIVE 3

Describe the role of the National Center for Complementary and Alternative Medicine.

CONCEPTS FOR LECTURE

1. The Office of Alternative Medicine (OAM) was established in 1992 by the National Institutes of Health. The purpose of the OAM is to promote research into complementary and alternative therapies and the provision of this information to consumers. A new National Center for Complementary and Alternative Medicine (NCCAM) was established in 1998 and expanded the mission of the original center by supporting the use of rigorous science to explore complementary and alternative therapies, training CAM researchers, and disseminating information to the public and professionals and recognizing a new domain of integrative medicine, combining conventional medicine with complementary therapy for which there is scientific evidence of safety and effectiveness.

POWERPOINT LECTURE SLIDES

(NOTE: The number on each PPT Lecture Slide directly corresponds with the Concepts for Lecture.)

1 National Center for Complementary and Alternative Medicine
- Established in 1998 at National Institutes of Health (NIH)
- Rigorous research on CAM
- Training CAM researchers
- Disseminating information to public and professionals
- Integrative medicine

SUGGESTIONS FOR CLASSROOM ACTIVITIES

Have students explore the NCCAM Web site at *http://nccam.nih.gov/*

LEARNING OBJECTIVE 4

Explain the role of complementary and alternative therapies in promoting wellness, disease prevention, and holistic healing.

CONCEPTS FOR LECTURE

1. Benefits of complementary and alternative therapies include the following: they maintain wellness and prevent illness; they utilize a holistic approach; and they may be less expensive and more accessible. The emphasis of these therapies is wellness and prevention of illness. These therapies use a holistic approach to heal the client's psyche, spirit, body, and even the community. They are often less expensive and readily available; however, most insurance companies do not cover the costs for these types of therapies.

POWERPOINT LECTURE SLIDES

(NOTE: The number on each PPT Lecture Slide directly corresponds with the Concepts for Lecture.)

 Benefits of CAM
- Emphasizes maintenance of wellness and prevention of illness
- Utilizes a holistic approach
- May be less expensive
- May be more accessible

SUGGESTIONS FOR CLASSROOM ACTIVITIES

Discuss the difference in approaches between conventional and complementary therapies to health.

LEARNING OBJECTIVE 5

Delineate the risks of using complementary and alternative therapies.

CONCEPTS FOR LECTURE

1. Risks of complementary and alternative therapies include lack of standardization, lack of regulation and research substantiating safety and effectiveness, inadequate training and certification of some healers, and financial and health risks of unproven methods. Herbs, dietary supplements, and other non-Food and Drug Administration (FDA)-approved ingested remedies may vary dramatically from one manufacturer to another, making them less trustworthy to the consumer.

POWERPOINT LECTURE SLIDES

(NOTE: The number on each PPT Lecture Slide directly corresponds with the Concepts for Lecture.)

 Risks of CAM
- Lack of standardization
- Lack of regulation and research
- Inadequate training and certification of some healers
- Financial and health risks of unproven methods

SUGGESTIONS FOR CLASSROOM ACTIVITIES

1. Have students review this Web site from NCCAM: *http://nccam.nih.gov/health/decisions/index.htm*
2. Have a group discussion about risks to consumers using CAM.

SUGGESTIONS FOR CLINICAL ACTIVITIES

Have students conduct a class for a group of healthcare consumers on deciding to use CAM using the information from the Web site noted under Suggestions for Classroom Activities.

LEARNING OBJECTIVE 6

Compare the basic principles and components of naturopathy, homeopathy, traditional Chinese medicine, and ayurvedic medicine.

CONCEPTS FOR LECTURE

1. Homeopathy is a system of healing that attempts to use like to cure like. Homeopathic substances are very small dilutions of substances that, if taken in larger amounts, would produce effects similar to the symptoms of the affliction being treated.

POWERPOINT LECTURE SLIDES

(NOTE: The number on each PPT Lecture Slide directly corresponds with the Concepts for Lecture.)

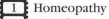 Homeopathy
- Healing system that uses like to cure like
- Remedies are minute dilutions of substances.

2. Naturopathy or natural medicine is a healing system that combines traditional, safe effective means of treating diseases with modern medicine.
3. Traditional Chinese medicine strives to ensure the balance of energy, which is called *chi* or *qi* (pronounced "chee"). Chi is defined as the invisible flow of energy in the body that maintains health and energy. Chi flows along certain pathways or meridians. Traditional Chinese medicine also embraces the concepts of *yin* and *yang,* opposing internal and external forces that represent the whole.
4. Hindu medicine, known as ayurveda, uses the five elements of ether, wind, fire, water, and earth. These elements take form in the body as three tendencies, called *doshas:* vata, pitta, and kapha. Each person has a combination of these three doshas. The objective of ayurveda medicine is to balance the doshas and achieve harmony and holism.

2 Naturopathy
- Is referred to as natural medicine
- Combines traditional with modern medicine
- Uses a variety of techniques

3 Traditional Chinese Medicine (Figure 3.1)
- Ensures a balance of energy.
- Chi is invisible flow of energy in the body.
- Chi flows along pathways or meridians.
- Yin and yang
  - Opposing pathways that form the whole

3a See Figure 3.1

4 Ayurveda
- Five elements
  - Ether, wind, fire, water, and earth
- Three tendencies, called *doshas*
  - Vata, pitta, and kapha
- Goal is to balance the doshas

SUGGESTIONS FOR CLASSROOM ACTIVITIES

Have groups of students present each of these types of CAM.

SUGGESTIONS FOR CLINICAL ACTIVITIES

Have students observe one of these types of CAM in clinical practice and discuss their observations.

LEARNING OBJECTIVE 7

Describe the use of mind-body therapies in promoting the well-being of childbearing families.

CONCEPTS FOR LECTURE

1. Mind-body therapies used in childbearing families include hypnosis, which is a state of great mental and physical relaxation during which the person is open to suggestions; biofeedback in which individuals learn to control their physiologic responses; visualization in which a person goes into a relaxed state and focuses on positive images; guided imagery during which the person is in an intense focused state of concentration to produce mental images; and meditation and prayer.

POWERPOINT LECTURE SLIDES

(NOTE: The number on each PPT Lecture Slide directly corresponds with the Concepts for Lecture.)

1 Mind-Body Therapies
- Hypnosis
- Biofeedback
- Visualization
- Guided imagery
- Meditation
- Prayer

SUGGESTIONS FOR CLASSROOM ACTIVITIES

Demonstrate the use of these types of therapies for use in childbearing in class.

SUGGESTIONS FOR CLINICAL ACTIVITIES

Have students teach pregnant clients about the use of one of these types of CAM.

LEARNING OBJECTIVE 8

Contrast the different manipulative and body-based therapies.

CONCEPTS FOR LECTURE

1. Chiropractice medicine is a manipulative technique used to manage backache and physical stress that results from spinal realignment. Craniosacral therapists believe that the bones of the skull do not fuse completely during childhood and rhythmic impulses can be detected. The therapist uses light tough to test for restrictions. This touch assists the hydraulic forces in the craniosacral system to improve the body's internal environment and strengthen its ability to heal itself.

   The Alexander technique focuses on proper alignment of the head, neck, and trunk. Touch is used along with instructions and activities to guide clients to correctly use their bodies. The Feldenkrais method attempts to establish new connections between the brain and body through movement reeducation to improve health. Clients develop alternate ways of moving that improve posture, flexibility, and range of motion, as well as physical performance and well-being.

2. In massage therapy, the soft tissues of the body are manipulated to reduce stress and tension, increase circulation, diminish pain, and promote a sense of well-being. Reflexology involves the application of pressure to designated points or reflexes on the client's feet, hands, or ears using the thumb and fingers. The benefits of hydrotherapy include relaxing muscles, promoting rest, decreasing pain, reducing swelling, promoting healing, cleansing wounds and burns, reducing fever, lessening cramps, and improving well-being.

   Hatha yoga is commonly practiced for wellness, illness prevention, and healing. The client moves through a series of gentle stretches and postures (called *asanas*), coordinated with deep, rhythmic breathing techniques that promote oxygenation of all body tissues. Regular physical exercise also plays an important role in maintaining health and fitness. The benefits of exercise include maintaining muscle tone and strength, controlling weight, promoting cardiovascular health, improving digestion and elimination, reducing stress, promoting sleep, preventing a variety of chronic health problems, and providing an overall sense of fitness and well-being.

POWERPOINT LECTURE SLIDES

(NOTE: The number on each PPT Lecture Slide directly corresponds with the Concepts for Lecture.)

1 Manipulative and Body-Based Therapies
- Chiropractic medicine
  - Based on concepts of manipulation
- Craniosacral therapy
  - Based on belief that bones of skull do not fuse completely and rhythmic pulses can be detected
  - Uses light touch to test for restrictions
  - Assists hydraulic forces to heal

1a Manipulative and Body-Based Therapies
- Alexander technique
  - Alignment of head, neck, and trunk
  - Use touch, instructions, and activities to guide client
- Feldenkrais method
  - Is a movement-oriented therapy
  - Improves health through new connections between brain and body
  - Improves posture, flexibility, and range of motion
  - Improves physical performance and well-being

2 Manipulative and Body-Based Therapies
- Massage therapy
- Reflexology
- Hydrotherapy
- Hatha Yoga
- Exercise

SUGGESTIONS FOR CLASSROOM ACTIVITIES

Bring in guest speakers to demonstrate these types of therapies to the class.

SUGGESTIONS FOR CLINICAL ACTIVITIES

Have students observe a manipulative or body-based therapy and discuss their observations.

LEARNING OBJECTIVE 9

Explain the advantages and disadvantages to childbearing women of therapies involving ingestion of substances such as foods, dietary supplements, herbs, and homeopathic remedies.

CONCEPTS FOR LECTURE

1. The contribution of nutrition for health and well-being has been well documented. Dietary supplements, or natural food supplements, are used to achieve specific purposes. Pregnant women should discuss the use of supplements with their health care provider. Herbal therapy has also been used to treat symptoms of an ailment. Pregnant and lactating women should consult with their health care provider before using any herbs.

POWERPOINT LECTURE SLIDES

(NOTE: The number on each PPT Lecture Slide directly corresponds with the Concepts for Lecture.)

1 Nutrition and Herbs
- Nutritive value of foods
- Dietary supplements
- Herbal medicine

SUGGESTIONS FOR CLASSROOM ACTIVITIES

Have students interview their families about the use of nutrition, dietary supplements, or herbal medicine during childbearing. Ask them to share their findings in class.

LEARNING OBJECTIVE 10

Distinguish between acupressure and acupuncture.

CONCEPTS FOR LECTURE

1. Acupressure (sometimes called Chinese massage) uses pressure from the fingers and thumbs to stimulate pressure points. Acupuncture, considered the stronger technique, uses very fine (hairlike) stainless steel needles to stimulate specific points depending on the client's medical assessment and condition. A treatment typically involves the placement of 6 to 12 needles.

POWERPOINT LECTURE SLIDES

(NOTE: The number on each PPT Lecture Slide directly corresponds with the Concepts for Lecture.)

1 Energy Therapies
- Acupressure
  - Pressure from thumbs and fingers
  - Stimulates pressure points
- Acupuncture
  - Fine stainless steel needles
  - Applied to specific sites

SUGGESTIONS FOR CLASSROOM ACTIVITIES

Have a practitioner who uses acupressure or acupuncture visit class to discuss their health beliefs and the therapy they provide.

LEARNING OBJECTIVE 11

Distinguish between Reiki and Therapeutic Touch.

CONCEPTS FOR LECTURE

1. Reiki is a form of hand-mediated therapy designed to promote healing, reduce stress, and encourage relaxation. Reiki is practiced by the placement of hands on or above problem areas and transferring energy from the practitioner to the client to restore balance in the client's energy field.
2. Therapeutic Touch is based on the belief that people are a system of energy with a self-healing potential. The Therapeutic Touch practitioner modulates his or her energy field with that of the client's, directing it in a specific way to promote well-being and healing.

POWERPOINT LECTURE SLIDES

(NOTE: The number on each PPT Lecture Slide directly corresponds with the Concepts for Lecture.)

1 Reiki
- Hand-mediated therapy
- Promotes healing, reduces stress, encourages relaxation
- Places hands on problem area
- Restores balance of client's energy field

2 Therapeutic Touch
- Modulates energy field with client energy
- Promotes well-being and healing

LEARNING OBJECTIVE 12

Discuss complementary therapies appropriate for the nurse to use with childbearing families.

CONCEPTS FOR LECTURE

1. The use of CAM therapies by nurses should include those methods that are within the scope of nursing practice. Nurses should use only those therapies that are evidence-based, safe and effective.
2. Nurses working with a pregnant woman could recommend the use of acupressure wristbands for the treatment of nausea, progressive relaxation, exercise and movement, Therapeutic Touch, visualization and guided imagery, prayer, meditation, music therapy, massage, hydrotherapy, storytelling, aromatherapy, and journaling.

POWERPOINT LECTURE SLIDES

(NOTE: The number on each PPT Lecture Slide directly corresponds with the Concepts for Lecture.)

 Complementary Therapies in Childbearing
- Scope of practice
- Documentation of intervention
- Use mainstream modalities
- Evidence of safety and effectiveness

 Examples of Nursing Use of CAM
- Progressive relaxation
- Exercise and movement
- Therapeutic Touch
- Visualization and guided imagery
- Prayer and meditation
- Music therapy

 Examples of Nursing Use of CAM
- Massage
- Hydrotherapy
- Storytelling
- Aromatherapy
- Journaling

CHAPTER 4
WOMEN'S HEALTH ACROSS THE LIFESPAN

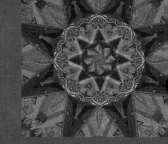

RESOURCE LIBRARY

PRENTICE HALL NURSING MEDIALINK DVD-ROM

Audio Glossary
NCLEX Review

COMPANION WEBSITE

Additional NCLEX Review
Case Study: *Premenstrual Girl*
Care Plan Activity: *Bone Injuries in Postmenopausal Woman*
Applications: *Teaching Adolescents How to Keep a Period Calendar; Menopause*
Critical Thinking

📖 IMAGE LIBRARY

Figure 4.1 Regular exercise is an important part of therapy for dysmenorrhea.
Figure 4.2 Tattoos vary greatly in size, complexity, and meaning to the individual.
Figure 4.3 For osteoporosis assessment, published studies demonstrate that up to 30% of clients

needing treatment are missed using BMD results of the spine and hip alone.
Figure 4.4 Regular exercise is important, especially for post-menopausal women.

LEARNING OBJECTIVE 1

Discuss the key points a nurse should consider in taking a sexual history.

CONCEPTS FOR LECTURE

1. Nurses play an important role in caring for women across their lifespan. Nurses must be skilled at obtaining an accurate sexual health history in a nonjudgmental manner. In order for a nurse to obtain an accurate sexual health history, she or he must be secure about her or his own sexuality; develop awareness about feelings, values, and attitudes about sexuality; be knowledgeable about the structure and function of both the male and female reproductive systems; and have accurate and up-to-date information.

2. Key aspects of taking a sexual health history include explaining the purpose of the interview, using direct eye contact, asking open-ended questions, clarifying terminology, proceeding from easier to more difficult topics, being alert to body language, listening and reacting in a nonjudgmental manner, using teachable moments to educate, not assuming that every woman is a heterosexual, and being respectful.

POWERPOINT LECTURE SLIDES

(NOTE: The number on each PPT Lecture Slide directly corresponds with the Concepts for Lecture.)

1 The Nurse's Role
- Is secure about own sexuality
- Develops an awareness of feelings, values, and attitudes about sexuality
- Has knowledge about the structure and function of female and male reproductive systems
- Has accurate and up-to-date information

2 Taking a Sexual History
- Explain purpose of interview
- Use direct eye contact unless it is culturally unacceptable
- Ask open-ended questions
- Clarify terminology
- Proceed from easier to more difficult topics
- Be alert to body language

2a Taking a Sexual History
- Listen and react in a nonjudgmental manner
- Use teachable moments to educate
- Do not assume the woman is heterosexual
- Be respectful

LEARNING OBJECTIVE 2

Summarize information that women may need in order to implement appropriate self-care measures for dealing with menstruation.

CONCEPTS FOR LECTURE

1. The onset of menarche is between the ages of 8 and 16 with an average age of 12.5 years. Accurate information is important for women to have in helping them care for themselves. The nurse can be an excellent source of information. Information that should be provided should include knowledge about cycle length, amount of flow, length of menses, and self-care measures such as the use of pads and tampons, the use of vaginal sprays, and douching and cleansing the perineum.

POWERPOINT LECTURE SLIDES

(NOTE: The number on each PPT Lecture Slide directly corresponds with the Concepts for Lecture.)

1 Menarche
- Onset of menstruation
- Occurs between the ages of 8–16 (average age 12.5 years)

1a Counseling Women About Self-Care Measures
- Cycle length
- Amount of flow
- Length of menses
- Variations are normal.

1b Educational Topics About Self-Care
- Pads and tampons
- Vaginal sprays and douching
- Cleansing the perineum

SUGGESTIONS FOR CLASSROOM ACTIVITIES

Ask students to develop a course outline for a class instructing adolescent girls about menarche, menstruation, and self-care.

LEARNING OBJECTIVE 3

Identify causes of amenorrhea.

CONCEPTS FOR LECTURE

1. Amenorrhea is defined as the absence of menses. It is classified as either primary or secondary. Primary amenorrhea occurs when menstruation has not been established by the age of 16. Secondary amenorrhea occurs when established menses of longer than 3 months ceases.

2. Amenorrhea may be related to hypothalamic dysfunction caused by systemic stress related to marked weight loss, excessive exercise, and severe or prolonged stress. It may also be caused by a tumor or failure of the central structures of the hypothalamus to develop. Pituitary dysfunction changing prolactin levels may also cause amenorrhea. Conditions such as pituitary tumors, medications, pituitary failure, Sheehan's syndrome, head trauma, and cancer may cause changes in the prolactin levels, resulting in amenorrhea. Chronic anovulation or

POWERPOINT LECTURE SLIDES

(NOTE: The number on each PPT Lecture Slide directly corresponds with the Concepts for Lecture.)

1 Amenorrhea
- Absence of menses
- Primary: menstruation has not been established by 16 years of age
- Secondary: when an established menses (of longer than three months) ceases

2 Causes of Amenorrhea
- Hypothalmic dysfunction
- Pituitary dysfunction
- Chronic anovulation or ovarian failure
- Anatomic abnormalities

ovarian failure related to Turner's syndrome, polycystic ovarian syndrome, thyroid disorders, exposure to radiation or chemotherapy, viral infection, or surgical removal of the ovary may be a cause of amenorrhea. Additionally, anatomic abnormalities, such as congenital absence of the ovaries, uterus, or vagina; congenital obstruction; and an imperforate hymen, may result in amenorrhea

SUGGESTIONS FOR CLINICAL ACTIVITIES

Have students interview a client who has experienced amenorrhea about her menstrual history. Assess for causes of the amenorrhea.

LEARNING OBJECTIVE 4

Contrast dysmenorrhea and premenstrual syndrome.

CONCEPTS FOR LECTURE

1. Dysmenorrhea is defined as painful menstruation that occurs at or a day before the onset of menstruation and disappears by the end of menses.
2. Dysmenorrhea can be classified as either primary or secondary. Primary dysmenorrhea is defined as cramps without underlying disease. The primary cause is increased production of prostaglandins F_2 and $F_2\alpha$, which increase uterine contractility and decrease uterine artery blood flow, causing ischemia. Secondary dysmenorrhea occurs due to pathology of the reproductive tract and occurs after menstruation has been established.
3. The treatment of primary dysmenorrhea includes the use of contraceptives, which inhibit ovulation; nonsteroidal anti-inflammatory drugs (NSAIDs), which act as prostaglandin inhibitors; and self-care measures such as regular exercise, rest, application of heat, and good nutrition.
4. Treatment of secondary dysmenorrhea may include continuous oral contraceptive therapy, which does not allow ovulation or menstruation to occur, and hysterectomy, if there are anatomic disorders and childbearing is not desired. Presacral neurectomy may control severe dysmenorrhea caused by endometriosis.
5. Nutritional self-care for dysmenorrhea should include vitamin supplements. Vitamin B_6 may help relieve the premenstrual bloating and irritability some women experience. Vitamin E, which is a mild prostaglandin inhibitor, may help decrease menstrual discomfort. Calcium carbonate is often effective in reducing physical and psychologic symptoms. Magnesium supplements of 200 mg daily may help reduce fluid retention and breast tenderness. Changes in diet may also help decrease the pain and symptoms of dysmenorrhea. These changes should include restricting intake of foods containing methylxanthines, such as chocolate, cola, and coffee; restricting intake of alcohol, nicotine, red meat, animal fats, and foods containing salt and

POWERPOINT LECTURE SLIDES

(NOTE: The number on each PPT Lecture Slide directly corresponds with the Concepts for Lecture.)

1 Dysmenorrhea
- Painful menstruation
- Occurs at the onset of menstruation
- Disappears by the end of menses

2 Dysmenorrhea
- Primary
  - Cramps without underlying disease
  - Caused by increased production of prostaglandins
  - Ischemia
- Secondary
  - Occurs after menstruation is established

3 Treatment of Primary Dysmenorrhea
- Oral contraceptives (which inhibit ovulation)
- Nonsteroidal anti-inflammatory drugs
- Self-care measures
- Regular exercise and rest
- Application of heat
- Good nutrition

4 Treatment of Secondary Dysmenorrhea
- Continuous oral contraceptive therapy
- Hysterectomy
- Presacral neurectomy

5 Nutritional Self-Care for Dysmenorrhea
- Restriction of foods containing methylxanthines:
  - Chocolate, cola, and coffee
- Restriction of:
  - Alcohol and nicotine
  - Red meat and animal fats
  - Foods containing salt and sugar

sugar; increasing intake of complex carbohydrates (such as whole grains, brown rice, oatmeal), protein, fruits, vegetables, and vegetable oils; and increasing the frequency of meals. Avoiding salt can decrease discomfort from fluid retention.

6. Premenstrual syndrome (PMS) is experienced by 20% to 40% of women. It is a symptom complex associated with the luteal phase of the menstrual cycle (2 weeks before onset of menses). In order to be diagnosed with PMS, at least one affective (emotional) or somatic (physical) symptom must be present that occurs after ovulation and before the onset of menses in three consecutive menstrual cycles.

7. Premenstrual dysphoric disorder (PMDD) is diagnosed when five or more symptoms are present in the given time frame, which are relieved with menstruation and have occurred during most cycles during the previous year.

 Nutritional Self-Care for Dysmenorrhea
- Increase intake of complex carbohydrates and protein
  - Fruits, vegetables and vegetable oils
- Nutritional supplements
  - Vitamins B6 and E
  - Calcium carbonate
  - Magnesium

 Premenstrual Syndrome
- Experienced by 20% to 40% of women
- Luteal phase of the menstrual cycle
- Affective or somatic symptoms
- Occurs after ovulation
- Occurs before menses
- Occurs in three consecutive menstrual cycles

 Premenstrual Dysphoric Disorder (PMDD)
- Experienced by 3% to 8% of women
- Five or more symptoms
- Symptoms are relieved with menstruation
- Symptoms occur during most cycles

SUGGESTIONS FOR CLASSROOM ACTIVITIES

Have groups of students develop a care plan for a woman with dysmenorrhea and present the care plan to the class.

SUGGESTIONS FOR CLINICAL ACTIVITIES

Have students teach a woman with dysmenorrhea about self-care measures. Have them ask the woman to keep a diary documenting measures and results.

LEARNING OBJECTIVE 5

Delineate the physical and psychologic aspects of menopause.

CONCEPTS FOR LECTURE

1. Menopause is defined as the absence of menstruation for 1 full year. It usually occurs between the ages of 45 and 52 with the current median age of 51.3 in the United States. Menopause occurs when estrogen levels fall due to a cessation of ovarian function. Onset is influenced by the woman's health, weight, nutrition, lifestyle, culture and genetic factors.

2. Psychologic adaptation to menopause involves many factors and may be complicated by other life events such as children leaving the household or caring for aging parents. Factors that influence the woman's ability to cope with menopause include self-concept, physical health, marital stability, relationship with others, and cultural values.

3. Physical changes of menopause include a cessation of ovulation, a rise in follicle-stimulating hormone (FSH), and a cessation of the production of estrogen by the ovarian follicles,. As estrogen levels decrease, the endometrium thins and the myometrium, fallopian tubes and ovaries atrophy. The vaginal mucosa becomes thinner and smoother and loses elasticity and dryness of the mucous membranes of the vagina occur because of

POWERPOINT LECTURE SLIDES

(NOTE: The number on each PPT Lecture Slide directly corresponds with the Concepts for Lecture.)

 Menopause
- Absence of menstruation for one full year
- Age of onset influenced by:
  - Overall health
  - Weight and nutrition
  - Lifestyle and culture
  - Genetic factors

 Psychologic Aspects of Menopause
- "Empty nest"
- Caring for aging parents
- Acceptance or lack of acceptance
- Personal factors affecting ability to cope
- Fatigue from insomnia and/or night sweats

Menopausal Changes
- Anovulation
- Irregular menstruation
- Amenorrhea
- Follicle-stimulating hormone (FSH) levels rise
- Estrogen decreases

CONCEPTS FOR LECTURE *continued*

the loss of cervical gland function. There is an increase in the vaginal pH level as the number of Döderlein's bacilli decreases, which can lead to atrophic vaginitis and an increased risk for vaginal infections. The pubic hair thins, turns gray or white, and may disappear while the labia shrink and lose pigmentation. Pelvic fascia and muscles also atrophy, which results in decreased pelvic support.

Vasomotor disturbances, often called hot flashes are described as a feeling of heat rising from the chest spreading to the neck and face. These are often accompanied by sleep difficulties and profuse sweating. Musculoskeletal changes associated with a decrease in estrogen include osteoporosis, a decrease in bone strength related to diminished bone density and bone quality, a weakness of skin collagen and elastin, and a change in body fat distribution.

4. The loss of the protective effects of estrogen is associated with an increase in risk for hypertension, coronary artery disease, and stroke. A decrease in estrogen levels may also be a risk for a lost of cognitive function.

POWERPOINT LECTURE SLIDES *continued*

- Endometrium thins and myometrium, fallopian tubes, and ovaries atrophy

3a Menopausal Changes
- Thinning and dryness of vaginal mucosa
- Vaginal pH increases
- Pubic hair thins and turns gray or white
- Labia shrink and lose pigmentation
- Pelvic fascia and muscles atrophy
- Breasts become pendulous

4 Menopausal Changes
- Vasomotor symptoms
- Increase in risk for:
  ○ Hypertension
  ○ Coronary artery disease
  ○ Stroke
- Changes in cognitive function
- Musculoskeletal

SUGGESTIONS FOR CLASSROOM ACTIVITIES

Have a group discussion about relatives of students who may be experiencing menopause. Have them share their observations of symptoms and management.

SUGGESTIONS FOR CLINICAL ACTIVITIES

Have students teach a class on menopause to a group of women in a clinical setting.

LEARNING OBJECTIVE 6

Explain the relationship between menopause and osteoporosis.

CONCEPTS FOR LECTURE

1. Osteoporosis is a decrease in bone strength due to decreased bone density and quality. Bone mineral density (BMD) testing is an effective risk screening tool for identifying individuals who are at risk for osteoporosis and is recommended for all woman age 65 or older and postmenopausal women with risk factors. Additionally, the height of the woman should be measured at each visit because a loss of height is often an early sign of vertebrae compression due to reduced bone mass.

2. The primary goal is prevention of osteoporosis. Prevention measures include the following: that women over age 50 have a daily calcium intake of 1000 mg while on hormone therapy (HT), and if no HT is being used, 1500 mg daily; take a vitamin D supplement; participate in weight-bearing exercise; consume only modest quantities of alcohol and caffeine; and stop smoking. Medications that have been shown to be helpful in preventing and treating osteoporosis include bisphosphonates which reduce bone resorption and bone loss by inhibiting osteoclast activity; Selective estrogen receptor modulator; Salmon calcitonin; parathyroid hormone; and ultra-low dose estrogen patches.

POWERPOINT LECTURE SLIDES

(NOTE: The number on each PPT Lecture Slide directly corresponds with the Concepts for Lecture.)

1 Assessment of Osteoporosis
- Bone mineral density testing (BMD) is recommended for:
  ○ All postmenopausal women aged 65 or older
  ○ All postmenopausal women with fractures
  ○ Postmenopausal women under age 65 with one or more risk factors
- Height

2 Prevention of Osteoporosis
- Women over age 50 have a daily calcium intake of 1000 mg while on hormone therapy (HT). If no HT is being used, 1500 mg daily.
- Vitamin D supplement
- Weight-bearing exercise
- Consume only modest quantities of alcohol and caffeine.
- Stop smoking.

2a Medication Therapy
- Bisphosphonates
- Selective estrogen receptor modulator
- Salmon calcitonin
- Parathyroid hormone
- Ultra-low dose estrogen patches

SUGGESTIONS FOR CLASSROOM ACTIVITIES

Have students develop a risk assessment plan for osteoporosis for the home of a woman experiencing menopause.

SUGGESTIONS FOR CLINICAL ACTIVITIES

Have students administer the risk assessment developed in class in the home of a woman experiencing menopause. Have them identify at-risk elements and develop interventions to decrease risk.

LEARNING OBJECTIVE 7

Identify medical and complementary therapies to alleviate the discomforts of menopause.

CONCEPTS FOR LECTURE

1. Hormone therapy (HT) refers to the administration of specific hormones to alleviate symptoms associated with the changes of menopause. Estrogen therapy (ET) and combined estrogen-progestogen therapy (EPT) are the individual types currently in use. HT can be prescribed in a number of ways including orally; transdermally (patch); topically as a gel, lotion, or vaginal cream; and through a vaginal ring. It is given in a continuous manner (daily administration of both estrogen and progestogen), or as a cyclic or sequential therapy (with estrogen use daily and a progestogen added on a set sequence).

2. Alternative or complementary treatemtne of the ailments of the perimenopause and menopause include nutrition supplements, such as a diet rich in calcium and vitamins E, D, and B complex, phytoestrogens, and herbal supplements including black cohosh, dong quai, red clover, soy isoflavones, ginseng, and kava. Examples of foods rich in phytoestrogens include carrots, yams, and soy products.

POWERPOINT LECTURE SLIDES

(NOTE: The number on each PPT Lecture Slide directly corresponds with the Concepts for Lecture.)

 1 Hormone Therapy (HT)
- Estrogen therapy
- Estrogen-progestogen therapy
- Administered orally; transdermally (patch); topically, gel, lotion, vaginal creams, or vaginal ring
- Continuous daily cyclic or sequential therapy

 2 Complimentary Therapies
- Phytoestrogens
  - Carrots
  - Yams
  - Soy products
- Herbal supplements

SUGGESTIONS FOR CLASSROOM ACTIVITIES

Review current publications on HT and discuss current findings in class. Discuss the dilemma for women in the face of changing clinical information on HT.

SUGGESTIONS FOR CLINICAL ACTIVITIES

Have students interview a woman experiencing menopause about her management of symptoms.

CHAPTER 5
WOMEN'S HEALTH: FAMILY PLANNING

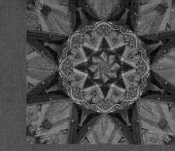

RESOURCE LIBRARY

🔘 PRENTICE HALL NURSING MEDIALINK DVD-ROM

Audio Glossary
NCLEX Review
Oral Contraceptive Animation
Videos: *Vasectomy; Through the Eyes of a Nurse—Welcoming the New Arrival at the First Postpartal Visit*

📖 IMAGE LIBRARY

Figure 5.1 Sample basal body temperature chart.
Figure 5.2 *A*, An unrolled condom with reservoir tip. *B*, Correct use.
Figure 5.3 *A*, The female condom. *B*, Remove condom and applicator from wrapper by pulling up on the ring. *C*, Insert condom slowly by gently pushing the applicator toward the small of the back. *D*, When properly inserted, the outer ring should rest on the folds of skin around the vaginal opening, and the inner ring (closed end) should fit loosely against the cervix.

COMPANION WEBSITE

Additional NCLEX Review
Case Study: *Family Planning*
Care Plan Activity: *Fertility Awareness*
Applications: *Abstinence Support Resources; Contraceptive Services for Minors*
Critical Thinking

Figure 5.4 Inserting the diaphragm.
Figure 5.5 A cervical cap.
Figure 5.6 The contraceptive sponge is moistened well with water and inserted into the vagina with the concave portion positioned over the cervix.
Figure 5.7 The Mirena Intrauterine System, which releases levonorgestrel gradually, may be left in place for up to 5 years.
Figure 5.8 The NuvaRing vaginal contraceptive ring.

LEARNING OBJECTIVE 1

Describe the reasons why women and couples choose to use contraception.

CONCEPTS FOR LECTURE

1. Approximately 62 million women in the United States are of childbearing age. Sixty-two percent of these women practice contraception. Nearly half of all pregnancies are unintended and of these, 4 out of 10 are terminated. Among all women having abortions, 52% of them are under the age of 25.
2. Family planning is an important component of women's health. Benefits of family planning include improved health; lower rates of abortions, fewer unwanted pregnancies and births; and the opportunity to get more education and to find jobs.
3. The choice of a contraceptive method may either be made by the woman or jointly by the couple. In order to make a good decision, women/couples should be educated about the advantages, disadvantages, effectiveness, side effects, contraindications, and long term effects. Factors that influence choice of contraception include cultural practices, religious beliefs, personality, cost, effectiveness, availability, misinformation, practicality of method, and self-esteem.

POWERPOINT LECTURE SLIDES

(NOTE: The number on each PPT Lecture Slide directly corresponds with the Concepts for Lecture.)

1 Overview of Family Planning
- 62 million U.S. women are of childbearing age
- 62% of these women practice contraception
- 50% of all pregnancies are unplanned
- Four out of 10 are terminated
- 52% of these women are under 25

2 Benefits of Family Planning
- Improved health of women
- Lower rates of induced abortions
- Fewer unwanted pregnancies and births
- Improved socioeconomic status

3 Choosing a Contraceptive Method
- Awareness of:
  - Advantages
  - Disadvantages
  - Side effects
  - Contraindications
  - Long-term effects

Choosing a Contraceptive Method
- Choice will be influenced by:
  - Cultural practices and religious beliefs
  - Personality
  - Cost and effectiveness
  - Availability
  - Misinformation
  - Practicality of method
  - Self-esteem

SUGGESTIONS FOR CLASSROOM ACTIVITIES

Have students develop an assessment questionnaire to help couples decide on a contraceptive method.

SUGGESTIONS FOR CLINICAL ACTIVITIES

Have students interview clients about the reasons why they chose a particular type of contraceptive.

LEARNING OBJECTIVE 2

Discuss approaches to fertility awareness-based methods such as natural family planning.

CONCEPTS FOR LECTURE

1. Fertility awareness-based (FAB) methods use knowledge about the changes that occur during a woman's menstrual cycle to identify fertile days. FAB takes into account the lifespan of sperm (2 to 7 days) and the ovum (1 to 3 days) in the female reproductive tract. Fertility awareness-combined methods refers to the use of a barrier method along with FAB during fertile days. Abstinence during fertile days is called natural family planning (NFP).

2. The basal body temperature (BBT) method allows the woman to record and determine her fertile days. BBT is also used with the symptothermal method. The BBT method uses temperature changes during the menstrual cycle to detect changes in fertility. The woman must take her temperature every morning before any activity and record the temperature on a graph. Examination of subsequent monthly graphs allows the woman to predict when ovulation will occur. The ovulation method (OM), sometimes called the cervical mucus method (or the Billings method), uses an assessment of cervical mucus changes that occur during the menstrual cycle due to the influence of estrogen and progesterone. The calendar rhythm method (CRM) is based on the assumptions that ovulation tends to occur 14 days (plus or minus 2 days) before the start of the next menstrual period, that sperm are viable for up to 7 days, and that the ovum is viable for up to 3 days. The symptothermal method consists of assessments about the cycle length; frequency and timing of coitus; cervical mucus changes; secondary signs of ovulation such as increased libido, abdominal bloating, mittelschmerz (midcycle abdominal pain); and change in BBT. The standard days method (SDM) is an appropriate method for women with regular cycles between 26 and 32 days. Intercourse should be avoided, or a barrier method used, between cycle days 8 through 19. The lactational amenorrhea method (LAM) is based on

POWERPOINT LECTURE SLIDES

(NOTE: The number on each PPT Lecture Slide directly corresponds with the Concepts for Lecture.)

 Fertility Awareness-Based Methods
- Fertility awareness, combined methods
  - Use of a barrier method during fertile days
- Natural family planning
  - Abstinence during fertile days

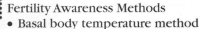 Fertility Awareness Methods
- Basal body temperature method
- Ovulation method
- Calendar rhythm method
- Symptothermal method
- Standard days method
- Lactational amenorrhea

a woman's breastfeeding exclusively for the first 6 months after childbirth. High levels of prolactin in the woman's body during breastfeeding prevent ovulation.

SUGGESTIONS FOR CLASSROOM ACTIVITIES

Have a group discussion about the advantages and disadvantages of natural family planning. Discuss how nurses can help couples be more successful with these methods.

SUGGESTIONS FOR CLINICAL ACTIVITIES

Have students teach a client about one of the natural family planning methods.

LEARNING OBJECTIVE 3

List the spermicides currently available in the United States.

CONCEPTS FOR LECTURE

1. The spermicide that is approved for use in the United States, nonoxynol-9 (N-9), is available as a cream, jelly, foam, vaginal film, and suppository. The spermicide is inserted into the vagina before intercourse and it works by destroying sperm by disrupting the cell membrane.

POWERPOINT LECTURE SLIDES

(NOTE: The number on each PPT Lecture Slide directly corresponds with the Concepts for Lecture.)

1 Spermicides
- Nonoxynl-9 (N-9) available as
  - Jelly
  - Foam
  - Vaginal film
  - Suppository

SUGGESTIONS FOR CLASSROOM ACTIVITIES

Show students examples of the different types of spermicides used in the United States. Discuss important elements to consider when teaching clients about using these spermicides.

SUGGESTIONS FOR CLINICAL ACTIVITIES

Have students develop and implement a teaching plan for the use of spermicides.

LEARNING OBJECTIVE 4

Compare the barrier methods of contraception with regard to correct use and advantages and disadvantages.

CONCEPTS FOR LECTURE

1. Barrier methods provide contraceptive benefits by blocking the transport of sperm to the ovum, immobilizing sperm, or are lethal against them. These methods are often used with a spermacide. The male condom is very effective when used consistently and correctly. The Reality female condom covers the cervix, the vagina and a portion of the perineum. The diaphragm consists of a steel band that forms a ring and is covered with rubber so that the cervix is covered. It is used with spermicidal cream or jelly. The cervical cap is a latex cup-shaped device, used with spermicidal cream or jelly, that fits snugly over the cervix. The cap may be left in place for up to 48 hours, and repeated acts of intercourse do not require additional spermicide. The vaginal sponge is available without a prescription. It is a pillow-shaped, soft, absorbent synthetic sponge containing a spermicide. It is designed to fit over the

POWERPOINT LECTURE SLIDES

(NOTE: The number on each PPT Lecture Slide directly corresponds with the Concepts for Lecture.)

1 Barrier Methods
- Male condom (Figure 5.2A, 5.2B)
- Female condom (Figure 5.3A)
- Diaphragm (Figure 5.4A–D)
- Cervical cap (Figure 5.5)
- Vaginal sponge (Figure 5.6)

1a See Figure 5.2A

1b See Insert Figure 5.2B

1c See Figure 5.3A

1d See Figure 5.4 A–D

cervix and has a loop to permit easy removal. The sponge releases the spermicide N-9 gradually over a 24-hour period.

[1e] See Figure 5.5

[1f] See Figure 5.6

SUGGESTIONS FOR CLASSROOM ACTIVITIES

Show students examples of each of the types of barrier methods. Have groups of students explain instructions for use for each of these types.

SUGGESTIONS FOR CLINICAL ACTIVITIES

Have students develop and implement a high school education plan for barrier methods of contraceptives.

LEARNING OBJECTIVE 5

Summarize the key points women who use combined oral contraceptives should know, including the correct procedure for taking pills, common side effects, warning signs, and noncontraceptive benefits.

CONCEPTS FOR LECTURE

1. Hormonal contraceptives work by preventing the release of an ovum, creating an unfavorable endometrial environment for implantation, and by maintaining a thick cervical mucus that impedes sperm transport. The combined oral contraceptive (COC) is a combination of a synthetic estrogen and progestin. This type of contraceptive is safe, highly effective and easily reversible. Contraindications include pregnancy, previous history of thrombophlebitis or thromboembolic disease, acute or chronic liver disease of cholestatic type with abnormal function, presence of estrogen-dependent carcinomas, undiagnosed uterine bleeding, heavy smoking, gallbladder disease, hypertension, diabetes, mirgraine with visual disturbances, hypercoagulable disorders, and hyperlipidemia. Women with migraine headaches without visual disturbances, epilepsy, depression, oligomenorrhea, and amenorrhea may use COCs; however, they should be monitored closely.

2. COCs are taken daily for 21 days, following one of these methods:
   Day 1 start. The woman begins taking the pill on the first day of her menstrual cycle. This method prevents ovulation in the first cycle, so no backup method of contraception is needed.
   Sunday start. The woman begins taking the pill on the Sunday after the first day of the menstrual cycle and ending on a Saturday. In most cases, a hormonally mediated menses (known as a "withdraw" bleed) will occur 1 to 4 days after the last pill is taken. However, a backup method of contraception is necessary during the first 7 days of use.
   Quick start. The woman begins taking the pill in the practitioner's office if she is reasonably certain she is not pregnant. A backup method is necessary for 7 days.

3. The side effects of of COCs that are primarily related to the estrogen include alterations in lipid metabolism, breast tenderness, fluid retention, weight gain, headache, hypertension, nausea, thromboembolic

POWERPOINT LECTURE SLIDES

(NOTE: The number on each PPT Lecture Slide directly corresponds with the Concepts for Lecture.)

[1] Combined Oral Contraceptives (COC)
- Contains estrogen and progestin
- Methods of administration
  - Day one start
  - Sunday start
  - Quick start

[2] Contraindications
- Previous history of thromboembolic disease
- Acute or chronic liver disease
- Presence of estrogen-dependent carcinomas
- Undiagnosed uterine bleeding
- Heavy smoking
- Gallbladder disease

[2a] Contraindications
- Hypertension, diabetes
- Migraine with visual disturbances
- Hypercoagulable disorders
- Hyperlipidemia

[3] Side Effects of COC Due to Estrogen
- Alterations in lipid metabolism
- Breast tenderness
- Fluid retention, weight gain
- Headache and hypertension
- Nausea
- Thromboembolic complications

[3a] Side Effects of COC Due to Progestin
- Acne
- Breast tenderness
- Decreased libido
- Decreased high-density lipoprotein (HDL)
- Depression and fatigue
- Hirsutism, weight gain, an amenorrhea

[4] Non-Contraceptive Benefits
- Relief of menstrual symptoms and premenstrual syndrome

 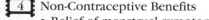

complications. Side effects primarily related to progestin include acne, breast tenderness, decreased libido, decreased HDL, depression, fatigue, hirsutism, weight gain, and amenorrhea.

4. The noncontraceptive benefits of COCs may include relief of menstrual symptoms and premenstrual syndrome; decreased incidence of functional ovarian cysts; and reduction in the incidence of ectopic pregnancy, PID, ovarian cancer, endometrial cancer, colorectal cancer, iron deficiency anemia, and benign breast disease.

- Decreased incidence of functional ovarian cysts
- Reduction in the incidence of:
  ○ Ectopic pregnancy and pelvic inflammatory disease (PID)
  ○ Ovarian, endometrial, and colorectal cancer
  ○ Iron deficiency anemia and benign breast disease

SUGGESTIONS FOR CLASSROOM ACTIVITIES

Have students develop a care plan for teaching women about COCs.

SUGGESTIONS FOR CLINICAL ACTIVITIES

Have students interview friends who use COCs about their patterns of use. Identify trends of use and potential risks in the use of this type of contraceptive.

LEARNING OBJECTIVE 6

Compare other hormonal methods of birth control, including Depo-Provera, NuvaRing, Ortho Evra, and the minipill.

CONCEPTS FOR LECTURE

1. Additional methods of hormonal contraception include the contraceptive skin patch, Ortho Evra, which is used weekly for 3 weeks on one of four sites: the abdomen, buttocks, upper outer arm, or trunk. The NuvaRing vaginal contraceptive ring is a flexible, soft vaginal ring that is inserted monthly. The ring is left in place for 21 days and then removed for 7 days. Depot-medroxyprogesterone acetate (DMPA) (Depo-Provera 150 mg), provides highly effective birth control for 3 months (every 10 to 14 weeks) when administered as a single IM injection of 150 mg. It acts by suppressing ovulation. The minipill contains only progestin and is used primarily by nursing mothers, as it does not interfere with breast milk production. This type of oral contraceptive is slightly less effective than the COC and must be taken at a consistent time every day.

POWERPOINT LECTURE SLIDES

(NOTE: The number on each PPT Lecture Slide directly corresponds with the Concepts for Lecture.)

1. Other Hormonal Contraceptives
   - Combination estrogen-progesterone
     ○ Transdermal
     ○ Vaginal Ring
     ○ NuvaRing
   - Progestin only
     ○ Minipill
     ○ Long-acting injectable progestin
     ○ Depo-Provera

SUGGESTIONS FOR CLASSROOM ACTIVITIES

Have students identify clients who would benefit from these types of contraceptives.

LEARNING OBJECTIVE 7

Identify the appropriate time frame for initiating postcoital emergency contraception (EC).

CONCEPTS FOR LECTURE

1. Postcoital emergency contraception (EC) is used when a woman is worried about pregnancy because of unprotected intercourse, sexual assault, or possible contraceptive failure. Two hormonal regimens for EC include a combined hormonal approach (levonorgestrel and ethinyl estradiol) and Plan B, a progestin-only approach (levonorgestrel).

POWERPOINT LECTURE SLIDES

(NOTE: The number on each PPT Lecture Slide directly corresponds with the Concepts for Lecture.)

 Emergency Contraception
   - Combined oral contraceptive
     ○ May cause nausea and vomiting
     ○ 72 hours of unprotected intercourse

The woman takes her first dose as soon after intercourse as possible and a second dose 12 hours later. The combined hormonal approach uses high-dose oral contraceptives and may result in nausea and vomiting. Plan B (progestin-only) is more effective than the combined hormonal EC and has a much lower incidence of associated nausea and vomiting. Another type of EC involves the placement of the Copper IUD within 5 days after unprotected intercourse.

- Progestin-only contraceptive (Plan B)
  - More effective than combined postcoital emergency contraception (EC)
  - 72 hours of unprotected intercourse
- Intrauterine device (IUD)
  - Must be placed within five days of unprotected intercourse

---

SUGGESTIONS FOR CLASSROOM ACTIVITIES

Have a discussion about the current controversy about EC and pharmaceutical distribution over the counter. Discuss implications for clients and healthcare providers.

LEARNING OBJECTIVE 8

Delineate the advantages and disadvantages of an IUD as a method of contraception.

CONCEPTS FOR LECTURE

1. The Copper IUD (ParaGARD T380A) provides contraception for 10 years, whereas the Mirena Levonorgestrel Intrauterine System (LNG-IUS) provides 5 years of protection. The LNG-IUS secretes progestin, etonogestrel which make the endometrium atrophic and the cervical secretions thick. Both types act by immobilizing sperm or by impeding their progress to the fallopian tubes and providing a local inflammatory effect.
2. Advantages of both types of IUDs include high rate of effectiveness, continuous contraceptive protection, non-coitus-related activity, and relative inexpensiveness over time. Potential adverse reactions to the IUD include discomfort to the wearer, increased bleeding during menses, increased risk of pelvic infection for about 3 weeks following insertion, perforation of the uterus during insertion, intermenstrual bleeding, dysmenorrhea, and expulsion of the device.

POWERPOINT LECTURE SLIDES

(NOTE: The number on each PPT Lecture Slide directly corresponds with the Concepts for Lecture.)

1 Intrauterine Devices
- Copper IUD (ParaGARD T380A)
  - Provides protection for 10 years
- Mirena Levonorgestrel Intrauterine System (LNG-IUS)
  - Provides protection for five years

2 Advantages of the IUD
- High rate of effectiveness
- Continuous contraceptive protection
- Noncoitus-related activity
- Relative inexpensiveness over time

2a Possible Adverse Reactions
- Increased and intermenstrual bleeding
- Increased risk of pelvic infection
- Perforation of the uterus during insertion
- Dysmenorrhea
- Expulsion of the device

SUGGESTIONS FOR CLASSROOM ACTIVITIES

Show students models of IUDs. Discuss the advantages and disadvantages of IUDs.

LEARNING OBJECTIVE 9

Contrast the forms of sterilization—tubal ligation, Essure, and vasectomy—with regard to risk, effectiveness, advantages, and disadvantages.

CONCEPTS FOR LECTURE

1. Surgical procedures that permanently prevent pregnancy include the vasectomy for the man and the tubal ligation for the woman. A vasectomy involves surgically severing the vas deferens in both sides of the

POWERPOINT LECTURE SLIDES

(NOTE: The number on each PPT Lecture Slide directly corresponds with the Concepts for Lecture.)

scrotum. The full contraceptive benefit is not realized until about 4 to 6 weeks and 6 to 36 ejaculations in-which the remaining sperm are cleared from the vas deferens. Tubal ligation may be done at any time, how-ever, the postpartal period is an ideal time to perform a tubal ligation because the uterus is enlarged and the tubes are easy to locate. The tubes are ligated, clipped, electrocoagulated, banded, or plugged, which inter-rupts the patency of the fallopian tube. The Essure method of permanent sterilization by Conceptus re-quires no surgical incision. It is done under hys-teroscopy whereby a stainless steel microinsert is placed into each proximal section of the fallopian tube. Within 3 months, these microinserts create tissue response that occludes the fallopian tubes. Occulusion is confirmed by hysterosalpingogram.

 Sterilization
- Operative
  - Vasectomy
  - Tubal ligation
- Nonoperative
  - Essure

SUGGESTIONS FOR CLINICAL ACTIVITIES

Have students teach a woman or man who is considering sterilization about the procedure.

LEARNING OBJECTIVE 10

Compare medical and surgical approaches to pregnancy termination.

CONCEPTS FOR LECTURE

1. The technique used for surgical abortion in the first trimester (less than 13 weeks' gestation) is vacuum curettage. Second trimester abortions are done using dilation and evacuation (D & E).

2. In 2000, the Food and Drug Administration (FDA) ap-proved mifepristone (Mifeprex), originally called RU 486. Mifepristone blocks the action of progesterone, thereby altering the endometrium and inhibiting implantation. After the length of the woman's gestation is confirmed, she takes a dose of oral mifepristone in her caregiver's office. One to 3 days (depending upon gestation) later she returns to her caregiver and takes an oral or vaginal dose of the prostaglandin misoprostol, which induces contractions that expel the embryo/fetus. The woman is seen about 14 days after taking the misoprostol to con-firm the successful abortion. Although methotrexate is not labeled for medical abortion, it is used in the first 7 weeks of pregnancy to stop cell division. Methotrexate may be given with misoprostol.

POWERPOINT LECTURE SLIDES

(NOTE: The number on each PPT Lecture Slide directly corresponds with the Concepts for Lecture.)

 Surgical Pregnancy Termination
- First trimester
  - Safer than second trimester
  - Vacuum curretage
- Second trimester
  - Dilatation and evacuation
- Nursing management
  - Support
  - Education

 Medical Pregnancy Termination
- Mifepristone (RU-486)/misoprostol
- First seven weeks of pregnancy
- Methotrexate
  - First seven weeks of pregnancy
  - Not currently approved for this use

SUGGESTIONS FOR CLASSROOM ACTIVITIES

Have a group discussion about the risks of each type of pregnancy termination. Discuss the nurse's role in pregnancy termination.

SUGGESTIONS FOR CLINICAL ACTIVITIES

Develop a care plan for a woman undergoing preg-nancy termination.

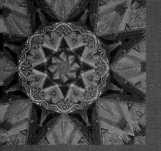

CHAPTER 6
WOMEN'S HEALTH: COMMONLY OCCURRING INFECTIONS

RESOURCE LIBRARY

 PRENTICE HALL NURSING MEDIALINK DVD-ROM

Audio Glossary
NCLEX Review

COMPANION WEBSITE

Additional NCLEX Review
Case Study: *Pediculosis Pubis*
Care Plan Activity: *Gynecologic Infection*
Applications: *Sexually Transmitted Infections;
Preventing Urinary Tract Infections*
Critical Thinking

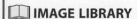 **IMAGE LIBRARY**

Figure 6.1 The characteristic "clue cells" seen in bacterial vaginosis.
Figure 6.2 Hyphae and spores of *Candida albicans*.
Figure 6.3 Microscopic appearance of *Trichomonas vaginalis*.

Figure 6.4 Condylomata acuminata on the vulva.
Figure 6.5 The nurse counsels the woman about measures for preventing urinary tract infection.

LEARNING OBJECTIVE 1

Compare vulvovaginal candidiasis and bacterial vaginosis.

CONCEPTS FOR LECTURE

1. The most common form of vaginal infections in the United States is bacterial vaginosis (BV). It results from an alteration in the normal vaginal bacterial flora, which causes an overgrowth of anaerobic bacteria. Risk factors include frequent sexual intercourse without condom use, trauma from douching, and an upset in normal vaginal flora. Symptoms may include an excessive amount of thin, watery, white or gray vaginal discharge with a foul odor. BV is treated with metronidazole (Flagyl) orally or intravaginally.

2. Another common vaginal infection is vulvovaginal candidiasis (VVC), also known as candidiasis, or fungal and yeast infection. Symptoms include thick, white vaginal discharge, severe itching, dysuria, and dyspareunia. Males who are infected with VVC may experience a rash or excoriation of the skin of the penis, and possibly pruritus. Women infected with VVC are treated with intravaginal butoconazole, clotrimazole, miconazole, nystatin, terconazole, or tioconazole cream, tablets, or suppositories. Women may also be treated orally with fluconazole. Male partners are generally not treated.

POWERPOINT LECTURE SLIDES

(NOTE: The number on each PPT Lecture Slide directly corresponds with the Concepts for Lecture.)

1 Bacterial Vaginosis (BV)
- Overgrowth of normal vaginal flora
- Thin, watery, white-gray discharge
- "Fishy" odor
- Treatment: Flagyl

2 Vulvovaginal Candidiasis (VVC)
- Fungal or yeast infection
- Thick, white vaginal discharge
- Severe itching, dysuria, and dyspareunia
- Treatment: miconazole cream

LEARNING OBJECTIVE 2

Summarize modes of transmission, treatments, and descriptions of the most commonly occurring sexually transmitted infections (STIs).

CONCEPTS FOR LECTURE

1. A commonly occurring sexually transmitted disease is caused by *Trichomonas vaginalis*. The infection usually occurs through sexual intimacy; however, fomite transmission may also occur through shared bath facilities, wet towels, or wet swimsuits. Most women are asymptomatic or have only mild symptoms. Symptoms may include a yellow-green, frothy, odorous discharge and vulvar itching, dysuria, and dyspareunia. Treatment for trichomoniasis is with oral metronidazole (Flagyl). Both partners should be treated and should avoid intercourse until they are cured.

2. The most common bacterial STI in the United States is caused by *Chlamydia trachomatis*. Transmission occurs through vaginal intercourse. Asymptomatic infection is common in women and men. If symptomatic, the symptoms may include thin or mucopurulent discharge, cervical ectopia, friable cervix (bleeds easily), burning and frequency of urination, and lower abdominal pain. Infection in women can affect the fallopian tubes, cervix, urethra, and Bartholin's glands. Long-term sequelae may include pelvic inflammatory disease (PID), infertility, and ectopic pregnancy. Chlamydial infection in men may result in epididymitis and infertility. Chlamydia is treated with azithromycin.

3. The second most commonly reported STI is gonorrhea, an infection caused by the bacterium *Neisseria gonorrhoeae*. Transmission occurs through vaginal, anal, or oral sex. Most women are asymptomatic; however, when symptoms occur, they may include a purulent, greenish-yellow vaginal discharge, dysuria, urinary frequency, vulvar inflammation, cervical inflammation and foul-smelling discharge, and bilateral lower abdominal or pelvic pain. This infection is treated with antibiotics such as cefixime, ciprofloxacin, ofloxacin, or levofloxacin orally (or ceftriaxone administered intramuscularly). Combined antibiotic treatment for gonorrhea and chlamydia should be considered as these two infections frequently occur together. Sexual partners must be treated and both should be treated until the infection is cured.

4. Recurrent genital herpes is most often caused by herpes simplex virus-2. It is transmitted through vaginal, anal, or oral sex, and through skin-to-skin contact with an infected site. The primary episode (first outbreak) is characterized by the development of single or multiple blisterlike vesicles, which usually occur in the genital area and sometimes affect the vaginal walls, cervix, urethra, and anus. These vesicles rupture spontaneously to form very painful, open, ulcerated lesions. Secondary effects may include difficult urination and urinary retention due to inflammation and pain. The inguinal lymph nodes may be enlarged, and flulike symptoms and

POWERPOINT LECTURE SLIDES

(NOTE: The number on each PPT Lecture Slide directly corresponds with the Concepts for Lecture.)

1 Trichomoniasis
- Bacterial organism: *Trichomonas vaginalis*
- Transmission: sexual intimacy
- Symptoms: asymptomatic or mild
  - Yellow-green, frothy, odorous discharge
  - Vulvar itching
- Treatment: metronidazole

2 Chlamydia
- Bacterial organism: *Chlamydia trachomatis*
- Transmission: vaginal sex
- Symptoms: 70% of women are asymptomatic
- Treatment: azithromycin or doxycycline

3 Gonorrhea
- Bacterial organism: *Neisseria gonorrhoeae*
- Transmission: vaginal, anal, or oral sex
- Symptoms: 80% of women are asymptomatic
- Treatment: antibiotic therapy

4 Herpes Simplex
- Viral organism: HSV-1 and HSV-2
- Transmission
  - Vaginal, anal, or oral sex
  - Skin-to-skin contact with an infected site

4a Herpes Simplex
- Symptoms: primary outbreak
  - Single or multiple blisterlike vesicles
  - Difficult urination and urinary retention
  - Enlargement of inguinal lymph nodes
  - Flulike symptoms, genital pruritus, or tingling
- Treatment: oral acyclovir

5 Syphilis
- Bacterial organism: *Treponema pallidum*
- Transmission
  - Vaginal, oral, or anal sex
  - Exposure to exudate from infected individual
  - Transplacental
- Treatment: penicillin G

5a Syphilis
- Symptoms: Early stage
  - Chancre appears, fever, weight loss, malaise
- Symptoms: Secondary stage
  - Condylomata lata on vulva, acute arthritis
  - Enlargement of liver and spleen, enlarged lymph nodes
  - Chronic sore throat with hoarseness

genital pruritus or tingling may also occur. The lesions heal spontaneously in 2 to 4 weeks and the virus enters a dormant phase, resting in the nerve ganglia of the affected area. Recurrences are usually less severe than the initial episode and may be triggered by emotional stress, menstruation, ovulation, pregnancy, frequent or vigorous intercourse, poor health status or a generally run-down physical condition, tight clothing, or overheating. There is no known cure for herpes; however, medications are available to provide pain relief and prevent complications. Recommended treatment includes oral acyclovir, valacyclovir, or famciclovir.

5. The spirochete *Treponema pallidum* causes syphilis. Transmission is through vaginal, oral, or anal sex; or, less commonly, nonsexual exposure to exudates from an infected individual. Syphilis can also be transmitted congenitally through the placenta. In the early stage (primary), a chancre (painless ulcer) appears at the site where the *Treponema pallidum* organism entered the body. Early symptoms may include slight fever, loss of weight, and malaise. The chancre disappears after about 4 weeks. Secondary symptoms appear in 6 weeks to 6 months. During this time, skin eruptions called condylomata lata may appear on the vulva. Additional symptoms may include acute arthritis, enlargement of the liver and spleen, nontender enlarged lymph nodes, iritis, and a chronic sore throat with hoarseness. Syphilis transmitted transplacentally may cause intrauterine growth restriction, preterm birth, and stillbirth. Treatment is with penicillin G.

6. Veneral warts (condylomata acuminata) is a common sexually transmitted infection caused by the human papilloma virus (HPV). Transmission occurs through vaginal, oral, or anal sex. Symptoms may include a single or multiple soft, grayish pink, cauliflower-like lesions in the genital area. The warts may be asymptomatic or they may cause itching, be friable, or be painful. Treatment varies depending on the client and provider and may include client-applied therapies such as podofilox solution or gel or imiquimod cream, or provider-administered therapies such as cryotherapy with liquid nitrogen or cryoprobe; topical podophyllin; trichloroacetic acid (TCA); bichloroacetic acid (BCA); or surgical removal by tangential scissors excision, shave excision, curettage, or electrosurgery.

7. Phthirus, a grayish, parasitic "crab" louse causes pediculosis pubis. The eggs attach to the hair shaft. Transmission occurs primarily by sexual contact, although transmission through shared towels and bed linens may occur. The most prevalent symptom is itching. Treatment includes the application of a 1% permethrin cream rinse to the affected area and washing it off after 10 minutes. The sexual partner must also be treated. Bed linens, towels, and clothing should be machine washed and dried in hot water and dried in a hot dryer, dry-cleaned, or removed from body contact for at least 72 hours.

 Genital Warts
- Viral organism: human papilloma virus (HPV)
- Transmission: vaginal, oral, or anal sex
- Symptoms:
  - Painless genital warts
  - Pruritus
- Treatment: client or provider therapies for wart removal

 Pediculosis Pubis
- Parasite: Phthirus
- Transmission: intimate sexual contact, shared towels and bed linens
- Symptoms:
  - Itching in pubic area
- Treatment: 1% permethrin cream, wash and dry linens, towels, and clothing

 Scabies
- Parasite: *Sarcoptes scabiei*
- Transmission: intimate sexual contact in adults
- Symptoms:
  - Itching and erythematous, papular lesions or furrows
- Treatment: 5% permethrin cream
  - Wash and dry linens, towels, and clothing

8. The parasitic itch mite, *Sarcoptes scabiei* burrows under the skin to deposit her eggs. Transmission is through intimate sexual contact in adults but not in children. Symptoms may include itching that worsens at night or when the individual is warm, and erythematous, papular lesions or furrows. Treatment includes the application of permethrin cream 5% to all body areas from the neck down and washing it off 8 to 14 hours later. Clothing and bed linens should be washed and dried in a hot dryer or dry-cleaned.

SUGGESTIONS FOR CLASSROOM ACTIVITIES

Show students slides from the CDC of symptomatology of the infections. Have a group discussion about strategies to prevent STIs.

SUGGESTIONS FOR CLINICAL ACTIVITIES

Have students teach a class in a high school about the recognition, treatment, and prevention of STIs.

LEARNING OBJECTIVE 3

Summarize the health teaching that a nurse needs to provide to a woman with an STI.

CONCEPTS FOR LECTURE

1. Health teaching that a nurse needs to provide to a woman with an STI includes information about the infection, methods of transmission, implications for pregnancy or future fertility, and importance of thorough treatment. Additionally, the woman should be made aware that her partner may need to be treated to prevent reinfection and that she may need to abstain from sexual activity during treatment. She should be taught preventive strategies for the future, such as planning ahead and developing strategies to say no to sex, limiting the number of sexual contacts and practicing monogamy, using a condom, negotiating condom use with a partner, reducing high-risk behaviors that lead to sexual risk-taking, and refraining from oral sex if the partner has active sores in the mouth, vagina, anus, or on the penis. She should also be taught to seek care as soon as symptoms are noticed if she develops STIs in the future and that she should take all medications until they are completed. She should be advised that she should have more frequent Pap screening for certain genital infections.

POWERPOINT LECTURE SLIDES

(NOTE: The number on each PPT Lecture Slide directly corresponds with the Concepts for Lecture.)

1 Health Teaching
- Planning ahead and developing strategies to say no to sex
- Limiting the number of sexual contacts and practicing monogamy
- Using a condom and negotiating condom use with a partner
- Reducing high-risk behaviors such as alcohol and recreational drugs
- Refraining from oral sex if partner has active sores in mouth, vagina, anus, or on penis
- Seeking care as soon as symptoms are noticed

1a Health Teaching
- Disappearance of symptoms does not mean treatment is unnecessary
- Take all prescribed medications completely
- More frequent Pap screening for certain genital infections

SUGGESTIONS FOR CLASSROOM ACTIVITIES

Have students develop a care plan for teaching a client with one of the STIs.

SUGGESTIONS FOR CLINICAL ACTIVITIES

Ask students to teach a client in a clinical setting about treatment for an STI. Have the students note the client response to teaching.

Learning Objective 4

Relate the implications of pelvic inflammatory disease (PID) for future fertility to its pathologic origin, signs and symptoms, and treatment.

Concepts for Lecture

1. A clinical syndrome of inflammation of the upper genital tract describes pelvic inflammatory disease (PID). It may include any combination of endometritis, salpingitis, tubo-ovarian abscess, pelvic abscess, and pelvic peritonitis. One of the most concerning sequelae is tubal damage, which is closely associated with infertility. *Chlamydia trachomatis* and *Neisseria gonorrhoeae*, which often occur together, are common causes of PID. Although some women may be asymptomatic, symptoms may include bilateral sharp, cramping pain in the lower quadrants, fever greater than 101F, chills, mucopurulent cervical or vaginal discharge, irregular bleeding, cervical motion tenderness during intercourse, malaise, nausea, and vomiting. These women are treated with intravenous (IV) fluids, pain medication, and administration of IV antibiotics.

PowerPoint Lecture Slides

(NOTE: The number on each PPT Lecture Slide directly corresponds with the Concepts for Lecture.)

1 Pelvic Inflammatory Disease (PID)
- Inflammation of upper female genital tract
- *Chlamydia trachomatis* and *Neisseria gonorrhoeae*
- Postinfection tubal damage associated with infertility
- Treatment:
  - IV fluids, pain medication, IV antibiotics

1a Symptoms of PID
- Bilateral sharp, cramping pain in the lower quadrants
- Fever greater than 101F, chills
- Mucopurulent cervical or vaginal discharge
- Irregular bleeding
- Cervical motion tenderness during intercourse
- Malaise, nausea, and vomiting

Suggestions for Classroom Activities

Form small groups in the classroom to discuss strategies for prevention of STIs and PID in adolescents.

Learning Objective 5

Contrast cystitis and pyelonephritis.

Concepts for Lecture

1. Risk factors for cystitis include sexual intercourse, the use of a diaphragm and a spermicide, delayed postcoital micturition, pregnancy, and a history of a recent urinary tract infection (UTI). Symptoms are often acute and include dysuria, specifically at the end of urination; as well as urgency and frequency, suprapubic or low back pain, a low-grade fever, and hematuria. Antibiotic treatment is based on the causative pathogen.

2. Pyelonephritis is often preceded by lower UTI. Symptoms include a sudden onset with chills, high temperature of 39.6C to 40.6C (103F to 105F), and costovertebral angle tenderness or flank pain, which may be unilateral or bilateral. The woman may also experience nausea, vomiting, and general malaise. She may also experience frequency, urgency, and burning with urination and a decrease in urinary output with severe colicky pain, vomiting, dehydration, and ileus of the large bowel. Treatment is hospitalization for IV hydration, antibiotic therapy, urinary analgesics such as Pyridium, pain management, and medication to manage fever.

PowerPoint Lecture Slides

(NOTE: The number on each PPT Lecture Slide directly corresponds with the Concepts for Lecture.)

1 Cystitis: Risk Factors
- Sexual intercourse
- Use of a diaphragm and a spermicide
- Delayed postcoital micturition
- Pregnancy
- History of a recent UTI

1a Cystitis
- Symptoms
  - Dysuria, urgency, and frequency
  - Suprapubic or low back pain
  - Low-grade fever
  - Hematuria
- Treatment: antibiotic therapy

2 Pyelonephritis: Symptoms
- Sudden onset with chills, high temperature, and costovertebral angle tenderness or flank pain

- Nausea, vomiting, and malaise
- Frequency, urgency, and burning with urination
- Decreased urinary output
- Severe colicky pain, vomiting, dehydration, and ileus of the large bowel

 Pyelonephritis: Treatment
- IV antibiotics
- IV hydration
- Urinary analgesics such as Pyridium
- Pain management and medication to manage fever

SUGGESTIONS FOR CLINICAL ACTIVITIES

Have students who care for clients with pyelonephritis do a physical assessment to observe for the symptoms of pyelonephritis. Have them document their observations.

LEARNING OBJECTIVE 6

Compare the different types of viral hepatitis.

CONCEPTS FOR LECTURE

1. An inflammatory process of the liver caused by an infection of one of five viruses, A, B, C, D, and E, is hepatitis. Symptoms of hepatitis A include jaundice, anorexia, nausea, vomiting, malaise, and fever, and the infection is acute rather than chronic. Prevention of hepatis A is possible by administering a vaccine. Symptoms of hepatits B, C, and D are similar to those of hepatitis A and may also include arthralgias, arthritis, and skin eruptions or rash; however, these infections are chronic. Hepatitis E is similar to hepatits A and occurs primarily in South Central Asia and the Middle East.

POWERPOINT LECTURE SLIDES

(NOTE: The number on each PPT Lecture Slide directly corresponds with the Concepts for Lecture.)

 Hepatitis A
- Transmission: fecal-oral, contaminated food/water
- Incubation: 15–50 days
- Not chronic
- Immunization available

 Hepatits B
- Transmission: blood/body fluids
- Incubation: 45–160 days
- Chronic
- Immunization available

 Hepatits C
- Transmission: blood/blood products
- Incubation: 14–180 days
- Chronic
- Immunization not available

 Hepatits D
- Transmission: blood/body fluids
- Incubation: 45–160 days
- Chronic
- Immunization not available

 Hepatits E
- Transmission: fecal-oral
- Incubation: 15–60 days
- Not chronic
- Immunization not available

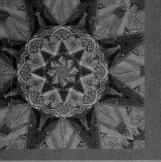

Chapter 7
Women's Health Problems

Resource Library

⊙ PRENTICE HALL NURSING MEDIALINK DVD-ROM

Audio Glossary
NCLEX Review
Video: *Breast Self-Examination*

🌐 COMPANION WEBSITE

Additional NCLEX Review
Case Study: *Toxic Shock Syndrome*
Care Plan Activity: *Irregular Bleeding in Perimenopausal Woman*
Applications: *Preparing an Adolescent for Her First Pelvic Examination; Cystocele*
Critical Thinking

📖 IMAGE LIBRARY

Figure 7.1 Positions for inspection of the breasts.
Figure 7.2 Procedure for breast self-examination.
Figure 7.3 Recommended position for mammogram.

Figure 7.4 Steps to follow to perform vulvar self-examination.
Figure 7.5 The nurse provides information for the woman during preoperative teaching.

Learning Objective 1

Contrast the common benign and malignant breast disorders.

Concepts for Lecture

1. Fibrocystic breast changes, fibroadenomas, galactor-rheas, intraductal papillomas, and duct ectasias are all benign breast disorders. The most common benign disorder is fibrocystic breast changes, which result from hormonal fluctuations, may produce an asymptomatic mass, and are often accompanied by pain or tenderness and sometimes nipple discharge. An asymptomatic, mobile, well-defined, painless, palpable mass with a rubbery texture is a fibroadenoma. Galactorrhea is nipple discharge not associated with lacation and may be physiologic, drug induced, idiopathic, or pathologic. Tumors growing in the terminal portion of a duct or, sometimes, throughout the duct system within a section of the breast are intraductal tumors. Associated symptoms may include a unilateral mass or a spontaneous, and often bloody, nipple discharge, and discharge from the nipple that may be serosanguineous or brownish green because of old blood. An inflammation of the ducts behind the nipple that commonly occurs during or near the onset of menopause is duct ectasia. Symptoms include a thick, sticky nipple discharge of various colors, and burning pain, pruritus, and inflammation.
2. Malignant breast disorders originate either in a duct or in the epithelium of the breast lobes. Approximately half of breast cancers originate in the upper outer quadrant and spread, or metastasize, to the axillary lymph

PowerPoint Lecture Slides

(NOTE: The number on each PPT Lecture Slide directly corresponds with the Concepts for Lecture.)

1 Benign Breast Disorders
- Fibrocystic breast change
- Fibroadenoma
- Galactorrhea
- Intraductal papillomas
- Duct ectasia

2 Malignant Breast Disorders
- Originates in duct or epithelium of lobes
- About 50% originate in upper outer quadrant
- Common sites of metastasis
  ○ Lymph nodes, lungs, liver, brain, and bone

2a Malignant Breast Disorders: Symptoms
(See Figure 7.3)
- Dimpling of breast tissue
- Recent or acute nipple inversion
- Change in breast size or shape
- Increase of size in breast mass
- Skin erosion or ulceration
- Presence of axillary lump

2b See Figure 7.3

nodes. Metastasis may occur in the lymph nodes, lungs, liver, brain, and bone. A physical assessment revealing dimpling of the breast tissue, recent or acute nipple inversion, change in breast size or shape, increase of size in breast mass, skin erosion or ulceration, or presence of axillary lump may indicate a higher risk for malignant breast disorders.

SUGGESTIONS FOR CLASSROOM ACTIVITIES

Bring in breast examination models to demonstrate how to do a breast exam and palpate for masses.

LEARNING OBJECTIVE 2

Briefly describe the emotional reactions a woman may experience in regard to a diagnosis of breast cancer.

CONCEPTS FOR LECTURE

1. Women who have a diagnosis of breast cancer experience emotional reactions that may lead to adjustment. This course of adjustment has been described in four phases: shock, reaction, recovery, and reorientation. Women are in the shock phase from the discovery of the lump to the diagnosis. When the treatment begins, reaction occurs as the woman is compelled to face what has occurred and begins to take in what has happened. Recuperation following medical treatment leads the woman to the recovery phase wherein her anxiety diminishes, she begins to look to the future again, and she resumes her former activities. If a woman is unable to complete this phase successfully, depression and social isolation occur. The final phase is reorientation. This phase follows recovery and is unending. This woman acknowledges the fact that breast cancer is part of her life, yet returns to her normal fullness of life.

POWERPOINT LECTURE SLIDES

(NOTE: The number on each PPT Lecture Slide directly corresponds with the Concepts for Lecture.)

1 Psychologic Adjustment to Breast Cancer
- Four phases
  - Shock
  - Reaction
  - Recovery
  - Reorientation

SUGGESTIONS FOR CLINICAL ACTIVITIES

Have students interview clients with a breast cancer diagnosis and identify the phase of psychologic adjustment that they are in.

LEARNING OBJECTIVE 3

Discuss the signs and symptoms, medical therapy, and implications for fertility of endometriosis.

CONCEPTS FOR LECTURE

1. The presence of endometrial tissue outside of the uterine cavity is classified as endometriosis. Although endometriosis can be found most anywhere in the body, the most common location is outside of the pelvis. Hormonal changes during the menstrual cycle will cause this tissue to bleed in a cyclic fashion, resulting in inflammation, scarring of the peritoneum, and

POWERPOINT LECTURE SLIDES

(NOTE: The number on each PPT Lecture Slide directly corresponds with the Concepts for Lecture.)

1 Endometriosis
- Presence of endometrial tissue outside the uterus
- Most common location is pelvis

CONCEPTS FOR LECTURE *continued*

formation of adhesions. The most common symptom is pelvic pain although it can also be asymptomatic. Dyspareunia (painful intercourse) and abnormal uterine bleeding may also occur. Surgical treatment may be conservative (laparoscopy) or definitive (hysterectomy). Medical treatment attempts to interrupt cyclic ovarian hormone production. A combination of therapies may also be used. Women with mild disease and symptoms may only require analgesics and non-steroidal anti-inflammatory drugs (NSAIDs). If pregnancy is desired, a suppression of estrogen synthesis is usually required to cause an atrophy of endometrial implants.

POWERPOINT LECTURE SLIDES *continued*

- Symptoms
  - Pelvic pain
  - Dyspareunia
  - Abnormal uterine bleeding

 Endometriosis
- Treatment
  - Medical—interruption of cyclic ovarian hormone production
  - Surgical—laparoscopy, hysterectomy

SUGGESTIONS FOR CLASSROOM ACTIVITIES

Discuss the psychologic effects of endometriosis on a woman and identify appropriate nursing interventions.

SUGGESTIONS FOR CLINICAL ACTIVITIES

Have students do a health history on a woman with a history of endometriosis, identifying the impact of the disease on her life.

LEARNING OBJECTIVE 4

Discuss the signs and symptoms, diagnosis criteria, treatment options, and health implications of polycystic ovarian syndrome.

CONCEPTS FOR LECTURE

1. Clinical signs of polycystic ovarian syndrome (PCOS) include menstrual dysfunction, androgen excess, obesity, hyperinsulinemia, and infertility. Elevated serum androgen levels, specifically testosterone and androsterone, can lead to clinical manifestations such as acne, alopecia (male-patterned hair loss), hirsutism, deepening voice, increased muscle mass, and menstrual irregularities. Many women with PCOS experience infertility related to anovulation. Diagnosis is made through a thorough history, physical examination, laboratory studies, and imaging. Treatment goals include decreasing the effects of hyperandrogenism, restoring reproductive functioning for women desiring pregnancy, protecting the endometrium, and reducing long-term risks, specifically type 2 diabetes and cardiovascular disease. Menstrual irregularities can be treated with a combined oral contraceptive or cyclic progesterone. The most common drug used to decrease circulating insulin is metformin (Glucophage®). Additionally, lifestyle changes such as weight loss, regular exercise, balanced diet, and cessation of smoking should be made. Women with PCOS are at an increased risk of developing overt type 2 diabetes, dyslipidemia, hypertension, cardiovascular disease, endometrial cancer, breast cancer, and ovarian cancer. These women may also experience emotional strain related to issues such as body image, infertility, problematic menses, and depression.

POWERPOINT LECTURE SLIDES

(NOTE: The number on each PPT Lecture Slide directly corresponds with the Concepts for Lecture.)

 Polycystic Ovarian Syndrome (PCOS)
- Symptoms
  - Menstrual dysfunction
  - Androgen excess
  - Obesity
  - Hyperinsulinemia
  - Infertility

 Polycystic Ovarian Syndrome (PCOS)
- Treatment goals
  - Decreasing the effects of hyperandrogenism
  - Restoring reproductive functioning
  - Protecting the endometrium
  - Reducing long-term risks

 Polycystic Ovarian Syndrome (PCOS)
- Risks
  - Type 2 diabetes
  - Dyslipidemia
  - Hypertension and cardiovascular disease
  - Endometrial, breast, and ovarian cancer
  - Emotional distress

CONCEPTS FOR LECTURE

1. Spotting between periods, missing several cycles followed by a heavy bleed, or menses that occur every 2 to 3 months can be classified as abnormal uterine bleeding (AUB). The mnemonic PHIMIC (*p*regnancy, *h*ormones, *i*atrogenic, *m*echanical, *i*nfection, and *c*ancer) can be used to help focus evaluation. Hormonal disorders such as thyroid, prolactin, chronic anovulation, and coagulation disorders may be causative factors. Iatrogenic causes are usually related to the effects of medications such as heparin, coumadin, prednisone, tamoxifen, and Depo-Provera. Mechanical causes of AUB may include leiomyomata (fibroids), endometrial polyps, or adenomyosis. Infection that results in endocervicitis, herpes, or endometritis can also be a cause of AUB. Endometrial and cervical cancers may also result in AUB. Treatment goals include controlling bleeding, preventing or treating anemia, preventing endometrial hyperplasia or cancer, and restoring quality of life.

2. Anovulatory cycles with abnormal uterine bleeding that does not appear to have an organic cause is classified as dysfunctional uterine bleeding (DUB). Examples of DUB include oligomenorrhea, polymenorrhea, menorrhagia, metrorrhagia, menometrorrhagia, and intermenstrual bleeding.

3. Masses found in the ovaries, fallopian tubes, broad ligament, or bowel, or even a lateral mass of the uterus are referred to as adnexal masses. Most of these masses are benign cysts. Women with ovarian masses may be asymptomatic or they may experience a sensation of fullness or cramping in the lower abdomen (often unilateral), dyspareunia, irregular bleeding, or delayed menstruation. Ovarian masses are diagnosed based on a palpable mass with or without symptoms. Overgrowths of the endometrium can result in endometrial polyps. Smooth muscle cells that are present in whorls and arise from uterine muscles and connective tissue are fibroids. These women may be asymptomatic or experience lower abdominal pain, fullness or pressure, menorrhagia, metrorrhagia, or have increased dysmenorrhea. Most of these masses do not require treatment and will resolve after menopause. Endometrial cancer generally occurs in postmenopausal women exhibiting the hallmark sign of vaginal bleeding without hormone replacement therapy (HRT). Endometrial cancer is diagnosed by Pap smear, by endometrial biopsy, by transvaginal ultrasound, or by posthysterectomy pathologic examination of the uterus. An exploratory laparotomy is usually performed to determine the stage of the cancer. The treatment for all types of endometrial cancer is total abdominal hysterectomy (TAH) and bilateral salpingo-oophorectomy (BSO).

POWERPOINT LECTURE SLIDES

(NOTE: The number on each PPT Lecture Slide directly corresponds with the Concepts for Lecture.)

1 Abnormal Uterine Bleeding (AUB)
- Pregnancy
- Hormonal disorders
- Iatrogenic causes
- Mechanical causes
- Infection
- Cancer

2 Dysfunctional Uterine Bleeding (DUB)
- Oligomenorrhea
- Polymenorrhea
- Menorrhagia
- Metrorrhagia
- Menometrorrhagia
- Intermenstrual bleeding

3 Masses
- Adnexal mass
- Endometrial polyps
- Endometrial cancer

LEARNING OBJECTIVE 6

Identify the implications of an abnormal finding during a pelvic examination.

CONCEPTS FOR LECTURE

1. Abnormal findings from a pelvic examination may involve tissues of the vulva, vagina, or cervix; abnormal uterine bleeding; or ovarian or uterine masses. Atrophic vaginitis is caused by a lack of estrogen stimulation to the vulva and vagina. The Bartholin's gland may also become infected resulting from inflammation of the gland. A depigmentation of the vulvar skin resulting in white patchy areas because of the absence of melanin is called vitiligo. A benign disorder of the vulva is lichen sclerosus in which bluish white papules coalesce and become white plaques, the skin becomes thin, and small fissures or ulcerations develop. Vestibulitis is a local irritation and inflammation of the vulvar vestibule with severe pain with vaginal penetration (tampons or intercourse), burning and itching, and sometimes urinary frequency or dysuria. Vulvar cancer occurs most commonly in postmenopausal women. These women present with pruritus, a lump, or a flat lesion, or may be relatively asymptomatic. Cervical inflammation can be caused by *Neisseria gonorrhoeae, Chlamydia trachomatis, Candida, Gardnerella vaginalis, Trichomonas,* herpes, staphylococci, or enterococci. Other causes of cervical inflammation may include use of intravaginal feminine hygiene products, frequent tampon use, frequent intercourse, or presence of a foreign body. Women present with a yellowish white vaginal discharge or copious purulent discharge that is sometimes malodorous, dyspareunia, pelvic heaviness, and urinary symptoms such as urgency, frequency, and burning.

POWERPOINT LECTURE SLIDES

(NOTE: The number on each PPT Lecture Slide directly corresponds with the Concepts for Lecture.)

1 Abnormal Pelvic Findings
- Atrophic vaginitis
- Infection of the Bartholin's gland
- Vitiligo
- Lichen sclerosus

1a Abnormal Pelvic Findings
- Vulvar vestibulitis
- Cancer of the vulva
- Cervicitis

LEARNING OBJECTIVE 7

Summarize behaviors that help to minimize recurrence of some of the common lesions of the vulva.

CONCEPTS FOR LECTURE

1. Women can be taught behaviors that help to minimize recurrence of some of the common lesions of the vulva. These include self-examination of the vulva to permit early detection of abnormalities and avoidance of irritating substances, synthetic clothing that traps moisture, tight clothing, some repetitive motion exercise such as running, frequent shaving of the perineum,

POWERPOINT LECTURE SLIDES

(NOTE: The number on each PPT Lecture Slide directly corresponds with the Concepts for Lecture.)

1 Minimizing Vulvar Lesions
- Vulvar self-exam (see Figure 7.4)
- Avoidance of irritants
  - Synthetic clothing that traps moisture
  - Tight clothing
  - Some repetitive motion exercises such as running

frequent intercourse or intercourse without lubrication, and deodorant menstrual products.

- ○ Frequent shaving of the perineum
- ○ Frequent intercourse or intercourse without lubrication
- ○ Deodorant menstrual products

 See Figure 7.4

SUGGESTIONS FOR CLASSROOM ACTIVITIES

Bring a vulvar model to class and teach the students how to do a self-exam.

SUGGESTIONS FOR CLINICAL ACTIVITIES

Have students develop a teaching plan for vulvar self-care for women in the clinical setting.

LEARNING OBJECTIVE 8

Discuss the importance of annual Pap smear evaluation, the implication of an abnormal finding, and appropriate follow-up.

CONCEPTS FOR LECTURE

1. The Papanicolaou smear (Pap smear) is done annually to screen for the presence of cellular abnormalities in the cervix and the endocervical canal, which can identify precancerous and cancerous conditions, as well as atypical findings and inflammatory changes. Because cervical cancer has a long preinvasive length, it is considered a preventable disease. A colposcopy and/or endocervical curettage (ECC) may be needed to be done for further diagnostic evaluation based upon the results of the Pap smear. Treatment for premalignant and malignant lesions involves surgery from a simple biopsy of the cervix to radical surgery of the pelvic organs dependent upon the extent of the disease.

POWERPOINT LECTURE SLIDES

(NOTE: The number on each PPT Lecture Slide directly corresponds with the Concepts for Lecture.)

 Cervical Cancer
- • Preventable, lengthy preinvasive state
- • Pap smear
- • Other diagnostics
  - ○ Colposcopy
  - ○ Endocervical curettage
- • Surgical treatment

SUGGESTIONS FOR CLASSROOM ACTIVITIES

Have a group discussion about the barriers for women to receive regular Pap smears and potential ways to overcome those barriers.

SUGGESTIONS FOR CLINICAL ACTIVITIES

Have students care for a woman with an abnormal Pap smear finding, identifying the diagnosis and extent of the disease and the treatment received. Discuss nursing interventions appropriate in caring for the woman.

LEARNING OBJECTIVE 9

Briefly discuss the role that human papilloma virus plays in abnormal Pap smears.

CONCEPTS FOR LECTURE

1. Human papilloma virus (HPV) has been linked to cervical dysplasia and carcinoma. Eleven specific types of HPV strains are now considered intermediate risk for high-grade cervical dysplasia, and cervical cancer and two strains are strongly associated with those disorders. Recently, a vaccine that is effective in preventing HPV-16 and HPV-18 has been developed.

POWERPOINT LECTURE SLIDES

(NOTE: The number on each PPT Lecture Slide directly corresponds with the Concepts for Lecture.)

 HPV
- • Increased risk for cervical dysplasia and cervical cancer
  - ○ Eleven types have an intermediate risk
  - ○ HPV-16 and HPV-18 are strongly associated
- • Vaccine available for prevention of HPV-16 and HPV-18

LEARNING OBJECTIVE 10

Delineate the psychosocial responses a woman may experience when facing any of the common gynecologic procedures.

CONCEPTS FOR LECTURE

1. Women facing common gynecologic procedures may have general concerns about treatment including fear of anesthesia, fear of death or disability, concerns about normal functioning, financial coverage for treatment and welfare of family members. Women may also face issues related to body image due to the loss of reproductive function and the resulting effect on childbearing and sexuality.

POWERPOINT LECTURE SLIDES

(NOTE: The number on each PPT Lecture Slide directly corresponds with the Concepts for Lecture.)

 1 Psychosocial Response
- Concerns about treatment
- Body image
  - Weight gain
  - Loss of sexuality
  - Inability to bear children

CHAPTER 8
WOMEN'S CARE: SOCIAL ISSUES

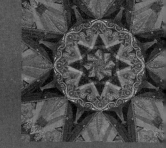

RESOURCE LIBRARY

💿 PRENTICE HALL NURSING MEDIALINK DVD-ROM

Audio Glossary
NCLEX Review

🌐 COMPANION WEBSITE

Additional NCLEX Review
Case Study: *Social Issues Affecting Women*
Care Plan Activity: *Pregnancy in a Disabled Client*
Applications: *How to Find Good Day Care; Elder Abuse*
Critical Thinking

📖 IMAGE LIBRARY

Figure 8.1 Two thirds of Americans living in poverty are women and children.

Figure 8.2 Some women rely on the father to provide full-time child care at home while they pursue their career.

Figure 8.3 Childhood education centers provide preschoolers with advanced skills for early education and provide care while parents work outside of the home.

Figure 8.4 Some mothers are able to combine professional careers with motherhood by telecommuting from a home office.

Figure 8.5 Older women are more likely to have multiple medical conditions that require medication.

Figure 8.6 Mental retardation is the most common developmental disability.

Figure 8.7 Lesbian families face discrimination that more traditional families do not commonly encounter.

LEARNING OBJECTIVE 1

Define the phrase *feminization of poverty*.

CONCEPTS FOR LECTURE

1. The feminization of poverty reflects the fact that more women live in poverty when compared with men. Children who live in female-headed households and are of an ethnic minority have the highest rates of poverty. This results in lower literacy levels and educational attainment for these women and children.

2. Issues that contribute to poverty include divorce, lower wages than men, public assistance, and homelessness. Divorced women have a decrease in their standard of living due to decreased earning potential and insufficient child support.

3. The Personal Responsibility and Work Opportunity Reconciliation Act was enacted in 1996. The act, while providing assistance to needy families, promotes job preparation, work, and marriage. An additional goal of the act is to encourage the formation of two-parent families and prevent out-of-wedlock pregnancies.

POWERPOINT LECTURE SLIDES

(NOTE: The number on each PPT Lecture Slide directly corresponds with the Concepts for Lecture.)

1 Feminization of Poverty
- Most in poverty are women
- 17% of children live in poverty
- More women are declaring bankruptcy
- Lower literacy rate than men

2 Social Issues Affecting Women in Poverty
- Divorce
- Lower wages compared with men
- Public assistance
- Homelessness (Figure 8.1)

2a See Figure 8.1

3 Temporary Assistance for Needy Families (TANF)
- Provides assistance for childcare
- Promotes job preparation, work, and marriage
- Reduces the incidence of unplanned pregnancies
- Encourages two-parent families

LEARNING OBJECTIVE 2

Identify factors that contribute to the wage gap between women and men.

CONCEPTS FOR LECTURE

1. Although women make up 40% of the US workforce, they do not earn as much as men for the same work.
2. The gap between wages of men and women is due to deliberate wage discrimination, undervaluing women's work, and socialization issues related to women's roles in the workplace and the world.

POWERPOINT LECTURE SLIDES

(NOTE: The number on each PPT Lecture Slide directly corresponds with the Concepts for Lecture.)

1. Wage Gap
   - 40% of US workforce consists of women (2004)
   - Expanded career options for women
   - Male-to-female earnings ratio is 76.5% (2004)
   - Widest gap between well-educated women and men

2. Causes of Wage Gap
   - Deliberate wage discrimination against women
   - Undervaluing of women's work
   - Women's socialization

LEARNING OBJECTIVE 3

Discuss poverty's effect on women's health care.

CONCEPTS FOR LECTURE

1. Factors that have played a role in poverty related to health care include a decrease in funding for many programs for women's and children's health, the movement of women receiving Medicaid to managed care, and a decrease in the private health insurance coverage for women.

POWERPOINT LECTURE SLIDES

(NOTE: The number on each PPT Lecture Slide directly corresponds with the Concepts for Lecture.)

1. Poverty's Effect on Women's Health
   - Medicaid
   - Managed care
   - Lack of health insurance

LEARNING OBJECTIVE 4

Discuss the impact of the Family and Medical Leave Act (FMLA) of 1993 on maternity and paternity leave.

CONCEPTS FOR LECTURE

1. Employees benefit from the FMLA of 1993 by permitting up to 12 weeks of unpaid leave after the birth or adoption of a child or the placement of a foster child. Employees who have a serious illness or must care for a spouse, child, or parent with a serious illness receive the same benefit. Although they do not receive pay

POWERPOINT LECTURE SLIDES

(NOTE: The number on each PPT Lecture Slide directly corresponds with the Concepts for Lecture.)

1. Family and Medical Leave Act (1993)
   - 12 weeks of unpaid leave following
     - Birth or adoption of a child
     - Placement of a foster child

during this leave, they receive health benefits and are assured of their former position or a comparable one when they return.

- Also applies to:
  - Serious illness
  - Illness of a spouse, child, or parent

LEARNING OBJECTIVE 5

Identify environmental hazards that may be present in the workplace or home of woman of childbearing age.

CONCEPTS FOR LECTURE

1. Environmental hazards to the health of women and their children may include air pollution, chemicals at work, and chemicals at home. Chemicals at work may include paints, varnishes, sealants, dry-cleaning chemicals, synthetic perfumes, hair or clothing dyes, and organic solvents. Chemicals at home may include plastics when heated, beauty products, pesticides, contaminated foods, produce, meat, and fish. Additionally, women in health care may be exposed to toxoplasmosis, rubella, cytomegalovirus, herpes simples, hepatitis B, HIV, and they may develop latex allergies.

POWERPOINT LECTURE SLIDES

(NOTE: The number on each PPT Lecture Slide directly corresponds with the Concepts for Lecture.)

1 Environmental Hazards
- Air pollution
- Chemicals at work
- Chemicals at home

1a Environmental Hazards in Health Care
- Exposure to TORCH viruses
- Exposure to HIV infection
- Latex allergy

SUGGESTIONS FOR CLASSROOM ACTIVITIES

Have students create an assessment tool to evaluate the home environment of a pregnant woman.

SUGGESTIONS FOR CLINICAL ACTIVITIES

Have students use the assessment tool to evaluate the home environment of a client who is pregnant or wants to become pregnant. Students should educate the client about the risks.

LEARNING OBJECTIVE 6

Identify factors that contribute to older women's economic vulnerability.

CONCEPTS FOR LECTURE

1. The economic vulnerability of women is due to their longer life expectancy, their weaker earning power, their economic dependence on men, their lack of pension benefits, less educational preparation, a smaller social security benefit, and more family caregiving responsibilities. Because of this they are more likely to live in poverty.

POWERPOINT LECTURE SLIDES

(NOTE: The number on each PPT Lecture Slide directly corresponds with the Concepts for Lecture.)

1 Economic Vulnerability of Older Women
- Women tend to outlive men
- Less educational preparation than men
- Economic dependency on men
- Limited or no pension benefits
- Fewer social security and retirement benefits
- Family caregiving responsibilities

SUGGESTIONS FOR CLASSROOM ACTIVITIES

Have a group discussion about the economic vulnerability of older women. Have them share examples of women they know.

Identify five different categories of elder abuse.

CONCEPTS FOR LECTURE

1. There are five categories of elder abuse: psychologic abuse, physical abuse (including sexual abuse), neglect (by self or caregiver), financial abuse, and abandonment. These may occur individually or at the same time.

POWERPOINT LECTURE SLIDES

(NOTE: The number on each PPT Lecture Slide directly corresponds with the Concepts for Lecture.)

 Elder Abuse
- Categories of abuse
  - Psychologic abuse
  - Physical abuse (including sexual abuse)
  - Neglect (by self or caregiver)
  - Financial abuse
  - Abandonment

SUGGESTIONS FOR CLASSROOM ACTIVITIES

Have students discuss the implications of elder abuse for healthcare providers. Have them discuss the role of the nurse in preventing, identifying, and reporting elder abuse.

LEARNING OBJECTIVE 8

Discuss the implications of aging on women's health and health care.

CONCEPTS FOR LECTURE

1. Common health problems of older women include: hypertension, coronary artery disease, arthritis, diabetes, osteoporosis, dementia, and depression. Approximately 50% of women have two or more of these chronic diseases. Women over 65 are most likely to die from heart disease, cancer, or stroke. The leading causes of death for women older than 65 are heart disease, cancer, and stroke, and minority and/or low income women are more likely to have serious health problems.

2. Barriers to healthcare experience by older women include: lack of transportation to healthcare facilities, lack of private health insurance coverage, and the inability to pay excessive medical costs not covered by Medicare. These women may have to choose between buying medicine and buying food. Polypharmacy is also a problem, as many of these women are on many medications for different illnesses, causing untoward effects.

POWERPOINT LECTURE SLIDES

(NOTE: The number on each PPT Lecture Slide directly corresponds with the Concepts for Lecture.)

 Effect of Aging on Women's Health: Common Problems
- Hypertension
- Coronary artery disease
- Arthritis, diabetes
- Osteoporosis
- Dementia
- Depression

 Effect of Aging on Women's Health
- 50% of women over 65 will have two or more chronic diseases.
- Leading causes of death for women greater or more than 65 years old
  - Heart disease
  - Cancer
  - Stroke
- Minority and low-income women are more at risk.

 Barriers to Health Care
- Lack of transportation
- Lack of private health insurance coverage
- Excessive medical costs
  - Choose between buying food and medicine
- Polypharmacy

LEARNING OBJECTIVE 9

Explain the implications of homophobia for lesbian and bisexual women's health care.

CONCEPTS FOR LECTURE

1. Discrimination in health care experienced by lesbian and bisexual women may include the lack of health insurance due to ineligibility for partner's benefits, perceived or actual antigay sentiments by healthcare providers, and lack of knowledge by healthcare providers regarding issues relevant to them.

POWERPOINT LECTURE SLIDES

(NOTE: The number on each PPT Lecture Slide directly corresponds with the Concepts for Lecture.)

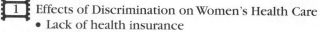 Effects of Discrimination on Women's Health Care
  - Lack of health insurance
  - Fear of antigay health provider sentiments
  - Reluctance to disclose sexual orientation
  - Lack of knowledge about lesbian/bisexual health issues

LEARNING OBJECTIVE 10

List the five main types of disability.

CONCEPTS FOR LECTURE

1. The five types of disabilities include: developmental, learning, neurologic, psychiatric, and sensory disabilities.

POWERPOINT LECTURE SLIDES

(NOTE: The number on each PPT Lecture Slide directly corresponds with the Concepts for Lecture.)

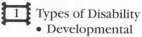 Types of Disability
  - Developmental
  - Learning
  - Neurological
  - Psychiatric
  - Sensory

LEARNING OBJECTIVE 11

Discuss ways in which a woman's disability may affect her health care.

CONCEPTS FOR LECTURE

1. Disabled women may have limited access to economic stability due to a limited ability to work full-time, lack of transportation to employment, and lack of access in the workplace. Their earning potential is less than that of a nondisabled woman and they are more likely to be a crime victim.
2. Access to health care is also an issue for these women. They may have difficulty getting onto examination tables, healthcare providers may be insensitive to the issues created by the disability, and as a sexual life may be assumed to be a nonissue with the disabled, they may not receive screening for sexually

POWERPOINT LECTURE SLIDES

(NOTE: The number on each PPT Lecture Slide directly corresponds with the Concepts for Lecture.)

1 Effects of Disability
  - Limited income potential due to:
    - Limited ability to work full-time
    - Lack of transportation
    - Lack of access in workplace
  - Do not earn as much as nondisabled
  - More likely to be a crime victim

2 Effects of Disability on Health Care
  - Difficulty getting onto examination tables
  - Lack of empathy from physician

transmitted infections (STIs), education regarding STI prevention, contraceptive counseling, and preconception counseling.

- Lack of
  - Screening for sexually transmitted infections (STI)
  - Education regarding STI prevention
  - Contraceptive and preconceptual counseling

LEARNING OBJECTIVE 12

Identify types of discrimination commonly faced by lesbian and bisexual women.

CONCEPTS FOR LECTURE

1. Discrimination that is experienced by lesbian and bisexual women includes employment and housing discrimination, discrimination involving domestic life and parenting issues, general social discrimination based on the stigma associated with homosexuality, and perceived or actual healthcare provider discrimination.

POWERPOINT LECTURE SLIDES

(NOTE: The number on each PPT Lecture Slide directly corresponds with the Concepts for Lecture.)

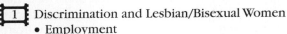 Discrimination and Lesbian/Bisexual Women
- Employment
- Housing
- Domestic life
- Parenting issues
- General social discrimination
- Healthcare provider discrimination

SUGGESTIONS FOR CLASSROOM ACTIVITIES

Have a group discussion about perceived and actual discrimination of lesbian and bisexual women.

LEARNING OBJECTIVE 13

Discuss the cultural implications of female genital mutilation.

CONCEPTS FOR LECTURE

1. The removal of all or part of a woman's genitalia for cultural reasons is termed genital mutilation. Resulting health problems may include: bleeding, infection, infertility, painful intercourse, and difficulties related to childbearing.
2. Female genital mutilation is done between the ages of 5 and 12 in male-dominated societies with patriarchal authority and control over the woman's body and fertility.

POWERPOINT LECTURE SLIDES

(NOTE: The number on each PPT Lecture Slide directly corresponds with the Concepts for Lecture.)

1 Female Genital Mutilation
- Removing all or parts of a girl's or woman's genitalia
- Health problems
  - Bleeding and infection
  - Infertility
  - Painful intercourse
  - Difficulties related to childbearing

2 Cultural Implications of Female Genital Mutilation
- Practiced in male-dominated societies
  - Patriarchal authority
  - Control of women's bodies
  - Control of fertility
- Done between 5 and 12 years of age

SUGGESTIONS FOR CLASSROOM ACTIVITIES

Have students select an article about female genital mutilation and present the article in class.

CHAPTER 9
VIOLENCE AGAINST WOMEN

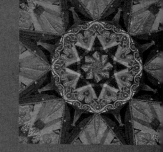

RESOURCE LIBRARY

 PRENTICE HALL NURSING MEDIALINK DVD-ROM

Audio Glossary
NCLEX review
Videos: *Spousal Abuse*; *Parental Sexual Abuse*; *Going Back?*

COMPANION WEBSITE

Additional NCLEX Review
Case Study: *Teenage Rape Victim*
Care Plan Activity: *Suspicious Injury and Bruises*
Applications: *Domestic Violence*; *Rohypnol*
Critical Thinking

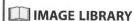 **IMAGE LIBRARY**

Figure 9.1 The power and control wheel.
Figure 9.2 Abuse assessment screen.

Figure 9.3 Screening for domestic violence should be done privately.

LEARNING OBJECTIVE 1

List the social, psychologic, political, and cultural factors that contribute to the occurrence of domestic violence and sexual assault.

CONCEPTS FOR LECTURE

1. Changes in healthcare policy and practices have occurred over the last three decades that have addressed the growing issue of violence against women. In 1990, the Joint Commission on the Accreditation of Hospitals and Healthcare Organizations (JCAHO) mandated the development of protocols for the identification and treatment of women who have been abused by their intimate partners. Additionally, Healthy People 2010 identified violence prevention and intervention as a national priority. The American Nurses Association (ANA) published a position statement advocating education for all nurses in identifying and preventing violence against women.

2. Women have been victims of violence for thousands of years in patriarchal societies. Wives have been considered as the property of husbands and the husband had the right and/or duty to keep the wife in line, to have sex on demand, and to even kill her. Over time, the legal status of women has improved in many cultures; however, male dominance in marriage or intimate relationships still exists in some cultures. Additionally, rape outside of marriage was traditionally not viewed as an act of a man against a woman, but as an act of aggression against another man who was considered her "owner."

POWERPOINT LECTURE SLIDES

(NOTE: The number on each PPT Lecture Slide directly corresponds with the Concepts for Lecture.)

1 Political Factors in Domestic Violence
- 1990 – JCAHO mandates identification and treatment protocols
- Healthy People 2010—intervention and prevention as a priority
- 1991—ANA position statement advocating education for nurses

2 Cultural Factors
- Patriarchal societies
- Women are property of husbands
- "Keep her in line"
- Male dominance
- Rape as an act of aggression against another man

SUGGESTIONS FOR CLASSROOM ACTIVITIES

Have a group discussion about student observations of male dominance in family behavior patterns and how that might play a role in domestic violence.

SUGGESTIONS FOR CLINICAL ACTIVITIES

Have students observe family interaction in the clinical setting, assessing for signs of family patterns that might put them at increased risk for domestic violence.

LEARNING OBJECTIVE 2

Describe ways in which psychologic, physical, and sexual abuse are used by batterers to maintain power and control in abusive relationships.

CONCEPTS FOR LECTURE

1. Batterers attempt to maintain control over their partner's behavior and the relationship through the following types of abuse: psychologic abuse, physical abuse, sexual abuse, threats of physical or sexual violence, and stalking. Psychologic abuse includes behaviors such as emotional abuse; isolation; obfuscation; using others against her; treating her like a servant, making all the household decisions; economic abuse; coercion threats; and intimidation. Physical and sexual abuse may include pushing, shoving, slapping, hitting the woman with a fist or object, kicking, choking, threatening with a gun or knife, or using a gun or knife against her. Sexual abuse is defined as any time the batterer forces or tries to force sex, the forced use of objects, or forcing a woman to have sex with someone else against her will.

POWERPOINT LECTURE SLIDES

(NOTE: The number on each PPT Lecture Slide directly corresponds with the Concepts for Lecture.)

1. Psychologic Abuse
   - Emotional abuse
   - Isolation
   - Obfuscation
   - Using others
   - Male privilege

1a. Psychologic Abuse
   - Economic abuse
   - Coercion threats
   - Intimidation

1b. Physical Abuse
   - Pushing
   - Shoving and slapping
   - Hitting with fist or object
   - Kicking
   - Choking
   - Threatening with gun or knife

1c. Sexual Abuse
   - Forces or tries to force sex
   - Forced use of objects
   - Forcing a women to have sex with someone else

SUGGESTIONS FOR CLASSROOM ACTIVITIES

Give the students examples of domestic violence in case situations and ask them to identify the abusive behaviors. Contrast emotional abuse with physical abuse.

LEARNING OBJECTIVE 3

Identify factors that contribute to domestic violence.

CONCEPTS FOR LECTURE

1. Factors that contribute to domestic violence include a complex and dynamic interaction of social, cultural, political, and psychologic factors. Children who witness or experience abuse and battering are more likely to become batterers or to be abused. Male economic and decision-making authority in the family is one of

POWERPOINT LECTURE SLIDES

(NOTE: The number on each PPT Lecture Slide directly corresponds with the Concepts for Lecture.)

1. Factors Contributing to Violence
   - Childhood experiences
   - Male dominance in the family

CONCEPTS FOR LECTURE *continued*

the strongest predictors of societies with a high rate of violence against women. High levels of conflict in relationships are associated with domestic violence. This is particularly more common in families with low incomes and unemployed men. Cultural definitions of manhood as dominant, tough, with an emphasis on male honor are associated with an increased likelihood of violence against women.

POWERPOINT LECTURE SLIDES *continued*

- Marital conflict
- Unemployment/low socioeconomic status
- Traditional definitions of masculinity

SUGGESTIONS FOR CLASSROOM ACTIVITIES

Ask students to list factors that they perceive as contributing to domestic violence. Discuss their lists as a group.

SUGGESTIONS FOR CLINICAL ACTIVITIES

Have students assess the family situation of women experiencing domestic violence for contributing factors and ask them to share these findings in postconference.

LEARNING OBJECTIVE 4

Dispel the common myths about domestic violence and sexual assault.

CONCEPTS FOR LECTURE

1. Myths about domestic violence and sexual assault include the following: that battering occurs in a small percentage of the population; women who are abused provoke men to beat them; alcohol and drug abuse cause battering; battered women can easily leave the situation; domestic violence is a low-income or minority issue; and battered women will be safer when they are pregnant.

POWERPOINT LECTURE SLIDES

(NOTE: The number on each PPT Lecture Slide directly corresponds with the Concepts for Lecture.)

 Common Myths
- Battering occurs in a small percentage of the population
- Women who are abused provoke men to beat them
- Alcohol and drug abuse cause battering
- Battered women can easily leave the situation
- Domestic violence is a low-income or minority issue
- Battered women will be safer when they are pregnant

SUGGESTIONS FOR CLASSROOM ACTIVITIES

Ask students to share their own perceptions about domestic violence and identify those perceptions that are myths.

SUGGESTIONS FOR CLINICAL ACTIVITIES

Have students interview friends or family about their perceptions of domestic violence and identify perceptions that are myths. Have them share their findings in postconference.

LEARNING OBJECTIVE 5

Identify the phases of the cycle of violence.

CONCEPTS FOR LECTURE

1. The three phases of the cycle of violence developed by Walker (1984) include: the tension-building phase, the acute battering incident, and the tranquil phase. The tension-building phase is one in which there is anger, arguing, blaming of the woman, and, possibly, minor battering. The acute battering incident is usually triggered by an external event or internal state of

POWERPOINT LECTURE SLIDES

(NOTE: The number on each PPT Lecture Slide directly corresponds with the Concepts for Lecture.)

 Cycle of Violence (Walker, 1984)
- Tension-building phase
- Acute battering incident
- Tranquil phase (honeymoon period)

---

the batterer and the batterer blames the woman for the abuse. The tranquil phase is characterized by extremely loving, kind, and contrite behaviors by the batterer as he attempts to make up with the woman. Without intervention, the cycle repeats.

SUGGESTIONS FOR CLASSROOM ACTIVITIES

Ask students to identify nursing interventions that would be appropriate during each phase of the cycle of violence.

SUGGESTIONS FOR CLINICAL ACTIVITIES

Have students identify the phase of the cycle of violence in which clients in the clinical setting experiencing domestic violence are in? Ask them to describe the assessment data supporting their assessment.

LEARNING OBJECTIVE 6

Summarize the characteristics of batterers and perpetrators of sexual assault.

CONCEPTS FOR LECTURE

1. The characteristics of batterers may include feelings of insecurity, inferiority, powerlessness, and helplessness that conflict with their assumptions of male supremacy. They tend to be emotionally immature and aggressive, and therefore, they have a tendency to express their feelings of inadequacy through violence. They tend to be very jealous and possessive and express their ambivalence by alternating beatings with periods of loving attention. The men lack respect toward women in general and usually come from homes where they witnessed abuse of their mothers or were abused themselves. They adopt "macho" values, yet they may appear childlike, dependent, seductive, manipulative, and in need of nurturing when they are not angry or aggressive. They have a low tolerance for frustration and poor impulse control, which leads them to strike out at the perceived inequities of life by abusing women.

POWERPOINT LECTURE SLIDES

(NOTE: The number on each PPT Lecture Slide directly corresponds with the Concepts for Lecture.)

1   Characteristics of Batterers
- Insecurity
- Inferiority
- Powerlessness
- Helplessness
- Male supremacy
- Emotionally immature

1a   Characteristics of Batterers
- Agressive
- Express overwhelming feelings through violence

SUGGESTIONS FOR CLASSROOM ACTIVITIES

Have students list the characteristics of their perception of a batterer. Combine student responses and look for similarities and differences as well as misconceptions. Discuss the findings as a group.

SUGGESTIONS FOR CLINICAL ACTIVITIES

Ask students to identify the characteristics of a batterer of a client in the clinical setting experiencing domestic violence. Have them share their findings in postconference.

LEARNING OBJECTIVE 7

Delineate the role of the nurse in caring for women who have experienced battering.

CONCEPTS FOR LECTURE

1. The role of the nurse caring for women experiencing battering includes assessment and documentation of abuse, counseling, safety planning, and referral. The goal is to empower the women by providing them with information that assists them in making decisions

POWERPOINT LECTURE SLIDES

(NOTE: The number on each PPT Lecture Slide directly corresponds with the Concepts for Lecture.)

1   Nurse's Role
- Recognizing and documenting abuse
- Intervention

and provides them with the assistance they need in safety planning for themselves and their children.

　　　○ Counseling
　　　○ Safety planning
　　　○ Referral

SUGGESTIONS FOR CLASSROOM ACTIVITIES

Role-play with students in the classroom a case of domestic violence where one student is the victim and the other is the nurse. Ask the nurse to identify interventions that would be appropriate in the care of the client.

SUGGESTIONS FOR CLINICAL ACTIVITIES

Have students interview nurses in the clinical setting about their role in caring for victims of domestic violence. Discuss the perceived roles and opportunities for education.

LEARNING OBJECTIVE 8

Articulate proper procedures for the screening, assessment, and documentation of abuse.

CONCEPTS FOR LECTURE

1. Screening tools are helpful in identifying women experiencing abuse. The screening should be done privately in a safe and quiet place. Reassurance must be given that all responses will be kept confidential. The nurse must be aware of signs that may not be related to a woman's presenting injuries that may indicate the possibility that the woman is in an abusive relationship. Information about the woman's history of abuse is also important to get a sense of the pattern of abuse and assess the degree of danger to the woman. An assessment of the presence of weapons in the home and a history of the batterer's threats to use these weapons is important. The nurse should also assess the presence of sexual abuse within the relationship. The woman's strengths should be assessed, such as her education, employment history, activities in the home, community involvement, and her ability to cope with past problems. Her support system should also be assessed and may include her family, friends, neighbors, and community agencies or organizations.

2. Documentation of physical abuse should include the extent of the injuries, the incident as described in the woman's own words, and the diagnosis of probable battering. Photographs should be taken of the injuries. To protect the woman's confidentiality and safety, domestic violence or abuse should not be referred to on any discharge papers.

POWERPOINT LECTURE SLIDES

(NOTE: The number on each PPT Lecture Slide directly corresponds with the Concepts for Lecture.)

 Screening for Domestic Abuse
- Screening tool
- Assessment of signs of abuse
- History of abuse
- Pattern of abuse
- Presence of weapons
- Strengths and support systems

2 Documentation of Abuse
- Extent of injuries
- The woman's exact words
- Describe the incident with a diagnosis of probable battering
- Take pictures as evidence
- Do not refer to domestic violence or abuse on any discharge papers

SUGGESTIONS FOR CLASSROOM ACTIVITIES

Have students do mock interviews of suspected victims of violence with their classmates using a screening tool. Give students feedback on their interview techniques.

SUGGESTIONS FOR CLINICAL ACTIVITIES

Ask students to observe an experienced nurse doing an assessment of a woman who is suspected of being a victim of violence and record their observations.

LEARNING OBJECTIVE 9

Specify physical and psychologic signs that may indicate a woman is in an abusive relationship.

CONCEPTS FOR LECTURE

1. Although no single sign may indicate abuse, the combination of several signs indicates an at-risk diagnosis. Neurologic signs that may indicate risk include headaches, dizziness, paresthesias, unexplained stroke from strangulation, hearing loss, or a detached retina. Gynecologic signs that may indicate risk include dyspareunia, sexually transmitted infections, frequent vaginal infections, sexual dysfunction, menstrual disorders, or pelvic pain. Obstetric signs that may indicate risk include late onset of prenatal care, premature labor, low-birth-weight infant, excessive concern over fetal well-being, recurrent therapeutic abortions, or recurrent spontaneous abortions. Gastrointestinal signs that may indicate risk include dyspepsia, irritable bowel syndrome, or globus. Musculoskeletal signs that may indicate risk include arthralgias, chronic pain, osteoarthritis, or fibromyalgia. Constitutional signs that may indicate risk include fatigue, weight loss, weight gain, multiple somatic complaints, contusions, abrasions, sleep and appetite disturbances, decreased concentration, or frequent use of pain medication or tranquilizers. Psychiatric signs may include anxiety, panic, post-traumatic stress disorders, depression, suicide attempts, somatization, eating disorders, substance abuse, or child abuse and neglect. Trauma may also indicate risk, including any injury to the female organs; an extensive accident history; old fractures; or sexual trauma. Other signs that may indicate risk include a history of missed or frequently changed appointments and low self-esteem.

2. A woman seeking care for an injury may exhibit the following cues of abuse: hesitation in providing detailed information about the injury and how it occurred; inappropriate affect for the situation; defensive injuries; delayed reporting of symptoms or of seeking care for injuries; pattern of injury consistent with abuse, including multiple injury sites involving bruises, abrasions, or contusions to the head, throat, chest, breast, abdomen, or genitals; inappropriate explanation for the injuries, such as being "accident prone"; vague complaints without accompanying pathology; lack of eye contact; and signs of increased anxiety in the presence of the possible batterer, who frequently does most of the talking or hovers around the woman.

POWERPOINT LECTURE SLIDES

(NOTE: The number on each PPT Lecture Slide directly corresponds with the Concepts for Lecture.)

1 Signs of Abuse
- Neurologic signs
- Gynecologic signs
- Obstetric signs
- Gastrointestinal signs
- Musculoskeletal signs
- Psychiatric signs

1a Signs of Abuse
- Constitutional signs
- Trauma
- Other signs

2 Cues of Abuse
- Hesitation in providing detailed information about the injury
- Inappropriate affect
- Defensive injuries
- Delayed reporting of symptoms
- Pattern of injury consistent with abuse
- Inappropriate explanation for the injuries

2a Cues of Abuse
- Vague complaints without accompanying pathology
- Lack of eye contact
- Signs of increased anxiety in the presence of the possible batterer

SUGGESTIONS FOR CLASSROOM ACTIVITIES

Discuss the difficulties in assessing injuries due to violence in the clinical setting. Discuss appropriate interventions if a nurse is unclear about the origin of the injury.

LEARNING OBJECTIVE 10

Discuss strategies for providing more culturally aware, competent care to survivors of domestic violence or sexual assault survivors.

CONCEPTS FOR LECTURE

1. In some cultural communities, women have difficulty seeking help outside of their families. This should be taken into consideration when providing care for women experiencing abuse. Because language can be a barrier to communication, translators should be available to translate. Additionally, information should be provided about culturally appropriate community resources. It is also important to assist women by finding creative interventions that do not ask a woman to choose between deeply held religious and spiritual conviction and legal interventions. Nurses should also avoid cultural stereotyping and create a safe space for the woman to share her needs, concerns, fears, and any cultural barriers that she must overcome.

POWERPOINT LECTURE SLIDES

(NOTE: The number on each PPT Lecture Slide directly corresponds with the Concepts for Lecture.)

 Culturally Competent Care
- Lack of ability to seek help outside the family
- Language is a barrier to communication
- Inaccurate perceptions of the legal system
- Potential threat of deportation
- Religious beliefs conflicting with legal remedies
- Avoid cultural stereotyping

SUGGESTIONS FOR CLASSROOM ACTIVITIES

Ask students to discuss any cultural barriers that they perceive in their own backgrounds that would be significant in caring for victims of domestic violence.

SUGGESTIONS FOR CLINICAL ACTIVITIES

Ask students to interview nurses who have cared for victims of violence about the barriers that they have faced when dealing with different cultures and how they altered their interventions based upon their cultural assessment.

LEARNING OBJECTIVE 11

Describe the needs that women with abusive partners and their children may have beyond the healthcare setting.

CONCEPTS FOR LECTURE

1. Women who have been abused may need medical treatment for injuries; temporary shelter to provide a safe environment for herself and her children; legal assistance for protection or prosecution of the batterer; financial assistance to provide shelter, food, and clothing; job training or employment counseling; and counseling to raise her self-esteem and help her understand the dynamics of domestic violence or an ongoing support group for herself and her children.

POWERPOINT LECTURE SLIDES

(NOTE: The number on each PPT Lecture Slide directly corresponds with the Concepts for Lecture.)

 Needs of Abused Women
- Medical treatment for injuries
- Temporary shelter
- Legal assistance for protection or prosecution of the batterer
- Financial assistance
- Job training or employment counseling
- Counseling

SUGGESTIONS FOR CLASSROOM ACTIVITIES

Ask students to identify local and national resources available to women who are victims of violence. Compile the lists from all of the students to share with the class.

SUGGESTIONS FOR CLINICAL ACTIVITIES

Upon assessing a woman who is a victim of domestic violence, ask the students to identify potential needs and potential resources for that woman.

LEARNING OBJECTIVE 12

Compare the types of sexual assault.

CONCEPTS FOR LECTURE

1. Sexual assault is defined as unwanted sexual touching or penetration without consent, from unwanted sexual contact or touching of an intimate part of another person to forced anal, oral, or genital penetration.

POWERPOINT LECTURE SLIDES

(NOTE: The number on each PPT Lecture Slide directly corresponds with the Concepts for Lecture.)

 Sexual Assault
- Touching or penetration without consent
- Unwanted sexual contact
- Unwanted touching of an intimate part
- Forced anal, oral, or genital penetration

SUGGESTIONS FOR CLASSROOM ACTIVITIES

Conduct a group discussion about unwanted sexual contact and implications for dating.

LEARNING OBJECTIVE 13

Identify the phases of the rape trauma syndrome.

CONCEPTS FOR LECTURE

1. Rape trauma syndrome has as many as four phases: the acute phase; the adjustment, or reorganization, phase; the intermediate, outward adjustment phase; and the integration and recovery phase. During the acute phase, the woman experiences fear, shock, disbelief, and sometimes denial. She may feel humiliated, guilty, unclean, angry, and powerless. During the adjustment phase, she may return to work or school and resumes her usual roles; however, she is coping by denial and suppression. Once these coping mechanisms deteriorate, she becomes depressed and anxious and wants to talk about the rape. She alters her self-concept and resolves her feelings about the rape.

POWERPOINT LECTURE SLIDES

(NOTE: The number on each PPT Lecture Slide directly corresponds with the Concepts for Lecture.)

 Rape Trauma Syndrome
- Acute phase
- Outward adjustment phase (denial)
- Reorganization
- Integration and recovery

SUGGESTIONS FOR CLINICAL ACTIVITIES

Ask students to identify the phase of recovery of a woman who has experienced unwanted sexual contact and identify the behaviors that support their assessment.

LEARNING OBJECTIVE 14

Identify drugs commonly used in drug-facilitated sexual assault.

CONCEPTS FOR LECTURE

1. Drugs used in sexual assault to sedate the intended victim include flunitrazepam (Rohypnol), gamma hydroxybutyrate (GHB), ketamine, MDMA (Ecstasy), clonazepam, and scopolamine. These drugs frequently

POWERPOINT LECTURE SLIDES

(NOTE: The number on each PPT Lecture Slide directly corresponds with the Concepts for Lecture.)

 Drug-Facilitated Sexual Assault
- Flunitrazepam (Rohypnol)

produce amnesia, making prosecution more difficult because the woman may be unable to remember the details.

- Gamma hydroxybutyrate (GHB)
- Ketamine
- MDMA (Ecstasy)
- Clonazepam
- Scopolamine

SUGGESTIONS FOR CLINICAL ACTIVITIES

Have students develop an educational program to teach adolescents about drug-facilitated sexual assault and ways to prevent it.

LEARNING OBJECTIVE 15

Explain the reasons why nurses who care for survivors of sexual assault and domestic violence should explore their personal values and beliefs.

CONCEPTS FOR LECTURE

1. Caregivers' values, attitudes, and beliefs affect the competence and focus of care. Therefore, nurses must understand their own beliefs about sexual assault and sexual assault survivors and resolve any conflicts that may exist. Also, nurses should be aware of the cultural or ethnic issues that may play a role in their care.

POWERPOINT LECTURE SLIDES

(NOTE: The number on each PPT Lecture Slide directly corresponds with the Concepts for Lecture.)

1 Nurses Caring for Sexual Assault Survivors
- Must understand own attitudes and beliefs about sexual assault
- Resolve any existing conflicts
- Be aware of potential for cultural implications of care

SUGGESTIONS FOR CLASSROOM ACTIVITIES

Conduct small group discussions regarding personal beliefs about sexual assault and violence.

LEARNING OBJECTIVE 16

Discuss the nurse's role as client advocate and counselor with domestic violence and sexual assault survivors.

CONCEPTS FOR LECTURE

1. As an advocate and counselor for sexual assault survivors the nurse should strive for the following outcomes: the survivor receives prompt, compassionate, respectful, and individualized medical attention; the woman recovers from the physical effects of the sexual assault; the woman is able to verbalize her recognition that sexual assault is a crime of violence expressed sexually; the woman is able to identify culturally appropriate community resources available to her as she works to adjust psychologically to the assault; the woman makes a decision about whether to prosecute her assailant; and if a survivor decides to prosecute her assailant, all necessary forensic evidence will have been collected, leading to a more successful investigation and prosecution.

POWERPOINT LECTURE SLIDES

(NOTE: The number on each PPT Lecture Slide directly corresponds with the Concepts for Lecture.)

1 Expected Outcomes of Nursing Care
- Client receives prompt, compassionate, respectful, and individualized medical attention
- Recovery from physical effects
- Recognition that sexual assault is a crime of violence
- Identification of culturally appropriate community resources
- Decision about prosecution of assailant
- If prosecuting, all forensic evidence is collected

LEARNING OBJECTIVE 17

Summarize the procedures for collecting and preserving physical evidence of sexual assault.

CONCEPTS FOR LECTURE

1. The procedures for collecting and preserving physical evidence of sexual assault include the following: An explanation of the procedures should be given and informed consent obtained from the woman. The chain of evidence must be preserved to ensure that all physical evidence remain in the hands of a professional until they are turned over to a police officer. After a thorough physical examination, a colposcope with photographic capability is used to document injuries to the genitalia. Clothing and foreign material dislodged from the clothing is marked, placed in an individual paper bag, sealed, and labeled. Body stains and secretions are swabbed and analyzed for semen or sperm. Cultures are obtained for detection of gonorrhea and chlamydia. Fingernail clippings or scrapings are examined for blood or tissue. Hair samples are obtained from the head and pubic areas to identify foreign hair. Pubic hair is also examined to check for loose hairs from the rapist. Serologic testing for syphilis and the woman's blood type is done. If a drug-facilitated sexual assault is suspected, urine should be collected. The injured areas should be photographed after consent is obtained.

POWERPOINT LECTURE SLIDES

(NOTE: The number on each PPT Lecture Slide directly corresponds with the Concepts for Lecture.)

1 Collecting Evidence of Sexual Assault
- Purpose
  - Confirm recent sexual contact
  - Show that force or coercion was used
  - Identify the assailant
  - Corroborate the survivor's story

1a Collecting Evidence of Sexual Assault
- Clothing
- Swabs of stains and secretions
- Hair and scrapings
- Blood samples
- Urine samples
- Photographs

SUGGESTIONS FOR CLASSROOM ACTIVITIES

Ask a local prosecutor to come to class to discuss the role of the nurse in collecting evidence for sexual assault prosecution.

SUGGESTIONS FOR CLINICAL ACTIVITIES

Ask students to interview emergency room nurses about their role in caring for victims of sexual assault.

LEARNING OBJECTIVE 18

Discuss the legal responsibilities of the community to prevent and address violence against women.

CONCEPTS FOR LECTURE

1. Sexual assault is considered a crime against the state rather than against the community. Therefore, prosecution is a community responsibility. The district attorney acts on the victim's behalf. However, the victim must initiate the process by reporting the crime and pressing charges.

POWERPOINT LECTURE SLIDES

(NOTE: The number on each PPT Lecture Slide directly corresponds with the Concepts for Lecture.)

1 Legal Responsibilities
- Crime against the state
- Prosecution is community responsibility
- Victim must report and press charges

SUGGESTIONS FOR CLASSROOM ACTIVITIES

Invite a local prosecutor to come to class to discuss the role of the state in prosecuting sex offenders.

CHAPTER 10
THE REPRODUCTIVE SYSTEM

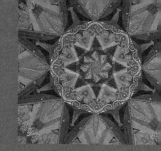

RESOURCE LIBRARY

🔘 PRENTICE HALL NURSING MEDIALINK DVD-ROM

Audio Glossary
NCLEX Review
Activities: *Female Reproductive System*
labeling exercise; *Female Reproductive System*
matching exercise; *Male Reproductive System*
labeling exercise; *Male Reproductive System*
matching exercise

📖 IMAGE LIBRARY

Figure 10.1 Embryonic differentiation of male and female internal reproductive organs.

Figure 10.2 Physiologic changes leading to onset of puberty.

Figure 10.3 Female external genitals, longitudinal view.

Figure 10.4 Female internal reproductive organs.

Figure 10.5 Structures of the uterus.

Figure 10.6 Blood supply to internal reproductive organs.

Figure 10.7 Uterine muscle layers.

Figure 10.8 Changes in squamocolumnar junction (arrows) at various stages of life.

Figure 10.9 Uterine ligaments.

Figure 10.10 Fallopian tube and ovaries.

Figure 10.11 Pelvis.

Figure 10.12 Muscles of the pelvic floor.

Figure 10.13 Female pelvis.

Figure 10.14 Pelvic angle of inclination while the woman is standing.

🌐 COMPANION WEBSITE

Additional NCLEX Review
Case Study: *Sex Education for Teens*
Care Plan Activity: *Irregular Menses in a Client with Anxiety*
Applications: *Pelvic Structures; Ovarian Cycle*
Critical Thinking

Figure 10.15 Comparison of Caldwell-Moloy pelvic types.

Figure 10.16 Anatomy of the breast.

Figure 10.17 Lymphatic vessels draining the breast.

Figure 10.18 Female reproductive cycle.

Figure 10.19 Various stages of development of the ovarian follicles.

Figure 10.20 Blood supply to the endometrium (cross-sectional view of the uterus).

Figure 10.21 Scanning electron micrographs of the uterine lining during different phases of the uterine cycle.

Figure 10.22 Scanning electron micrograph of the inner lining of the uterus at the time of blastocyst implantation.

Figure 10.23 Male reproductive system, sagittal view.

Figure 10.24 The testes.

Figure 10.25 Schematic illustration of a mature spermatozoon.

LEARNING OBJECTIVE 1

Describe the differentiation of the male and female reproductive organs during embryonic development.

CONCEPTS FOR LECTURE

1. Female differentiation takes place by about the 10th week when the cortex will develop into an ovary and the medulla will regress. Production of oogonia, which will become oocytes (primitive eggs), occurs through the process of oogenesis.

2. The fallopian tubes form from the unfused portions of the paramesonephric ducts, whereas the epithelium and uterine glands form from the fused portions. The endometrial stroma and the myometrium are developed

POWERPOINT LECTURE SLIDES

(NOTE: The number on each PPT Lecture Slide directly corresponds with the Concepts for Lecture.)

1 Embryonic Development of Ovaries (Figure 10.1)
- In 10th week, the cortex develops into an ovary
- Oogonia produce oocytes
- Process is called oogenesis

2 Internal Female Structure Development (Figure 10.1)
- Paramesonephric ducts
  ◦ Fallopian tubes

from the mesenchyme, whereas the vaginal epithelium develops from the endoderm of the urogenital sinus.

3. The medulla develops into a testis and the cortex will regress during the 7th and 8th weeks in males. Through the process of spermatogenesis, the testis will produce sperm.

4. The mesonephric ducts develop into the male genital tract after stimulation by testosterone. They further differentiate into the efferent ductile, vas deferens, epididymis, seminal vesicle, and ejaculatory duct. Suppression of the development of the paramesonephric ducts (which would cause development of the female genital tract) is due to müllerian regression factor.

- Mesenchyme
  ○ Endometrial stroma and myometrium
- Urogenital sinus
  ○ Vaginal epithelium

3 Embryonic Development of Testes (Figure 10.1)
- During 7th and 8th weeks, medulla develops into a testis.
- Spermatozoa are produced.
- Process is called spermatogenesis.
- Mature sperm are produced in puberty.

4 Internal Male Structure Development (Figure 10.1)
- Mesonephric ducts
  ○ Male genital tract
  ○ Stimulated by testosterone
- Müllerian regression factor
  ○ Stimulates regression of paramesonephric duct

4a See Figure 10.1

LEARNING OBJECTIVE 2

Summarize the major changes in the reproductive system that occur during puberty.

CONCEPTS FOR LECTURE

1. Puberty is the period of development between childhood and the development of sexual characteristics and functioning. Boys usually go through puberty about 2 years later than girls. The period of puberty generally lasts about 1.5 to 5 years and involves physic, psychologic, and emotional changes.

2. During puberty, girls' hips will broaden, breasts will bud, pubic and axillary hair will appear, and menstruation will begin.

3. During puberty, boys will experience linear growth spurts; external genitals will increase in size; pubic, axillary, and facial hair will appear; the voice will deepen; and nocturnal seminal emissions occur without sexual stimulation.

POWERPOINT LECTURE SLIDES

(NOTE: The number on each PPT Lecture Slide directly corresponds with the Concepts for Lecture.)

1 Puberty
- Attainment of mature sexual characteristics
- Lasts 18 months to 5 years
- Occurs 2 years later in boys

2 Female Puberty
- Broadening of the hips
- Budding of the breasts
- Appearance of pubic and axillary hair
- Onset of menstruation
  ○ Called *menarche*

3 Male Puberty
- Linear growth spurts
- Increase in the size of the external genitals
- Appearance of pubic, axillary, and facial hair
- Deepening of the voice
- Nocturnal seminal emissions

SUGGESTIONS FOR CLASSROOM ACTIVITIES

Have students share their experiences during puberty.

SUGGESTIONS FOR CLINICAL ACTIVITIES

Have students develop and implement a teaching plan about puberty for a group of middle school students.

CONCEPTS FOR LECTURE

1. The external genitalia of the female, which is called the vulva includes: the mons pubis, the labia majora, the labia minora, the clitoris, the urethral meatus and the opening of the paraurethral (Skene's) glands, the vaginal vestibule (vaginal orifice, vulvovaginal glands, hymen, and fossa navicularis), and the perineal body. The superficial area between the vagina and the anus is called the perineum.

2. Female internal reproductive organs include the vagina, the uterus, the fallopian tubes, and the ovaries. The uterus is comprised of two parts; the upper portion is the corpus and the lower portion is the cervix.

3. The body or corpus of the uterus is made of three layers. The outermost layer, which is comprised of the peritoneum, is the perimetrium. The middle muscular layer is the myometrium. The inner glandular layer is the endometrium.

4. The cervix is a protective portal for the body of the uterus. It has an inner os that opens to the body of the uterus and an external os that opens to the vagina. It has three functions: to provide lubrication, to act as a bacteriostatic agent, and to provide an alkaline environment to protect sperm from the acidic environment of the vagina.

5. The function of the uterine ligaments is to support and stabilize the reproductive organs. They include the broad ligament, the round ligaments, the ovarian ligaments, the cardinal ligaments, the infundibulopelvic ligament, and the uterosacral ligaments.

6. The fallopian tubes arise from each side of the uterus and are divided into three parts: the isthmus, the ampulla, and the infundibulum or fimbria. The functions of the fallopian tube include transporting the ovum to the uterus, providing a site for fertilization, and providing a nourishing environment for the ovum or zygote.

7. The ovaries function to store and mature the woman's follicles. The ovaries also secrete estrogen and progesterone.

8. The breasts are specialized sebaceous glands whose primary function is lactation. The nipple becomes prominent during the menstrual cycle, sexual excitation, pregnancy, and lactation. The area around the nipple is the areola. Both structures contain small papillae called tubercles of Montgomery. These secrete a fatty substance that lubricates and protects the breast. The lobe of each breast is made up of several lobules that are made up of many clusters of alveoli around ducts. The ducts come together to form larger lactiferous ducts, which then join together to form the lactiferous sinuses that serve to store milk.

9. The male genitals function to produce and transport sperm through and out of the genital tract into the female genital tract. Male external structures include

POWERPOINT LECTURE SLIDES

(NOTE: The number on each PPT Lecture Slide directly corresponds with the Concepts for Lecture.)

1 Female External Genitals (Figure 10.3)
- Mons pubis
- Labia majora and minora
- Clitoris
- Urethral meatus
- Vaginal vestibule
- Perineal body

1a See Figure 10.3

2 Female Internal Reproductive Organs (Figure 10.4)
- Vagina
- Uterus
  - Corpus
  - Cervix

2a See Figure 10.4

3 Uterine Corpus (Figure 10.5)
- Perimetrium
  - Peritoneum
- Myometrium
  - Muscle layer
- Endometrium
  - Mucosal layer

3a See Figure 10.5

4 Cervix
- Internal os
- External os
- Function
  - Lubrication of vagina
  - Acts as bacteriostatic agent
  - Provides an alkaline environment

5 Uterine Ligaments (Figure 10.9)
- Broad
- Round
- Ovarian
- Cardinal
- Infundibulopelvic
- Uterosacral

5a See Figure 10.9

6 Fallopian Tubes (Figure 10.10)
- Isthmus
- Ampulla
- Fimbria
- Transport of the ovum to the uterus
- Site for fertilization
- Nourishing environment for ovum/zygote

6a See Figure 10.10

the penis and the scrotum. Internal male reproductive organs include the gonads (testes or testicles), a system of ducts (epididymis, vas deferens, ejaculatory duct, and urethra), and accessory glands (seminal vesicles, prostate gland, bulbourethral glands, and urethral glands).

7 Ovaries (Figure 10.10)
- Store and mature follicles
- Secrete hormones
  - Estrogen
  - Progesterone

8 Breasts (Figure 10.16)
- Nipple
- Areola
- Tubercles of Montgomery
- Alveoli
- Lactiferous ducts
- Lactiferous sinuses

8a See Figure 10.16

9 Male Reproduction (Figure 10.23)
- External genitals
  - Penis
  - Scrotum

9a Male Reproduction (Figure 10.23)
- Internal organs
  - Testes
  - Epididymis
  - Vas deferens
  - Ejaculatory ducts
  - Urethra
  - Accessory glands

9b See Figure 10.23

SUGGESTIONS FOR CLASSROOM ACTIVITIES

Give students an outlined picture of female and male internal and external reproductive characteristics. Have them identify the structure and function of each.

LEARNING OBJECTIVE 4

Discuss the significance of specific female reproductive structures during pregnancy and childbirth.

CONCEPTS FOR LECTURE

1. The functions of the female bony pelvis include supporting and protecting the pelvic contents and the formation of a relatively fixed axis of the birth passage. Four bones make up the pelvis: two innominate bones, the sacrum, and the coccyx (or tailbone). The pelvis resembles a bowl or basin; its sides are the innominate bones, and its back is composed of the sacrum and coccyx. The pelvic cavity is comprised of the false pelvis and the true pelvis. The function of the false pelvis is to support the weight of the pregnant uterus and direct the presenting fetal part into the true pelvis. The function of the true pelvis is fetal passage during labor and birth. There are four types of bony pelves: gynecoid, android, anthropoid, and platypelloid.

POWERPOINT LECTURE SLIDES

(NOTE: The number on each PPT Lecture Slide directly corresponds with the Concepts for Lecture.)

1 Female Bony Pelvis
- Solid passageway for descent of fetus
- Pelvic types
  - Gynecoid
  - Android
  - Anthropoid
  - Platypelloid

LEARNING OBJECTIVE 5

Identify the actions of the hormones that affect reproductive functioning.

CONCEPTS FOR LECTURE

1. Female hormones that play a role in reproduction include gonadotropin-releasing hormone (GnRH), which when stimulated by low levels of estrogen and progesterone, is secreted by the hypothalamus. The GnRH sends a message to the anterior pituitary gland to release follicle-stimulating hormone (FSH), which stimulates the maturation of an immature follicle, and luteinizing hormone (LH), which triggers the release of the follicle from the ovary.

2. The function of estrogen is the development of female secondary sex characteristics, follicle maturation, and proliferation of the endometrial mucosa. The function of progesterone is to decrease uterine motility and contractility, to build up the endometrium, the proliferation of the vaginal endometrium, and the secretion of thick viscous mucus by the cervix. Prostaglandins promote smooth muscle relaxation.

POWERPOINT LECTURE SLIDES

(NOTE: The number on each PPT Lecture Slide directly corresponds with the Concepts for Lecture.)

1 Hormonal Function in Reproduction
- GnRH: causes anterior pituitary to release FSH and LH
- FSH: maturation of follicle
- LH: release of mature follicle

2 Hormonal Function in Reproduction
- Estrogen
- Progesterone
- Prostaglandins

SUGGESTIONS FOR CLASSROOM ACTIVITIES

Have students identify pelvic types and the implications of childbirth for each type.

LEARNING OBJECTIVE 6

Identify the two phases of the ovarian cycle and the changes that occur in each phase.

CONCEPTS FOR LECTURE

1. There are two phases of the ovarian cycle: the *follicular phase* (days 1 to 14) and the *luteal phase* (days 15 to 28 in a 28-day cycle). The immature follicle will mature during the follicular phase in response to FSH. The graafian follicle appears on day 14 under the influence of FSH and LH. The ovum leaves the follicle and under the influence of LH, the corpus luteum develops from the ruptured follicle. This is the beginning of the luteal phase. If fertilization does not occur, the corpus luteum degenerates and estrogen and progesterone levels fall, triggering the hypothalamus.

POWERPOINT LECTURE SLIDES

(NOTE: The number on each PPT Lecture Slide directly corresponds with the Concepts for Lecture.)

1 Ovarian Cycle (Figure 10.18)
- Follicular phase (days 1 to 14)
- Graafian follicle appears by day 14
- Luteal phase (Days 14 to 28)

1a See Figure 10.18

SUGGESTIONS FOR CLASSROOM ACTIVITIES

Have students create a circular ovarian cycle that they can use to visualize changes during the cycle.

SUGGESTIONS FOR CLINICAL ACTIVITIES

Have students teach a group of women about the ovarian cycle.

LEARNING OBJECTIVE 7

Describe the phases of the menstrual cycle, their dominant hormones, and the changes that occur in each phase.

CONCEPTS FOR LECTURE

1. There are four phases of the menstrual cycle: the menstrual phase, the proliferative phase, the secretory phase, and the ischemic phase. During the menstrual phase, menstruation occurs in response to low levels of estrogen and progesterone. During the proliferative phase, the the endometrial glands enlarge in response to increasing estrogen levels. During the secretory phase, the endometrium undergoes slight cellular growth due to estrogen, and progesterone cause marked swelling and growth. The ischemic phase begins if fertilization does not occur. The corpus luteum degenerates and estrogen and progesterone levels fall.

POWERPOINT LECTURE SLIDES

(NOTE: The number on each PPT Lecture Slide directly corresponds with the Concepts for Lecture.)

 Menstrual Cycle
- Menstrual phase
- Proliferative phase
- Secretory phase
- Ischemic phase

SUGGESTIONS FOR CLASSROOM ACTIVITIES

Have students add the menstrual cycle to the ovarian model they created earlier.

SUGGESTIONS FOR CLINICAL ACTIVITIES

Have students teach a client about the menstrual cycle.

Chapter 11
Conception and Fetal Development

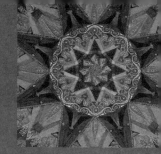

Resource Library

💿 PRENTICE HALL NURSING MEDIALINK DVD-ROM

Audio Glossary
NCLEX Review
Animations: *Cell Division; Oogenesis; Spermatogenesis; Oogenesis and Spermatogenesis Compared; Conception; Development of Placenta; Fetal Circulation; Embryonic Heart Formation and Circulation*
Activities: *Oogenesis and Spermatogenesis* matching exercise; *Oogenesis and Spermatogenesis* labeling exercise
Video: *Through the Eyes of a Nurse—The First Trimester*

🌐 COMPANION WEBSITE

Additional NCLEX Review
Case Study: *Teaching about Pregnancy*
Care Plan Activity: *Client Fearful of Multiple Gestations*
Applications: *Fraternal or Identical Twins; Fetal Development*
Critical Thinking

📖 IMAGE LIBRARY

Figure 11.1 *A*, Chromosomes contain two longitudinal halves called *chromatids*. *B*, One pair of homologous chromosomes with similar (homozygous) genes and dissimilar (heterozygous) genes.
Figure 11.2 Comparison of mitosis and meiosis.
Figure 11.3 Gametogenesis involves meiosis within the ovary and testis.
Figure 11.4 Sperm penetration of an ovum.
Figure 11.5 During ovulation, the ovum leaves the ovary and enters the fallopian tube.
Figure 11.6 Formation of primary germ layers.
Figure 11.7 Endoderm differentiates to form the epithelial lining of the digestive and respiratory tracts and associated glands.
Figure 11.8 Early development of primary embryonic membranes.
Figure 11.9 Summary of the significant pathways of water and solute exchange between the amniotic fluid and fetus.

Figure 11.10 *A*, Formation of fraternal twins. *B*, Formation of identical twins.
Figure 11.11 Maternal side of placenta (Dirty Duncan)
Figure 11.12 Fetal side of placenta (Shiny Schultz).
Figure 11.13 Longitudinal section of placental villus.
Figure 11.14 Vascular arrangement of the placenta.
Figure 11.15 Fetal circulation.
Figure 11.16 The actual size of a human conceptus from fertilization to the early fetal stage.
Figure 11.17 The embryo at 4 weeks.
Figure 11.18 The embryo at 5 weeks.
Figure 11.19 The embryo at 7 weeks.
Figure 11.20 The embryo at 8 weeks.
Figure 11.21 The fetus at 9 weeks.
Figure 11.22 The fetus at 14 weeks.
Figure 11.23 The fetus at 20 weeks.

LEARNING OBJECTIVE 1

Explain the differences between mitotic cellular division and meiotic cellular division.

CONCEPTS FOR LECTURE

1. Cell division that results in exact copies of the original cell is mitosis. The process of cell division that leads to the development of eggs and sperm that are essential to producing a new organism is meiosis.

POWERPOINT LECTURE SLIDES

(NOTE: The number on each PPT Lecture Slide directly corresponds with the Concepts for Lecture.)

 Cell Division (Figure 11.2)
   • Mitosis
      ○ Exact copies of original cell

2. Mitosis is divided into five stages: interphase, prophase, metaphase, anaphase, and telophase. The chromosomes condense during prophase. The chromosomes then line up at the equator of the spindles during metaphase. During anaphase, the two chromatids of each chromosome separate and move to opposite ends of the spindle, where they cluster at the two poles. During telophase, a nuclear membrane forms, which separates the newly formed nucleus from the cytoplasm. The spindle then disappears and the centrioles relocate outside of each new nucleus; within the nucleus, the chromosomes lengthen and become threadlike. A furrow then develops in the cell cytoplasm and divides it into two daughter cells.

3. In meiosis, there are two successive cell divisions. During the first division, the chromosomes replicate and pair up with similar chromosomes, becoming intertwined. There is a physical exchange of genetic material between the chromatids. The pairs then separate, with each member moving to an opposite side of the cell. The cell then divides, forming two daughter cells with 23 double-structure chromosomes. The chromatids separate and move to opposite poles of the daughter cells. The result is four cells, each containing 23 single chromosomes.

- Meiosis
  - Production of new organism

 See Figure 11.2

Mitosis
- Interphase
- Prophase
- Metaphase
- Anaphase
- Telophase

Meiosis
- First division
  - Chromosomes replicate, pair, and exchange information.
  - Chromosome pairs separate, cell divides.
- Second division
  - Chromatids separate and move to opposite poles.
  - Cells divide, forming four daughter cells.

SUGGESTIONS FOR CLASSROOM ACTIVITIES

Have students review the cell division animation from the Prentice Hall Nursing MediaLink DVD-ROM.

LEARNING OBJECTIVE 2

Compare the processes by which ova and sperm are produced.

CONCEPTS FOR LECTURE

1. Through the process of oogenesis, female gametes (ovum) are produced. Oogonial cells from the ovary develop into oocytes. Before the birth of a female child, meiosis begins in all oocytes but stops before the first division is complete and does not resume until puberty. At the time of puberty, the primary oocyte continues the first meiotic division in the graafian follicle.

2. At the time of puberty in the male, the germinal epithelium in the seminiferous tubules begin spermatogenesis, which produces the male gametes, sperm. Spermatogona are called the primary spermatocytes as they begin the first meiotic division. During this division, the spermatogonium replicates and forms two haploid cells called secondary spermatocytes. At the time of the second division, they divide to form four spermatids.

POWERPOINT LECTURE SLIDES

(NOTE: The number on each PPT Lecture Slide directly corresponds with the Concepts for Lecture.)

 Oogenesis (Figure 11.3A)
- Ovary gives rise to oogonial cells.
- Develop into oocytes.
- Meiosis begins and stops before birth.
- Cell division resumes at puberty.
- Development of graafian follicle.

 Spermatogenesis (Figure 11.3B)
- Production of sperm
- First meiotic division
  - Primary spermatocyte replicates and divides.
- Second meiotic division
  - Secondary spermatocytes replicate and divide.
  - Produce four spermatids.

 See Figures 11.3A & B

LEARNING OBJECTIVE 3

Describe the process of fertilization.

CONCEPTS FOR LECTURE

1. The creation of a zygote occurs when an ovum and sperm unite. Ova are available for fertilization for 12 to 24 hours after ovulation, whereas sperm remain viable in the female reproductive tract for 48 to 72 hours (sperm are believed to be healthy and fertile for only the first 24 hours). Fertilization takes place in the outer third or ampulla of the fallopian tube. The sperm move up the reproductive tract by using flagellar motion.

2. In order for fertilization to occur, the sperm must undergo two processes; capacitation and the acrosomal reaction. During capacitation, the plasma membrane and glycoprotein coat covering the spermatozoa's acrosomal area is removed and seminal plasma proteins are lost. During the acrosomal reaction, the acrosome caps of the sperm surrounding the ovum release their enzymes, which break down the hyaluronic acid that hold the elongated cells of the corona radiata of the ovum.

3. When the ovum is penetrated by the sperm, the zona pellucida undergoes a reaction to prevent additional sperm from entering the ovum. After the sperm enters the ovum, the oocyte is signaled to complete the second meiotic division, which forms the nucleus of the ovum and ejects the second polar body. At this time, the nuclei of the ovum and the sperm swell and approach each other. True fertilization occurs as the nuclei unite, their individual nuclear membranes disappear, and their chromosomes pair up to produce the diploid zygote.

POWERPOINT LECTURE SLIDES

(NOTE: The number on each PPT Lecture Slide directly corresponds with the Concepts for Lecture.)

1 Fertilization
- Uniting sperm and ovum form a zygote
- Ova are fertile for 12 to 24 hours
- Sperm are fertile for 72 hours
- Takes place in the ampulla of fallopian tube

2 Changes in Sperm (Figure 11.4A)
- Capacitation
  - Removal of plasma membrane and glycoprotein coat
  - Loss of seminal plasma proteins
- Acrosomal Reaction
  - Release of enzymes
  - Allows entry through corona radiata

2a See Figure 11.4A

3 After Sperm Entry
- Zone pellucida blocks additional sperm
- Secondary oocyte completes second meiotic division
- Forms nucleus of ovum
- Nuclei of ovum and sperm unite
- Membranes disappear
- Chromosomes pair up

LEARNING OBJECTIVE 4

Identify the differing processes by which fraternal (dizygotic) and identical (monozygotic) twins are formed.

CONCEPTS FOR LECTURE

1. Fraternal twins arise from two separate ova fertilized by two separate spermatozoa. Identical twins (monozygotic) develop from a single ovum and sperm. Monozygotic twins originate at different stages of early development. If it occurs within 3 days of fertilization, two embryos, two amnions, and two chorions

POWERPOINT LECTURE SLIDES

(NOTE: The number on each PPT Lecture Slide directly corresponds with the Concepts for Lecture.)

1 Twins
- Fraternal—two ova and two sperm
- Identical—single fertilized ovum
  - Originate at different stages

develop. The placentas may be fused or distinct. If division occurs about 5 days after fertilization, the two embryos will have separate amniotic sacs, which will be covered by a common chorion. If division occurs 7 to 13 days after fertilization, the two embryos will have a common amniotic sac and chorion.

SUGGESTIONS FOR CLASSROOM ACTIVITIES

Have a group discussion about the parenting issues that arise from multiple births and strategies for addressing these issues.

LEARNING OBJECTIVE 5

Describe in order of increasing complexity the structures that form during the cellular multiplication and differentiation stages of intrauterine development.

CONCEPTS FOR LECTURE

1. As the zygote moves through the fallopian tube toward the uterus, cellular multiplication begins. This rapid period of mitotic divisions is called cleavage and the cells are called blastomeres. Eventually, the blastomeres form a morula, a solid ball of 12 to 16 cells. When the morula reaches the uterus, the intracellular fluid in the morula increases and a central cavity forms within the morula. Within this cavity, an inner solid mass of cells exists, which is called the blastocyst. Cells surrounding the cavity are called the trophoblast. The trophoblast will develop into the chorion and the blastocyst will develop into the embryonic disc. This disc will develop into the embryo and the amnion.

2. Implantation will occur between days 7 and 10 when the blastocyst implants itself by burrowing into the uterine lining until it is completely covered. Once implantation occurs, the endometrium is called the decidua.

3. Ten to 14 days after conception, the blastocyst differentiates into the primary germ layers: the ectoderm, the mesoderm, and the endoderm. The tissues, organs, and organ systems develop from these germ layers.

POWERPOINT LECTURE SLIDES

(NOTE: The number on each PPT Lecture Slide directly corresponds with the Concepts for Lecture.)

1 Preembryonic Stage
- Cleavage
- Blastomeres form morula
- Blastocyst
  - Develops into embryonic disc and amnion
- Trophoblast
  - Develops into chorion

2 Implantation
- 7 to 10 days after fertilization
- Blastocyst burrows into endometrium
- Endometrium now called *decidua*

3 Embryonic Development
- Primary germ layers
  - Ectoderm
  - Mesoderm
  - Endoderm

LEARNING OBJECTIVE 6

Describe the development, structure, and functions of the placenta during intrauterine life.

CONCEPTS FOR LECTURE

1. The function of the placenta is metabolic and nutrient exchange between the fetus and the mother. There are two parts of the placenta: the decidua basalis, which is the maternal portion, and the chorionic villi, which is the fetal portion. The amnion covers the placenta.

2. The chorionic villi form spaces in the tissue of the decidua basalis, which will be filled with maternal blood and chorionic villi. The chorionic villi then differentiate,

POWERPOINT LECTURE SLIDES

(NOTE: The number on each PPT Lecture Slide directly corresponds with the Concepts for Lecture.)

1 Placenta (Figure 11.14)
- Metabolic and nutrient exchange
- Maternal portion
  - Decidua

forming two trophoblastic layers: the synctium or outer layer, and the cytotrophoblast or inner layer. An inner layer of connective mesoderm develops in the chorionic villi, which form the anchoring villi. They will form the septa of the placenta. The septa divide the placenta into 15 to 20 segments called cotyledons. Within each of these, branching villi form a highly complex vascular system that provides compartmentalization for the uteroplacental circulation through which exchange of gases and nutrients takes place.

3. Attaching the embryo to the yolk sac is the body stalk, which contains blood vessels that extend into the chorionic villi. This fuses with the embryonic portion of the placenta to provide a circulatory pathway. In a fully developed placental umbilical cord, fetal blood will flow through two umbilical arteries to the capillaries of the villi and oxygen-rich blood flows from the umbilical vein to the fetus.

4. Placental functions include fetal respiration, nutrition, and excretion, and placental production of glycogen, cholesterol, and fatty acid for fetal use. The placenta also secretes the following hormones: human chorionic gonadotropin (hCG), human placental lactogen (hPL), estrogen, and progesterone. Transfer of nutrients occurs through simple diffusion, facilitated transport, active transport, and hydrostatic and osmotic pressures.

- Fetal portion
  - Chorionic villi
- Fetal surface covered by amnion

2 Placental Development (Figure 11.13)
- Chorionic villi form spaces in decidua basalis
- Spaces fill with maternal blood
- Chorionic villi differentiate
  - Synctium—outer layer
  - Cytotrophoblast—inner layer
- Anchoring villi form septa

2a See Figure 11.13

3 Umbilical Cord (Figure 11.14)
- Body stalk fuses with embryonic portion of the placenta.
- Provides circulatory pathway from chorionic villi to embryo
  - One vein
- Oxygenated blood to fetus
  - Two arteries

3a See Figure 11.14

4 Placental Functions
- Nutrition
- Excretion
- Fetal respiration
- Production of fetal nutrients
- Production of hormones

SUGGESTIONS FOR CLASSROOM ACTIVITIES

Have students review the formation of placenta animation from the Prentice Hall Nursing MediaLink DVD-ROM. Bring in a model of a placenta for students to view.

LEARNING OBJECTIVE 7

Summarize the significant changes in growth and development of the fetus at 4, 6, 12, 16, 20, 24, 28, 32, 36, and 38 weeks postconception.

CONCEPTS FOR LECTURE

1. At 4 weeks, the body is flexed, arm and leg buds are present, the gastrointestinal tract appears as a tubelike structure, all somites are present, the heart is beating at a regular rhythm and double heart chambers are visible, primary lung buds appear, and the eyes and ears appear as optic vessels and otocysts.

2. At 6 weeks, the body is straighter and the head structures are more highly developed. The trachea has developed and bifurcated. Blood cells are beginning to be produced by the liver. The arms and legs have developed digits. The tail begins to recede.

POWERPOINT LECTURE SLIDES

(NOTE: The number on each PPT Lecture Slide directly corresponds with the Concepts for Lecture.)

1 Fetal Development: Week 4
- Beginning development of GI tract
- Heart is developing
- Somites develop—beginning vertebrae
- Heart is beating and circulating blood
- Eyes and nose begin to form
- Arm and leg buds present

3. At 12 weeks, the eyelids are closed, toothbuds appear, fetal heart tones can be heard using electronic devices, and the limbs are long and slender. Genitals are well-differentiated and urine is produced. Spontaneous fetal movement occurs.

4. At 16 weeks, lanugo begins to develop, blood vessels are clearly developed, active movements are present, and the fetus makes sucking motions, swallows amniotic fluid, and produces meconium.

5. At 20 weeks, lanugo will cover the entire body, there are subcutaneous deposits of brown fat, nipples appear over the mammary glands, fetal movement is felt by the mother, and the fetal heartbeat is audible by fetoscope.

6. At 24 weeks, the eyes are structurally complete, skin is covered by vernix caseosa, and the alveoli in the lungs are beginning to form.

7. At 28 weeks, the brain develops rapidly, the eyelids are open, there are nails on fingers and toes, testes begin to descend into the scrotal sac in male fetuses, and the lungs are sufficiently developed to provide gas exchange.

8. At 32 weeks, the fetus has rhythmic breathing movements and the ability to partially control temperature. Bones are fully developed but soft and flexible.

9. At 36 weeks, the fetus gains weight with the deposits of subcutaneous fat. Lanugo begins to disappear and the nails reach the edge of the fingertips.

10. At 38 weeks, the fetus is considered to be mature. The skin appears polished, lanugo has disappeared except for lanugo in the upper arms and shoulders. Hair is now coarse and approximately 1 inch in length. The fetus is flexed and has developed its own body rhythms and responses.

2 Fetal Development: Week 6
- Trachea is developed
- Liver produces blood cells
- Trunk is straighter
- Digits develop
- Tail begins to recede

3 Fetal Development: Week 12
- Eyelids are closed
- Tooth buds appear
- Fetal heart tones can be heard
- Genitals are well-differentiated
- Urine is produced
- Spontaneous movement occurs

4 Fetal Development: Week 16
- Lanugo begins to develop
- Blood vessels are clearly developed
- Active movements are present
- Fetus makes sucking motions
- Swallows amniotic fluid
- Produces meconium

5 Fetal Development: Week 20
- Subcutaneous brown fat appears
- Quickening is felt by mother
- Nipples appear over mammary glands
- Fetal heartbeat is heard by fetoscope

6 Fetal Development: Week 24
- Eyes are structurally complete
- Vernix caseosa covers skin
- Alveoli are beginning to form

7 Fetal Development: Week 28
- Testes begin to descend
- Lungs are structurally mature

8 Fetal Development: Week 32
- Rhythmic breathing movements
- Ability to partially control temperature
- Bones are fully developed but soft and flexible

9 Fetal Development: Week 36
- Increase in subcutaneous fat
- Lanugo begins to disappear

10 Fetal Development: Week 38
- Skin appears polished
- Lanugo has disappeared except in upper arms and shoulders
- Hair is now coarse and approximately 1 inch in length
- Fetus is flexed

SUGGESTIONS FOR CLASSROOM ACTIVITIES

Have students review the embryonic heart formation and circulation and fetal circulation animations from the Prentice Hall Nursing MediaLink DVD-ROM. Bring in fetal development models for the students to view.

LEARNING OBJECTIVE 8

Identify the vulnerable periods during which malformations of the various organ systems may occur, and describe the resulting congenital malformations.

CONCEPTS FOR LECTURE

1. Factors that influence fetal development include the quality of the sperm or ovum, genetic code, the adequacy of the intrauterine environment, and teratogens. If the intrauterine environment is not favorable before cellular differentiation, all cells will be affected, resulting in slowed growth and spontaneous abortion. When differentiation is complete, the effect is on the cells undergoing the most rapid growth. The embryonic period is the most vulnerable period during which congenital malformations can occur because the organs are primarily formed during this period. Teratogens can be drugs, viruses, or chemicals. The maternal environment can also play a role in congenital malformations. Nutritional deficiencies can affect brain growth. Maternal hyperthermia in the first trimester can cause spontaneous abortion, CNS defects, and failure to close the neural tube.

POWERPOINT LECTURE SLIDES

(NOTE: The number on each PPT Lecture Slide directly corresponds with the Concepts for Lecture.)

 1 Factors Influencing Development
- Quality of sperm or ovum
- Genetic code
- Adequacy of intrauterine environment
- Teratogens

SUGGESTIONS FOR CLASSROOM ACTIVITIES

Have students join in groups to devise a teaching plan for new mothers or mothers considering pregnancy to avoid teratogens.

SUGGESTIONS FOR CLINICAL ACTIVITIES

Have students develop a teaching pamphlet on the avoidance of teratogens for a women's health clinic.

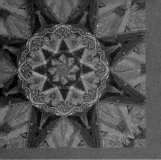

CHAPTER 12
SPECIAL REPRODUCTIVE CONCERNS: INFERTILITY AND GENETICS

RESOURCE LIBRARY

PRENTICE HALL NURSING MEDIALINK DVD-ROM

Audio Glossary
NCLEX Review
Activity: *Ovulation*
Video: *Through the Eyes of a Nurse—The First Trimester*

COMPANION WEBSITE

Additional NCLEX Review
Case Study: *Infertility*
Care Plan Activity: *Infertile Couple*
Applications: *Infertility Testing; In Vitro Fertilization*
Critical Thinking

IMAGE LIBRARY

Figure 12.1 Flow chart for management of the infertile couple.

Figure 12.2 Sequence of events in a normal reproductive cycle showing the relationship of hormone levels to events in the ovarian and endometrial cycles.

Figure 12.3 *A*, A monophasic, anovulatory basal body temperature (BBT) chart. *B*, A biphasic BBT chart illustrating probable time of ovulation, the different types of testing, and the time in the cycle that each would be performed.

Figure 12.4 *A*, Spinnbarkheit (elasticity). *B*, Ferning pattern. *C*, Lack of ferning pattern.

Figure 12.5 Sperm passage through cervical mucus.

Figure 12.6 *A*, A selection of commonly prescribed medications for ovulation induction. *B*, Derivation of gonadotropin medications.

Figure 12.7 *A*, Operating room setup for ultrasound-guided oocyte retrieval. *B*, Transvaginal ultrasound-guided oocyte retrieval.

Figure 12.8 Assisted reproductive techniques.

Figure 12.9 Assisted hatching of embryo.

Figure 12.10 Normal female karyotype.

Figure 12.11 Normal male karyotype.

Figure 12.12 Karyotype of a female who has trisomy 21, Down syndrome.

Figure 12.13 A boy with Down syndrome.

Figure 12.14 Karyotype of a male who has trisomy 18.

Figure 12.15 Karyotype of male with trisomy 13.

Figure 12.16 Diagram of various types of offspring when the mother has a balanced translocation between chromosomes 14 and 21 and the father has a normal arrangement of chromosomal material.

Figure 12.17 Infant with cri du chat syndrome resulting from deletion of part of the short arm of chromosome 5.

Figure 12.18 Infant with Turner syndrome at 1 month of age.

Figure 12.19 Autosomal dominant pedigree.

Figure 12.20 Autosomal recessive pedigree.

Figure 12.21 X-linked recessive pedigree.

Figure 12.22 *A*, Genetic amniocentesis for prenatal diagnosis is done at 14 to 16 weeks' gestation. *B*, Chorionic villus sampling is done at 8 to 10 weeks, and the cells are karyotyped within 48 to 72 hours.

Figure 12.23 Dermatoglyphic patterns of the hands in *A*, a normal individual and *B*, a child with Down syndrome.

Figure 12.24 Screening pedigree.

LEARNING OBJECTIVE 1

Identify the components of fertility.

CONCEPTS FOR LECTURE

1. The components of fertility that are essential for the female partner include: favorable cervical mucous, clear passage between the cervix and the fallopian tubes, patent fallopian tubes with normal motility, ovulation and the release of the ova, no obstruction between the ovary and the fallopian tube, favorable endometrial environment for implantation, and adequate reproductive hormones.

POWERPOINT LECTURE SLIDES

(NOTE: The number on each PPT Lecture Slide directly corresponds with the Concepts for Lecture.)

 1 Essential Components of Fertility: Female
- Favorable cervical mucus
- Clear passage between cervix and tubes
- Patent tubes with normal motility
- Ovulation and release of ova

2. The components of fertility that are essential for the male partner include: normal semen analysis, unobstructed genital tract, normal genital tract secretions, and ejaculated spermatozoa deposited at the cervix.

1a Essential Components of Fertility: Female
- No obstruction between ovary and tubes
- Endometrial preparation
- Adequate reproductive hormones

2 Essential Components of Fertility: Male
- Normal semen analysis
- Unobstructed genital tract
- Normal genital tract secretions
- Ejaculated spermatozoa deposited at the cervix

LEARNING OBJECTIVE 2

Describe the elements of the preliminary investigation of infertility.

CONCEPTS FOR LECTURE

1. Both partners will undergo a thorough history and physical examination as well as several tests to identify cause of infertility. The woman's ovulatory function and the structure and function of the cervix, uterus, fallopian tubes, and ovaries will be assessed. In the male, a semen analysis for sperm quality, quantity, and motility is the most important assessment.

POWERPOINT LECTURE SLIDES

(NOTE: The number on each PPT Lecture Slide directly corresponds with the Concepts for Lecture.)

1 Preliminary Investigation of Infertility
- Ovulation (Figure 12.2)
- Cervix
- Uterine structures
- Tubal patency
- Semen analysis

1a See Figure 12.2

SUGGESTIONS FOR CLASSROOM ACTIVITIES

Show students pictures of a BBT chart. Discuss the implications of temperature change in fertility.

LEARNING OBJECTIVE 3

Summarize the indications for the tests and associated treatments, including assisted reproductive technologies, that are done in an infertility work-up.

CONCEPTS FOR LECTURE

1. If a woman has ovulatory problems, the diagnostic tests that are most appropriate would be BBT, hormonal assessments (including FSH, LH, progesterone, TSH, and androgen levels), an endometrial biopsy to assess endometrial receptivity, and a transvaginal ultrasound to monitor follicles. Pharmacologic treatment to induce or improve ovulation and donor oocytes would be instituted. If the woman has cervical problems, the diagnostic test that is most appropriate is cervical mucous analysis. This problem would best be treated by therapeutic insemination (THI), in vitro fertilization (IVF) and gamete intrafallopian transfer (GIFT). The woman with problems involving the uterine structures or tubal patency would benefit most from assessment techniques including hysterosalpingography, hysteroscopy, and laparoscopy. The most appropriate treatments may include in vitro fertilization, gamete intrafallopian

POWERPOINT LECTURE SLIDES

(NOTE: The number on each PPT Lecture Slide directly corresponds with the Concepts for Lecture.)

1 Treatment of Infertility Problems
- Ovulatory
  - Pharmacologic treatment
  - Donor oocytes
- Cervical
  - THI, IVF, GIFT (Figure 12.8)

1a Treatment of Infertility Problems
- Uterine/Tubal
  - IVF, GIFT (Figure 12.8)
  - Donor oocytes or gestational carrier
- Sperm
  - THI, IVF, GIFT (Figure 12.8)
  - Micromanipulation

1b See Figure 12.8

transfer, donor oocytes, and in vitro fertilization using a gestational carrier. If infertility is related to a semen problem, analysis of the quality and quantity of the semen would be most appropriate, and treatment may include therapeutic insemination, in vitro fertilization, gamete intrafallopian transfer, and micromanipulation techniques.

SUGGESTIONS FOR CLASSROOM ACTIVITIES

Have students break up into groups and give each group a case study with one type of infertility problem. Ask them to list the diagnostic workups and treatment that would be appropriate for this couple and to explain why.

SUGGESTIONS FOR CLINICAL ACTIVITIES

Have students observe one of the infertility tests mentioned above in the clinical setting and review the client indications for that test and the implications of the outcomes of the test.

LEARNING OBJECTIVE 4

Summarize the physiologic and psychologic effects of infertility.

CONCEPTS FOR LECTURE

1. Infertility often taxes a couple's financial, physical, and emotional resources. Their marriage may be stressed and their relationship affected by the intrusiveness of the testing. They may experience guilt, frustration, anger, or shame. They may experience loss of control, feelings of reduced competency and defectiveness, loss of status and ambiguity as a couple, a sense of social stigma, stress on the marital and sexual relationship, and a strained relationship with healthcare providers.

POWERPOINT LECTURE SLIDES

(NOTE: The number on each PPT Lecture Slide directly corresponds with the Concepts for Lecture.)

 Physiologic and Psychologic Effects
- Marriage may be stressed
- Relationship affected by intrusiveness
- Guilt
- Frustration
- Anger
- Shame

1a Physiologic and Psychologic Effects
- Loss of control
- Feelings of reduced competency and defectiveness
- Loss of status and ambiguity as a couple
- A sense of social stigma
- Stress on the marital and sexual relationship
- A strained relationship with healthcare providers

SUGGESTIONS FOR CLASSROOM ACTIVITIES

Have students discuss their perception of the effects of infertility on couples that they know.

SUGGESTIONS FOR CLINICAL ACTIVITIES

Have students do a psychosocial assessment on a couple experiencing infertility and discuss their findings.

LEARNING OBJECTIVE 5

Describe the nurse's roles as counselor, educator, and advocate during infertility evaluation and treatment.

CONCEPTS FOR LECTURE

1. The nurse's role in caring for couples with infertility is that of a counselor, educator, and advocate. The nurse counsels the couple about treatment options and provides education about the treatment. Additionally, the nurse counsels them to help give them control and negotiate the treatment process.

POWERPOINT LECTURE SLIDES

(NOTE: The number on each PPT Lecture Slide directly corresponds with the Concepts for Lecture.)

1 Nursing Management of Infertility
- Counselor
- Educator
- Advocate

SUGGESTIONS FOR CLASSROOM ACTIVITIES

Ask students to role-play in the class, where two students are a couple with infertility and the other student is the nurse. Have the student playing the nurse interview the couple about their infertility, and note the role of the nurse in that interaction.

SUGGESTIONS FOR CLINICAL ACTIVITIES

Have students follow an infertility nurse in a clinic setting. Have them observe his/her interactions with the clients and discuss the role of the nurse.

LEARNING OBJECTIVE 6

Discuss the indications for preconceptual genetic counseling and prenatal testing.

CONCEPTS FOR LECTURE

1. Indications for preconceptual genetic counseling and prenatal testing may include: women age 35 or over, couples with a chromosomal abnormality, a family history of known or suspected Mendelian genetic disorders, couples with a previous child with a chromosomal abnormality, couples in which either partner or a previous child is affected by (or in which both partners are carriers for) a diagnosable metabolic disorder, a family history of birth defects and/or mental retardation, ethnic groups at increased risk for specific disorders, couples with a history of two or more first trimester spontaneous abortions, women with an abnormal MSAFP, and women with a teratogenic risk secondary to an exposure or maternal health condition.

POWERPOINT LECTURE SLIDES

(NOTE: The number on each PPT Lecture Slide directly corresponds with the Concepts for Lecture.)

1 Indications for Preconceptual Genetic Testing
- Maternal age 35 or over
- Family history
  - Known or suspected Mendelian genetic disorder
  - Birth defects and/or mental retardation

1a Indications for Preconceptual Genetic Testing
- Previous pregnancies
  - Previous child with chromosomal anomaly
  - Previous child with metabolic disorder
  - Two or more first trimester spontaneous abortions

1b Indications for Preconceptual Genetic Testing
- Parental genetics
  - Couples with a balanced translocation
  - Couples who are carriers for a metabolic disorder
- Abnormal MSAFP
- Women with teratogenic risk

SUGGESTIONS FOR CLINICAL ACTIVITIES

Have students assess prenatal client histories for risk factors that indicate the need for genetic testing.

LEARNING OBJECTIVE 7

Identify the characteristics of autosomal dominant, autosomal recessive, and X-linked (sex-linked) recessive disorders.

CONCEPTS FOR LECTURE

1. Multiple generations are affected by autosomal dominant disorders, with affected individuals having a 50% chance of passing on the abnormal gene to each of their children. Males and females are equally affected, and fathers can pass on the abnormal gene to their sons.

2. An individual may have an autosomal recessive disorder passed to them through clinically normal parents who are carriers of the gene. Each carrier has a 25% chance of passing on the abnormal gene to a child. There is a 25% chance with each pregnancy that there will be an affected child. There is a 50% chance that an unaffected child will be a carrier. Males and females are equally affected. Males cannot pass on the abnormal gene in an X-linked recessive disorder because it is carried on the X chromosome. A carrier mother has a 50% chance of passing the abnormal gene to each of her sons who will become affected. She also has a 50% chance of passing the abnormal gene to each of her daughters who will become affected. Affected fathers will pass on the gene to all of their daughters.

POWERPOINT LECTURE SLIDES

(NOTE: The number on each PPT Lecture Slide directly corresponds with the Concepts for Lecture.)

`1` Autosomal Dominant Disorders (Figure 12.19)
- Multigenerational
- 50% chance of passing on the gene
- Males and females equally affected
- Varying degrees of presentation

`1a` See Figure 12.19

`2` Autosomal Recessive Disorders (Figure 12.20)
- Carrier parents
- 25% chance of passing on abnormal gene
- 25% chance of an affected child
- If child is clinically normal, 50% chance child is carrier
- Males and females equally affected

`2a` See Figure 12.20

`2b` X-Linked Recessive Disorders (Figure 12.21)
- No male-to-male transmission
- 50% chance carrier mother will pass the abnormal gene to sons (affected)
- 50% chance carrier mother will pass the abnormal gene to daughters (carrier)

`2c` See Figure 12.21

SUGGESTIONS FOR CLASSROOM ACTIVITIES

Have students do a pedigree for case studies illustrating each type of disorder to understand the genetic relationships.

LEARNING OBJECTIVE 8

Compare prenatal and postnatal diagnostic procedures used to determine the presence of genetic disorders.

CONCEPTS FOR LECTURE

1. Prenatal diagnostic procedures that may be done to assess the fetus for genetic disorders include: ultrasound at 18 to 20 weeks, amniocentesis, chorionic villus sampling (CVS), and maternal serum AFP (MSAFP). Postnatal diagnostic procedures include: a detailed family history, a thorough physical examination including dermatoglyphic analysis, and laboratory analysis (including chromosome analysis, enzyme assay for inborn errors of metabolism, DNA studies, and antibody titers for infectious teratogens).

POWERPOINT LECTURE SLIDES

(NOTE: The number on each PPT Lecture Slide directly corresponds with the Concepts for Lecture.)

`1` Genetic Testing
- Genetic ultrasound
- Genetic amniocentesis (Figure 12.21A)
- Chorionic villus sampling (Figure 12.21B)
- Percutaneous umbilical blood sampling
- MSAFP

`1a` See Figure 12.22A

`1b` See Figure 12.22B

LEARNING OBJECTIVE 9

Explore the emotional impact on a couple undergoing genetic testing or coping with the birth of a baby with a genetic disorder, and explain the nurse's role in supporting the family undergoing genetic counseling.

CONCEPTS FOR LECTURE

1. The emotional impact on a couple undergoing genetic testing involves their decision to have the child affected with a genetic disorder or to abort. If abortion is not an option, couples may not choose to have genetic testing; however, other couples may choose to have the testing in order to prepare themselves for the birth of a child with special needs. The nurse should prepare the family for genetic counseling and act as a resource person and an advocate for the family.

POWERPOINT LECTURE SLIDES

(NOTE: The number on each PPT Lecture Slide directly corresponds with the Concepts for Lecture.)

 Nurse's Role
- Educate about tests
- Provide support
- Refer for counseling
- Resource during and after counseling

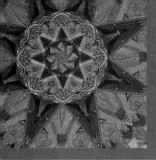

CHAPTER 13
PREPARATION FOR PARENTHOOD

RESOURCE LIBRARY

PRENTICE HALL NURSING MEDIALINK DVD-ROM

Audio Glossary
NCLEX Review
Videos: *Through the Eyes of a Nurse—The First Trimester; Through the Eyes of a Nurse—The Third Trimester*

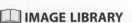 IMAGE LIBRARY

Figure 13.1 Pregnancy decision tree.
Figure 13.2 Birth plan for childbirth choices.
Figure 13.3 In a group setting with a nurse-instructor, expectant parents share information about pregnancy and childbirth.
Figure 13.4 It is especially important that siblings be well prepared when they are going to be present at the birth.

COMPANION WEBSITE

Additional NCLEX Review
Case Study: *Preparing for Pregnancy*
Care Plan Activity: *Preconception Counseling*
Applications: *Benefits of Having a Doula; Lamaze*
Critical Thinking

Figure 13.5 To help the woman practice relaxing in the presence of discomfort, the coach can induce discomfort by "twisting" the skin of her upper arm or by pinching her inner thigh.
Figure 13.6 Effleurage is light stroking of the abdomen with the fingertips.

LEARNING OBJECTIVE 1

Apply the nursing process to help couples prepare for childbirth.

CONCEPTS FOR LECTURE

1. The nurse can apply the nursing process by helping the childbearing family make the decisions that are part of pregnancy and birth, seek preconceptual counseling, select a healthcare provider, find prenatal classes that meet their needs, and make informed choices. The nurse can help the family work through the decisions and take on the parenting role.

POWERPOINT LECTURE SLIDES

(NOTE: The number on each PPT Lecture Slide directly corresponds with the Concepts for Lecture.)

1 Nursing Role in Childbirth Preparation
  • Helping the childbearing family:
    ○ Make decisions that are part of pregnancy and birth
    ○ Seek preconceptual counseling
    ○ Select a healthcare provider
    ○ Find prenatal classes that meet their needs
    ○ Make informed choices

1a Nursing Role in Childbirth Preparation
  • Affirm decision-making abilities
  • Affirm ability to take on parenting role

LEARNING OBJECTIVE 2

Identify the various issues related to preconception counseling, pregnancy, labor, and birth that require decision making by parents.

CONCEPTS FOR LECTURE

1. Some of the decisions that the childbearing family must consider include the decision to have a baby, choice of care provider, type of childbirth preparation, place of birth, activities during the birth, method of infant feeding, and choices surrounding the care of the newborn.

POWERPOINT LECTURE SLIDES

(NOTE: The number on each PPT Lecture Slide directly corresponds with the Concepts for Lecture.)

1 Decision Making in Pregnancy (see Figure 13.1)
  • Choice of care provider
  • Type of childbirth preparation

2. A couple may choose to use a birth plan to identify aspects of the childbearing experience that are important to them and those they wish to avoid. The plan serves as a tool for communication between the parents and healthcare providers.

- Place of birth
- Activities during birth
- Method of infant feeding
- Choices about care of the newborn

| 1a | See Figure 13.1

| 2 | Purposes of a Birth Plan
- Identify aspects of the childbearing most important to family
- Identify available options
- Communication tool
- Specify options to avoid
- Set priorities

SUGGESTIONS FOR CLASSROOM ACTIVITIES

Have students develop a questionnaire to help childbearing families develop a birth plan. Ask them to discuss why they included the items they chose.

SUGGESTIONS FOR CLINICAL ACTIVITIES

Have students review the birth plans of childbearing families in labor.

LEARNING OBJECTIVE 3

Discuss the basic goals of childbirth education.

CONCEPTS FOR LECTURE

1. The goals of childbirth education are to provide opportunities to share information about pregnancy, childbirth, coping mechanisms, and choices available for the woman and her support person. Childbirth preparation can have a positive effect on the labor and delivery experience.

POWERPOINT LECTURE SLIDES

(NOTE: The number on each PPT Lecture Slide directly corresponds with the Concepts for Lecture.)

| 1 | Goals of Childbirth Education (See Figure 13.3)
- Provide information about:
  ○ Pregnancy
  ○ Childbirth
  ○ Coping mechanisms
  ○ Choices available for the woman and her support person

| 1a | See Figure 13.3

SUGGESTIONS FOR CLINICAL ACTIVITIES

Have students attend a childbirth education class and discuss their observations.

LEARNING OBJECTIVE 4

Summarize the role of the doula/labor companion during labor and birth.

CONCEPTS FOR LECTURE

1. A doula/labor companion will provide support—emotional, physical, and informational—during labor. The doula also acts as an advocate for the woman and the family by facilitating communication between the woman and family and the healthcare providers. Benefits of labor support include facilitation of the birth process, enhancement of the mother's memory of the experience, strengthening of the mother-infant bonding

POWERPOINT LECTURE SLIDES

(NOTE: The number on each PPT Lecture Slide directly corresponds with the Concepts for Lecture.)

| 1 | Role of a Doula/Labor Companion
- Provides emotional, physical, and informational support
- Acts as an advocate by verbalizing the wishes of the family

process, breastfeeding success, and a significant reduction in medical intervention during the childbirth experience. The doula may also provide support during the postpartum period.

 Benefits of a Doula/ Labor Companion
- Facilitates birth
- Enhances the mother's memory of the experience
- Strengthens mother-infant bonding
- Increases breastfeeding success

SUGGESTIONS FOR CLASSROOM ACTIVITIES

Invite a doula to class to speak to the students about her role in childbearing.

LEARNING OBJECTIVE 5

Describe the types of prenatal education programs available to expectant couples and their families.

CONCEPTS FOR LECTURE

1. Prenatal education programs may include classes aimed at childbirth choices, preparation of the mother for pregnancy and birth, preparation for cesarean birth, preparation for vaginal birth after cesarean-preparation for couples who desire an unmedicated birth, and preparation of specific people, such as grandparents or siblings, for the birth.

2. Classes in the early prenatal period may cover early gestational changes; self-care during pregnancy; fetal development and environmental dangers for the fetus; sexuality in pregnancy; birth settings and types of care providers; nutrition, rest, and exercise suggestions; common discomforts of pregnancy and relief measures; psychologic changes in pregnancy for the woman and man; and getting the pregnancy off to a good start by following a healthful lifestyle, learning methods of coping with stress, and avoiding alcohol and smoking. Information about risk for preterm labor and infant feeding should also be presented.

3. The later classes focus on preparation for the birth, infant care and feeding, postpartum self-care, birth choices (episiotomy, medications, fetal monitoring, perineal prep, enema, and so forth), and newborn safety issues.

POWERPOINT LECTURE SLIDES

(NOTE: The number on each PPT Lecture Slide directly corresponds with the Concepts for Lecture.)

 Prenatal Education
- Childbirth choices available today
- Preparation of the mother for pregnancy and birth
- Preparation for cesarean birth
- Preparation for vaginal birth after cesarean
- Preparation for couples who desire an unmedicated birth
- Preparation of specific people such as grandparents or siblings for the birth (see Figure 13.4)

 See Figure 13.4

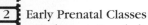 Early Prenatal Classes
- Early gestational changes
- Self-care during pregnancy
- Fetal development and environmental dangers
- Sexuality in pregnancy
- Birth settings and types of care providers
- Nutrition, rest, and exercise suggestions

 Early Prenatal Classes
- Common discomforts of pregnancy and relief measures
- Psychologic changes in pregnancy for the woman and man
- Healthful lifestyle issues
- Risk factors for preterm labor
- How to recognize symptoms of preterm labor
- The advantages and disadvantages of formula-feeding or breastfeeding

 Later Prenatal Classes
- Preparation for the birth
- Infant care and feeding
- Postpartum self-care
- Birth choices
- Newborn safety issues

SUGGESTIONS FOR CLASSROOM ACTIVITIES

Have students develop a teaching plan for a particular type of childbirth education class. Have them share their teaching plans with their peers.

SUGGESTIONS FOR CLINICAL ACTIVITIES

Have students attend different types of childbirth education classes and discuss their observations.

LEARNING OBJECTIVE 6

Delineate the childbirth educator's role in promoting relaxation for pregnant women.

CONCEPTS FOR LECTURE

1. The childbirth educator teaches couples about the techniques and benefits of relaxation exercises including progressive relaxation, touch, disassociation, controlled breathing, and effleurage. Relaxation allows the woman to conserve energy and the uterine muscles to work more efficiently. Additional methods that may be used to promote relaxation in labor include guided imagery, hypnosis, meditation, music, massage, aromatherapy, therapeutic touch, biofeedback, transcutaneous electrical nerve stimulation (TENS) unit, acupressure, and acupuncture.

POWERPOINT LECTURE SLIDES

(NOTE: The number on each PPT Lecture Slide directly corresponds with the Concepts for Lecture.)

1 Relaxation During Labor
- Purpose (see Figure 13.5)
  - Conserve energy
  - Allows uterine muscles to work more efficiently

1a See Figure 13.5

1b Relaxation Exercises
- Touch
- Disassociation
- Effleurage (see Figures 13.16 A and B)

1c See Figures 13.6A and B

1d Promotion of Relaxation
- Guided imagery
- Hypnosis
- Meditation
- Music
- Massage
- Aromatherapy

1e Promotion of Relaxation
- Therapeutic touch
- Biofeedback
- Transcutaneous electrical nerve stimulation unit (TENS unit)
- Acupressure and acupuncture
- Controlled breathing

SUGGESTIONS FOR CLASSROOM ACTIVITIES

Have students practice relaxation exercises in class and describe their response to the exercises.

SUGGESTIONS FOR CLINICAL ACTIVITIES

Ask students to share some of the exercises that they learned in class with women in labor and observe the client response.

LEARNING OBJECTIVE 7

Compare methods of childbirth preparation.

CONCEPTS FOR LECTURE

1. The most common methods of childbirth preparation are Lamaze (psychoprophylactic), Kitzinger (sensory memory), Bradley (partner-coached childbirth), and HypnoBirthing. All of these programs help eliminate fear and teach coping mechanisms, teach relaxation techniques, prepare the participants for what to expect during labor and birth, and teach exercises to condition muscles and use breathing patterns needed in labor. The biggest differences are the theories of why each type works and the relaxation techniques and breathing patterns.

POWERPOINT LECTURE SLIDES

(NOTE: The number on each PPT Lecture Slide directly corresponds with the Concepts for Lecture.)

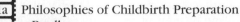 Methods of Childbirth Preparation
- Lamaze (psychoprophylactic)
- Kitzinger (sensory memory)
- Bradley (partner-coached childbirth)
- HypnoBirthing

1a Philosophies of Childbirth Preparation
- Bradley
  - Have the best, safest, most rewarding birth experience
- Lamaze
  - Empowers women to make informed choices
  - Empowers women to assume responsibility for health
  - Trust in inner wisdom

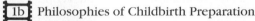 Philosophies of Childbirth Preparation
- Kitzinger
  - Have information to make informed choices
  - Benefits of home birth for low-risk women
- HypnoBirthing
  - Eliminating fear, stress-free, calm, gentle environment
  - Environment resembles nature's design

CHAPTER 14
PHYSICAL AND PSYCHOLOGIC CHANGES OF PREGNANCY

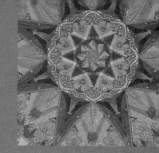

RESOURCE LIBRARY

⊙ PRENTICE HALL NURSING MEDIALINK DVD-ROM

Audio Glossary
NCLEX Review
Videos: *Through the Eyes of a Nurse—
The First Trimester; Through the Eyes of a Nurse—
The Second Trimester; Through the Eyes of a Nurse—
The Third Trimester; Through the Eyes of a Nurse—
Welcoming the NewArrival at the Postpartum Visit*

📖 IMAGE LIBRARY

Figure 14.1 Vena caval syndrome.
Figure 14.2 Linea nigra.
Figure 14.3 Postural changes during pregnancy.
Figure 14.4 Hegar's sign, a softening of the isthmus of the uterus, can be determined by the examiner during a vaginal examination.

COMPANION WEBSITE

Additional NCLEX Review
Case Study: *Prenatal Education*
Care Plan Activity: *Preparing Siblings for New Baby*
Applications: *Endocrine Hormones; Internet Pregnancy Information*
Critical Thinking

Figure 14.5 Early uterine changes of pregnancy.
Figure 14.6 Approximate height of the fundus at various weeks of pregnancy.

LEARNING OBJECTIVE 1
Identify the anatomic and physiologic changes that occur during pregnancy.

CONCEPTS FOR LECTURE

1. Hypertrophy of the myometrial cells of the uterus is the cause of uterine enlargement during pregnancy. Estrogen and progesterone cause the uterine walls to thicken and there is an increase in the uterine vascular and lymphatic systems.
2. Cell number is increased in the glandular tissue of the cervix. A mucous plug forms due to the secretion of thick mucus by the endocervical glands to prevent bacteria or other substances from entering the uterus. Goodell's sign, a softening of the cervix, occurs, as well as an increase in vascularization, which causes a bluish-purple discoloration called Chadwick's sign.
3. Under the influence of estrogen, the vaginal epithelium hypertrophies, increases vascularization, and undergoes hyperplasia. Because of this, the mucosa thickens, the connective tissue loosens, and there is an increase in vaginal secretions. Glandular hyperplasia and hypertrophy result in an increase in breast size, with superficial veins becoming prominent, the nipples becoming more erect, striae may develop, and the areola becoming more deeply pigmented. Colostrum may be expressed by the 12th week of pregnancy.
4. Tidal volume increases as pregnant women slightly hyperventilate. To meet the demands of the mother and the fetus, oxygen consumption increases as well as

POWERPOINT LECTURE SLIDES

(NOTE: The number on each PPT Lecture Slide directly corresponds with the Concepts for Lecture.)

1 Uterine Changes
- Enlargement due to hypertrophy (Figure 14.6)
- Thickening of the walls
- Increase in vascular and lymphatic system

1a See Figure 14.6

2 Cervical Changes
- Development of mucous plug
- Goodell's sign—softening
- Chadwick's sign—bluish-purple discoloration

3 Vaginal Changes
- Hypertrophy, increased vascularization, hyperplasia due to estrogen
- Increase in secretions, loosening of connective tissue

3a Breast Changes
- Glandular hyperplasia and hypertrophy
- Areolae darken, superficial veins prominent
- Striae may develop
- Colostrum is secreted

vital capacity. Lung compliance and pulmonary diffusion remain constant. The pregnant woman changes her breathing from abdominal to thoracic. Nasal stuffiness and congestion are a common complaint of pregnant women due to the vascular congestion of the nasal mucosa. Pressure on the diaphragm by the growing uterus pushes the heart upward and to the left. There is an increase in blood volume to between 40% and 45% above nonpregnant levels due to an increase in plasma and erythrocytes. Systemic and pulmonary vascular resistance both decrease, which maintains normal blood pressures with larger blood volumes. There is an increase in cardiac output to about 30% to 50% above nonpregnant levels. Supine hypotensive syndrome may occur due to pressure of the growing uterus on the inferior vena cava.

5. Women often experience nausea and vomiting during the first trimester due to human chorionic gonadotropin (hCG) secretion and a change in carbohydrate metabolism. Hyperemia, softening, and bleeding of the gums also occurs. Heartburn, delayed gastric emptying time, and delayed intestinal motility also occur. Smooth muscle relaxation and increased electrolyte and water reabsorption in the large intestine also contribute to the development of constipation. Hemorrhoids are caused by pressure on the vessels below the level of the uterus.

6. Urinary frequency in the first trimester is caused by pressure on the bladder. In the third trimester, pressure of the presenting part on the bladder causes frequency. Pregnant women are at an increased risk for urinary tract infections due to a dilatation of the kidneys and ureters. During pregnancy there is also an increase in glomerular filtration rate and renal plasma flow.

7. Skin hyperpigmentation occurs on the following areas: areolae, nipples, vulva, perianal area, and the linea alba. Linea nigra is the darkening of the linea alba. Facial chloasma also may occur. Stretch marks, also called striae, often occur on the abdomen, the breasts, and the thighs. The chest, face, neck, arms, and legs may be affected by vascular spider nevi. Hair growth may decrease during pregnancy and the number of hair follicles in the resting phase may decrease. Because of the subsequent increase in the number of hair follicles in the resting phase after birth, excessive hair shedding may occur for 1 to 4 months. Hyperactive sweat and sebaceous glands are present during pregnancy.

8. Pelvic joint relaxation, which occurs in the latter part of pregnancy due to hormonal changes, will change the woman's gait. The change in the center of gravity results in an accentuated lumbodorsal spinal curve and a posture change, which often result in a low backache. The rectus abdominus muscle may separate due to pressure from the enlarging uterus.

9. There is a decrease in the intraocular pressure due to an increase in vitreous outflow. The cornea thickens slightly due to fluid retention. Cognitively, pregnant

4 Respiratory Changes
- Tidal volume increases
- Oxygen consumption increases
- Breathing changes from abdominal to thoracic
- Vascular congestion of nasal mucosa

4a Cardiac Changes
- Blood volume increases 40% to 45%
- Decrease in systemic and pulmonary vascular resistance
- Increase in cardiac output

5 GI Changes
- Nausea and vomiting
- Hyperemia, softening and bleeding of gums
- Constipation
- Heartburn
- Hemorrhoids

6 Urinary Changes
- Pressure on bladder causes frequency
- Dilatation of kidneys and urine
- Increased GFR and renal plasma flow

7 Skin Changes
- Hyperpigmentation
- Striae
- Chloasma
- Vascular spider nevi
- Decreased hair growth
- Hyperactive sweat and sebaceous glands

8 Musculoskeletal Changes
- Pelvic joints relax
- Center of gravity changes
- Separation of rectus abdominus

9 Eye, Cognitive and Metabolic Changes
- Decreased intraocular pressure
- Thickening of cornea
- Reports of decreased attention, concentration, and memory
- Extra water, fat, and protein are stored
- Fats are more completely absorbed

10 Endocrine Changes
- T_4 and BMR increase, TSH decreases
- Concentration of parathyroid hormone increases
- Thyrotropin and adrenotropin alter maternal metabolism
- Prolactin is responsible for lactation
- Secretion of oxytocin and vasopressin
- Increased aldosterone

women often describe a decrease in attention, concentration, and memory. Extra water, fat, and protein are stored as maternal reserves. There is an increase in serum lipids, lipoproteins, and cholesterol due to more complete absorption of fats. Pregnant women often experience intermittent glycosuria as well.

10. The influence of pregnancy on the thyroid gland includes an increase in total serum thyroxine (T_4), a decrease in thyroid-stimulating hormone (TSH), and an increase in the basal metabolic rate (BMR). There is an increase in the size of the parathyroid gland and a concentration of the parathyroid hormone to parallel fetal calcium requirements. Thyrotropin and adrenotropin change maternal metabolism to support the pregnancy. The hormone responsible for lactation is prolactin. Oxytocin and vasopressin are secreted by the posterior pituitary. Oxytocin promotes uterine contractility and the stimulation of milk ejection from the breasts. Vasoconstriction resulting in increased blood pressure is the result of vasopressin, which also has an antidiuretic effect. Increased levels of aldosterone are secreted by the adrenals in the second trimester as a protective response to the increase in sodium excretion associated with progesterone.

LEARNING OBJECTIVE 2

Relate the physiologic and anatomic changes that occur in the body systems during pregnancy to the signs and symptoms that develop in the woman.

CONCEPTS FOR LECTURE

1. Braxton Hicks contractions occur intermittently throughout pregnancy. Hyperactivity of the glandular tissue in the cervix results in an increase in vaginal discharge. Pregnant women are at an increased risk for developing vaginal infections due to the acidic environment in the vaginal epithelium. In response to the secretion of prolactin, colostrum may leak from the breasts during the last trimester of pregnancy. An increase in the awareness of the need to breathe is due to the increase in tidal volume causing a slight decrease in PCO_2. Due to the influence of estrogen, nasal stuffiness and nosebleeds are common. Stagnation of the blood in the lower extremities causes edema and an increase in varicose vein formation in the legs, vulva, and rectum. Pregnant women may experience symptoms of postural hypotension such as dizziness due to an increase in blood volume in the lower extremities. Pressure on the vena cava by the enlarging uterus results in supine hypotensive syndrome. Nausea and vomiting in the first trimester are associated with hCG secretion and a change in carbohydrate metabolism. Bleeding of the gums may occur due to the influence of estrogen. Pregnant women may experience constipation due to a decrease in gastric emptying time and a delay in intestinal motility. Pregnant women are also at risk for

POWERPOINT LECTURE SLIDES

(NOTE: The number on each PPT Lecture Slide directly corresponds with the Concepts for Lecture.)

1 Physical Symptoms of Pregnancy
- Braxton Hicks
- Increased vaginal discharge and risk of infection
- Leaking of colostrum
- Hyperventilation
- Nasal stuffiness and nosebleeds
- Lower extremity edema

1a Physical Symptoms of Pregnancy
- Postural hypotension
- Supine hypotensive syndrome (Figure 14.1)
- Nausea and vomiting
- Bleeding of gums
- Constipation and hemorrhoids
- Pruritus

1b See Figure 14.1

1c Physical Symptoms of Pregnancy
- Urinary frequency
- Hyperpigmentation (Figure 14.2)
- Striae
- Vascular spider nevi
- Decreased rate of hair growth
- Heavy perspiration, night sweats, acne

the development of hemorrhoids due to constipation and/or pressure from the enlarged uterus on the vessels. Retained bile salts may cause pruritus. Pressure of the growing uterus on the bladder may result in urinary frequency. Hyperpigmentation occurs due to the influence of estrogen. Linea nigra, chloasma, striae, and vascular spider nevi are manifestations of this. There is a decrease in hair growth rate and the number of hair follicles in the resting phase. Excessive perspiration, night sweats, and/or the development of acne may occur. A waddling gait is due to pelvic joint relaxation. A change in posture and low backache may occur due to a change in the center of gravity. There is a difficulty in wearing contact lenses due to a decrease in intraocular pressure and a slight thickening of the cornea.

1d See Figure 14.2

1e Physical Symptoms of Pregnancy
- Waddling gait
- Backache
- Difficulty wearing contact lenses

SUGGESTIONS FOR CLASSROOM ACTIVITIES

Have a group discussion about the symptoms and discomforts of pregnancy and potential nursing interventions.

SUGGESTIONS FOR CLINICAL ACTIVITIES

Have students develop a care plan for a nursing diagnosis for one of the discomforts of pregnancy.

LEARNING OBJECTIVE 3

Compare subjective (presumptive), objective (probable), and diagnostic (positive) changes of pregnancy.

CONCEPTS FOR LECTURE

1. The following are presumptive signs of pregnancy: amenorrhea, nausea and vomiting, excessive fatigue, urinary frequency, breast changes, and quickening.
2. The following are probable signs of pregnancy: changes in the pelvic organs: Goodell's sign, Chadwick's sign, Hegar's sign, uterine enlargement, Braun von Fernwald's sign, Piskacek's sign; enlargement of the abdomen; Braxton Hicks contractions; uterine souffle; changes in the pigmentation of the skin: chloasma, linea nigra, and nipples/areolae; abdominal striae; balottement; positive pregnancy tests; and palpation of fetal outline.
3. The following are positive signs of pregnancy: auscultation of fetal heartbeat, fetal movement, and visualization of the fetus.

POWERPOINT LECTURE SLIDES

(NOTE: The number on each PPT Lecture Slide directly corresponds with the Concepts for Lecture.)

1 Presumptive Signs of Pregnancy
- Amenorrhea
- Nausea and vomiting
- Excessive fatigue
- Urinary frequency
- Breast changes
- Quickening

2 Probable Signs of Pregnancy
- Changes in the pelvic organs (Figures 14.4 and 14.5)
- Enlargement of the abdomen
- Braxton Hicks contractions
- Abdominal striae
- Uterine souffle
- Changes in the pigmentation of the skin

2a See Figure 14.4

2b See Figure 14.5

2c Probable Signs of Pregnancy
- Ballottement
- Positive pregnancy tests

3 Positive Signs of Pregnancy
- Auscultation of fetal heartbeat
- Fetal movement
- Visualization of the fetus

LEARNING OBJECTIVE 4

Contrast the various types of pregnancy tests.

CONCEPTS FOR LECTURE

1. A hemagglutination-inhibition test is a urine pregnancy test that uses hCG-sensitized red blood cells of sheep. The latex agglutination test is also a urine pregnancy test that is based on the fact that latex particle agglutination is inhibited in the presence of hCG. A very accurate serum pregnancy test is β-subunit radioimmunoassay (RIA), which uses an antiserum with specificity for the β-subunit of hCG in blood plasma. It permits diagnosis of pregnancy a few days after implantation. Another serum pregnancy test is the immunoradiometric assay (IRMA), which uses a radioactive antibody to identify the presence of hCG in the serum. The enzyme-linked immunosorbent assay (ELISA) can detect hCG levels as early as 7 to 9 days after ovulation and conception. Another serum pregnancy test is the fluoroimmunoassay (FIA) that uses an antibody tagged with a fluorescent label to detect serum hCG.

2. Home pregnancy tests are quite sensitive and detect even low levels of hCG in urine. There is a low false-positive rate and a higher false-negative result.

POWERPOINT LECTURE SLIDES

(NOTE: The number on each PPT Lecture Slide directly corresponds with the Concepts for Lecture.)

1 Pregnancy Tests
- Hemagglutination-inhibition (HI) test
- Latex agglutination test
- β-subunit radioimmunoassay (RIA)
- Immunoradiometric assay (IRMA)
- Enzyme-linked immunosorbent assay (ELISA)
- Fluoroimmunoassay (FIA)

2 Home Pregnancy Tests
- Enzyme immunoassay tests
- False-positive results low
- False-negative results higher

LEARNING OBJECTIVE 5

Discuss the emotional and psychologic changes that commonly occur in a woman, her partner, and her family during pregnancy.

CONCEPTS FOR LECTURE

1. The emotional responses to pregnancy may include ambivalence, acceptance, introversion, mood swings, and changes in body image. Although a pregnancy may be planned, surprise and/or ambivalence may occur. A woman may become introverted during pregnancy, and those who were once active, may now be more focused on the self and the need for rest. This assists the woman with planning, adjusting, building, and drawing strength in preparation for the birth. Mood swings are common from great joy to despair. Pregnant women may become tearful for no reason. Emotions related to body image changes also play a role.

2. The four tasks of pregnancy as identified by Rubin (1984) include ensuring safe passage through pregnancy, labor, and birth; seeking of acceptance of this child by others; seeking of commitment and acceptance of self as mother to the infant (binding-in); and learning to give of oneself on behalf of one's child.

POWERPOINT LECTURE SLIDES

(NOTE: The number on each PPT Lecture Slide directly corresponds with the Concepts for Lecture.)

1 Mother's Response to Pregnancy
- Ambivalence
- Acceptance
- Introversion
- Mood swings
- Changes in body image

2 Rubin's (1984) Tasks of Pregnancy
- Ensuring safe passage through pregnancy, labor, and birth
- Seeking of acceptance of this child by others
- Seeking of commitment and acceptance of self as mother to the infant (binding-in)
- Learning to give of oneself on behalf of one's child

3. The expectant father may feel left out of the pregnancy. He may be confused by the expectant mother's mood changes and his responses to her changing body. Resentment over the attention that the mother receives may occur. Changes in the relationship due to the woman's fatigue and decreased interest in sex may negatively affect him. Expectant fathers also need to confront their own conflicts about fathering. As the pregnancy reaches the third trimester, the couple may grow closer as the father has a more clearly defined role and they prepare together for the birth of the baby. The father may express concern about the risks to the expectant mother and the baby during childbirth. Expectant fathers may develop couvade, which is the unintentional development of physical symptoms, such as fatigue, increased appetite, difficulty sleeping, depression, headache, or backache by the partner of the pregnant woman.

4. Sibling rivalry may occur with the introduction of a new baby into the family, which results from a child's fear of change in the relationship with his or her parents. A closer relationship between the expectant couple and their parents may occur even if conflicts previously existed.

3. Father's Response to Pregnancy
   - Confused by partner's mood changes
   - Feels left out of pregnancy
   - Resents attention given to the woman
   - Resents changes in their relationship
   - Needs to resolve conflicts about fathering
   - Couvade

4. Family Response to Pregnancy
   - Siblings
     - Rivalry
     - Fear of changing parent relationships
   - Grandparents
     - Closer relationship with expectant couple
     - Increasingly supportive of couple

SUGGESTIONS FOR CLASSROOM ACTIVITIES

Have a group discussion about the psychologic changes that a family goes through during pregnancy.

SUGGESTIONS FOR CLINICAL ACTIVITIES

Have students interview a woman in a prenatal clinic about her family's adjustment to the pregnancy.

LEARNING OBJECTIVE 6

Summarize cultural factors that may influence a family's response to pregnancy.

CONCEPTS FOR LECTURE

1. An important aspect of prenatal care is a cultural assessment in which the nurse needs to identify family beliefs, values, and behaviors that relate to pregnancy and childbearing. Information about ethnic groups, patterns of decision making, religious preferences, language, communication style, and common etiquette practices are important, as well as expectations of the healthcare system.

POWERPOINT LECTURE SLIDES

(NOTE: The number on each PPT Lecture Slide directly corresponds with the Concepts for Lecture.)

1. Cultural Factors
   - Identify beliefs, values, and behaviors
     - Ethnic background
     - Patterns of decision making
     - Religious preferences, language, communication style
     - Common etiquette practices
     - Expectations of healthcare system

SUGGESTIONS FOR CLASSROOM ACTIVITIES

Ask students to share some of their cultural traditions regarding childbirth and childbearing.

CHAPTER 15
ANTEPARTAL NURSING ASSESSMENT

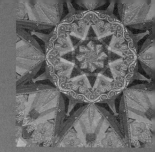

RESOURCE LIBRARY

PRENTICE HALL NURSING MEDIALINK DVD-ROM

Audio Glossary
NCLEX Review
Videos: *Through the Eyes of a Nurse—The First Trimester; Through the Eyes of a Nurse—The Second Trimester; Through the Eyes of a Nurse—The Third Trimester*

IMAGE LIBRARY

Figure 15.1 The TPAL approach provides more detailed information about the woman's pregnancy history.
Figure 15.2 Sample prenatal questionnaire.
Figure 15.3 The EDB wheel can be used to calculate the due date.
Figure 15.4 A cross-sectional view of fetal position when McDonald's method is used to assess fundal height.

 ### COMPANION WEBSITE

Additional NCLEX Review
Case Study: *Initial Prenatal Assessment*
Care Plan Activity: *Initial Assessment of Primigravida*
Application: *Ovulation Calculator*
Critical Thinking

Figure 15.5 Listening to the fetal heartbeat with a Doppler device.
Figure 15.6 Anteroposterior diameters of the pelvic inlet and their relationship to the pelvic planes.
Figure 15.7 Manual measurement of inlet and outlet.
Figure 15.8 Use of a closed fist to measure the outlet.
Figure 15.9 Evaluation of the outlet.

LEARNING OBJECTIVE 1

Summarize the essential components of a prenatal history.

CONCEPTS FOR LECTURE

1. Essential components of a prenatal history should include information about the current pregnancy, the past pregnancy history, gynecologic history, the current medical history, the past medical history, the family medical history, religious and cultural history, occupational history, partner history, and personal information about birth and infant feeding preference.

POWERPOINT LECTURE SLIDES

(NOTE: The number on each PPT Lecture Slide directly corresponds with the Concepts for Lecture.)

1. Prenatal History
   - Assessment of current and past pregnancies
   - Gynecologic history
   - Current and past medical history
   - Family medical history
   - Religious, cultural, and occupational history
   - Partner history

SUGGESTIONS FOR CLASSROOM ACTIVITIES

Have students practice doing a prenatal history on classmates. Give feedback about interview techniques.

SUGGESTIONS FOR CLINICAL ACTIVITIES

Have students do a prenatal health history on a woman in a prenatal clinic and summarize their results.

Define common obstetric terminology found in the history of maternity clients.

CONCEPTS FOR LECTURE

1. The following terms are used to document the obstetric history:
   - *Antepartum.* The time between conception and labor
   - *Intrapartum.* The time from labor until the birth of the infant and placenta
   - *Postpartum.* The time from birth until the return to the prepregnant condition
2. Gestational terms include:
   - *Gestation.* The number of weeks since the first day of the last menstrual period (LMP)
   - *Abortion.* A birth that occurs before 20 weeks' gestation or the birth of a newborn less than 500 g
   - *Term.* Normal duration of pregnancy from 38 to 42 weeks
3. Labor and delivery terms include:
   - *Preterm or premature labor.* The occurrence of labor after 20 weeks' but before 37 weeks' gestation
   - *Postterm labor.* The occurrence of labor after 42 weeks' gestation
   - *Stillbirth.* A fetus who is born dead after 20 weeks' gestation
4. Pregnancy terms include:
   - *Gravida.* Pregnancy, regardless of duration
   - *Nulligravida.* Never been pregnant
   - *Primigravida.* A first pregnancy
   - *Multigravida.* A second or subsequent pregnancy
5. Birth terms include:
   - *Para.* The birth after 20 weeks' gestation
   - *Nullipara.* Never given birth at more than 20 weeks' gestation
   - *Primipara.* One birth at more than 20 weeks' gestation
   - *Multipara.* Two or more births at more than 20 weeks' gestation
6. The terms "gravida" and "para" describe pregnancies, not number of fetuses.
   T: number of *term* infants born
   P: number of *preterm* infants born
   A: number of pregnancies ending in either spontaneous or therapeutic *abortion*
   L: number of currently living children.

POWERPOINT LECTURE SLIDES

(NOTE: The number on each PPT Lecture Slide directly corresponds with the Concepts for Lecture.)

1. Obstetric History Terminology
   - Antepartum
   - Intrapartum
   - Postpartum
2. Gestational Terminology
   - Gestation
   - Abortion
   - Term
3. Labor and Delivery Terminology
   - Preterm or premature labor
   - Postterm labor
   - Stillbirth
4. Pregnancy Terminology
   - Gravida
   - Nulligravida
   - Primigravida
   - Multigravida
5. Birth Terminology
   - Primipara
   - Para
   - Nullipara
   - Multipara
6. Pregnancy and Birth History (Figure 15.1)
   - G—the number of pregnancies including current pregnancy
   - T—the number of pregnancies that were delivered at 37 weeks or later
   - P—the number of pregnancies that were delivered between 20 and 37 weeks
   - A—the number of pregnancies ending in spontaneous or therapeutic abortion
   - L—the number of currently living children
6a. See Figure 15.1

SUGGESTIONS FOR CLASSROOM ACTIVITIES

Play a matching game in class with definitions and terms.

LEARNING OBJECTIVE 3

Identify factors related to the father's health that should be recorded on the prenatal record.

CONCEPTS FOR LECTURE

1. Information about the father's health that should be recorded in the prenatal record include the presence of genetic conditions or diseases in him or in his family history, his age, significant health problems, previous or present alcohol intake, drug use or tobacco use, his blood type and Rh factor, occupation, educational level, methods by which he learns best, and his attitude toward the pregnancy.

POWERPOINT LECTURE SLIDES

(NOTE: The number on each PPT Lecture Slide directly corresponds with the Concepts for Lecture.)

1 Factors Related to Father's Health
- Family history of genetic conditions
- Age
- Significant health problems
- Previous or present alcohol intake
- Drug and tobacco use
- Blood type and Rh factor

1a Factors Related to Father's Health
- Occupation
- Educational level
- Methods by which he learns best
- Attitude toward the pregnancy

SUGGESTIONS FOR CLASSROOM ACTIVITIES

Have a group discussion about implications of paternal risk factors for the infant and family.

LEARNING OBJECTIVE 4

Describe the normal physiologic changes one would expect to find when performing a physical assessment on a pregnant woman.

CONCEPTS FOR LECTURE

1. Normal skin changes in pregnancy may include spider nevi and pigmentation changes such as linea nigra, striae gravidarum, and melasma. The nose may be edematous during pregnancy. There may be hypertrophy of gingival tissue in the mouth. There is slight hyperplasia by the third month. The breasts are soft, symmetric, and have darker pigmentation of the nipples and the areolae. They increase in size, they become nodular, the superficial veins dilate and become more prominent, striae appear in multiparas, and the tubercles of Montgomery enlarge. Pregnant women report a tingling sensation in the first and third trimesters, and colostrum may be present after 12 weeks. During pregnancy, many women report cardiac palpitations and upon ausculation, a short systoic murmur may be heard. Purple or silver striae may be present over the abdomen and the linea nigra will appear. There is progressive abdominal enlargement, and diastasis of the rectus abdominus muscle may occur. During pregnancy, the lumbar spinal curve may be accentuated. Changes in the pelvis include an enlargement in the anteroposterior diameter, softening of the cervix (Goodell's sign), softening of the isthmus of the uterus (Hegar's sign), and bluishness of the cervix (Chadwick's sign). The uterus becomes pear shaped, mobile, and smooth.

POWERPOINT LECTURE SLIDES

(NOTE: The number on each PPT Lecture Slide directly corresponds with the Concepts for Lecture.)

1 Normal Changes in Pregnancy
- Skin
  - Spider nevi common
  - Pigmentaton changes—linea nigra, striae gravidarum, melasma
- Nose
  - May be edematous

1a Normal Changes in Pregnancy
- Mouth
  - May have hypertrophy of gingival tissue
- Thyroid
  - Slight hyperplasia by third month

1b Normal Changes in Pregnancy
- Breasts
  - Size increase noted in first 20 weeks
  - Become nodular
  - Tingling sensation in first and third trimesters
  - Pigmentation of nipples and areolae darken
  - Superficial veins dilate and become more prominent

1c Normal Changes in Pregnancy
- Breasts
  - Striae in multiparas
  - Tubercles of Montgomery enlarge
  - Colostrum may be present after 12 weeks

1d Normal Changes in Pregnancy
- Heart
  - Palpitations may occur
  - Short systolic murmurs

1e Normal Changes in Pregnancy
- Abdomen
  - Purple or silver striae may be present
  - Linea nigra
  - Diastasis of the rectus muscle
  - Progressive enlargement
  - Ballottement

1f Normal Changes in Pregnancy
- Spine
  - Lumbar spinal curve may be accentuated
- Pelvis
  - Enlargement in anteroposterior diameter
  - Softening of cervix (Goodell's sign), softening of isthmus of uterus (Hegar's sign), cervix takes on bluish coloring (Chadwick's sign)
  - Uterus is pear shaped, mobile, and smooth

SUGGESTIONS FOR CLINICAL ACTIVITIES

Have students do a prenatal physical examination on a woman and summarize the results.

LEARNING OBJECTIVE 5

Explain the use of Nägele's rule to determine the estimated date of birth.

CONCEPTS FOR LECTURE

1. To estimate the date of birth (EDB), Nägele's rule is used. To derive a date, begin with the first day of the LMP, subtract 3 months, and add 7 days.

POWERPOINT LECTURE SLIDES

(NOTE: The number on each PPT Lecture Slide directly corresponds with the Concepts for Lecture.)

1 Näegle's Rule (Figure 15.3)
- First day of last menstrual period—3 months + 7 days = EDB

1a See Figure 15.3

SUGGESTIONS FOR CLASSROOM ACTIVITIES

Give students LMP dates to practice calculation of EDB.

LEARNING OBJECTIVE 6

Develop an outline of the essential measurements that can be determined by clinical pelvimetry.

CONCEPTS FOR LECTURE

1. Clinical pelvimetry can provide essential measurements to assist the healthcare provider in making clinical birth decisions. Important anteroposterior diameters of the inlet for childbearing are the diagonal conjugate; the obstetric conjugate; and the conjugata vera, or true conjugate. The important midpelvic measurements include the plane of least dimension, or midplane, and transverse diameter. The important pelvic outlet measurements include the anteroposterior diameter and the transverse diameter. Estimation of the suprapubic angle and the length and shape of the pubic rami are also important. The height and inclination of the symphysis pubis and the contour of the pubic arch are important measurements as well.

POWERPOINT LECTURE SLIDES

(NOTE: The number on each PPT Lecture Slide directly corresponds with the Concepts for Lecture.)

1 Assessment of Pelvic Adequacy (Figures 15.6, 15.7A–D, 15.8, 15.9A–D)
- Pelvic inlet
- Midpelvis
- Pelvic outlet

1a See Figure 15.6

1b See Figure 15.7 A–D

1c See Figure 15.8

1d See Figure 15.9 A–D

SUGGESTIONS FOR CLASSROOM ACTIVITIES

Bring in a pelvic model to illustrate the pelvic measurements.

LEARNING OBJECTIVE 7

Describe areas that should be evaluated as part of the initial assessment of psychosocial factors related to a woman's pregnancy.

CONCEPTS FOR LECTURE

1. Psychosocial factors that should be considered in the assessment of the pregnant woman should include any history of emotional or physical deprivation or abuse of herself or her children; history of emotional problems, specifically about depression in general, postpartum depression, and anxiety; support systems; overuse or underuse of the healthcare system; acceptance of pregnancy—intended or unintended; personal preferences about the birth; plans for care of child following birth and feeding preference for the baby.

POWERPOINT LECTURE SLIDES

(NOTE: The number on each PPT Lecture Slide directly corresponds with the Concepts for Lecture.)

1 Psychosocial Assessment
- History of emotional or physical abuse
- History of emotional problems
  - Depression and anxiety in general
  - Postpartum depression
- Support systems

1a Psychosocial Assessment
- Overuse or underuse of healthcare system
- Acceptance of pregnancy, intended or unintended
- Personal preferences about the birth
- Plans for care of child following birth
- Feeding preference for the baby

SUGGESTIONS FOR CLASSROOM ACTIVITIES

Have students identify cues in the prenatal health history that might help them identify potential or actual psychosocial issues.

LEARNING OBJECTIVE 8

Relate the danger signs of pregnancy to their possible causes.

CONCEPTS FOR LECTURE

1. Danger signs of pregnancy include a sudden gush of fluid from the vagina, which may be due to ruptured membranes; vaginal bleeding, which may be due to abruptio placentae, placenta previa, vaginal or cervical lesions, or bloody show; abdominal pain, which may be due to premature labor or abruptio placentae; temperature above 38.3C and chills, which may be due to infection; dizziness, blurring or double vision, or spots before the eyes, which may be due to hypertension or preeclampsia; persistent vomiting, which may be due to hyperemesis gravidarum; severe headache, which may be due to hypertension or preeclampsia; edema of the hands, face, legs, and feet, which may be due to preeclampsia; muscular irritability or convulsions, which may be due to preeclampsia or eclampsia; epigastric pain, which may be due to preeclampsia or ischemia in the major vessels; oliguria, which may be due to renal impairment or decreased fluid intake; dysuria, which may be due to a urinary tract infection; or absence of fetal movement, which may be due to maternal medication, obesity, or fetal death.

POWERPOINT LECTURE SLIDES

(NOTE: The number on each PPT Lecture Slide directly corresponds with the Concepts for Lecture.)

 Danger Signs of Pregnancy
- Gush of fluid from vagina
- Vaginal bleeding
- Abdominal pain
- Fever
- Dizziness, blurred vision, spots before eyes
- Persistent vomiting

 Danger Signs of Pregnancy
- Edema
- Muscular irritability or convulsions
- Epigastric pain
- Oliguria
- Dysuria
- Absence of fetal movement

SUGGESTIONS FOR CLINICAL ACTIVITIES

Have students teach a prenatal class on the warning signs in pregnancy.

Chapter 16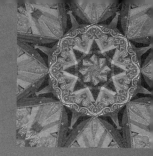
The Expectant Family: Needs and Care

Resource Library

PRENTICE HALL NURSING MEDIALINK DVD-ROM

AudioGlossary
NCLEX Review
Videos: *Through the Eyes of a Nurse—The First
Trimester; Through the Eyes of a Nurse—The Second
Trimester; Through the Eyes of a Nurse—The
Third Trimester*

COMPANION WEBSITE

Additional NCLEX Review
Case Study: *First Trimester Client*
Care Plan Activity: *Common Discomforts of Pregnancy*
Applications: *Teaching Resources for Pregnant
Couples; Exercise During Pregnancy; Smoking
Cessation Plan; Fetal Alcohol Syndrome*
Critical Thinking

IMAGE LIBRARY

Figure 16.1 The Empathy Belly is a pregnancy simulator that allows males and females to experience some of the symptoms of pregnancy.

Figure 16.2 The culturally competent nurse respects the culture and values of the pregnant woman.

Figure 16.3 Acupressure wristbands are sometimes used to help relieve nausea during early pregnancy.

Figure 16.4 Swelling and discomfort from varicosities can be decreased by lying down with the legs and one hip elevated (to avoid compression of the vena cava).

Figure 16.5 When picking up objects from floor level or lifting objects, the pregnant woman must use proper body mechanics.

Figure 16.6 The expectant father can help relieve the woman's painful leg cramps by flexing her foot and straightening her leg.

Figure 16.7 An adaptation of the Cardiff Count-to-Ten scoring card for fetal movement assessment.

Figure 16.8 *A,* When not stimulated, normal and inverted nipples often look alike. *B,* When stimulated, the normal nipple protrudes. *C,* When stimulated, the inverted nipple retracts.

Figure 16.9 This breast shield is designed to increase the protractility of inverted nipples.

Figure 16.10 Position for relaxation and rest as pregnancy progresses.

Figure 16.11 *A,* Starting position when the pelvic tilt is done on hands and knees. *B,* A prenatal yoga instructor offers pointers for proper positioning for the first part of the tilt. *C,* The instructor helps the woman assume the correct position for the next part of the tilt. *D,* Proper posture.

Figure 16.12 The pregnant woman can strengthen her abdominal muscles by doing partial sit-ups.

Figure 16.13 Kegel exercises.

Figure 16.14 For many older couples, the decision to have a child may be a very rewarding one.

Learning Objective 1

Describe the significance of using the nursing process to promote health in the woman and her family during pregnancy.

Concepts for Lecture

1. Because of the time intervals between prenatal visits, it is essential that a written care plan be in place to ensure continuity of care. For women with low-risk pregnancies, there are expected nursing diagnoses that will be made more frequently than others.

PowerPoint Lecture Slides

(NOTE: The number on each PPT Lecture Slide directly corresponds with the Concepts for Lecture.)

 Nursing Process
- Assessment data every 4 to 6 weeks
- Ensure continuity of care
- Expected nursing diagnoses, goals, and interventions

LEARNING OBJECTIVE 2

Describe actions the nurse can take to help maintain the well-being of the expectant father and siblings during a family's pregnancy.

CONCEPTS FOR LECTURE

1. The primary nursing interventions in the prenatal period are providing support and prenatal education. The goals are that family members will have greater problem-solving ability, self-esteem, self-confidence, and ability to participate in health care.

2. The role of the father in the mother's life must be assessed and if he is part of her support system, the nurse must provide anticipatory guidance to him. The nurse should provide information about the changes of pregnancy and in the postpartum period, the effect of pregnancy on sexuality, and feelings he might experience. The nurse must also address the father's intention to participate during labor and birth and his knowledge of what to expect. Involving the siblings in antepartal visits is also helpful to make the pregnancy more real to them. An emphasis on open communication between parents and children should be made in order to make children feel less neglected and more secure.

POWERPOINT LECTURE SLIDES

(NOTE: The number on each PPT Lecture Slide directly corresponds with the Concepts for Lecture.)

1 Goals for Family Management
- Improvement in
  - Problem-solving ability
  - Self-esteem
  - Self-confidence
  - Ability to participate in health care

2 Nurse-Family Interventions
- Father
  - Assess role
  - Anticipatory guidance
  - Provide information about pregnancy changes
  - Guidance about couple's sexuality during pregnancy

2a Nurse-Family Interventions
- Siblings
  - Encourage involvement in pregnancy
  - Emphasize open parent-child communication

LEARNING OBJECTIVE 3

Discuss the significance of cultural considerations in managing nursing care during pregnancy.

CONCEPTS FOR LECTURE

1. The healthcare assessment should include a cultural assessment to determine the specific needs of the client. A transcultural nursing diagnosis can be formulated to meet these needs. Recognizing the impact of culture and life experience on the childbearing family is the foundation of culturally competent care.

POWERPOINT LECTURE SLIDES

(NOTE: The number on each PPT Lecture Slide directly corresponds with the Concepts for Lecture.)

1 Cultural Considerations
- Cultural assessment
  - Adapt to client needs
- Using nursing process
  - Transcultural nursing diagnosis
- Cultural competence
  - Recognition of influence of culture and life experiences

LEARNING OBJECTIVE 4

Explain the causes of the common discomforts of pregnancy.

CONCEPTS FOR LECTURE

1. Discomforts of the first trimester include nausea and vomiting, urinary frequency, fatigue, breast sensitivity, leukorrhea, nasal stuffiness and discharge, nosebleeds and pytalism. Nausea and vomiting may be due to a rise in human chorionic gonadotropin (hCG) and estrogen levels, carbohydrate metabolism, fatigue, and emotional factors. Due to the pressure of the enlarging uterus on the bladder, urinary frequency will occur early in pregnancy and again during the third trimester. Fatigue often occurs in early pregnancy and is considered a presumptive sign of pregnancy. It may be due to increased levels of progesterone and awakening at night to urinate. Breast sensitivity is due to increased levels of estrogen and progesterone. Leukorrhea occurs as the result of hyperplasia of vaginal mucosa and increased production of mucus by the endocervical glands. The increased acidity of these secretions encourages the growth of *Candida albicans*, making the woman more susceptible to monilial vaginitis. Nasal stuffiness, nasal discharge, obstruction (rhinitis of pregnancy), or epistaxis (nosebleed) may also result.

2. Common discomforts in the second and third trimesters include heartburn, ankle edema, varicose veins, flatulence, hemorrhoids, constipation, backache, leg cramps, feeling faint, shortness of breath, sleep disturbances, and round ligament pain. Displacement of the stomach by the enlarging uterus, an increase in progesterone levels, and a decrease in gastrointestinal motility cause heartburn. An increase in the difficulty of venous return from the lower extremities may cause ankle edema in the last part of pregnancy. A weakening of the walls of the veins or faulty function valves may result in varicose veins. This is further aggravated by the weight of the gravid uterus on the pelvic veins. Decreased gastrointestinal motility, air swallowing, and pressure on the large intestine by the uterus results in flatulence. Hemorrhoids may develop due to pressure of the uterus on the veins and interference with venous circulation and straining accompanying constipation. General bowel sluggishness caused by increased progesterone and steroid metabolism, displacement of the intestines, and oral iron supplements predisposes the pregnant woman to constipation. Backache occurs primarily due to the increased curvature of the lumbosacral vertebrae that occurs as the uterus enlarges and becomes heavier and a softening and relaxation of pelvic joints due to

POWERPOINT LECTURE SLIDES

(NOTE: The number on each PPT Lecture Slide directly corresponds with the Concepts for Lecture.)

1 Common Discomforts: First Trimester
- Nausea and vomiting
- Urinary frequency
- Fatigue
- Breast sensistivity
- Leukorrhea
- Nasal stuffiness and discharge

1a Common Discomforts: First Trimester
- Nosebleeds
- Pytalism

2 Common Discomforts: Second and Third Trimesters
- Heartburn
- Ankle edema
- Varicose veins
- Flatulence
- Hemorrhoids
- Constipation

2a Common Discomforts: Second and Third Trimesters
- Backache
- Leg cramps
- Feeling faint
- Shortness of breath
- Sleep disturbances
- Round ligament pain

circulating steroid hormones. Pressure from the enlarged uterus on pelvic nerves or blood vessels leading to the legs may cause leg cramps. A combination of changes in blood volume and postural hypotension may cause faintness. As the uterus rises into the 1abdomen and causes pressure on the diaphragm, shortness of breath may occur. Women also have sleep disturbances due to discomfort at night related to the pregnancy. Round ligament pain is due to the stretching of these ligaments as the uterus rises up in the abdomen.

SUGGESTIONS FOR CLASSROOM ACTIVITIES

Have groups of students present a common discomfort of pregnancy to the class, including the causes and management of the discomfort.

LEARNING OBJECTIVE 5

Summarize appropriate measures to alleviate the common discomforts of pregnancy.

CONCEPTS FOR LECTURE

1. Nausea and vomiting may be alleviated by eating dry crackers before getting out of bed; getting out of bed slowly; eating small, frequent meals; avoiding spicy food; and drinking herbal tea. Napping may help to alleviate fatigue. Wearing a supportive bra may be helpful in alleviating breast tenderness. Daily bathing, wearing cotton underwear, and avoiding douching may help with the discomfort of increased vaginal discharge. Using a cool air vaporizer and normal saline spray may help with nasal stuffiness. To avoid heartburn, the pregnant woman should avoid fried and fatty foods; eat small, frequent meals; and maintain good posture. By avoiding prolonged sitting or standing, and keeping feet and legs elevated, ankle edema can be minimized. The risk of varicose veins can be minimized by getting regular exercise and avoiding prolonged sitting or standing. Avoidance of gas-forming foods and regular bowel habits can minimize flatulence. Hemorrhoids can be prevented by avoiding constipation. This is done by increasing fluids and roughage, daily exercise, and regular bowel habits. The discomfort of hemorrhoids can be minimized by gently self-reducing them. The discomfort of backache can be minimized by performing the pelvic tilt exercise, maintaining good posture, avoiding fatigue, and using good body mechanics when lifting. Massage, warm soaks, and stretching exercises can help with the leg cramps that occur in pregnancy. If a pregnant woman becomes faint, she should sit down and lower her head between her knees. She can avoid this by not standing in one place too long. Shortness of breath can be minimized by utilizing good posture when sitting and propping herself up in bed. Avoiding caffeine and maximizing comfort in bed can help with sleep difficulties.

POWERPOINT LECTURE SLIDES

(NOTE: The number on each PPT Lecture Slide directly corresponds with the Concepts for Lecture.)

1 Alleviating Discomforts
- Urinary frequency
  - Safety considerations at home
- Fatigue
  - Napping
- Breast tenderness
  - Wear supportive bra

1a Alleviating Discomforts
- Increased vaginal discharge
  - Daily bathing, cotton underwear, avoid douching
- Nasal stuffiness
  - Cool air vaporizers, normal saline nasal spray
- Heartburn
  - Avoid fried and fatty foods, eat small frequent meals, good posture

1b Alleviating Discomforts
- Ankle edema
  - Avoid prolonged sitting or standing, keep feet and legs elevated
- Varicose veins (Figure 16.4)
  - Regular exercise, avoid prolonged sitting or standing
- Flatulence
  - Avoid gas-forming foods, regular bowel habits

1c See Figure 16.4

1d Alleviating Common Discomforts
- Hemorrhoids
  - Avoid constipation, gently self-reduce hemorrhoid

- Constipation
  - Increase fluids and roughage, daily exercise, regular bowel habits
- Backache
  - Pelvic tilt exercise, good posture, avoid fatigue, good body mechanics when lifting

1e Alleviating Common Discomforts
- Leg cramps (Figure 16.6)
  - Massage, warm soaks, stretching exercises
- Faintness
  - Sit down and lower head between knees, avoid standing in one place too long

1f See Figure 16.6

1g Alleviating Discomforts
- Shortness of breath
  - Good posture when sitting, prop up in bed
- Difficulty sleeping
  - Avoid caffeine, maximize comfort in bed

SUGGESTIONS FOR CLINICAL ACTIVITIES

Have students teach a prenatal class in a clinic about management of the discomforts of pregnancy.

LEARNING OBJECTIVE 6

Delineate self-care actions a pregnant woman and her family can take to maintain and promote well-being during each trimester of pregnancy.

CONCEPTS FOR LECTURE

1. A woman can care for her breasts by providing proper support to promote comfort, retain breast shape, and prevent back strain. Soap should be avoided on the nipples to avoid the drying effect; however, cleanliness is important. Nipple preparation by nipple rolling distributes natural lubricants produced by Montgomery tubercles and prevents soreness during breastfeeding. Women should wear loose, nonconstricting clothing during pregnancy and those with large, pendulous abdomens may also benefit from a well-fitting supportive girdle to avoid backache. Pregnant women should also avoid high-heeled shoes as they may aggravate back discomfort by increasing the curvature of the spine. Increased perspiration and mucoid vaginal discharge necessitates daily bathing during pregnancy. Caution should be used during tub baths because of changes in balance as pregnancy progresses. If vaginal bleeding is present or the membranes are ruptured, tub baths should be avoided to prevent infection. Women can continue to work until they go into labor; however, women who engage in strenuous physical activity during pregnancy have an increased risk for having a baby with low birth weight. Women should be aware of any potential environmental hazards that may put the pregnancy at risk. Travel is not restricted in uncomplicated

POWERPOINT LECTURE SLIDES

(NOTE: The number on each PPT Lecture Slide directly corresponds with the Concepts for Lecture.)

1 Self-Care During Pregnancy
- Breast care
  - Supportive bra
  - Cleanliness
  - No soap on nipples
  - Nipple preparation (Figure 16.8A–C)
- Clothing
  - Loose and nonconstricting

1a See Figure 16.8A–C

1b Self-Care During Pregnancy
- Cleanliness
  - Daily bathing
  - Tub baths contraindicated with vaginal bleeding or ruptured membranes
  - Hyperthermia contraindicated in first trimester

1c Self-Care During Pregnancy
- Employment
  - Can work until labor starts
  - May be at risk for preterm birth or low birth weight with certain jobs
  - Must be aware of environmental hazards

pregnancies; however, they should take frequent opportunities to ambulate and wear a seat belt when riding in a car. Drinking plenty of fluids and avoiding caffeinated beverages will help them avoid dehydration. Exercise is encouraged during pregnancy to maintain maternal fitness and muscle tone. It also leads to improved self-image, an increase in energy, improved sleep, reduced tension; controls weight gain; promotes regular bowel function; and is associated with improved postpartum recovery. The pelvic tilt can help prevent or reduce back strain and strengthen muscle tone. Kegel exercises help strengthen perineal muscle tone. A cross-legged sitting position helps to stretch the muscles of the inner thighs in preparation for labor and birth.

- Travel
  - No restrictions unless complications

 Self-Care During Pregnancy
- Frequent breaks during car travel
- Use seat belt
- Flying safe up to 36 weeks
- Drink plenty of fluid
- Avoid caffeinated beverages
- Wear support hose while flying

 Benefits of Exercise
- Improved self-image
- Increases energy
- Improves sleep
- Relieves tension
- Helps control weight gain
- Promotes regular bowel function

 Pregnancy Exercises
- Pelvic tilt (Figure 16.11C)
- Abdominal exercise
- Kegel exercise (Figure 16.13)
- "Tailor-sit" stretch

 See Figure 16.11C

 See Figure 16.13

SUGGESTIONS FOR CLASSROOM ACTIVITIES	**SUGGESTIONS FOR CLINICAL ACTIVITIES**
Have students practice the different pregnancy exercises in class. Discuss the benefits of these exercises.	Have students teach a group of pregnant women in a clinic self-care measures during pregnancy.

LEARNING OBJECTIVE 7

Identify some of the concerns that an expectant couple may have about sexual activity.

CONCEPTS FOR LECTURE

1. Changes in sexual desire by the woman during pregnancy are related to the discomforts of pregnancy. As the discomforts lesssen in the second trimester and vascular congestion increases, the woman may experience greater sexual satisfaction. Sexual desire may decrease again in the third trimester as the discomforts and fatigue increase. Reduced mobility may also interfere with sexual activity. Couples could consider alternative coital positions and other methods of showing affection.

2. Changes in the sexual desires of men also occur during pregnancy. Factors that affect the man may include the previous relationship with the partner, acceptance of the pregnancy, attitudes toward the partner's change of appearance, and concern about hurting the expectant mother or baby. Withdrawal from sexual contact may occur because of a belief that sex with a

POWERPOINT LECTURE SLIDES

(NOTE: The number on each PPT Lecture Slide directly corresponds with the Concepts for Lecture.)

 Concerns About Sexual Activity
- Related to discomforts
  - First trimester—fatigue, nausea, and vomiting
  - Second trimester—fewer discomforts, vascular congestion
  - Third trimester—fatigue, shortness of breath, decreased mobility

 Father's Feelings About Sex
- Affected by
  - Previous relationship with the partner
  - Acceptance of the pregnancy
  - Attitudes toward the partner's change of appearance
  - Concern about hurting the expectant mother or baby

pregnant woman is immoral, particularly if the purpose of sex is viewed from the religious perspective of procreation. Role conflicts may exist as some men find it difficult to find their partner sexually appealing while adjusting to the concept of her role as a mother. The opposite may also be true, with an increase in arousal by the man because of the pregnancy.

LEARNING OBJECTIVE 8

Describe factors that have contributed to the increased incidence of pregnancy in women over age 35.

CONCEPTS FOR LECTURE

1. Factors that have contributed to the increase in pregnancies over age 35 include the availability of effective birth control methods; the expanded roles and career options available for women; the increased number of women obtaining advanced education; pursuing careers, and delaying parenthood until they are established professionally; the increased incidence of later marriage and second marriage; the high cost of living, which causes some young couples to delay childbearing until they are more secure financially; the increased number of women in this older reproductive age group because of the baby boom between 1946 and 1964; and the increased availability of specialized fertilization procedures, which offers opportunities for women who had previously been considered infertile

POWERPOINT LECTURE SLIDES

(NOTE: The number on each PPT Lecture Slide directly corresponds with the Concepts for Lecture.)

1. Factors Contributing to Pregnancies over 35
   - The availability of effective birth control methods
   - The career options available for women
   - The increased number of women
     - Obtaining advanced education
     - Pursuing careers
     - Delaying parenthood
   - The increased incidence of later marriage and second marriage
   - The high cost of living
   - The increased number of women in this older reproductive age group
   - The increased availability of specialized fertilization procedures

SUGGESTIONS FOR CLINICAL ACTIVITIES

Have students interview new mothers over the age of 35 about their pregnancy and parenting experience. Ask the students to share their findings in postconference.

LEARNING OBJECTIVE 9

Compare similarities and differences in the needs of expectant women in various age groups.

CONCEPTS FOR LECTURE

1. Advantages to having a first baby over the age of 35 are that these women tend to be well-educated, more financially secure; are more aware of the realities of having a child; have experienced fulfillment in their careers; feel secure enough to take on the added responsibility of a child; are ready to make a change in their lives; may desire to stay home with the baby; and are able to afford good child care.
2. There are significant risks for the mother over the age of 35. The mother is at increased risk for death, are more likely to have chronic medical conditions, and have a higher risk of having an infant with low birth weight. There is an increased risk of miscarriage and

POWERPOINT LECTURE SLIDES

(NOTE: The number on each PPT Lecture Slide directly corresponds with the Concepts for Lecture.)

1. Advantages of Older Mothers
   - Tend to be well educated and financially secure
   - More aware of the realities of having a child
   - Feel secure about taking on the added responsibility of a child
   - May be ready to stay home with a new baby
   - Can afford good child care

2. Risks for Older Mothers
   - More likely to have chronic medical conditions
   - Increased incidence of low-birth-weight and preterm infants

an increased risk for gestational diabetes mellitus, hypertension, placenta previa, difficult labor, newborn complications, cesarean birth rate, and an infant with Down syndrome.

- Increased rate of miscarriage
- Increased risk for cesarean delivery
- Increased risk for infant with Down syndrome

 Risks for Older Mothers
- Increased risk for
  - Gestational diabetes mellitus
  - Hypertension
  - Placenta previa
  - Difficult labor
  - Newborn complications

SUGGESTIONS FOR CLASSROOM ACTIVITIES

Have student interview pregnant women over the age of 35 about their readiness for pregnancy/motherhood and discuss their findings.

SUGGESTIONS FOR CLINICAL ACTIVITIES

Have students review the charts of mothers over the age of 35 for risk factors in pregnancy and labor and delivery.

CHAPTER 17
ADOLESCENT PREGNANCY

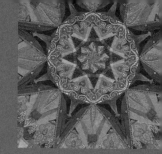

RESOURCE LIBRARY

PRENTICE HALL NURSING MEDIALINK DVD-ROM

Audio Glossary
NCLEX Review

COMPANION WEBSITE

Additional NCLEX Review
Case Study: *Late Detection of Adolescent Pregnancy*
Care Plan Activity: *Adolescent's Response to Pregnancy*
Applications: *Teen Pregnancy; Preeclampsia in an Adolescent Client*
Critical Thinking

IMAGE LIBRARY

Figure 17.1 Birth rates for teenagers by age: United States, 1990–2004.
Figure 17.2 The nurse gives a young mother an opportunity to listen to her baby's heartbeat.

Figure 17.3 Young adolescents may benefit from prenatal classes designed specifically for them.

LEARNING OBJECTIVE 1

Briefly discuss the physical and psychosocial changes of adolescence.

CONCEPTS FOR LECTURE

1. Physical changes in adolescence include a growth spurt, weight change, and the appearance of secondary sex characteristics. Psychosocial changes include the following developmental tasks: developing an identity, gaining autonomy and independence, developing intimacy in a relationship, developing comfort with one's own sexuality, and developing a sense of achievement.

POWERPOINT LECTURE SLIDES

(NOTE: The number on each PPT Lecture Slide directly corresponds with the Concepts for Lecture.)

 1 Physical Changes During Adolescence
  • Growth spurt
  • Weight change
  • Appearance of secondary sexual characteristics

1a Psychosocial Tasks of Adolescence
  • Developing an identity
  • Gaining autonomy and independence
  • Developing intimacy in a relationship
  • Developing comfort with one's own sexuality
  • Developing a sense of achievement

SUGGESTIONS FOR CLASSROOM ACTIVITIES

Discuss the developmental tasks of adolescence and their significance in relationship to sexual activity and risk-taking behaviors.

SUGGESTIONS FOR CLINICAL ACTIVITIES

Have students interview adolescents in the clinical setting and identify the developmental stages that they are in.

LEARNING OBJECTIVE 2

Compare the three stages of adolescence: early adolescence, middle adolescence, and late adolescence.

CONCEPTS FOR LECTURE

1. Early adolescence (age 14 and under) is a period of time during which there are rapid physical and psychosocial changes. The self-centered early adolescent initiates the struggle for independence, seeing authority as resting with the parent. Their perceived locus of control is external. They begin to leave the family by spending more time with their friends and conforming to their peer group in behavior and dress. They may also lack impulse control, resulting in risk-taking behaviors. They have a rich fantasy life, are very egocentric, are concrete thinkers, and have only a minimal ability to see themselves in the future or foresee the consequences of their behavior.

2. The period of middle adolescence is between ages 15 to 17. These adolescents challenge authority, experiment with drugs, alcohol, and sex. They seek independence by conforming to their peer group. They want to be treated as adults; however, fear of adult responsibility may cause a fluctuation in behavior. They are beginning to move from concrete thinking to formal operational thought but still can't anticipate long-term consequences.

3. Late adolescence is the period between ages 18 and 19. During this time, a young woman is more at ease with her individuality and decision-making ability. She now has the ability to think abstractly and can anticipate the consequences of her actions. She is more confident with her identity. She is capable of formal operational thought and is learning how to solve problems, conceptualize, and make decisions.

POWERPOINT LECTURE SLIDES

(NOTE: The number on each PPT Lecture Slide directly corresponds with the Concepts for Lecture.)

1 Early Adolescence (14 and under)
- Parents have authority
- Perceived external locus of control
- Spends more time with friends
- Conforms to peer group in behavior and dress
- May lack impulse control
- Has rich fantasy life

1a Early Adolescence (14 and under)
- Very egocentric
- Concrete thinker

2a Middle Adolescence (15–17 years)
- Challenges authority
- Experiments with drugs, alcohol, and sex
- Seeks independence by turning to peer group
- Wants to be treated as an adult
- Beginning to move from concrete thinking to formal operational thought
- Not yet able to anticipate the long-term implications of actions

3 Late Adolescence (18–19 years)
- More at ease with individuality and decision-making ability
- Can think abstractly and anticipate consequences
- Capable of formal operational thought
- Sees self as having control
- Understands and accepts the consequences of behaviors

SUGGESTIONS FOR CLASSROOM ACTIVITIES

Break students into three groups. Assign an early, middle, or late adolescent pregnancy case study to each of the groups, and ask students to discuss nursing interventions that may be appropriate for that adolescent.

SUGGESTIONS FOR CLINICAL ACTIVITIES

Have students that are working with pregnant adolescents or those that have just delivered identify the stage of adolescence that they are in and how that affects their pregnancy and/or transition to motherhood.

LEARNING OBJECTIVE 3

Summarize the developmental tasks of adolescence and the impact that pregnancy superimposes on these tasks.

CONCEPTS FOR LECTURE

1. The development of an identity is an important task in adolescence and one that is at risk if an adolescent becomes pregnant, particularly if the adolescent feels she cannot live up to her parents' expectations or she is in a dysfunctional family. Because of this, she may become rebellious and actively involved in risk-taking behaviors. Gaining independence is another important

POWERPOINT LECTURE SLIDES

(NOTE: The number on each PPT Lecture Slide directly corresponds with the Concepts for Lecture.)

1 Impact of Pregnancy on Developmental Tasks
- Developing an identity
  - Cannot live up to parents' expectations
  - Negative identity

developmental task in adolescence. If peers are involved in antisocial behavior, this will influence her behavior and all other developmental tasks. Sexual activity may be an expression of the adolescent's need for emotional intimacy. Early sexual involvement may not lead to comfort with individual sexuality and may result from peer pressure, pressure from an older male partner, rebellion against parents, and sexual abuse and its consequences. A sense of achievement is also essential to adolescents, and pregnancy may put an adolescent at risk because she may drop out of school prematurely and/or suffer economic stressors related to the pregnancy.

- Gaining autonomy and independence
  - Peer pressure to engage in antisocial behavior
- [1a] Impact of Pregnancy on Developmental Tasks
  - Developing intimacy in a relationship
    - Sexual activity may be an attempt to develop intimacy
  - Developing comfort with one's own sexuality
    - Engaging in sexual activity for wrong reasons
  - Developing a sense of achievement
    - Poor school performance

SUGGESTIONS FOR CLASSROOM ACTIVITIES

Have students list factors that may play a role in the completion of the developmental tasks and potential nursing interventions for assisting the pregnant adolescent client.

SUGGESTIONS FOR CLINICAL ACTIVITIES

Ask students who are working with pregnant adolescents to identify factors in the client's history that have played a role in the completion of developmental tasks.

LEARNING OBJECTIVE 4

Describe the major factors that contribute to teenage pregnancy.

CONCEPTS FOR LECTURE

1. Contributing factors to adolescent pregnancy include peer pressure to engage in sexual activity, lack of knowledge about sexuality and contraception, emotional factors, and socioeconomic factors. Emotional factors may include meeting relationship needs or age-related goals. Pregnancy may be seen as an escape from an undesirable home situation. The lack of future goals such as college or a career may contribute to adolescent pregnancy. Pregnancy also occurs more frequently in adolescents who are poor or near poor. The younger the adolescent is when she gets pregnant, the more likely she will get pregnant again. There is also an increase in the likelihood of repeat pregnancies if she lives with her sexual partner or she drops out of school. Their siblings are also at an increased risk.

POWERPOINT LECTURE SLIDES

(NOTE: The number on each PPT Lecture Slide directly corresponds with the Concepts for Lecture.)

- [1] Contributing Factors to Adolescent Pregnancy (Figure 17.1)
  - Peer pressure to engage in sexual activity
  - Lack of knowledge about sexuality and contraception
  - Emotional factors
  - Socioeconomic factors
- [1a] See Figure 17.1

SUGGESTIONS FOR CLASSROOM ACTIVITIES

Ask students to survey friends and family members about what they think causes teenage pregnancy. Have them share their findings in class, and then discuss the implications for these perceptions in devising community-based prevention strategies.

SUGGESTIONS FOR CLINICAL ACTIVITIES

Have students that are caring for pregnant adolescents interview the client to assess potential contributing factors to that pregnancy. Have the students share their findings in postconference.

LEARNING OBJECTIVE 5

Identify the impact of cultural factors on the desirability of early pregnancy.

CONCEPTS FOR LECTURE

1. Early pregnancy is desirable in some cultures. For example, in a country where Islam is the predominant religion, where large families are desired, where social change is slow in coming, and where most childbearing occurs within marriage, early pregnancy is valued.

POWERPOINT LECTURE SLIDES

(NOTE: The number on each PPT Lecture Slide directly corresponds with the Concepts for Lecture.)

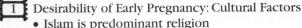 Desirability of Early Pregnancy: Cultural Factors
- Islam is predominant religion
- Large families are desired
- Social change is slow in coming
- Most childbearing occurs within marriage

SUGGESTIONS FOR CLASSROOM ACTIVITIES

Have a group discussion in class about student observations of planned early pregnancies in their communities and discuss the characteristics of those families.

LEARNING OBJECTIVE 6

Identify the physical, psychological, and sociologic risks faced by an adolescent who is pregnant.

CONCEPTS FOR LECTURE

1. Pregnant adolescents over the age of 15 have no additional risks if they receive early prenatal care; however, many do not seek early prenatal care, and those who do may not be compliant. These teens are more likely to smoke than older women and are less likely to gain sufficient weight. This poses the following risks for these women: preterm births, low-birth-weight (LBW) infants, preeclampsia-eclampsia and its sequelae, iron deficiency anemia, and cephalopelvic disproportion (CPD). These women also have a higher incidence of sexually transmitted infections, including the herpes virus, chlamydia, syphilis, and gonorrhea. Additionally, many of these women have problems with drug and alcohol use.

2. The primary psychological risk to the adolescent is the interruption of progress in the developmental tasks. Additionally, the adolescent must incorporate the tasks of pregnancy, which itself creates significant psychological hurdles to overcome. Additional risks for the adolescent mother include social and economic disadvantages when compared with a nonpregnant adolescent. She may have to take on adult roles before completing the developmental tasks of adolescence, which may result in a prolonged dependence on parents, lack of stable relationships with the opposite sex, and lack of economic and social stability.

POWERPOINT LECTURE SLIDES

(NOTE: The number on each PPT Lecture Slide directly corresponds with the Concepts for Lecture.)

1 Physiologic Risks
- Preterm births and LBW infants
- Preeclampsia-eclampsia
- Iron deficiency anemia
- Cephalopelvic disproportion (CPD)
- Effects of alcohol and drug use
- Sexually transmitted infections

2 Psychological Risks
- Interruption of progress in developmental tasks
- Prolonged dependence on parents
- Lack of stable relationships with the opposite sex
- Lack of economic and social stability

SUGGESTIONS FOR CLASSROOM ACTIVITIES

Have students develop a tool to assess an adolescent pregnancy for potential risk factors.

SUGGESTIONS FOR CLINICAL ACTIVITIES

Ask students to do a history and physical exam on a pregnant adolescent in the clinical setting and to identify risk factors.

LEARNING OBJECTIVE 7

Discuss the reactions of the adolescent's family and social support groups to her pregnancy.

CONCEPTS FOR LECTURE

1. The reaction to pregnancy by families who foster educational and career goals for their children may include shock, anger, shame, and sorrow. Peer relationships may change as well. Family and friends may be more supportive of adolescent parents in populations where adolescent pregnancy is more prevalent and socially acceptable. Friends and family may be involved in the adolescent mother's labor and delivery experience. These couples may have friends that are already adolescent parents. Pregnancy and the birth of a baby may be seen as a sign of adult status and increased sexual prowess by male partners of these young women.

POWERPOINT LECTURE SLIDES

(NOTE: The number on each PPT Lecture Slide directly corresponds with the Concepts for Lecture.)

1 Reactions of Family and Support Groups
- Families fostering educational and career goals
  - Shock
  - Anger
  - Shame
  - Sorrow

1a Reactions of Family and Support Groups
- Families where adolescent pregnancy is more socially acceptable
  - Supportive
  - Involved
  - May have friends who are teen parents
  - Father of baby—adult status, sense of pride

SUGGESTIONS FOR CLINICAL ACTIVITIES

Ask students to observe the family dynamics of families of pregnant adolescents in the clinical setting and to record their observations to share in post-conference.

LEARNING OBJECTIVE 8

Formulate a plan of care to meet the needs of a pregnant adolescent.

CONCEPTS FOR LECTURE

1. A nursing assessment should include a history of family health and personal physical health, developmental level and impact of pregnancy, and emotional and financial support. The assessment should also include the family and social support network and the father's degree of involvement in the pregnancy. While nursing diagnoses that are applicable to all pregnant women will also apply to the pregnant adolescent, there are additional nursing diagnoses that address her particular needs. The following are examples of these nursing diagnoses:
   - *Imbalanced Nutrition: Less than Body Requirements* related to poor eating habits
   - *Risk,* Early
   - *Risk for Situational Low Self-Esteem*

   Nursing interventions should include counseling and client teaching. Essential to this is safeguarding the client's confidentiality, winning her trust, and helping her build her self-esteem. The focus of this counseling and teaching should be on weight gain, nutrition counseling, assessing for high-risk conditions, testing for STIs and education about prevention, and education about substance use. Family adaptation should also be promoted by the nurse, and prenatal education should be facilitated.

POWERPOINT LECTURE SLIDES

(NOTE: The number on each PPT Lecture Slide directly corresponds with the Concepts for Lecture.)

1 Nursing Plan of Care
- Assessment
  - History of family and personal physical health
  - Developmental level and impact of pregnancy
  - Emotional and financial support
  - Family and social support network
  - Father's degree of involvement

1a Nursing Plan of Care
- Nursing Diagnoses
  - *Imbalanced Nutrition: Less than Body Requirements* related to poor eating habits
  - *Risk*, Early
  - *Risk for Situational Low Self-Esteem* related to unanticipated pregnancy

1b Nursing Interventions: Prenatal (Figure 17.2)
- Nutrition assessment and counseling
- Assessment for high-risk conditions
- Testing for and educating about prevention of STIs

2. During labor, the adolescent has the same needs as any pregnant woman; however, continuous presence of support is even more important for this woman. The nurse should answer any questions honestly and simply, and provide education to help the decision-making process. Additionally, the nurse should help the support people understand their roles in labor and birth.

3. It is vital for the nurse to help the teen mother understand the risk of becoming pregnant again in the postpartum period. Education about contraception is a primary nursing intervention at this time. The nurse should also make the adolescent mother aware of community resources available to assist her and her family. The nurse should also provide education about parenting and parenting skills.

- Education about substance use
- Promote family adaptation
- Facilitate prenatal education (Figure 17.3)

1c See Figure 17.2

1d See Figure 17.3

2 Nursing Interventions: Labor
- Sustained presence
- Education about choices
- Help support people understand role

3 Nursing Interventions: Postpartum
- Contraception education
- Availability of community resources
- Parenting

SUGGESTIONS FOR CLASSROOM ACTIVITIES

Have students develop a care plan for a pregnant adolescent and share those care plans in class.

SUGGESTIONS FOR CLINICAL ACTIVITIES

Have students who are caring for an adolescent in labor develop a care plan and document their evaluation of the outcomes.

LEARNING OBJECTIVE 9

Describe successful community approaches to adolescent pregnancy prevention.

CONCEPTS FOR LECTURE

1. When teens are given comprehensive information about sexual activity, the rates of sexually transmitted infections and pregnancy are decreased. A strong community-wide approach directed at multiple causes of the problem is the best approach. Access to contraceptive services is also important. Additionally, youth development programs that are aimed at cultivating individual talent and increasing self-worth can reduce sexual behaviors and unintended pregnancy. Programs should involve adolescents in planning, be long term and intensive, include role models from the same cultural and racial backgrounds, and focus on the adolescent male as well as the female.

POWERPOINT LECTURE SLIDES

(NOTE: The number on each PPT Lecture Slide directly corresponds with the Concepts for Lecture.)

1 Effective Community-Based Pregnancy Prevention
- Accurate, balanced, and realistic sexuality education
- Youth development programs that build on the assets and strengths of young people
- Confidential and low-cost access to contraceptive services
- Long term and intensive
- Involve adolescents in program planning

1a Effective Community-Based Pregnancy Prevention
- Include good role models from the same cultural and racial backgrounds
- Focus on the adolescent male as well as the female

SUGGESTIONS FOR CLASSROOM ACTIVITIES

Ask students to identify community resources available for pregnant adolescents and have them bring those resources to class to share with others.

SUGGESTIONS FOR CLINICAL ACTIVITIES

Have students interview a representative from an agency aimed at adolescent pregnancy prevention about the strategies they use and their outcomes.

CHAPTER 18
MATERNAL NUTRITION

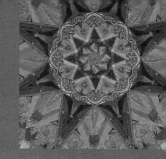

RESOURCE LIBRARY

 PRENTICE HALL NURSING MEDIALINK DVD-ROM

Audio Glossary
NCLEX Review
Video: *Through the Eyes of a Nurse—The First Trimester*

 COMPANION WEBSITE

Additional NCLEX Review
Case Study: *Maternal Weight Gain*
Care Plan Activity: *Maternal Nutritional Requirements*
Applications: *Nutritional Needs During Pregnancy; Pica*
Critical Thinking

 IMAGE LIBRARY

Figure 18.1 It is important to monitor a pregnant woman's weight over time.
Figure 18.2 MyPyramid: Steps to a Healthier You identifies the basic food groups and provides guidance about healthful eating.

Figure 18.3 The vegetarian food pyramid.
Figure 18.4 Cultural factors affect food preferences and habits.
Figure 18.5 Sample nutritional questionnaire used in nursing management of a pregnant woman.

LEARNING OBJECTIVE 1

Identify the role of specific nutrients in the diet of the pregnant woman.

CONCEPTS FOR LECTURE

1. Carbohydrates are essential for energy and bowel function. If carbohydrates are not available, protein is utilized for energy and then becomes unavailable for growth. Protein is essential during pregnancy for fetal development, blood volume expansion, and growth of maternal tissues. Fats are essential for energy and are more completely absorbed during pregnancy, which results in an increase in serum lipids, lipoproteins, and cholesterol, and a decreased elimination of fat through the bowel. Calcium and phosphorus play an important role in the mineralization of fetal bones and teeth, energy and cell production, and acid-base buffering. Calcium is also more efficiently used and absorbed during pregnancy. Iodine is also essential during pregnancy, and inorganic iodine is excreted in the urine during pregnancy. The thyroid gland may enlarge if there is not adequate dietary intake or supplement. Sodium is important for metabolism and regulation of fluid balance. Zinc is involved in protein metabolism and in the synthesis of deoxyribonucleic acid (DNA) and ribonucleic acid (RNA). It is also important for fetal growth and development and milk production. Magnesium is vital for cellular metabolism and structural growth. There is an increased need for iron during pregnancy because of growth demands by the fetus and the placenta and

POWERPOINT LECTURE SLIDES

(NOTE: The number on each PPT Lecture Slide directly corresponds with the Concepts for Lecture.)

1 Role of Nutrients
- Carbohydrates
  - Primary source of energy
  - Fiber
- Fats
  - Energy
  - More completely absorbed during pregnancy

1a Role of Nutrients
- Calcium and phosphorus
  - Mineralization of fetal bones and teeth
  - Energy and cell production
  - Acid-base buffering

1b Role of Nutrients
- Iodine
  - Essential for brain development
- Sodium
  - Metabolism
  - Regulation of fluid balance

1c Role of Nutrients
- Zinc
  - Protein metabolism
  - Synthesis of DNA and RNA

the expansion of maternal blood volume. Vitamin D is essential for the absorption and utilization of calcium and phosphorus for skeletal development. Vitamin E deficiency results in a long-term inability to absorb fats. Vitamin K plays a role in the production of prothrombin and is important for clotting. Vitamin C levels decline throughout pregnancy. Ascorbic acid concentrates in the placenta. It is important for the formation and development of connective tissue and the vascular system. B vitamins serve as important coenzyme factors in cell respiration, glucose oxidation, energy metabolism, and other reactions. The need for B vitamins increases during pregnancy.

- ○ Fetal growth
- ○ Lactation

 Role of Nutrients
- • Magnesium
  - ○ Cellular metabolism
  - ○ Structural growth
- • Iron
  - ○ Oxygen-carrying capability

 Role of Nutrients
- • Vitamin D
  - ○ Absorption and utilization of calcium and phosphorus
- • Vitamin E
  - ○ Fat absorption
- • Vitamin K
  - ○ Synthesis of prothrombin

Role of Nutrients
- • Vitamin C
  - ○ Development of connective tissue
  - ○ Development of vascular system
- • B vitamins
  - ○ Cell respiration and glucose oxidation
  - ○ Energy metabolism

SUGGESTIONS FOR CLASSROOM ACTIVITIES

Have students develop a dietary plan for a pregnant woman.

SUGGESTIONS FOR CLINICAL ACTIVITIES

Have students interview pregnant women about their current dietary intake and identify potential deficits.

LEARNING OBJECTIVE 2

Compare nutritional needs during pregnancy, postpartum, and lactation with nonpregnant requirements.

CONCEPTS FOR LECTURE

1. Needs that are unchanged during pregnancy include fat, vitamins A and K, iodine, and sodium. Caloric intake should be increased by 300 kcal/day. Protein should be increased to 1000 mg/day during pregnancy and lactation and 1300 mg/day if 18 years of age or less. Zinc should be increased to 11 mg/day during pregnancy and 12 mg/day during lactation. Magnesium should be increased to 320 mg/day during pregnancy and lactation. Iron and vitamin E, 15 mg/day; needs during pregnancy are increased to 27 mg/day. Vitamin D should be increased 5 mcg/day; vitamin C, 85 mg/day; thiamine, 1/4 mg/day; niacin, 18 mg/day; vitamin B_6, 1.9 mg/day; and vitamin B_{12}, 2.6 mcg/day.

POWERPOINT LECTURE SLIDES

(NOTE: The number on each PPT Lecture Slide directly corresponds with the Concepts for Lecture.)

 Changes in Nutritional Needs
- • No change
  - ○ Fat
  - ○ Vitamin A
  - ○ Vitamin K
  - ○ Iodine
  - ○ Sodium

Changes in Nutritional Needs
- • Increased needs:
  - ○ Calories
  - ○ Carbohydrates
  - ○ Protein
  - ○ Calcium
  - ○ Zinc
  - ○ Magnesium

1b Nutritional Needs During Pregnancy
- Iron—27 mg/day
- Vitamin D—5 mcg/ day
- Vitamin E—15 mg/day
- Vitamin C—85 mg/day
- Thiamine—1.4 mg/day
- Riboflavin—1.4 mg/day

1c Nutritional Needs During Pregnancy
- Niacin—18 mg/day
- Vitamin B$_6$—1.9
- Vitamin B$_{12}$—2.6 μg/day

SUGGESTIONS FOR CLASSROOM ACTIVITIES	SUGGESTIONS FOR CLINICAL ACTIVITIES
Have students identify foods that can help meet the nutritional needs of pregnancy.	Ask students to teach a prenatal class on maternal nutrition in pregnancy.

LEARNING OBJECTIVE 3

Discuss effects of maternal nutrition on fetal outcomes.

CONCEPTS FOR LECTURE

1. The nutritional status of the mother affects the fetus. Deficiencies can affect fetal cell and organ growth. Nutritional problems that interfere with cell division may have long-term consequences. Alternatively, if nutritional deficiencies occur when cells are enlarging, the changes are usually reversible.

POWERPOINT LECTURE SLIDES

(NOTE: The number on each PPT Lecture Slide directly corresponds with the Concepts for Lecture.)

1 Effects of Maternal Nutrition on Fetus
- Deficiencies can interfere with cell and organ growth
- If deficiencies occur during cell division—permanent consequences
- If deficiencies occur during cell enlargement—reversible

LEARNING OBJECTIVE 4

Evaluate adequacy and pattern of weight gain during different stages of pregnancy.

CONCEPTS FOR LECTURE

1. The optimal weight gain for a pregnant woman depends on the woman's weight for height body mass index (BMI) and her prepregnant nutritional state. Pattern of weight gain is also important. Inadequate weight gain during the second trimester results in low birth weight in the newborn. The recommended weight gain for normal weight women is 1.6 to 2.3 kg (3.5 to 5 lb) during the first trimester, followed by an average gain of 0.5 kg (1 lb) per week during the last two trimesters. The recommended weight gain in the second and third trimesters is slightly higher for underweight women and slightly lower for overweight women.

POWERPOINT LECTURE SLIDES

(NOTE: The number on each PPT Lecture Slide directly corresponds with the Concepts for Lecture.)

1 Weight Gain During Pregnancy
- Weight gain in terms of optimum ranges based on prepregnant body mass index (BMI)
- Pattern of weight gain
  - Normal weight—gain of 1.6 to 2.3 kg (3.5 to 5 lb) during the first trimester, followed by an average gain of 0.5 kg (1 lb) per week during the last two trimesters
  - Underweight—gain of 1.75 lb per week during the last two trimesters
  - Overweight—gain of 0.7 lb per week during the last two trimesters

LEARNING OBJECTIVE 5

Plan adequate prenatal vegetarian diets based on nutritional requirements of pregnancy.

CONCEPTS FOR LECTURE

1. A lacto-ovovegetarian pregnant woman can acquire adequate proteins from dairy products and eggs. The quality of plant protein may be improved if taken with these animal proteins. Calcium supplementation may be necessary if the diet contains fewer than four servings of milk and dairy products. Vegans have a slightly increased need for protein due to the exclusion of animal proteins. Consuming a varied diet with an adequate caloric intake and complementary amino acids can provide adequate dietary protein. Plant-based proteins such as beans and rice, peanut butter on whole grain bread, and whole grain cereal with soy milk can provide complete dietary proteins. Vegans often have difficulty taking in sufficient calories to achieve adequate weight gain because the diet tends to be higher in fiber and therefore more filling. Diets should be supplemented with energy-dense foods to help provide increased energy intake. Vegans require a daily supplement of 4 mg of vitamin B_{12} because of their lack of nutritional animal products; however, if soy milk is used, only partial supplementation may be required.

POWERPOINT LECTURE SLIDES

(NOTE: The number on each PPT Lecture Slide directly corresponds with the Concepts for Lecture.)

1 Vegetarian Diets
- Lacto-ovovegetarian—includes milk, dairy products, and eggs
- Lactovegetarian—includes dairy products but no eggs
- Vegetarian—consumes no animal products

1a Vegetarian Diets in Pregnancy
- Increase in protein needs because of the lower quality protein sources
  - Varied diet with adequate caloric intake and complementary amino acids
  - Complete proteins may be obtained by eating different types of plant-based proteins and whole-grain cereal with soy milk
- Difficulty obtaining sufficient calories because diet tends to be higher in fiber
  - Supplementation with energy-dense foods

1b Vegetarian Diets in Pregnancy
- Daily supplement of 4 mg of vitamin B_{12} is necessary
- Daily supplements of calcium and vitamin D are necessary
  - If soy milk is used, only partial supplementation may be needed

LEARNING OBJECTIVE 6

Describe ways in which various physical, psychosocial, and cultural factors can affect nutritional intake and status.

CONCEPTS FOR LECTURE

1. The cultural, ethnic, and, possibly, religious backgrounds of a woman can play a role in her food preferences and habits. Foods have a symbolic significance in culture that may be related to major life experiences or developmental milestones. Customs may differ among groups within the same region of the country, among families within that region, and among individuals within individual families. The sharing of food is

POWERPOINT LECTURE SLIDES

(NOTE: The number on each PPT Lecture Slide directly corresponds with the Concepts for Lecture.)

1 Food and Culture (Figure 18.4)
- Foods have symbolic significance
- Related to major life milestones
- Variations within cultural groups

often associated with friendliness, warmth, and social acceptance. Food is also part of caretaking that is reflected in the maternal role. Nutritional status may be reflective of the socioeconomic level. Families in poverty may be unable to afford quality food. Pregnant women with low incomes would then be at risk for nutritional deficits. Also, the attitudes and feelings of the expectant mother about the pregnancy may affect her nutritional status. As an example, food can be used as a substitute for expressing emotions.

- Symbol of friendliness, warmth, and social acceptance
- Taking care of the family

1a See Figure 18.4

1b Psychosocial Factors
- Socioeconomic factors may determine nutritional status
- Attitudes and feelings about pregnancy may influence diet
- May be used as a substitute for emotions

SUGGESTIONS FOR CLASSROOM ACTIVITIES

Ask students to share any cultural, religious, or family traditions that they have related to food.

LEARNING OBJECTIVE 7

Compare recommendations for weight gain and nutrient intakes in the pregnant adolescent with those for the mature pregnant adult.

CONCEPTS FOR LECTURE

1. Nutritional recommendations for pregnant adolescents are derived using the dietary reference intake (DRI) for nonpregnant adolescents and adding recommended nutrients for all pregnant women. For those adolescents who are mature (more than 4 years since menarche), the nutritional needs are closer to those of the pregnant adult. Adolescents who are pregnant less than 4 years after menarche are at risk because of their immaturity, and they are most likely growing.

2. Iron is of particular concern for pregnant adolescents because of the increasing maternal muscle mass and volume. Supplements of 30 to 60 mg are recommended. As inadequate intake of calcium is frequently a problem with adolescents, it is of particular concern in pregnancy because it is needed to support the normal growth and development of the fetus as well as the growth and maintenance of calcium stores in the adolescent. There has also been an association between inadequate calcium and maternal hypertension and preeclampsia. Adolescents also have irregular eating patterns. This should be considered in dietary counseling.

POWERPOINT LECTURE SLIDES

(NOTE: The number on each PPT Lecture Slide directly corresponds with the Concepts for Lecture.)

1 Adolescent Pregnancy Weight Gain
- Use dietary reference intakes (DRI) for nonpregnant teenagers
- Add nutrient amounts recommended for all pregnant women
- At risk because of their physiologic and anatomic immaturity
- Young adolescents need to gain more than older adolescents

2 Adolescent Dietary Issues
- Iron supplements are required
- Calcium supplements are required
- Irregular eating patterns must be assessed over time

LEARNING OBJECTIVE 8

Describe basic factors a nurse should consider when offering nutritional counseling to a pregnant adolescent.

CONCEPTS FOR LECTURE

1. When counseling a pregnant adolescent about nutrition, a positive approach is more effective than a negative one. Nutrient-dense foods should be suggested so that she can get them in many places and at any time. The individual within the family who does most of the meal preparation should also be included in dietary counseling if it is

POWERPOINT LECTURE SLIDES

(NOTE: The number on each PPT Lecture Slide directly corresponds with the Concepts for Lecture.)

1 Nutritional Counseling for the Adolescent
- Positive approach
- Suggest nutrient-rich foods

agreeable to the pregnant adolescent. Including the father of the baby may also be helpful. The message should be that good nutrition is important for her health and that of the family and should focus on the foods rather than the nutrients. Peer classes may also be helpful.

- Include other family members involved in meal preparation
- Involve expectant father
- Emphasize benefits to her and her baby
- Peer classes

SUGGESTIONS FOR CLASSROOM ACTIVITIES

Have students role play counseling a pregnant adolescent about nutrition. Have them give each other feedback on their counseling techniques.

SUGGESTIONS FOR CLINICAL ACTIVITIES

Have students teach a class of pregnant adolescents about nutrition.

LEARNING OBJECTIVE 9

Compare nutritional counseling issues for breastfeeding and formula-feeding mothers.

CONCEPTS FOR LECTURE

1. The nutritional requirements of a mother who feeds her baby formula returns to prepregnant levels after the birth. She should be advised to reduce her daily caloric intake by about 300 kcal.

2. The woman who is breastfeeding should increase her caloric intake by 200 kcal over pregnancy requirements as an inadequate intake can reduce milk volume. Milk quality, however, is unaffected by caloric intake. Adequate protein is essential in the maternal diet as it is an important component of breast milk. The recommended intake is 65 g per day during the first 6 months of breastfeeding and 62 g per day after that. Calcium is also an essential element in milk production. Requirements remain the same as during pregnancy. Adequate liquid intake is also essential as inadequate levels may decrease milk volume.

POWERPOINT LECTURE SLIDES

(NOTE: The number on each PPT Lecture Slide directly corresponds with the Concepts for Lecture.)

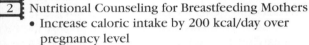 Nutritional Counseling for Formula-Feeding Mothers
- Dietary requirements return to prepregnancy levels
- Reduce caloric intake by 300 kcal/day

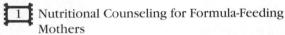 Nutritional Counseling for Breastfeeding Mothers
- Increase caloric intake by 200 kcal/day over pregnancy level
- Protein intake of 65 mg/day for first 6 months and then 62 mg/day thereafter
- Calcium intake of 1000 mg/day
- Adequate fluid intake

LEARNING OBJECTIVE 10

Formulate a nutritional care plan for pregnant women based on a diagnosis of nutritional problems.

CONCEPTS FOR LECTURE

1. The nursing diagnosis of a pregnant women may be ***Imbalanced Nutrition: Less than Body Requirements*** related to nausea and vomiting. In other women, the nursing diagnosis may be related to excessive weight gain. In these cases the diagnosis might be ***Imbalanced Nutrition: More than Body Requirements*** related to excessive calorie intake. Another nursing diagnosis may be ***Health-Seeking Behavior***, especially if the woman asks for information about nutrition.

POWERPOINT LECTURE SLIDES

(NOTE: The number on each PPT Lecture Slide directly corresponds with the Concepts for Lecture.)

1 Nursing Diagnoses
- ***Imbalanced Nutrition: Less than Body Requirements***, related to nausea and vomiting
- ***Imbalanced Nutrition: More than Body Requirements***, related to excessive calorie intake
- ***Health-Seeking Behavior***, if the woman asks for information about nutrition

SUGGESTIONS FOR CLASSROOM ACTIVITIES

Have students develop a care plan based on one of these nutritional nursing diagnoses.

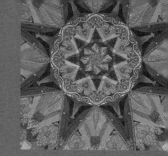

CHAPTER 19
PREGNANCY AT RISK: PREGESTATIONAL PROBLEMS

RESOURCE LIBRARY

 PRENTICE HALL NURSING MEDIALINK DVD-ROM

Audio Glossary
NCLEX Review

 COMPANION WEBSITE

Additional NCLEX Review
Case Study: *Client with Gestational Diabetes*
Care Plan Activity: *Antepartal Client at Risk*
Applications: *Gestational Diabetes; Iron Deficiency Anemia*
Critical Thinking

📖 IMAGE LIBRARY

Figure 19.1 Percentages of females ages 15 to 44 reporting past month use of any illicit drugs, by pregnancy status and age, 2003–2004.

Figure 19.2 Percentages of pregnant females ages 15 to 44 reporting past month alcohol use, by trimester, 2003–2004.

Figure 19.3 During labor the nurse closely monitors the blood glucose levels of the woman with diabetes mellitus.

Figure 19.4 The nurse teaches the pregnant woman with gestational diabetes mellitus how to do home glucose monitoring.

Figure 19.5 Health teaching is an important part of nursing care for the pregnant woman with sickle cell anemia.

Figure 19.6 When a woman with heart disease begins labor, the nursing students and instructor caring for her monitor her closely for signs of congestive heart failure.

Table 19.5 Less common medical conditions and pregnancy

LEARNING OBJECTIVE 1

Summarize the effects of alcohol and illicit drugs on the childbearing woman and her fetus/newborn.

CONCEPTS FOR LECTURE

1. Chronic alcohol abuse can have the following effects on pregnant women: malnutrition, bone marrow suppression, increased incidence of infections, and liver disease. The intrapartum woman may experience withdrawal seizures 12 to 48 hours after she stops drinking. The fetus and child of a mother who chronically abuses alcohol during pregnancy may be affected by Fetal Alcohol Spectrum disorders (FASD).

2. Cocaine use in pregnant women may result in: an increased incidence of spontaneous first trimester abortion, abruptio placentae, intrauterine growth restriction (IUGR), preterm birth, and stillbirth. Additionally, adverse effects may include seizures and hallucinations, pulmonary edema, respiratory failure, and cardiac problems. Neonatal complications include decreased birth weight and head circumference and feeding difficulties. Infants are exposed to cocaine via the breast milk and may experience extreme irritability, vomiting, diarrhea, dilated pupils, and apnea.

POWERPOINT LECTURE SLIDES

(NOTE: The number on each PPT Lecture Slide directly corresponds with the Concepts for Lecture.)

1 Alcohol Use in Pregnancy (Figure 19.2)
- Maternal effects
  - Malnutrition
  - Bone marrow suppression
  - Increased incidence of infections
  - Liver disease
- Neonatal effects
  - Fetal Alcohol Spectrum disorders (FASD)

1a See Figure 19.2

2 Cocaine Use in Pregnancy: Maternal Effects (Figure 19.1)
- Seizures and hallucinations
- Pulmonary edema
- Respiratory failure
- Cardiac problems

---

3. The effects of heroin on pregnant women include: an increased incidence of poor nutrition, iron deficiency anemia, preeclampsia-eclampsia, an increased rate of breech position, abnormal placental implantation, abruptio placentae, preterm labor, premature rupture of the membranes (PROM), and meconium staining. They are also at an increased risk of acquiring a sexually transmitted infection or HIV infection. Their fetuses are at risk for IUGR and withdrawal symptoms after birth.

4. The effect of marijuana use on a pregnant woman has been difficult to study; however, there has been no research that has demonstrated any teratogenic effects on the fetus. The risks of phencyclidine (PCP) for the pregnant woman include overdose or a psychotic response. The use of MDMA (methylenedioxymethamphetamine), better known as Ecstasy, has been associated with impairment of long-term memory and learning. Methadone is used to block withdrawal symptoms from heroin and the craving for street drugs, and it does cross the placenta. Studies have reported inconsistent effects on the newborn.

- Spontaneous first trimester abortion, abruptio placentae, intrauterine growth restriction (IUGR), preterm birth, and stillbirth

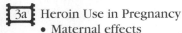 Cocaine Use in Pregnancy: Fetal Effects
- Decreased birth weight and head circumference
- Feeding difficulties
- Neonatal effects from breastmilk
  - Extreme irritability
  - Vomiting and diarrhea
  - Dilated pupils and apnea

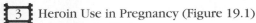 Heroin Use in Pregnancy (Figure 19.1)
- Maternal effects
  - Poor nutrition and iron deficiency anemia
  - Preeclampsia-eclampsia
  - Breech position
  - Abnormal placental implantation
  - Abruptio placentae
  - Preterm labor

3a Heroin Use in Pregnancy
- Maternal effects
  - Premature rupture of the membranes (PROM)
  - Meconium staining
  - Higher incidence of STIs and HIV
- Fetal effects
  - IUGR
  - Withdrawal symptoms after birth

4 Substance Use in Pregnancy: Maternal Effects (Figure 19.1)
- Marijuana—difficult to evaluate, no known teratogenic effects
- PCP—maternal overdose or a psychotic response
- MDMA (Ecstasy)—long-term impaired memory and learning

4a See Figure 19.1

SUGGESTIONS FOR CLASSROOM ACTIVITIES

Have students develop a teaching plan for a prenatal class on the risks of substance abuse to mothers and their infants.

SUGGESTIONS FOR CLINICAL ACTIVITIES

Have students do a physical and neurobehavioral exam on an infant who was exposed to drugs in utero. Ask them to identify those observations that are due to substance exposure.

LEARNING OBJECTIVE 2

Discuss the pathology, treatment, and nursing care of pregnant women with diabetes.

CONCEPTS FOR LECTURE

1. An inadequate production or utilization of insulin is the primary pathology involved in diabetes mellitus (DM). Fats and proteins are utilized as a source of energy as glucose is unavailable for this purpose. Wasting of fat and muscle tissue occurs due to protein breakdown,

POWERPOINT LECTURE SLIDES

(NOTE: The number on each PPT Lecture Slide directly corresponds with the Concepts for Lecture.)

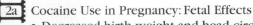 Pathology of Diabetes Mellitus (DM)
- Endocrine disorder of carbohydrate metabolism
- Results from inadequate production or utilization of insulin

and ketosis occurs because of fat metabolism. Cellular dehydration occurs as high levels of glucose in the blood pull water from the cells. Glucose eventually spills into the urine, and the high osmotic pressure of this glucose prevents reabsorption of water into the kidney tubules, which causes extracellular dehydration.

2. Gestational diabetes mellitus (GDM) has variable severity and occurs as a result of the pregnancy. It may be due to: (1) an unidentified preexistent disease, (2) the unmasking of a compensated metabolic abnormality by the added stress of pregnancy, or (3) a direct consequence of the altered maternal metabolism stemming from changing hormonal levels.

3. A rise in serum levels of estrogen, progesterone, and other hormones early in pregnancy stimulate maternal insulin production and increase tissue response to insulin. Placental secretion of human placental lactogen (hPL) and prolactin, as well as elevated levels of cortisol and glycogen, cause increased maternal peripheral resistance to insulin in the second half of pregnancy (to ensure that there is a sustained supply of glucose available for the fetus). This glucose crosses the placenta.

4. The following are maternal complications from DM: hydramnios, preeclampsia-eclampsia, ketoacidosis, dystocia, and increased susceptibility to infections.

5. The following are fetal/neonatal risks associated with maternal DM: increased risk for perinatal mortality, congenital anomalies, macrosomia, IUGR, RDS, polycythemia, hyperbilirubinemia, and hypocalcemia. Tight metabolic control of glucose can reduce the risk for these complications.

6. Risk assessment should begin at the first prenatal visit. Low risk women should be tested toward the end of the second trimester using a 1 hour, 50-g oral glucose test. Risk factors include: age over 40; family history of diabetes in a first-degree relative; a prior macrosomic, malformed, or stillborn infant; obesity; hypertension; or glucosuria. Women with these risk factors should be tested as early as possible in pregnancy. A level that is equal to or greater than 130 to 140 mg/dL indicates a need for further diagnostic testing. To diagnose gestational diabetes, a 3-hour, 100-g oral glucose tolerance test (OGTT) is done. If two or more of the following values are met or exceeded, gestational diabetes is diagnosed: Fasting: 95 mg/dL; 1 hour: 180 mg/dL; 2 hour: 155 mg/dL; and 3 hour: 140 mg/dL.

7. The treatment goals for a pregnant woman with diabetes are: (1) to maintain a physiologic equilibrium of insulin availability and glucose utilization during pregnancy, and (2) to ensure an optimally healthy mother and newborn. Diet therapy and regular exercise form the cornerstone of intervention for GDM. Dietary management is instituted first. If dietary management does not result in 1-hour postprandial blood glucose values of less than 130 to 140 mg/dL, a 2-hour postprandial level less than 120 mg/dL, or a fasting glucose less than 95 mg/dL, insulin therapy may be necessary.

- Cellular and extracellular dehydration
- Breakdown of fats and proteins for energy

2 Gestational Diabetes (GDM)
- Carbohydrate intolerance of variable severity
- Causes
  - An unidentified preexistent disease
  - The effect of pregnancy on a compensated metabolic abnormality
  - A consequence of altered metabolism from changing hormonal levels

3 Effect of Pregnancy on Carbohydrate Metabolism
- Early pregnancy
  - Increased insulin production and tissue sensitivity
- Second half of pregnancy
  - Increased peripheral resistance to insulin

4 Maternal Risks with DM
- Hydramnios
- Preeclampsia-eclampsia
- Ketoacidosis
- Dystocia
- Increased susceptibility to infections

5 Fetal/Neonatal Risks with DM
- Perinatal mortality
- Congenital anomalies
- Macrosomia
- IUGR
- RDS
- Polycythemia

5a Fetal/Neonatal Risks with DM
- Hyperbilirubinemia
- Hypocalcemia

6 Screening for DM in Pregnancy
- Assess risk at first visit
- Low risk—screen at 24–28 weeks
- High risk—screen as early as feasible

6a Risk Factors
- Age over 40
- Family history of diabetes in a first-degree relative
- Prior macrosomic, malformed, or stillborn infant
- Obesity
- Hypertension
- Glucosuria

6b Screening Tests
- One-hour glucose tolerance test
  - Greater than 130–140 mg/dL requires further testing
- Three-hour glucose tolerance test
  - GDM diagnosed if 2 levels are exceeded

7 Treatment Goals
- Maintain a physiologic equilibrium of insulin availability and glucose utilization

 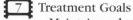

8. Assessment of fetal status is also important for the woman with diabetes. Maternal serum α-fetoprotein (AFP) screening is offered at weeks 16 to 20 of gestation because of the increase in risk for neural tube defects. Maternal fetal activity monitoring, nonstress testing (NST), biophysical profiles, and ultrasounds are important to assess fetal status.

9. Nursing care should include: assessment of glucose, nutrition counseling, education about the disease process and management, education about glucose monitoring and insulin administration, assessment of the fetus, and support.

- Ensure an optimally healthy mother and newborn
- Treatment
  ○ Diet therapy and exercise
  ○ Glucose monitoring (Figure 19.4)
  ○ Insulin therapy

7a See Figure 19.4

8 Fetal Assessment
- AFP
- Fetal activity monitoring
- NST
- Biophysical profile
- Ultrasound

9 Nursing Management
- Assessment of glucose
- Nutrition counseling
- Education about the disease process and management
- Education about glucose monitoring and insulin administration
- Assessment of the fetus
- Support

SUGGESTIONS FOR CLASSROOM ACTIVITIES

Have students develop a concept map for the assessment and treatment of a pregnant woman with gestational diabetes.

SUGGESTIONS FOR CLINICAL ACTIVITIES

Ask students to review the prenatal charts of a woman with diabetes and note the interventions and fetal assessment that occurred during that woman's pregnancy.

LEARNING OBJECTIVE 3

Discriminate among the four major types of anemia associated with pregnancy with regard to signs, treatment, and implications for pregnancy.

CONCEPTS FOR LECTURE

1. An expansion of plasma volume in pregnancy without the normal expansion of hemoglobin mass causes iron deficiency anemia. While she may be asymptomatic, this woman: is more susceptible to infection, may tire easily, has an increased chance of preeclampsia and postpartal hemorrhage, and tolerates poorly even minimal blood loss during birth. Neonatal risks include: an increased risk of low birth weight, prematurity, stillbirth, and neonatal death. The primary goal is prevention; however, if affected, the goal of treatment is to return iron and hemoglobin levels to normal. This type of anemia can be prevented by taking at least 27 mg of iron supplements daily, which is found in most prenatal vitamins, and to eat an iron-rich diet. Treatment of women with the disease is an increase in the amount of the supplement to 60 to 120 mg per day of iron.

POWERPOINT LECTURE SLIDES

(NOTE: The number on each PPT Lecture Slide directly corresponds with the Concepts for Lecture.)

1 Iron Deficiency Anemia
- Maternal complications
  ○ Susceptible to infection
  ○ May tire easily
  ○ Increased chance of preeclampsia and postpartal hemorrhage
  ○ Tolerates poorly even minimal blood loss during birth

1a Iron Deficiency Anemia
- Fetal complications
  ○ Low birth weight
  ○ Prematurity
  ○ Stillbirth
  ○ Neonatal death

2. Megaloblastic anemia during pregnancy is caused by folate deficiency. An associated fetal risk is the development of neural tube defects. Maternal symptoms include nausea, vomiting, and anorexia. Prevention of this type of anemia can be accomplished by taking a daily supplement of 0.4 mg of folate. If affected, the woman is treated with a 1 mg folic acid supplement. Iron deficiency anemia usually coexists with this type of anemia; therefore, the woman should also receive iron supplements.

3. A recessive autosomal disorder in which the normal adult hemoglobin, hemoglobin A (HbA), is abnormally formed is sickle cell anemia (HbSS). Women who are of African descent or are of Southeast Asian or Mediterranean origin are at increased risk. Symptoms include acute, recurring episodes of tissue, abdominal, and joint pain. Women who have sickle cell anemia are at an increased risk for nephritis, bacteriuria, and hematuria, and tend to become anemic during pregnancy. They may also develop congestive heart failure or acute renal failure. Fetal risks include fetal death during and immediately following an attack, prematurity, and intrauterine growth restriction (IUGR). Folic acid supplements of 1.0 mg/day should be taken to maintain hemoglobin levels. Vaso-occlusive crisis can occur with dehydration and fever; therefore, maternal infection should be treated promptly. Hospitalization during a crisis is important for rehydration with intravenous fluids; administration of oxygen, antibiotics and analgesics; and monitoring of fetal heart rate.

4. A group of autosomal recessive disorders characterized by a defect in the synthesis of the alpha or beta chains in the hemoglobin molecule is called thalassemia. Women from Greece, Italy, or southern China are at an increased risk. β-thalassemia minor is a mild anemia with small (microcytic) red cells. While pregnancy is rare in women with β-thalassemia major, if it occurs, the woman has severe anemia, needs transfusion therapy, and is at risk for congestive heart failure. Treatment is with folic acid supplements, not iron. Transfusion and chelation therapy may be necessary in women with thalassemia intermedia and thalassemia major.

1b Iron Deficiency Anemia
- Prevention and Treatment
  ○ Prevention: at least 27 mg of iron daily
  ○ Treatment: 60–120 mg of iron daily

2 Folate Deficiency
- Maternal complications
  ○ Nausea, vomiting, and anorexia
- Fetal complications
  ○ Neural tube defects
- Prevention: 4 mg folic acid daily
- Treatment: 1 mg folic acid daily plus iron supplements

3 Sickle Cell Anemia
- Maternal complications
  ○ Vaso-occlusive crisis
  ○ Infections
  ○ Congestive heart failure
  ○ Renal failure

3a Sickle Cell Anemia
- Fetal complications include fetal death, prematurity, IUGR
- Treatment
  ○ Folic acid
  ○ Prompt treatment of infections
  ○ Prompt treatment of vaso-occlusive crisis

4 Thalassemia
- Treatment
  ○ Folic acid
  ○ Transfusion
  ○ Chelation

SUGGESTIONS FOR CLINICAL ACTIVITIES

Have students do a physical assessment on a woman diagnosed with anemia in pregnancy and note their observations in relation to the diagnosis.

Learning Objective 4

Discuss acquired immunodeficiency syndrome (AIDS), including care of the pregnant woman with HIV/AIDS, neonatal implications, and ramifications for the childbearing family.

Concepts for Lecture

1. Pregnancy can accelerate the progression of HIV/AIDS if women have low CD4 counts; however, pregnancy is not believed to accelerate progression in women who are asymptomatic. Zidovudine (ZDV) used during pregnancy significantly reduces the risk of transmission of HIV to the fetus. Most medications used to treat HIV can be used safely in pregnancy. While HIV transmission can occur anytime during pregnancy and breastfeeding, most infection occurs during labor and birth. Women with HIV are at an increased risk for intrapartal or postpartal hemorrhage, postpartal infection, poor wound healing, and infections of the genitourinary tract.

2. Infants will have a positive antibody titer due to the passive transfer of maternal antibodies. These infants are usually asymptomatic at birth; however, they are likely to be premature, have low birth weight, and be small for gestational age (SGA). These complications may not be necessarily due to HIV, as they are also associated with several socioeconomic factors.

3. Treatment should include: counseling for women who test positive about the risks for themselves and their fetus, stabilizing the disease, preventing opportunistic infections and transmission of the virus from the mother to the fetus, and providing psychosocial and educational support. Antiretroviral therapy is recommended for all infected pregnant women to decrease the risk of perinatal transmission. Close monitoring of the fetus should be done through nonstress testing, biophysical profiles, and ultrasounds. A scheduled cesarean birth is recommended by the American College of Obstetricians and Gynecologists for all HIV-positive pregnant women as early as 38 weeks gestation to decrease the risk of rupture of membranes.

PowerPoint Lecture Slides

(NOTE: The number on each PPT Lecture Slide directly corresponds with the Concepts for Lecture.)

1 HIV in Pregnancy
- Asymptomatic women—pregnancy has no effect
- Symptomatic with low CD4—pregnancy accelerates the disease
- Zidovudine (ZDV) therapy diminishes risk of transmission to fetus
- Transmitted through breast milk
- Half of all infection occurs during labor and birth

1a HIV in Pregnancy: Maternal Risks
- Intrapartal or postpartal hemorrhage
- Postpartal infection
- Poor wound healing
- Infections of the genitourinary tract

2 HIV Effects on Fetus
- Infants will often have a positive antibody titer
- Infected infants are usually asymptomatic but are likely to be
  - Premature
  - Low birth weight
  - Small for gestational age (SGA)

3 Treatment During Pregnancy
- Counsel about implications of diagnosis on pregnancy
- Antiretroviral therapy
- Fetal testing
- Cesarean birth

Suggestions for Classroom Activities

Ask students to develop a care plan for a woman with HIV in pregnancy.

Suggestions for Clinical Activities

Have students interview prenatal health providers about their care of the woman with HIV and screening for all women for HIV in pregnancy.

Learning Objective 5

Describe the effects of various heart disorders on pregnancy, including their implications for nursing care.

Concepts for Lecture

1. Women with congenital heart defects that have been repaired, with no evidence of remaining organic heart disease, may become pregnant with confidence. Prophylactic antibiotic treatment is recommended to prevent subacute bacterial endocarditis at the time of birth.

PowerPoint Lecture Slides

(NOTE: The number on each PPT Lecture Slide directly corresponds with the Concepts for Lecture.)

1 Cardiac Disorders in Pregnancy
- Congenital heart disease
- Marfan syndrome

If the congenital disease is associated with cyanosis, the woman and her fetus are at increased risk and there is an increased risk that the fetus will inherit the disorder. The woman with mitral valve stenosis is at increased risk during pregnancy because of the increased blood volume during pregnancy and the increased need for cardiac output. Symptoms may include dyspnea, orthopnea, and pulmonary edema and an increased risk for congestive heart failure (CHF). An autosomal dominant disorder of connective tissue in which there may be serious cardiovascular involvement (usually dissection or rupture of the aorta) is Marfan syndrome. These women are at high risk for maternal mortality, and there is a 50% chance that the disease will be passed on to offspring. Dysfunction of the left ventricle that occurs in the last month of pregnancy or the first 5 months postpartum in a woman with no previous history of heart disease is peripartum cardiomyopathy. Symptoms may include: dyspnea, orthopnea, chest pain, palpitations, weakness, and edema. Although the cause is unknown, the symptoms may be due to chronic hypertension, mitral stenosis, obesity, or viral myocarditis. The usual presentation is anemia and infection. Treatment includes digitalis, diuretics, vasodilators, anticoagulants, sodium restriction, and strict bed rest. A complication that can develop as a result of other cardiac lesions causing left-to-right shunting is Eisenmenger syndrome. Progressive pulmonary hypertension may result. There is a high rate of maternal mortality associated with this complication. An asymptomatic condition that is found in as many as 12% to 17% of women of childbearing age is mitral valve prolapse. These women usually tolerate pregnancy well, and the prognosis is excellent. Symptoms may include: palpitations, chest pain, and dyspnea, which are usually due to arrhythmias. Treatment is the administration of propranolol hydrochloride (Inderal) and limiting caffeine intake.

- Peripartum cardiomyopathy
- Eisenmenger syndrome
- Mitral valve prolapse

SUGGESTIONS FOR CLASSROOM ACTIVITIES

Have students make a chart of various cardiac symptoms and potential diagnoses associated with those symptoms.

LEARNING OBJECTIVE 6

Compare the effects of selected gestational medical conditions on pregnancy.

CONCEPTS FOR LECTURE

1. Additional medical conditions that may impact pregnancy include: rheumatoid arthritis, epilepsy, hepatitis B, hyperthyroidism, hypothyroidism, maternal phenylketonuria, multiple sclerosis, systemic lupus erythematosus, and tuberculosis. The affected woman should be aware of the possible impact of the disease on her pregnancy.

POWERPOINT LECTURE SLIDES

(NOTE: The number on each PPT Lecture Slide directly corresponds with the Concepts for Lecture.)

1 Less Common Medical Conditions in Pregnancy
- Rheumatoid arthritis
- Epilepsy
- Hepatitis B
- Hyperthyroidism

- Hypothyroidism
- Maternal phenylketonuria

 Less Common Medical Conditions in Pregnancy
- Multiple sclerosis
- Systemic lupus erythematosus
- Tuberculosis

Suggestions for Classroom Activities

Have students review Table 19.5 in their book for maternal and fetal/neonatal implications for less common medical conditions in pregnancy.

CHAPTER 20
PREGNANCY AT RISK: GESTATIONAL ONSET

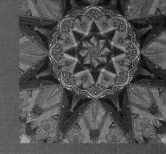

RESOURCE LIBRARY

PRENTICE HALL NURSING MEDIALINK DVD-ROM

Audio Glossary
NCLEX Review
Animation: *Early Preterm Labor*

COMPANION WEBSITE

Additional NCLEX Review
Case Study: *Client with Preeclampsia*
Care Plan Activity: *Client at Risk for Preterm Labor*
Applications: *Potential Pregnancy Complications;*
Preeclampsia and HELLP
Critical Thinking

📖 IMAGE LIBRARY

Figure 20.1 Types of spontaneous abortion.
Figure 20.2 Various implantation sites in ectopic pregnancy.
Figure 20.3 Hydatidiform mole.
Figure 20.4 A cerclage or purse-string suture is inserted in the cervix to prevent preterm cervical dilatation and pregnancy loss.
Figure 20.5 Endovaginal ultrasound of the cervix.
Figure 20.6 Clinical manifestations and possible pathophysiology of preeclampsia-eclampsia.
Figure 20.7 *A*, In a normal pregnancy, the passive quality of the spiral arteries permits increased blood flow to the placenta. *B*, In preeclampsia,

vasoconstriction of the myometrial segment of the spiral arteries occurs.
Figure 20.8 Correct position for eliciting patellar reflex: siting.
Figure 20.9 To elicit clonus, sharply dorsiflex the foot.
Figure 20.10 Rh alloimmunization sequence.
Figure 20.11 Ultrasound measurement of peak systolic velocity (PSV) of the middle cerebral artery.
Figure 20.12 Indications for intrapartum antibiotic prophylaxis to prevent perinatal GBS disease under a universal prenatal screening strategy based on combined vaginal and rectal cultures collected at 35 to 37 weeks' gestation from all pregnant women.

LEARNING OBJECTIVE 1

Contrast the etiology, medical therapy, and nursing interventions for the various bleeding problems associated with pregnancy.

CONCEPTS FOR LECTURE

1. Spontaneous abortion is embryonic death which results in the loss of human chorionic gonadotropin (hCG) and decreased progesterone and estrogen levels, a sloughing of the uterine decidua, irritability and contraction of the uterus, and expulsion of the embryo/fetus. The following are categories of spontaneous abortion: threatened abortion, imminent abortion, incomplete abortion, complete abortion, missed abortion, recurrent pregnancy loss, and septic abortion. Symptoms include pelvic cramping, backache, and bleeding. Treatment may include bed rest, abstinence from coitus, and perhaps sedation. If there is persistent bleeding and the abortion is imminent or incomplete, hospitalization may be necessary for IV therapy or blood transfusions and dilation and curettage (D&C) or suction evacuation to remove the remainder of the products of conception. Rh immune globulin (RhoGAM) is given if the woman is Rh negative and

POWERPOINT LECTURE SLIDES

(NOTE: The number on each PPT Lecture Slide directly corresponds with the Concepts for Lecture.)

 1 Spontaneous Abortion (Figure 20.1)
- Threatened abortion
- Imminent abortion
- Incomplete abortion
- Complete abortion

1a See Figure 20.1A–C

1b Spontaneous Abortion
- Missed abortion
- Recurrent pregnancy loss
- Septic abortion

1c Spontaneous Abortion: Treatment
- Bed rest
- Abstinence from coitus
- D&C or suction evacuation
- Rh immune globulin

not sensitized and there has been prior ultrasound documentation of fetal cardiac activity. Nursing interventions include assessment of vaginal bleeding and monitoring vital signs and degree of discomfort. In pregnancies 10 to 12 weeks or more, the fetal heart rate should be assessed by Doppler. Assessment of the responses of the woman and her family to this crisis and evaluation of their coping mechanisms is an important nursing intervention.

2. The implantation of a fertilized ovum in a site other than the endometrial lining of the uterus is an ectopic pregnancy. The following are risk factors: tubal damage caused by pelvic inflammatory disease; previous pelvic or tubal surgery; endometriosis; previous ectopic pregnancy; presence of an IUD; high levels of progesterone, which can alter the motility of the egg in the fallopian tube; congenital anomalies of the tube; use of ovulation-inducing drugs; primary infertility; smoking; and advanced maternal age. Ectopic pregnancy occurs when the fertilized ovum is prevented or slowed in its progress down the tube and implantation occurs somewhere other than the uterus. As the trophoblastic cells grow into the adjacent tissue, internal hemorrhage results. Fluctuations in hormone levels will fail to support the growing edometrium, causing vaginal bleeding. Rupture of the fallopian tube may occur if implantation occurs there, and the woman will experience one-sided lower abdominal pain or diffuse lower abdominal pain and vasomotor disturbances such as fainting or dizziness. Hypovolemic shock may occur if internal hemorrhage is profuse; however, more commonly the bleeding is slow and the abdomen gradually becomes rigid and tender. Treatment may include the administration of methotrexate to dissolve the pregnancy or a laparoscopic linear salpingostomy or salpingectomy. Nursing responsibilities include assessing the appearance and amount of vaginal bleeding, monitoring vital signs, assessing the woman's emotional status and coping abilities, and evaluating the couple's informational needs.

3. The pathologic proliferation of trophoblastic cells that includes a partial or complete hydatidiform mole, invasive mole, or choriocarcinoma is called gestational trophoblastic disease (GTD). This disease involves the loss of the pregnancy and the possibility of developing choriocarcinoma. Symptoms include: vaginal bleeding, anemia, passing of hydropic vesicles, uterine enlargement greater than expected for gestational age, absence of fetal heart sounds, elevated hCG, low levels of MSAFP, hyperemesis gravidarum, and preeclampsia. Treatment includes suction evacuation of the mole and curettage of the uterus to remove all fragments of the placenta. Nursing care includes identification of symptoms, monitoring vital signs and vaginal bleeding, and assessment of pain, emotional state, and coping ability.

4. An improper implantation of the placenta in the lower uterine segment is called placenta previa. Bleeding

 Spontaneous Abortion: Nursing Care
- Assess the amount and appearance of any vaginal bleeding
- Monitor the woman's vital signs and degree of discomfort
- Assess need for Rh immune globulin
- Assess fetal heart rate
- Assess the responses and coping of the woman and her family

 Ectopic Pregnancy: Risk Factors
- Tubal damage
- Previous pelvic or tubal surgery
- Endometriosis
- Previous ectopic pregnancy
- Presence of an IUD
- High levels of progesterone

 Ectopic Pregnancy: Risk Factors
- Congenital anomalies of the tube
- Use of ovulation-inducing drugs
- Primary infertility
- Smoking
- Advanced maternal age

 Ectopic Pregnancy: Treatment (Figure 20.2)
- Methotrexate
- Surgery

 See Figure 20.2

 Ectopic Pregnancy: Nursing Care
- Assess the appearance and amount of vaginal bleeding
- Monitors vital signs
- Assess the woman's emotional status and coping abilities
- Evaluate the couple's informational needs
- Post-operative care

Gestational Trophoblastic Disease: Symptoms (Figure 20.3)
- Vaginal bleeding
- Anemia
- Passing of hydropic vesicles
- Uterine enlargement greater than expected for gestational age
- Absence of fetal heart sounds
- Elevated hCG

 Gestational Trophoblastic Disease: Symptoms
- Low levels of MSAFP
- Hyperemesis gravidarum
- Preeclampsia

 Gestational Trophoblastic Disease: Treatment
- D&C
- Possible hysterectomy
- Careful follow-up

CONCEPTS FOR LECTURE *continued*

occurs as the lower uterine segment contracts and the cervix dilates in the later weeks of pregnancy and the placenta villi are torn from the uterine wall exposing the uterine sinuses at the placental site. The premature separation of a normally implanted placenta from the uterine wall is abruptio placentae. Characteristic signs are maternal pain disproportionate to the strength of uterine contractions that may or may not be accompanied by obvious bleeding.

POWERPOINT LECTURE SLIDES *continued*

 See Figure 20.3

3d Gestational Trophoblastic Disease: Nursing Care
- Monitor vital signs
- Monitor vaginal bleeding
- Assess abdominal pain
- Assess the woman's emotional state and coping ability

4 Bleeding Disorders
- Placenta previa—placenta is improperly implanted in the lower uterine segment
- Abruptio placentae—the premature separation of a normally implanted placenta from the uterine wall

---

SUGGESTIONS FOR CLASSROOM ACTIVITIES

Bring a pelvic model to class to demonstrate to students where the bleeding is originating from and why it is occurring.

SUGGESTIONS FOR CLINICAL ACTIVITIES

Ask students who are caring for women in the clinical setting to do a chart review to assess for risk factors contributing to that disease process.

LEARNING OBJECTIVE 2
Identify the medical therapy and nursing interventions indicated in caring for a woman with an incompetent cervix.

CONCEPTS FOR LECTURE

1. Treatments for an incompetent cervix include: serial cervical ultrasound assessments, bed rest, progesterone supplementation, antibiotics, anti-inflammatory drugs, and various types of cerclage procedures.

POWERPOINT LECTURE SLIDES

(NOTE: The number on each PPT Lecture Slide directly corresponds with the Concepts for Lecture.)

1 Cervical Incompetence: Treatment
- Serial cervical ultrasound assessments
- Bed rest
- Progesterone supplementation
- Antibiotics
- Anti-inflammatory drugs
- Cerclage procedures (Figure 20.4)

1a See Figure 20.4

SUGGESTIONS FOR CLASSROOM ACTIVITIES

Bring a dilatation model to class to demonstrate dilatation with an incompetent cervix. Discuss the psychological factors that the woman and her family will experience.

LEARNING OBJECTIVE 3
Discuss the medical therapy and nursing care of a woman with hyperemesis gravidarum.

CONCEPTS FOR LECTURE

1. Treatment goals for a woman suffering from hyperemesis include: controlling vomiting, correcting dehydration, restoring electrolyte balance, and maintaining adequate nutrition. Frequent small meals and the occasional use of antiemetics may help; however, if the woman does not respond, she may require intravenous

POWERPOINT LECTURE SLIDES

(NOTE: The number on each PPT Lecture Slide directly corresponds with the Concepts for Lecture.)

1 Hyperemesis Gravidarum: Treatment
- Control vomiting
- Correct dehydration

(IV) fluids or total parenteral nutrition. Nursing interventions include: assessing the amount and character of further emesis, intake and output, fetal heart rate, maternal vital signs, initial weight, evidence of jaundice or bleeding, and the woman's emotional state.

- Restore electrolyte balance
- Maintain adequate nutrition

 Hyperemesis Gravidarum: Nursing Care
- Assess the amount and character of further emesis
- Assess intake and output and weight
- Assess fetal heart rate
- Assess maternal vital signs
- Observe for evidence of jaundice or bleeding
- Assess the woman's emotional state

SUGGESTIONS FOR CLASSROOM ACTIVITIES

Ask students to develop a nutritional care plan for a woman experiencing hyperemesis.

SUGGESTIONS FOR CLINICAL ACTIVITIES

Have students caring for a woman with hyperemesis assess and discuss the psychological response to the disease process.

LEARNING OBJECTIVE 4

Discuss the nursing care for a woman experiencing premature rupture of the membranes or preterm labor.

CONCEPTS FOR LECTURE

1. The nursing care for a woman experiencing premature rupture of membranes (PROM) includes: determining the duration of the rupture of membranes, assessment of gestational age, observation for signs and symptoms of infection, assessment of fetal heart rate, evaluation of childbirth preparation and coping abilities of the woman and her partner, assessment of uterine activity and fetal response to the labor, provision of comfort measure, and maintenance of adequate hydration. Vaginal exams are not done unless absolutely necessary. Education of the couple about the implications of PROM and treatments are also important nursing interventions.

2. Identification of the woman at risk for preterm labor is an important nursing intervention. Continued assessment should include change in risk status for preterm labor, educational needs of the woman and her loved ones, and the woman's responses to medical and nursing interventions. The nurse should educate the woman about the importance of recognizing the onset of labor. Signs and symptoms of preterm labor include the following: uterine contractions that occur every 10 minutes or less with or without pain; mild menstrual-like cramps felt low in the abdomen; constant or intermittent feelings of pelvic pressure that may feel like the baby pressing down; rupture of membranes; a low, dull backache, which may be constant or intermittent; a change in the vaginal discharge; and abdominal cramping with or without diarrhea.

POWERPOINT LECTURE SLIDES

*(NOTE: **The number on each PPT Lecture Slide directly corresponds with the Concepts for Lecture.**)*

 Nursing Care of Clients with PROM
- Determine duration of PROM
- Assess gestational age
- Observe for signs and symptoms of infection
- Assess hydration status
- Assess fetal status
- Assess childbirth preparation and coping

 Nursing Clients with PROM
- Encourage resting on left side
- Comfort measures
- Education

 Nursing Care of Clients with Preterm Labor
- Identify risk for preterm labor
- Assess change in risk status for preterm labor
- Assess educational needs of the woman and her loved ones
- Assess the woman's responses to medical and nursing intervention
- Teach about the importance of recognizing the onset of labor

 Signs and Symptoms of Preterm Labor
- Uterine contractions occurring every 10 minutes or less
- Mild menstrual-like cramps felt low in the abdomen
- Constant or intermittent feelings of pelvic pressure

- Rupture of membranes
- Low, dull backache, which may be constant or intermittent

2b Signs and Symptoms of Preterm Labor
- A change in vaginal discharge
- Abdominal cramping with or without diarrhea

SUGGESTIONS FOR CLASSROOM ACTIVITIES	SUGGESTIONS FOR CLINICAL ACTIVITIES
Have students develop a teaching plan for women, educating them about the signs of premature labor.	Have students do an assessment of a woman with PROM and identify any risk factors for infection.

LEARNING OBJECTIVE 5

Describe the development and course of hypertensive disorders associated with pregnancy.

CONCEPTS FOR LECTURE

1. Hypertension in pregnancy is classified as preeclampsia-eclampsia, chronic hypertension, chronic hypertension with superimposed preeclampsia, and gestational hypertension. Preeclampsia is an increase in blood pressure after 20 weeks' gestation accompanied by proteinuria. The occurrence of a seizure in a woman with preeclampsia who has no other cause for seizure is eclampsia. Delivery is the only cure for this disease. An increase in the blood pressure to 140/90 or higher before pregnancy or before the 20th week of gestation or persisting 42 days after birth is chronic hypertension.

2. Findings in women with preeclampsia include: maternal vasospasm resulting in decreased perfusion to virtually all organs, a decrease in plasma volume, activation of the coagulation cascade, and alterations in the glomerular capillary endothelium. Edema may be more profound than in an uncomplicated pregnancy. The hematocrit rises because of the decreased intravascular volume which causes an increase in the viscosity of the blood. Hyperreflexia, headache, and eclamptic seizure may also occur. A rare occurrence is the development of a subcapsular hematoma of the liver, putting the woman at risk for rupture and potentially death. Hepatomegaly and peritoneal irritation may also exist.

3. Effects on the infants of women with preeclampsia include IUGR, placental abruption resulting in fetal hypoxia or death, and prematurity.

4. Home management of the woman with preeclampsia should include education about the condition to recognize the signs and symptoms of worsening preeclampsia, counting fetal movements, and encouragement to rest frequently, especially in the left lateral position. On a daily basis, the woman should monitor her blood pressure, weight, and urine protein. NST

POWERPOINT LECTURE SLIDES

(NOTE: The number on each PPT Lecture Slide directly corresponds with the Concepts for Lecture.)

1 Classification of Hypertension in Pregnancy
- Preeclampsia-eclampsia
- Chronic hypertension
- Chronic hypertension with superimposed preeclampsia
- Gestational hypertension

2 Characteristics of Preeclampsia
- Maternal vasospasm (Figure 20.7)
- Decreased perfusion to virtually all organs
- Decrease in plasma volume
- Activation of the coagulation cascade
- Alterations in glomerular capillary endothelium
- Edema

2a Characteristics of Preeclampsia
- Increased viscosity of the blood
- Hyperreflexia
- Headache
- Subcapsular hematoma of the liver

2b See Figure 20.7

3 Hypertensive Effects on Fetus
- Small for gestational age
- Fetal hypoxia
- Death related to abruption
- Prematurity

4 Home Management
- Monitoring for signs and symptoms of worsening condition
- Fetal movement counts
- Frequent rest in the left lateral position
- Monitoring of blood pressure, weight, and urine protein daily

---

may be done in the home to assess fetal status. Regular laboratory testing includes platelet counts, uric acid and BUN, liver enzymes, and 24-hour urine specimens for creatinine clearance and total protein.

5. When the woman's condition worsens, she should be hospitalized for potential delivery; be on bed rest; receive a high-protein, moderate-sodium diet; receive treatment with magnesium sulfate, corticosteroids, fluid and electrolyte replacement, and antihypertensive therapy. Antihypertensives are given for sustained systolic blood pressure of at least 160 to 180 mm Hg or diastolic blood pressures of 105 to 110 or above to maintain the diastolic blood pressure between 90 and 100 mm Hg to prevent a decrease in uterine blood flow.

6. Signs of impending eclampsia include: scotomata (which can appear as dark spots or flashing lights in the field of vision), blurred vision, epigastric pain, vomiting, persistent or severe headache (generally frontal in location), neurologic hyperactivity, pulmonary edema, or cyanosis. If eclampsia occurs, the nurse should assess the following: the time of onset, progress of the seizure, body involvement, duration, presence of incontinence, status of the fetus, and signs of placental abruption. Nursing interventions should include: maintenance of the airway, administration of oxygen, positioning to avoid aspiration, suctioning the airway, prevention of injury by keeping siderails up and padded, and administration of a bolus of 6 g magnesium sulfate intravenously over 15 to 20 minutes, followed by 2 g/hour IV infusion.

- NST
- Laboratory testing

 Management of Severe Preeclampsia
- Bed rest
- High-protein, moderate-sodium diet
- Treatment with magnesium sulfate
- Corticosteroids
- Fluid and electrolyte replacement
- Antihypertensive therapy

 Signs and Symptoms of Eclampsia
- Scotomata
- Blurred vision
- Epigastric pain
- Vomiting
- Persistent or severe headache
- Neurologic hyperactivity

 Signs and Symptoms of Eclampsia
- Pulmonary edema
- Cyanosis

 Management of Eclampsia
- Assess characteristics of seizure
- Assess status of the fetus
- Assess signs of placental abruption
- Maintain airway and oxygenation
- Position on side to avoid aspiration
- Suctioning to keep the airway clear

 Management of Eclampsia
- To prevent injury, side rails should be up and padded
- Administration of mag sulfate

SUGGESTIONS FOR CLASSROOM ACTIVITIES

Have students develop a nursing plan of care for women managed at home with preeclampsia.

SUGGESTIONS FOR CLINICAL ACTIVITIES

Have students care for a woman who has been hospitalized with preeclampsia. Have them do assessments for progression of the disease and discuss their findings.

LEARNING OBJECTIVE 6

Explain the cause and prevention of hemolytic disease of the newborn secondary to Rh incompatibility.

CONCEPTS FOR LECTURE

1. When an Rh-negative woman carries an Rh-positive fetus either to term or to termination by miscarriage or induced abortion, Rh alloimmunization (sensitization), also called isoimmunization, can occur. This condition can also occur if an Rh-negative nonpregnant woman receives an Rh-positive blood transfusion, experiences an Rh-positive tubal pregnancy, has an amniocentesis, or any other traumatic event that might allow Rh-positive fetal cells to enter her circulation. Maternal IgG antibodies in the fetus cause hemolysis which creates fetal anemia. Because of this, the fetus responds by

POWERPOINT LECTURE SLIDES

(NOTE: The number on each PPT Lecture Slide directly corresponds with the Concepts for Lecture.)

 Rh Incompatibility (Figure 20.10)
- Rh− mother, Rh+ fetus
- Maternal IgG antibodies produced
- Hemolysis of fetal red blood cells
- Rapid production of erythroblasts
- Hyperbilirubinemia

 See Figure 20.10

increasing red blood cell production. If left untreated, this anemia can also cause marked fetal edema, called hydrops fetalis, resulting in congestive heart failure. Hyperbilirubinemia and jaundice may also occur, which can lead to kernicterus.

2. An intramuscular injection of 300 mcg Rh immune globulin (RhoGAM, HypRho-D) is given within 72 hours to an Rh-negative mother who has no titer and who has given birth to an Rh-positive fetus so that she does not have time to produce antibodies to fetal cells that entered her bloodstream when the placenta separated. Rh immune globulin destroys fetal cells in the maternal circulation before sensitization occurs, blocking maternal antibody production. Rh immune globulin is also given after each spontaneous or induced abortion, ectopic pregnancy, chorionic villus sampling, multifetal pregnancy reduction, partial molar pregnancy, amniocentesis, PUBS, antepartum hemorrhage, or external version. A Kleihauer-Betke test can be performed to identify the need for Rh immune globulin administration following maternal trauma. A smaller (50 mcg) dose of Rh immune globulin (MICRhoGAM or Mini-Gamulin Rh) is used in the first trimester.

 Administration of Rh Immune Globulin
- After birth of an Rh + infant
- After spontaneous or induced abortion
- After ectopic pregnancy
- After invasive procedures during pregnancy
- After maternal trauma

SUGGESTIONS FOR CLASSROOM ACTIVITIES

Have students discuss a community education plan to make Rh− mothers aware of the risks for Rh sensitization and preventative measures.

SUGGESTIONS FOR CLINICAL ACTIVITIES

Have students administer RhoGAM in the prenatal or postpartum setting. Ask them to identify the purpose of the medication and the indications for administering it.

LEARNING OBJECTIVE 7

Compare Rh incompatibility to ABO incompatibility with regard to occurrence, treatment, and implications for the fetus/newborn.

CONCEPTS FOR LECTURE

1. A type O mother with a type A or B fetus may experience ABO incompatibility as a result of the maternal antibodies present in her serum and interaction between the antigen sites on the fetal red blood cells. Women may have naturally occurring anti-A and anti-B antibodies because of the foods that they eat and through exposure to infection by gram-negative bacteria. These antibodies then cross the placenta and produce hemolysis of fetal red blood cells.

POWERPOINT LECTURE SLIDES

(NOTE: The number on each PPT Lecture Slide directly corresponds with the Concepts for Lecture.)

 ABO Incompatibility
- Mom is type O
- Infant is type A or B
- Maternal serum antibodies present in serum
- Hemolysis of fetal red blood cells

SUGGESTIONS FOR CLINICAL ACTIVITIES

Have students assess an infant with ABO incompatibility and the neonatal effects.

LEARNING OBJECTIVE 8

Summarize the effects of surgical procedures on pregnancy, and explain ways in which pregnancy may complicate diagnosis of conditions that require surgery.

CONCEPTS FOR LECTURE

1. Surgery performed during the first trimester can increase the incidence of spontaneous abortion. There is an increase in the risk of vomiting during induction of anesthesia and during the postoperative period because of decreased intestinal motility and decreased free gastric acid secretion during pregnancy. To prevent this, a nasogastric tube is recommended before major surgery. To decrease the risk of injury to the bladder by preventing bladder distention and promoting ease of monitoring output, an indwelling urinary catheter should be placed. Pregnant women are at an increased risk for thrombophlebitis, so support stockings during and after surgery should be used to help prevent venous stasis. Assessment of the fetus by monitoring fetal heart tones must be monitored before, during, and after surgery. The woman should be positioned during and after surgery to allow optimal uteroplacental–fetal circulation. The preferred types of anesthesia are spinal or epidural anesthetics.

POWERPOINT LECTURE SLIDES

(NOTE: The number on each PPT Lecture Slide directly corresponds with the Concepts for Lecture.)

1. Surgery During Pregnancy
   - Incidence of spontaneous abortion increased in first trimester
   - Insert nasogastric tube prior to surgery
   - Insert indwelling catheter
   - Encourage patient to use support stockings
   - Assess fetal heart tones
   - Position to maximize utero-placental circulation

LEARNING OBJECTIVE 9

Discuss the implications of trauma due to accidents or battering for the pregnant woman and her fetus.

CONCEPTS FOR LECTURE

1. Complications that commonly accompany maternal trauma include shock, premature labor, and spontaneous abortion. Blood loss in pregnant women is greater when compared with a nonpregnant woman before evidence of shock is seen. This occurs because the woman is able to maintain hemodynamic stability temporarily by decreasing uteroplacental perfusion, thereby compromising fetal status. Pregnant women are more susceptible to hypoxemia with apnea because of the increase in minute ventilation and oxygen consumption. There is an increased risk of thrombosis after injury because of the normal increase in clotting factors during pregnancy. Severe trauma may also result in disseminating intravascular coagulation (DIC). Head trauma or hemorrhage are the injuries that are primarily responsible for maternal mortality. Separation of the placenta may occur even if the site of injury is not the abdomen, and this results in a high rate of fetal mortality. Rupture of membranes may occur during an accident, resulting in premature labor. Pelvic fractures can result in significant retroperitoneal hemorrhage.

2. Battering during pregnancy may result in psychological distress, loss of pregnancy, preterm labor, low-birth-weight infants, injury to the fetus, and fetal death. Maternal complications may include poor maternal weight gain, infection, anemia, and second and third trimester bleeding. Sexual abuse puts the woman

POWERPOINT LECTURE SLIDES

(NOTE: The number on each PPT Lecture Slide directly corresponds with the Concepts for Lecture.)

1. Trauma During Pregnancy
   - Greater volume of blood loss before signs of shock
   - More susceptible to hypoxemia with apnea
   - Increased risk of thrombosis
   - DIC
   - Traumatic separation of placenta
   - Premature labor

2. Battering During Pregnancy
   - Psychologic distress
   - Loss of pregnancy
   - Preterm labor
   - Low-birth-weight infants
   - Fetal death
   - Increased risk of STIs

CONCEPTS FOR LECTURE *continued*

at an increased risk of contracting sexually transmitted infections from her partner. Violence often escalates during pregnancy and the postpartum period.

SUGGESTIONS FOR CLASSROOM ACTIVITIES

Have a group discussion about community interventions to minimize trauma in pregnant women.

LEARNING OBJECTIVE 10

Describe the effects of infections on the woman and her unborn child.

CONCEPTS FOR LECTURE

1. Infections are most likely to cause harm to an embryo when exposed during the first trimester. When they occur later in pregnancy, the fetal effects may include growth restriction, nonimmune hydrops, and neurologic disturbances. The infections that have the most impact on the fetus during pregnancy include toxoplasmosis, rubella, cytomegalovirus, herpes simplex virus, group B streptococcus, and parvovirus B19.
2. The effect of toxoplasmosis may range from the very mild retinochoroiditis to the severe, including convulsions, coma, microcephaly, and hydrocephalus. Long term sequelae includes blindness, deafness, and severe retardation.
3. Congenital rubellas may result in congenital cataracts, sensorineural deafness, and congenital heart defects. Mental retardation or cerebral palsy may also occur.
4. Approximately 10% to 15% of fetuses affected by chlamydia will be SGA, have hemolysis, thrombocytopenia, and hepatosplenomegaly. Mental retardation and auditory deficits are also possible.
5. There is an increase in the risk of spontaneous abortion when a primary herpes simplex infection occurs in the first trimester. If the infection occurs in the second trimester or early third trimester, premature labor, intrauterine growth restriction, and neonatal infection are possible. The risk varies dependent upon the route of birth, the presence of a lesion, and whether the infection is primary or recurrent. Cesarean birth is warranted when there is a recent outbreak because of the serious nature of the disease in the newborn.
6. A perinatal infection with GBS may result in an infant being asymptomatic at birth but becoming symptomatic after an incubation period of 2 to 12 days. Symptoms may include fever (or hypothermia), jaundice, seizures, and poor feeding. Transmission rate is effected by the degree of colonization, the persistence of the positive culture, and the site of colonization. Infants with early-onset GBS may exhibit respiratory distress or pneumonia, apnea, and shock. Infants with late-onset GBS often develop meningitis.
7. Spontaneous abortion, fetal hydrops, and stillbirth are associated with fetal infection with human B-19 parvovirus.

POWERPOINT LECTURE SLIDES

(NOTE: The number on each PPT Lecture Slide directly corresponds with the Concepts for Lecture.)

1 Perinatal Infections
- Toxoplasmosis
- Rubella
- Cytomegalovirus
- Herpes simplex virus
- Group B streptococcus
- Human B-19 parvovirus

2 Fetal Risks: Toxoplasmosis
- Retinochoroiditis
- Convulsions
- Coma
- Microcephaly
- Hydrocephalus

3 Fetal Risks: Rubella
- Congenital cataracts
- Sensorineural deafness
- Congenital heart defects

4 Fetal Risks: Chlamydia
- Neurologic complications
- Anemia
- Hyperbilirubinemia
- Thrombocytopenia
- Hepatosplenomegaly
- SGA

5 Fetal Risks: Herpes
- Preterm labor
- Intrauterine growth restriction
- Neonatal infection

6 Fetal Risks: GBS
- Respiratory distress or pneumonia
- Apnea
- Shock
- Meningitis
- Long-term neurologic complications

7 Fetal Risks: Human B-19 Parvovirus
- Spontaneous abortion
- Fetal hydrops
- Stillbirth

© 2008 Pearson Education, Inc.

Chapter 20/Objective 10   **135**

SUGGESTIONS FOR CLASSROOM ACTIVITIES

Have students develop a class to educate women about the implications of exposure to perinatal infections and how to prevent them.

SUGGESTIONS FOR CLINICAL ACTIVITIES

Have students assess infants in the clinical setting that have been exposed to perinatal infection and discuss their assessments.

CHAPTER 21
ASSESSMENT OF FETAL WELL-BEING

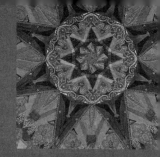

RESOURCE LIBRARY

PRENTICE HALL NURSING MEDIALINK DVD-ROM

Audio Glossary
NCLEX Review
Video: *Through the Eyes of a Nurse—The Third Trimester*

COMPANION WEBSITE

Additional NCLEX Review
Case Study: *Client Undergoing Contraction Stress Test*
Care Plan Activity: *Monitoring Well-Being of a Slow-Developing Fetus*
Applications: *Fetal Assessment; Fetal Lung Maturity*
Critical Thinking

IMAGE LIBRARY

Figure 21.1 Ultrasound scanning permits visualization of the fetus in utero.
Figure 21.2 Transvaginal ultrasound transducer.
Figure 21.3 Ultrasound of the fetal face.
Figure 21.11 Example of a reactive nonstress test (NST).
Figure 21.12 Example of a nonreactive NST.
Figure 21.13 Fetal acoustic stimulation testing.

Figure 21.14 Example of a negative CST (and reactive NST).
Figure 21.15 Example of a positive contraction stress test (CST).
Figure 21.18 Placental grading.
Figure 21.19 Amniocentesis.
Figure 21.20 During amniocentesis, amniotic fluid is aspirated into a syringe.

LEARNING OBJECTIVE 1

Describe the various psychologic responses to antenatal testing.

CONCEPTS FOR LECTURE

1. Although some antenatal tests are viewed as routine and an expected part of prenatal care, others may evoke fear and anxiety. Ultrasound provides confirmation of a viable pregnancy, may identify the sex of the fetus, and may promote psychologic preparation for attachment after the birth. More invasive testing, however, may create anxiety due to the risks to the fetus and the woman and the implications of the test results.

POWERPOINT LECTURE SLIDES

(NOTE: The number on each PPT Lecture Slide directly corresponds with the Concepts for Lecture.)

 Psychologic Response to Testing (Figure 21.1)
- Routine part of care
- Confirmation of viability
- Psychologic preparation for attachment
- Fear and anxiety

 See Figure 21.1

SUGGESTIONS FOR CLASSROOM ACTIVITIES

Have students role play a discussion between a practitioner and a couple discussing antenatal testing. Discuss the concerns and feelings of the couple.

LEARNING OBJECTIVE 2

Identify indications and interpret findings for ultrasound examinations performed in the first trimester.

CONCEPTS FOR LECTURE

1. A transvaginal or abdominal sonogram early in pregnancy can be done to establish an accurate gestational age using the crown-rump length if performed between 6 and 10 weeks' gestation. A combination of ultrasound and maternal serum testing called nuchal translucency testing is done to screen fetuses between 11 weeks and 1 day and 13 weeks and 6 days to assess fetal risk for chromosomal disorders such as Down syndrome.

POWERPOINT LECTURE SLIDES

(NOTE: The number on each PPT Lecture Slide directly corresponds with the Concepts for Lecture.)

 First Trimester Ultrasound
- Establish gestational age
  - Crown to rump length
  - Most accurate between 6 and 10 weeks
- Nuchal translucency testing
  - Combined ultrasound and serum testing
  - Risk for chromosomal disorder
  - Screened between 11 weeks and 1 day and 16 weeks and 7 days

SUGGESTIONS FOR CLINICAL ACTIVITIES

Have students view an ultrasound in a clinical facility and observe gestational age determination in a first trimester client.

LEARNING OBJECTIVE 3

Describe the procedures used in the first trimester to confirm fetal viability.

CONCEPTS FOR LECTURE

1. Viability is defined as the potential for a pregnancy to result in the birth of a live infant. First trimester viability can be ascertained through serial detection of the beta hCG hormone, progesterone-level testing, and ultrasound.

POWERPOINT LECTURE SLIDES

(NOTE: The number on each PPT Lecture Slide directly corresponds with the Concepts for Lecture.)

 First Trimester Viability Confirmation
- Serial quantitative serum beta hCG testing
- Progesterone
- Ultrasound

LEARNING OBJECTIVE 4

Delineate the use of ultrasound in the second trimester to assess fetal life, number, presentation, anatomy, age, and growth.

CONCEPTS FOR LECTURE

1. Ultrasound is used in the second trimester to identify multiple gestation and fetal position, to measure the amount of amniotic fluid, and to identify fetal abnormalities. Fetal measurement is done using the Hadlock method, which uses average measures of the biparietal diameter, head circumference, abdominal circumference, and femur length to estimate gestational age. Uterine anatomy can also be assessed during this time.

POWERPOINT LECTURE SLIDES

(NOTE: The number on each PPT Lecture Slide directly corresponds with the Concepts for Lecture.)

 Second Trimester Ultrasound
- Fetal life
- Fetal number
- Fetal presentation
- Fetal anatomy
- Gestational age
- Amniotic fluid index

 Second Trimester Ultrasound
- Placental position
- Uterus

SUGGESTIONS FOR CLASSROOM ACTIVITIES

Discuss the significance of finding of second trimester ultrasound testing for the client.

SUGGESTIONS FOR CLINICAL ACTIVITIES

Have students observe a second trimester ultrasound in the clinical setting.

Compare the indications and procedures for fetal movement awareness, the nonstress test, vibroacoustic stimulation, the contraction stress test, biophysical profile, and amniotic fluid index.

CONCEPTS FOR LECTURE

1. The assessment of fetal movement is a noninvasive, cost-effective method of fetal surveillance and serves as an indirect measure of fetal central nervous system integrity and function. Vigorous movement indicates fetal well-being. Decreased fetal movement is often associated with chronic complications that compromise the fetal status.

2. A nonstress test (NST) evaluates fetal well-being using an electronic fetal monitor to obtain a tracing of the fetal heart rate (FHR), observing for accelerations with fetal movement. Accelerations imply an intact central and autonomic nervous system that is not being affected by hypoxia. NSTs are reported as reactive (two or more fetal heart accelerations within a 20-minute period) or nonreactive. The acceleration must be at least 15 beats per minute above the baseline and last 15 seconds. Vibroacoustic stimulation (VAS) is used to stimulate movement in the fetus through the application of sound and vibration to the mother's abdomen. This is used in addition to the NST to stimulate the accelerations.

3. The contraction stress test (CST) is used to evaluate the respiratory function of the placenta by examining the response of the FHR to the stress of uterine contractions. If there is insufficient placental reserve, fetal hypoxia, depression of the myocardium, and a decrease of FHR will occur. Pitocin may be used to stimulate contractions; however, the most common method is breast self-stimulation. The results are reported as negative, positive, equivocal, or unsatisfactory.
   Negative The absence of late or significant variable decelerations.
   Positive The presence of late decelerations.
   Equivocal-suspicious The presence of intermittent late decelerations or significant variable decelerations should be viewed as a suspicious finding that merits follow-up testing.
   Equivocal-hyperstimulatory FHR decelerations may occur in the presence of contractions that occur more frequently than every 2 minutes or that last longer than 90 seconds.
   Unsatisfactory The CST cannot be interpreted if fewer than three contractions lasting 40 to 60 seconds occur in a 10-minute window of time.

4. Amniotic fluid volume assessment is done to assess for decreased uteroplacental perfusion, which may lead to diminished renal blood flow, decreased urination, and oligohydramnios. An amniotic fluid index (AFI) of 5 or less indicates risk.

5. A biophysical profile (BPP) assesses five fetal biophysical variables: FHR acceleration, fetal breathing, fetal movements, fetal tone, and amniotic fluid volume

POWERPOINT LECTURE SLIDES

(NOTE: The number on each PPT Lecture Slide directly corresponds with the Concepts for Lecture.)

1 Fetal Movement
- Noninvasive
- Cost-effective
- Indirect measure of the fetal central nervous system (CNS)
- Vigorous movement indicates fetal well-being
- Decreased movement is associated with chronic oxygen compromise

2 Nonstress Test (NST) (Figures 21.11 and 21.12)
- Accelerations imply an intact CNS
- Acceleration patterns are affected by gestational age
- Accelerations must be 15 beats per minute above baseline, lasting 15 seconds
- Reactive—two or more accelerations within 20 minutes
- Nonreactive—insufficient accelerations over 40 minutes

2a See Figure 21.11

2b See Figure 21.12

2c Vibroacoustic Stimulation (VAS) (Figure 21.13)
- Application of sound and vibration to stimulate fetal movement
- Used to facilitate NST

2d See Figure 21.13

3 Contraction Stress Test (CST)
- Evaluates uteroplacental function
- Identifies intrauterine hypoxia
- Observes FHR response to contractions
- If compromised, FHR will decrease

3a Interpretation of CST (Figures 21.14 and 21.15)
- Negative
- Positive
- Equivocal-suspicious
- Equivocal-hyperstimulatory
- Unsatisfactory

3b See Figure 21.14

3c See Figure 21.15

4 Amniotic Fluid Index (AFI)
- Decreased uteroplacental perfusion results in oligohydramnios
- AFI of five or less requires further evaluation

5 Biophysical Profile (BPP)
- Fetal heart rate acceleration
- Fetal breathing

using electronic fetal monitoring and ultrasound. Each normal variable is assigned a score of 2 and abnormal variables a score of 0 (zero). A score of 8 out of a possible 10 indicates fetal well-being.

- Fetal movements
- Fetal tone
- Amniotic fluid volume

SUGGESTIONS FOR CLASSROOM ACTIVITIES

Bring in sample fetal monitoring strips from NSTs and CSTs and ask students to interpret them.

SUGGESTIONS FOR CLINICAL ACTIVITIES

Have students observe an NST, a CST, and/or a BPP performed on a client in the clinical setting. Ask students to interpret the findings and implications for the client and her baby.

LEARNING OBJECTIVE 6

Explain the purpose of maternal serum alpha-fetoprotein testing and the implications of abnormal values.

CONCEPTS FOR LECTURE

1. Maternal serum alpha-fetoprotein (MSAFP) is part of the quadruple check that utilizes multiple markers including alpha fetoprotein (AFP), hCG, diameric inhibin-A, and estriol to screen pregnancies for neural tube defect (NTD), trisomy 21 (Down syndrome), and trisomy 18. The test is done between 15 and 22 weeks' gestation. High levels indicate a higher risk for a fetus with a neural tube deficit. Low levels indicate a higher risk for a fetus with Down syndrome or a trisomy.

POWERPOINT LECTURE SLIDES

(NOTE: The number on each PPT Lecture Slide directly corresponds with the Concepts for Lecture.)

 Maternal Serum Alpha-Fetoprotein
- Component of quadruple check
- Screening test for
  - Neural tube defects
  - Trisomy 21 (Down syndrome)
  - Trisomy 18
- Performed between 15 and 22 weeks of gestation

SUGGESTIONS FOR CLASSROOM ACTIVITIES

Discuss the psychosocial implications of an abnormal MSAFP and ways that nurses can address client concerns.

LEARNING OBJECTIVE 7

Contrast the use of amniocentesis and chorionic villus sampling in detecting a fetus with a chromosomal disorder.

CONCEPTS FOR LECTURE

1. An amniocentesis is used for genetic diagnosis. It is done by obtaining a small amount of amniotic fluid through a sterile needle inserted into the uterine cavity under ultrasound guidance so that genetic testing can be performed. It is done between 15 and 20 weeks' gestation. Complications, although infrequent, may include transient vaginal spotting, cramping, or amniotic fluid leakage. The complication and pregnancy loss rate is higher when the amniocentesis is performed early (11 to 14 weeks).

2. Chorionic villi sampling (CVS) is also used to detect genetic, metabolic, and DNA abnormalities. Under ultrasound guidance, a small sample (5 to 40 mg) of chorionic villi from the edge of the developing placenta is retrieved. The advantage of a CVS is that an earlier diagnosis can be obtained; however, CVS cannot detect neural tube defects. There is a higher risk of spontaneous abortion with CVS and limb reduction may occur when the CVS is performed before $9\frac{1}{2}$ weeks' gestation.

POWERPOINT LECTURE SLIDES

(NOTE: The number on each PPT Lecture Slide directly corresponds with the Concepts for Lecture.)

 Amniocentesis (Figure 21.19)
- Used to detect genetic, metabolic, and DNA abnormalities
- Can detect neural tube defects
- Amniotic fluid obtained through needle aspiration
- Complications include
  - Vaginal spotting and cramping
  - Mild fluid leaking

[1a] See Figure 21.19

[2] Chorionic Villus Sampling (CVS)
- Used to detect genetic, metabolic, and DNA abnormalities
- Needle aspiration of chorionic villi from placenta

- Earlier diagnosis than amniocentesis
- Cannot detect neural tube defects
- Pregnancy loss is twice as high as with amniocentesis
- Potential for limb reduction

SUGGESTIONS FOR CLINICAL ACTIVITIES

Have students observe an amniocentesis and/or CVS in the clinical setting.

LEARNING OBJECTIVE 8

Discuss fetal fibronectin and transvaginal measurement of cervical length as predictors of preterm labor.

CONCEPTS FOR LECTURE

1. The presence of fetal fibronectin (fFN) in the cervix or vagina between 20 and 34 weeks' gestation has been shown to be a strong predictor of preterm delivery due to spontaneous preterm labor or premature rupture of membranes. fFN levels may be measured in combination with an ultrasound assessment to measure cervical length and dilatation of the internal cervical os. A shortened cervix and dilated internal os have been associated with preterm birth. Transvaginal assessment of cervical length and dilatation alone may result in a false-positive result.

POWERPOINT LECTURE SLIDES

(NOTE: The number on each PPT Lecture Slide directly corresponds with the Concepts for Lecture.)

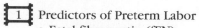 Predictors of Preterm Labor
- Fetal fibronectin (fFN)
  - Presence between 20 and 34 weeks is predictor of preterm delivery
- Cervical length and internal os
  - Measured by ultrasound
  - Shortened cervix and dilated internal os can predict preterm birth
  - False-positive common

LEARNING OBJECTIVE 9

Discuss how the lecithin/sphingomyelin ratio of the amniotic fluid and phosphatidylglycerol (PG) can be used to assess fetal lung maturity.

CONCEPTS FOR LECTURE

1. As assessment of fetal lung maturity can be done by determining the ratio of two components of surfactant—lecithin and sphingomyelin—in the amniotic fluid. A ratio of 2 to 1 indicates that respiratory distress syndrome (RDS) is unlikely. An assessment for the presence of phosphatidylglycerol (PG) can also be done. PG is also abundant in surfactant and appears at about 36 weeks' gestation. The presence of PG indicates a low risk for RDS.

POWERPOINT LECTURE SLIDES

(NOTE: The number on each PPT Lecture Slide directly corresponds with the Concepts for Lecture.)

Fetal Lung Maturity
- Lecithin/sphingomyelin ratio
  - Ratio of 2 to 1 indicates fetal lung maturity
- Phosphatidylglycerol (PG)
  - Presence indicates fetal lung maturity

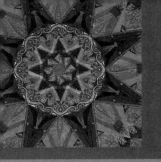

CHAPTER 22
PROCESSES AND STAGES OF LABOR AND BIRTH

RESOURCE LIBRARY

PRENTICE HALL NURSING MEDIALINK DVD-ROM

Audio Glossary
NCLEX Review
Videos: *Fetal Lie; First Stage of Labor; First Stage of Labor—Transition; Second Stage of Labor; Third Stage of Labor—Part 1; Third Stage of Labor—Part 2; Third Stage of Labor—Part 3; Through the Eyes of a Nurse—The Third Trimester*
Animations: *Rupturing Membranes; Placental Delivery*

COMPANION WEBSITE

Additional NCLEX Review
Case Study: *Client in First Stage of Labor*
Care Plan Activities: *Teenage Client in Uncomplicated Labor; Labor Progress in the First Stage of Labor*
Applications: *Normal Labor and Delivery; Breech Presentation*
Critical Thinking

IMAGE LIBRARY

Figure 22.1 Superior view of the fetal skull.
Figure 22.2 Lateral view of the fetal skull identifying the landmarks that have significance during birth.
Figure 22.3 *A,* Anteroposterior diameters of the fetal skull. *B,* Transverse diameters of the fetal skull.
Figure 22.4 Fetal attitude.
Figure 22.5 Cephalic presentation.
Figure 22.6 Process of engagement in cephalic presentation.
Figure 22.7 Measuring the station of the fetal head while it is descending.
Figure 22.8 Categories of presentation.
Figure 22.9 Characteristics of uterine contractions.

Figure 22.10 Effacement of the cervix in the primigravida.
Figure 22.11 The birth sequence.
Figure 22.12 Mechanisms of labor.
Figure 22.13 Placental separation and expulsion.
Figure 22.14 Pain pathway from uterus to spinal cord.
Figure 22.15 Area of reference of labor pain during the first stage.
Figure 22.16 Distribution of labor pain during the later phase of the first stage and early phase of the second stage.
Figure 22.17 Distribution of labor pain during the later phase of the second stage and actual birth.

LEARNING OBJECTIVE 1

Examine the five critical factors that affect the labor process.

CONCEPTS FOR LECTURE

1. There are five factors that are important in the process of labor and birth, including the birth passageway (birth canal), the passenger (fetus), the physiologic forces of labor, the position of the mother, and the woman's psychosocial considerations. These factors are dependent on each other.
2. Critical interacting factors of the passenger are: the fetal head, fetal attitude, fetal lie, fetal presentation, and fetal position.
3. The relation of the fetal body parts to one another is the fetal attitude. Flexion is the normal attitude of the fetus.
4. The relationship of the long, or cephalocaudal, axis (spinal column) of the fetus to the long, or cephalocaudal, axis of the mother is fetal lie. It may either be a longitudinal (vertical) or a transverse (horizontal) lie.

POWERPOINT LECTURE SLIDES

(NOTE: The number on each PPT Lecture Slide directly corresponds with the Concepts for Lecture.)

1 Factors Affecting Labor Progress
- The birth passageway (birth canal)
- The passenger (fetus)
- The physiologic forces of labor
- The position of the mother
- The woman's psychosocial considerations

2 Passenger
- Fetal head
- Fetal attitude
- Fetal lie
- Fetal presentation
- Fetal position

5. The body part of the fetus that enters the maternal pelvis first and leads through the birth canal during labor is fetal presentation. It may be cephalic (head first), breech (buttocks or feet first), or shoulder. When the largest diameter of the presenting part reaches or passes through the pelvic inlet, the fetus is engaged. The relationship of the presenting part to an imaginary line drawn between the ischial spines of the maternal pelvis is the station. A negative number is assigned if the presenting part is higher than the ischial spines. The midpelvis is zero station and the fetus progressively moves to positive stations during labor.

6. The relationship of the landmark on the presenting fetal part to the anterior, posterior, or sides (right or left) of the maternal pelvis is fetal position.

3 Fetal Attitude
- The relation of the fetal body parts to one another (Figure 22.4)
- Normal attitude is flexion

3a See Figure 22.4

4 Fetal Lie
- The relationship of spinal column of the fetus to that of the mother
- Longitudinal or transverse

5 Fetal Presentation
- Engagement
- Station (Figure 22.7)
- Ischial spines are zero station
- Presenting part moves from − to +

5a See Figure 22.7

6 Fetal Position
- Right (R) or left (L) side of the maternal pelvis
- Landmark: occiput (O), mentum (M), sacrum (S), or acromion (scapula[Sc]) process (A)
- Anterior (A), posterior (P), or transverse (T)

SUGGESTIONS FOR CLASSROOM ACTIVITIES

Bring models or charts to class depicting fetal attitude, fetal lie, and fetal position to help students understand the concepts.

LEARNING OBJECTIVE 2

Describe the physiology of labor.

CONCEPTS FOR LECTURE

1. The physiology of labor involves primary and secondary forces. The primary force is the uterine contractions. The secondary force is the involvement of the abdominal muscles to push during the second stage of labor.

2. Uterine contractions can be described in terms of frequency, duration, and intensity. The frequency is the timing between the beginning of one contraction to the beginning of the next contraction. Duration is measured from the beginning to the end of the contraction. The strength of the uterine contraction during the acme is intensity.

3. Softening, stretching, and thinning of the cervix are caused by uterine muscle contractions stimulated by estrogen, the breakdown of collagen fibers by collagenase and elastase, and an increase in the water content of the cervix. The physiologic retraction ring is the division of the uterus in true labor into two portions. As

POWERPOINT LECTURE SLIDES

(NOTE: The number on each PPT Lecture Slide directly corresponds with the Concepts for Lecture.)

1 Physiology of Labor
- Primary force is uterine muscular contractions
- Secondary force is pushing during the second stage of labor

2 Uterine Contractions (Figure 22.9)
- Frequency
- Duration
- Intensity

2a See Figure 22.9

3 Causes of Cervical Effacement
- Estrogen
  - Stimulates uterine muscle contractions
- Collagen fibers in the cervix are broken down
- Increase in the water content of the cervix

---

labor progresses, the upper portion, which is the contractile segment, becomes thicker. The passive lower segment expands and thins out as labor progresses. Each contraction causes the muscles of the upper uterine segment to shorten and exert a longitudinal traction on the cervix, causing effacement.

 Cervical Effacement (Figure 22.10)
- Physiologic retraction ring
- Upper uterine segment thickens and pulls up
- Lower segment expands and thins out
- Effacement

 See Figure 22.10

SUGGESTIONS FOR CLASSROOM ACTIVITIES

Bring fetal monitoring strips in for students to review contraction patterns. Bring in a cervical dilatation chart for students to view cervical changes.

SUGGESTIONS FOR CLINICAL ACTIVITIES

Have students review uterine contraction patterns on the fetal monitor and discuss the clinical implications.

LEARNING OBJECTIVE 3

Discuss premonitory signs of labor.

CONCEPTS FOR LECTURE

1. Premonitory signs of labor include lightening, Braxton Hicks contractions, ripening, bloody show, a sudden burst of energy, and rupture of membranes. As the fetus begins to settle into the pelvic inlet (engagement), lightening occurs. Before the onset of labor, irregular, intermittent contractions that have been occurring throughout the pregnancy (Braxton-Hicks) become more uncomfortable. Softening of the cervix under the influence of hormonal factors is called ripening. Passage of the mucous plug with a small amount of blood from exposed cervical capillaries occurs because of this. This discharge is called bloody show. Membranes may rupture (ROM) before the onset of labor and most of these women will experience spontaneous labor in 24 hours. There may be a sudden burst of energy approximately 24 to 48 hours before labor. Additional signs include the following: weight loss of 2.2 to 6.6 kg (1 to 3 lb) resulting from fluid loss and electrolyte shifts produced by changes in estrogen and progesterone levels, increased backache and sacroiliac pressure from the influence of relaxin hormone on the pelvic joints, and diarrhea, indigestion, or nausea and vomiting just before the onset of labor.

POWERPOINT LECTURE SLIDES

(NOTE: The number on each PPT Lecture Slide directly corresponds with the Concepts for Lecture.)

 Premonitory Signs of Labor
- Lightening
- Braxton Hicks contractions
- Bloody show
- Rupture of membranes (ROM)
- Sudden burst of energy
- Weight loss

 Premonitory Signs of Labor
- Backache
- Nausea and vomiting
- Diarrhea

SUGGESTIONS FOR CLINICAL ACTIVITIES

Have students teach a class in a prenatal setting about premonitory signs of labor.

LEARNING OBJECTIVE 4

Differentiate between false and true labor.

CONCEPTS FOR LECTURE

1. In true labor, contractions produce progressive dilatation and effacement of the cervix. These contractions occur regularly and increase in frequency, duration, and intensity. Labor pain usually starts in the back and radiates around to the abdomen and is not relieved by ambulation.

2. In false labor, contractions do not produce progressive cervical effacement and dilatation. They are irregular and do not increase in frequency, duration, and intensity. Pain from these contractions occurs mainly in the lower abdomen and the groin and may be relieved by ambulation, changes of position, resting, or a hot bath or shower.

POWERPOINT LECTURE SLIDES

(NOTE: The number on each PPT Lecture Slide directly corresponds with the Concepts for Lecture.)

1 True Labor
- Progressive dilatation and effacement
- Regular contractions increasing in frequency, duration, and intensity
- Pain usually starts in the back and radiates to the abdomen
- Pain is not relieved by ambulation or by resting

2 False Labor
- Lack of cervical effacement and dilatation
- Irregular contractions do not increase in frequency, duration, and intensity
- Contractions occur mainly in the lower abdomen and groin
- Pain may be relieved by ambulation, changes of position, resting, or a hot bath or shower

LEARNING OBJECTIVE 5

Describe the characteristics of the four stages of labor and their accompanying phases.

CONCEPTS FOR LECTURE

1. The first stage of labor is divided into the latent, active, and transition phases. The onset of regular contractions is the latent phase, with an increase in the frequency, duration, and intensity. In the active phase, the cervix dilates from about 4 to 7 cm and fetal descent is progressive. During the transition phase, cervical dilatation slows as it progresses from 8 to 10 cm and the rate of fetal descent increases.

2. From complete cervical dilatation to the birth of the infant is the second stage of labor.

3. The period of time from the birth of the infant until the completed delivery of the placenta is the third stage of labor.

4. The time from 1 to 4 hours after birth in which physiologic readjustment of the mother's body begins is the fourth stage of labor. There will be a cessation of nausea and vomiting, she may be thirsty and hungry, she may experience a shaking chill, and the bladder is often hypotonic due to trauma during the second stage and/or the administration of anesthetics. The uterus is contracted and midline and the fundus is usually midway between the symphysis pubis and umbilicus.

POWERPOINT LECTURE SLIDES

(NOTE: The number on each PPT Lecture Slide directly corresponds with the Concepts for Lecture.)

1 First Stage of Labor: Latent Phase
- Beginning cervical dilatation and effacement
- No evident fetal descent
- Uterine contractions increase in frequency, duration, and intensity
- Contractions are usually mild

1a First Stage of Labor: Active Phase
- Cervical dilatation from 4 to 7 cm
- Progressive fetal descent
- Contractions more frequent and intense

1b First Stage of Labor: Transition
- Cervical dilatation from 7 to 10 cm
- Progressive fetal descent
- Contractions more frequent and intense

2 Second Stage of Labor (Figure 22.12)
- Begins with complete dilatation (10 cm)
- Ends with birth of the baby

2a See Figure 22.12

3 Third Stage of Labor
- From birth of infant to delivery of placenta

POWERPOINT LECTURE SLIDES *continued*

 4 Fourth Stage of Labor
- First 4 hours after birth
- Physiologic readjustment
- Thirsty and hungry
- Shaking
- Bladder is often hypotonic
- Uterus remains contracted

SUGGESTIONS FOR CLASSROOM ACTIVITIES

Play the videos on the CD for the first stage of labor and transition, the second and third stages of labor, and the placental delivery animation.

SUGGESTIONS FOR CLINICAL ACTIVITIES

Have students observe a woman in labor and document the physical and psychologic changes experienced by the woman.

LEARNING OBJECTIVE 6

Describe the physiologic and psychosocial changes that are indicative of the maternal progress during each of the stages of labor.

CONCEPTS FOR LECTURE

1. During the latent phase of labor, the woman feels able to cope with the discomfort and she may be relieved that labor has finally started. Although she may be anxious, she is able to express those feelings of anxiety. During the active phase, anxiety increases as the contractions and pain intensify. She may also fear a loss of control and will use a variety of coping mechanisms. In the transition phase, the woman may withdraw into herself and may doubt her ability to cope with labor. She may be apprehensive and irritable and she may not want anyone to talk to her or touch her even though she is terrified of being alone. During the second stage of labor, a childbirth-prepared woman feels relieved that the acute pain she felt during the transition phase is over and that the birth is near and she can now push. She may feel a sense of control now that she can be actively involved. If she has not had childbirth preparation, she may become frightened and fight each contraction and instructions to push.

POWERPOINT LECTURE SLIDES

(NOTE: The number on each PPT Lecture Slide directly corresponds with the Concepts for Lecture.)

 1 Psychologic Adaptations: Latent Phase
- Feels able to cope with the discomfort
- May be relieved that labor has finally started
- Is able to recognize and express feelings of anxiety

1a Psychologic Adaptations: Active Phase
- Anxiety increases
- Fears loss of control
- May have decreased ability to cope

 1b Psychologic Adaptations: Transition Phase
- Withdraws into herself
- Doubts ability to cope
- Apprehensive and irritable
- Terrified of being alone
- Does not want anyone to talk to her or touch her

 1c Second Stage
- Relieved acute pain is over
- Relieved she can push
- Sense of control because actively involved
- May become frightened

SUGGESTIONS FOR CLASSROOM ACTIVITIES

Have a group discussion about nursing interventions to assist a woman during the various phases of labor.

SUGGESTIONS FOR CLINICAL ACTIVITIES

Have students assist a woman in labor, noting the psychologic changes and identifying interventions that were effective in assisting the woman.

LEARNING OBJECTIVE 7

Summarize maternal systemic responses to labor.

CONCEPTS FOR LECTURE

1. Nearly every major body system is affected by labor. There is a significant increase in cardiac output due to stress by uterine contractions, pain, and anxiety. This will also cause an increase in blood pressure. Intrathoracic pressure rises during bearing-down in the second stage. This is due to the Valsalva maneuver that is used when she holds her breath and pushes against a closed glottis. As this pressure increases, venous return is interrupted and venous pressure increases. When the woman stops pushing, intrathoracic pressure decreases and venous return increases, resulting in recovery of the cardiac output and stroke volume. Cardiac output peaks immediately after birth and then in the first 10 minutes, it decreases and continues to decrease in the first hour after birth. Diaphoresis occurs because of muscle activity during labor, which elevates the body temperature, thus increasing sweating and evaporation from the skin. There is also an evaporative water loss because of a rise in respiratory rate. There is an increase in oxygen demand and consumption at the onset of labor because of the presence of uterine contractions. A mild metabolic acidosis compensated by respiratory alkalosis occurs by the end of the first stage of labor. During the second stage of labor, the $PaCO_2$ levels may rise along with blood lactate levels and a mild respiratory acidosis occurs. At the end of the second stage, a metabolic acidosis uncompensated by respiratory alkalosis exists. During labor, polyuria is common due to an increase in cardiac output, causing an increase in the glomerular filtration rate and renal plasma flow. Some women may also experience proteinuria. Impairment of the blood and lymph drainage from the base of the bladder may also occur due to pressure from the presenting part.

There is a reduction in the gastric motility during labor, and gastric emptying time is prolonged. There is an increase in the white blood cell (WBC) count to 25,000/mm^3 to 30,000/mm^3 during labor and early postpartum due to increased neutrophils resulting from a physiologic response to stress. During labor, maternal blood glucose levels decrease and this leads to a decrease in insulin requirements. During the first stage of labor, pain comes from (1) dilatation of the cervix, (2) hypoxia of the uterine muscle cells during contraction, (3) stretching of the lower uterine segment, and (4) pressure on adjacent structures. Pain in the second stage of labor come from (1) hypoxia of the contracting uterine muscle cells, (2) distention of the vagina and perineum, and (3) pressure on adjacent structures including the lower back, buttocks, and thighs. During the third stage of labor, pain comes from uterine contractions and cervical dilatation as the placenta is expelled.

POWERPOINT LECTURE SLIDES

(NOTE: The number on each PPT Lecture Slide directly corresponds with the Concepts for Lecture.)

 Systemic Responses to Labor
- Changes in cardiac output
- Diaphoresis
- Hyperventilation
- Changes in ABG levels
- Polyuria
- Slight proteinuria

 Systemic Responses to Labor
- Reduced gastric motility
- Increased WBCs
- Decreased maternal blood glucose
- Pain

LEARNING OBJECTIVE 8

Describe fetal adaptations to labor.

CONCEPTS FOR LECTURE

1. A normal fetus will have no adverse effects from labor. Decelerations of the fetal heart rate can occur with intracranial pressures of 40 to 55 mm Hg. The fetal pH may decrease as the blood flow to the fetus is slowed during the acme of the contraction. A drop in fetal oxygen saturation and an increase in fetal base deficit and $PaCO_2$ occurs. Behavioral states are unchanged during labor.

POWERPOINT LECTURE SLIDES

(NOTE: The number on each PPT Lecture Slide directly corresponds with the Concepts for Lecture.)

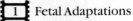 Fetal Adaptations
- Fetal heart rate decelerations due to intracranial pressure
- Quiet and awake state
- Aware of pressure sensations

SUGGESTIONS FOR CLINICAL ACTIVITIES

Have students review fetal monitoring strips to identify and discuss fetal heart rate changes and the potential physiologic causes of those changes.

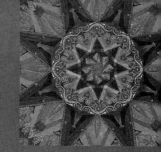

CHAPTER 23
INTRAPARTAL NURSING ASSESSMENT

RESOURCE LIBRARY

PRENTICE HALL NURSING MEDIALINK DVD-ROM

Audio Glossary
NCLEX Review
Videos: Leopold's Maneuvers *Monitoring a Fetal Heart Rate; through the eyes of a Nurse—The Third Trimester*
Critical Thinking

COMPANION WEBSITE

Additional NCLEX Review
Case Study: *Maternal Assessment During Labor*
Care Plan Activity: *Client with Decelerations*
Applications: *Fetal monitoring; Fetal Bradycardia*

IMAGE LIBRARY

Figure 23.1 Woman in labor with external monitor applied.

Figure 23.2 The beltless tocodynamometer system features remote telemetry.

Figure 23.3 INTRAN Plus intrauterine pressure catheter.

Figure 23.4 To gauge cervical dilatation, the nurse places the index and middle fingers against the cervix and determines the size of the opening.

Figure 23.5 Palpation of the presenting part (the portion of the fetus that enters the pelvis first).

Figure 23.6 Descent of the fetus through the maternal pelvis can be assessed by determining station (the relationship of the presenting part to an imaginary line between the maternal ischial spines).

Figure 23.7 Leopold's maneuvers for determining fetal head position, presentation, and lie.

Figure 23.8 *A*, When the fetal heart rate is picked up by the electronic monitor, the sound of the heartbeat can be heard by all persons in the room. *B*, The nurse uses a Doppler to assess the fetal heart rate.

Figure 23.9 Location of FHR in relation to the more commonly seen fetal positions.

Figure 23.10 Top, An FHR tracing obtained by internal monitoring.

Figure 23.11 Sinusoidal pattern.

Figure 23.12 *A* and *B*, Moderate variability. *C*, Minimal variability. *D*, Absent variability.

Figure 23.13 Marked variability.

Figure 23.14 Types of accelerations.

Figure 23.15 Types and characteristics of early, late, and variable decelerations.

Figure 23.16 Mechanism of early deceleration (head compression).

Figure 23.17 Early decelerations.

Figure 23.18 Mechanism of late deceleration.

Figure 23.19 Late decelerations.

Figure 23.20 Variable decelerations with overshoot.

Figure 23.21 Mechanism of variable deceleration.

Figure 23.22 Atypical variable decelerations.

Figure 23.23 The prolonged deceleration depicted lasts approximately 160 seconds.

LEARNING OBJECTIVE 1

Summarize intrapartal physical, psychosocial, and cultural assessments necessary for optimum maternal-fetal outcome.

CONCEPTS FOR LECTURE

1. A patient history and screening for intrapartal risk factors is the first step in optimizing maternal-fetal outcome. Historical data include the patient's demographic and socioeconomic information as well as the medical, surgical, family, obstetrical, and gynecological histories. A psychosocial assessment is a critical component of an intrapartal nursing assessment. The woman's ideas, knowledge, and fears about childbearing should be assessed. It is also important to assess the adequacy of resources, such as housing, transportation, utilities, and access to social services. A cultural assessment will

POWERPOINT LECTURE SLIDES

(NOTE: The number on each PPT Lecture Slide directly corresponds with the Concepts for Lecture.)

 Intrapartal Assessment
- Historical data
- Physical assessment
- Psychosocial history and status
- Cultural assessment

 Physical Assessment
- Vital signs and weight
- Lungs
- Fundus

provide information about the patient's values, beliefs, and customs related to childbearing.

2. The physical assessment should include: assessment of vital signs, weight, lungs, the location of the fundus, signs of dependent edema, hydration, and mucous discharge and bloody show.

3. Assessment of the labor status includes: contraction pattern, cervical dilatation and effacement, fetal descent, and the status of the membranes.

4. Assessment of the fetus should include: FHR, presentation, position, and fetal activity.

5. A psychosocial assessment should include assessment of: preparation for childbirth, response to labor, feelings of anxiety, and available support system.

- Edema
- Hydration
- Perineum

 Labor Status
- Uterine contractions
- Cervical dilatation
- Cervical effacement
- Fetal descent
- Membranes

 Fetal Status
- FHR
- Presentation
- Position
- Activity

Psychosocial Assessment
- Preparation for childbirth
- Response to labor
- Anxiety
- Support system

SUGGESTIONS FOR CLASSROOM ACTIVITIES

Have students role play doing admission assessment interviews with each other. Give them feedback on their interviewing techniques.

SUGGESTIONS FOR CLINICAL ACTIVITIES

Have students observe the admission assessment of a woman admitted to Labor and Delivery and document their observations.

LEARNING OBJECTIVE 2

Define the outer limits of normal progress of each of the phases and stages of labor.

CONCEPTS FOR LECTURE

1. During the latent phase of labor, contractions will initially occur every 10–30 minutes, lasting 20–40 seconds with mild intensity; then, the contractions will progress to every 5–7 minutes, lasting 30–40 seconds with moderate intensity. During the active phase of labor, contractions will occur every 2–3 minutes, last 40 seconds, and be moderate to strong in intensity. During the transition phase of labor, contractions will occur every $1\frac{1}{2}$–2minutes, last 60–90 seconds, and be strong in intensity.

POWERPOINT LECTURE SLIDES

(NOTE: The number on each PPT Lecture Slide directly corresponds with the Concepts for Lecture.)

 Labor Progress
- Latent phase contractions
  - Every 10–30 minutes × 30–40 seconds, mild
  - Progresses to every 5–7 minutes × 30–40 seconds, moderate
- Active phase contractions
  - Every 2–3 minutes × 40–60 seconds, moderate to strong

 Labor Progress
- Transition phase contractions
  - Every $1\frac{1}{2}$–2 minutes × 60–90 seconds, strong

SUGGESTIONS FOR CLASSROOM ACTIVITIES

Have students draw a labor chart to designate changes that will occur during the phases of labor.

SUGGESTIONS FOR CLINICAL ACTIVITIES

Ask students to review the labor progress chart of a woman who delivered. Have them note the physical changes that occurred with each phase.

LEARNING OBJECTIVE 3

Compare the various methods of monitoring fetal heart rate and contractions, giving advantages and disadvantages of each.

CONCEPTS FOR LECTURE

1. Monitoring uterine contractions by palpation allows the nurse to assess relative frequency, duration, and a subjective assessment of contraction strength and uterine resting tone. The advantages of palpation include the following: palpation is noninvasive and does not increase the risk for infection or patient injury; it is readily accessible, requiring no equipment; it increases the "hands on" care of the patient that can be reassuring to the patient; and it allows the mother freedom from restricting and sometimes uncomfortable abdominal belts. Limitations to palpation include the following: palpation does not provide an actual quantitative measure of uterine pressure, there is no permanent record, and direct palpation may be difficult due to maternal size and adipose tissue.

2. External electronic uterine monitoring is done using a tocodynamometer or tocotransducer (toco). Advantages of external electronic uterine monitoring are that it is noninvasive, easy to place, may be used both before and following rupture of membranes, and provides a permanent record. Limitations of external electronic uterine monitoring include: potential inaccurate graphic tracing due to incorrect placement of the tocotransducer, belts may cause patient discomfort, and patient movement may be limited.

3. Internal electronic monitoring of UCs can be done using an intrauterine pressure catheter (IUPC). The benefits of internal uterine monitoring include the provision of a near-exact pressure measurement for contraction intensity and uterine resting tone, increased sensitivity allows for very accurate timing of UCs, and it provides a permanent record. Limitations and risks of internal uterine monitoring include the need for adequate cervical dilation for insertion, invasiveness, and increased risk of uterine infection or uterine perforation or trauma.

4. Assessment of the fetal heart rate can be done by auscultation. Benefits of auscultation include a minimal use of instrumentation, portability, and maximum maternal movement. Disadvantages of auscultation include limited data and lack of a permanent record. The only data that this method can provide is baseline fetal heart rate (BL FHR), rhythms of the FHR, and obvious increases and decreases that can be monitored.

5. A continuous tracing of the FHR is provided using external electronic fetal monitoring (EFM). An ultrasound (US) transducer is used for external EFM. Benefits of external EFM include: the provision of a continuous graphic recording; availability of baseline information, baseline variability, and changes in the FHR; it is noninvasive; and it does not require rupture of membranes or minimal cervical dilation. Limitations of external EFM include: susceptibility to interference from

POWERPOINT LECTURE SLIDES

(NOTE: The number on each PPT Lecture Slide directly corresponds with the Concepts for Lecture.)

1 Palpation: Advantages
- Noninvasive
- Readily accessible, requiring no equipment
- Increases the "hands on" care of the patient
- Allows the mother freedom

1a Palpation: Disadvantages
- Does not provide actual quantitative measure of uterine pressure
- No permanent record
- Maternal size and positioning may prevent direct palpation

2 External Electronic Uterine Monitoring: Advantages
- Noninvasive
- Easy to place
- May be used before and following rupture of membranes
- Can be used intermittently
- Provides a permanent, continuous recording

2a External Electronic Uterine Monitoring: Disadvantages
- The nurse must compare subjective findings with monitor
- The belt may become uncomfortable
- The belt may require frequent readjustment
- The mother may feel inhibited to move

3 Internal Electronic Uterine Monitoring: Advantages (Figure 23.3)
- Provides pressure measurements for contraction intensity and uterine resting tone
- Allows for very accurate timing of UCs
- Provides a permanent record of the uterine activity

3a Internal Electronic Uterine Monitoring: Disadvantages
- Membranes must be ruptured and adequate cervical dilation must be achieved
- Invasive
- Increases the risk of uterine infection or perforation
- Contraindicated in cases with active infections
- Use with a low-lying placenta can result in placenta puncture

3b See Figure 23.3

4 Auscultation: Advantages
- Uses minimum instrumentation
- Is portable

maternal and fetal movement and the tracing may become sketchy and difficult to interpret.

6. A fetal scalp electrode (FSE) is used for internal fetal heart rate monitoring. A fine surgical spiral wire is attached to the fetal scalp or other presenting part. Benefits of this type of monitoring include clearer tracings and the provision of information about short-term variability. The major disadvantages are the risk for infection and injury.

- Allows for maximum maternal movement
- Convenient and economical

 Auscultation: Disadvantages
- Can only provide the baseline fetal heart rate, rhythms, and obvious increases and decreases
- Does not provide a permanent record

 External Electronic Fetal Heart Monitoring Advantages
- Produces a continuous graphic recording
- Can show the baseline, baseline variability, and changes in the FHR
- Noninvasive
- Does not require rupture of membranes

 External Electronic Fetal Heart Monitoring Disadvantages
- Is susceptible to interference from maternal and fetal movement
- May produce a weak signal
- Tracing may become sketchy and difficult to interpret

 Internal Electronic Fetal Heart Monitoring Advantages
- Clearer tracings
- Provides information about short-term variability

 Internal Electronic Fetal Heart Monitoring Disadvantages
- Infection
- Injury
- Requires ruptured membranes and sufficient cervical dilatation

---

SUGGESTIONS FOR CLASSROOM ACTIVITIES

Bring in an ultrasound transducer, a tocodynamometer, belts, and a pregnant belly model to demonstrate to the students how the equipment is used.

SUGGESTIONS FOR CLINICAL ACTIVITIES

Have students do an assessment of a fetal heart rate using first auscultation and then the ultrasound transducer and compare the results. Have students assess the uterine contractions using palpation and the tocodynamometer and compare the results.

LEARNING OBJECTIVE 4

Describe the procedure for performing Leopold's maneuvers and the information that can be obtained.

CONCEPTS FOR LECTURE

1. A systematic way of evaluating the maternal abdomen is called Leopold's maneuvers. In the first maneuver, while facing the woman, the nurse palpates the upper abdomen to determine what part of the fetus occupies the fundus. The nurse then palpates for the fetal back and determines whether it is on the right or left side. The second maneuver involves the palpation of the abdomen with deep but gentle pressure using the palms to explore both sides of the uterus. The third maneuver

POWERPOINT LECTURE SLIDES

(NOTE: The number on each PPT Lecture Slide directly corresponds with the Concepts for Lecture.)

 Leopold's Maneuvers (Figure 23.7)
- Is the fetal lie longitudinal or transverse?
- What is in the fundus? Am I feeling buttocks or head?
- Where is the fetal back?
- Where are the small parts or extremities?

involves determining what fetal part is lying above the inlet by grasping the lower part of the abdomen with the thumb and fingers of the right hand. In the fourth maneuver, the nurse attempts to locate the cephalic prominence or brow by facing the woman's feet and moving the fingers of both hands gently down the sides of the uterus toward the pubis. The brow is found where there is greatest resistance to the fingers.

- What is in the inlet? Does it confirm what I found in the fundus?
- Is the presenting part engaged, floating, or dipping into the inlet?

 See Figure 23.7

SUGGESTIONS FOR CLASSROOM ACTIVITIES

Bring a pregnant abdominal model to class and demonstrate to the students how to do Leopold's maneuvers. Have them practice with the model.

SUGGESTIONS FOR CLINICAL ACTIVITIES

Have students assess the fetal position of a pregnant woman in clinical using Leopold's maneuvers.

LEARNING OBJECTIVE 5

Differentiate between baseline and periodic changes in the fetal heart rate.

CONCEPTS FOR LECTURE

1. The mean FHR during a 10-minute period rounded to increments of 5 beats per minute (bpm) is the baseline rate. This excludes periodic or episodic changes in FHR, periods of marked FHR variability, or segments of baseline (BL) that differ by more than 25 bpm. A minimum of 2 minutes of the baseline must be observed in any 10-minute segment in either 2 consecutive minutes or two 1 minute segments. Intermittent or transient deviations or changes from the baseline are commonly referred to as accelerations and decelerations. These may be episodic or periodic. Those that are not associated with uterine contractions are episodic. Changes occurring with uterine contractions are periodic.

POWERPOINT LECTURE SLIDES

(NOTE: The number on each PPT Lecture Slide directly corresponds with the Concepts for Lecture.)

 Fetal Heart Rate (FHR) (Figure 23.10)
- Baseline FHR
  - Mean FHR during 10-minute period
  - Must be observed for 2 minutes
- Changes in FHR
  - Episodic—not associated with uterine contractions
  - Periodic—associated with uterine contractions

 See Figure 23.10

SUGGESTIONS FOR CLASSROOM ACTIVITIES

Bring in sample electronic fetal monitoring strips for students to practice assessing baseline fetal heart rate.

SUGGESTIONS FOR CLINICAL ACTIVITIES

Have students assess the fetal tracing of a woman in labor for baseline fetal heart rate and the presence of episodic or periodic changes.

LEARNING OBJECTIVE 6

Identify the differences between fetal tachycardia and fetal bradycardia.

CONCEPTS FOR LECTURE

1. A FHR baseline greater than 160 bpm for at least a 10-minute period is defined as tachycardia. A FHR baseline less than 110 bpm for at least a 10-minute period is defined as bradycardia.

POWERPOINT LECTURE SLIDES

(NOTE: The number on each PPT Lecture Slide directly corresponds with the Concepts for Lecture.)

 Changes in FHR Baseline
- Fetal tachycardia
  - Baseline greater than 160 bpm for at least a 10-minute period
- Fetal bradycardia
  - Baseline less than 110 bpm for at least a 10-minute period

LEARNING OBJECTIVE 7

Identify fetal heart rates and patterns using National Institute of Child Health and Human Development (NICHD) terminology.

CONCEPTS FOR LECTURE

1. A smooth, unsteady baseline that fluctuates in the normal baseline range without variability is called a wandering baseline. A FHR pattern consisting of a series of cycles that are extremely smooth and regular in amplitude and duration is a sinusoidal baseline. An acceleration is an increase in the BL FHR, with an onset-to-peak of less than 30 seconds beginning at the most recent calculated baseline. Accelerations can be either episodic or periodic. A reliable indicator of fetal cardiac and neurological function and well-being is baseline variability (BV). BV is defined as baseline fluctuations of 2 cycles per minute or greater, and it is classified by the visually quantified amplitude of peak-to-trough in beats per minute. It is classified into four categories: (1) absent (amplitude undetected); (2) minimal (amplitude range detectable but $\leq$ 5 bpm); (3) moderate (amplitude range of 6–25 bpm); and (4) marked (amplitude greater than 25 bpm).

2. Decelerations are defined as decreases in the FHR below the baseline. They are classified by their shape, appearance, rate of descent, and timing in relationship to uterine contractions. Decelerations are classified into two types based on the rate at which the fetal heart rate descends after it leaves the FHR baseline. Abrupt decelerations occur in less than 30 seconds. Gradual decelerations require 30 seconds or longer. Decelerations can be episodic or periodic. Classification of periodic decelerations is determined by their timing in respect to the uterine contractions. Decelerations that occur simultaneously with UCs are early decelerations; these are due to vagal nerve stimulation caused by the fetal head. The onset, nadir, and recovery of late decelerations occur after the beginning, peak, and end of the contraction, respectively; these are due to placental insufficiency. Variable decelerations anytime within the uterine contraction can occur either early or late with respect to a UC; these are due to cord compression.

POWERPOINT LECTURE SLIDES

(NOTE: The number on each PPT Lecture Slide directly corresponds with the Concepts for Lecture.)

1 NICHD Classification: Baseline FHR
- Tachycardia
- Bradycardia
- Accelerations (Figure 23.14)
- Sinusoidal

1a See Figure 23.14

1b NICHD Classification: Baseline Variability (BV) (Figure 23.12)
- Absent—amplitude undetected
- Minimal—amplitude range detectable but $\leq$ 5 bpm
- Moderate—amplitude range of 6–25 bpm
- Marked—amplitude greater than 25 bpm

1c See Figure 23.12 A–B

2 NICHD Classifications: Decelerations
- Rate of descent
- Episodic
- Periodic
  - Early (Figure 23.17)
  - Late (Figure 23.19)
  - Variable (Figure 23.20)

2a See Figure 23.17

2b See Figure 23.19

2c See Figure 23.20

LEARNING OBJECTIVE 8

Outline the steps to be performed in the systematic evaluation of fetal heart rate tracings.

CONCEPTS FOR LECTURE

1. To assess the uterine contraction pattern, first determine the uterine resting tone, and then assess the contractions for frequency, duration, and intensity. To evaluate the fetal heart tracing the following steps should be used: (1) determine the baseline, (2) determine FHR variability, (3) determine whether a sinusoidal pattern is present, and (4) determine whether there are periodic changes. The FHR tracing should then be classified as reassuring or nonreassuring.

POWERPOINT LECTURE SLIDES

(NOTE: The number on each PPT Lecture Slide directly corresponds with the Concepts for Lecture.)

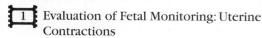 Evaluation of Fetal Monitoring: Uterine Contractions
- Determine the uterine resting tone
- Assess the contractions
  - What is the frequency?
  - What is the duration?
  - What is the intensity (if internal monitoring)?

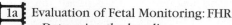 Evaluation of Fetal Monitoring: FHR
- Determine the baseline
- Determine FHR variability
- Determine whether a sinusoidal pattern is present
- Determine whether there are periodic changes

SUGGESTIONS FOR CLINICAL ACTIVITIES

Have students do a systematic assessment of a fetal monitoring strip using the steps mentioned above.

LEARNING OBJECTIVE 9

List factors to consider in evaluation of abnormal findings on a fetal heart rate tracing.

CONCEPTS FOR LECTURE

1. The following are characteristics on nonreassuring patterns: (1) variable decelerations dropping below 70 bpm for longer than 30 to 45 seconds and accompanied by rising baseline or decreasing variability, (2) late decelerations of any magnitude, (3) absence of variability, (4) prolonged deceleration lasting 2 minutes but less than 10 minutes, and (5) severe bradycardia of 70 bpm or less.

POWERPOINT LECTURE SLIDES

(NOTE: The number on each PPT Lecture Slide directly corresponds with the Concepts for Lecture.)

Nonreassuring Patterns
- Variable decelerations
- Late decelerations of any magnitude
- Absence of variability
- Prolonged deceleration
- Severe (marked) bradycardia

SUGGESTIONS FOR CLASSROOM ACTIVITIES

Bring examples of both reassuring and nonreassuring strips to class and ask students to identify them as such.

LEARNING OBJECTIVE 10

Identify the interventions that are indicated when a nonreassuring fetal heart rate pattern is identified.

CONCEPTS FOR LECTURE

1. The following are nursing interventions for moderate variable decelerations: report findings to physician/CNM and document in chart, provide explanation to the woman and her partner, change maternal position, discontinue oxytocin if it is being administered, perform a vaginal examination to assess for prolapsed cord or change in labor progress, and monitor FHR continuously

POWERPOINT LECTURE SLIDES

(NOTE: The number on each PPT Lecture Slide directly corresponds with the Concepts for Lecture.)

Nursing Interventions for Nonreassuring Patterns
- Notify MD/Midwife and document
- Change position
- Increase IV fluids
- Provide oxygen

CONCEPTS FOR LECTURE *continued*

to assess current status and changes. If variables are severe oxygen should also be administered and the woman should be prepared for a cesarean or vacuum birth. All of these interventions should also be performed for late decelerations along with maintaining the maternal position on the left side, maintaining hydration with IV fluids, and monitoring for signs of hypotension. If decelerations are prolonged, tocolytics may also need to be administered if hypertonus is noted.

POWERPOINT LECTURE SLIDES *continued*

- Tocolytics
- Prepare for cesarean or vacuum birth

SUGGESTIONS FOR CLASSROOM ACTIVITIES

Do the care plan activity, Client with Decelerations, in class together and discuss the appropriate interventions and documentation for a nonreassuring electronic fetal monitoring strip.

SUGGESTIONS FOR CLINICAL ACTIVITIES

Have students observe the nursing interventions performed by a nurse caring for a woman in labor with a nonreassuring electronic fetal monitoring strip, and identify the purpose of those interventions.

LEARNING OBJECTIVE 11

Discuss the steps used to perform fetal scalp stimulation.

CONCEPTS FOR LECTURE

1. The use of direct stimulation to the fetal scalp in utero to elicit an acceleration when auscultating or when interpreting a nonreassuring EFM pattern is scalp stimulation. It is done by applying direct digital pressure to the fetal scalp during a vaginal examination.

POWERPOINT LECTURE SLIDES

(NOTE: The number on each PPT Lecture Slide directly corresponds with the Concepts for Lecture.)

 Scalp Stimulation
- Direct stimulation to fetal scalp to elicit an acceleration
- Uncompromised fetuses will elicit acceleration of at least 15 bpm for 15 seconds

SUGGESTIONS FOR CLINICAL ACTIVITIES

Observe the technique for fetal scalp stimulation being performed in the clinical setting and the fetal response.

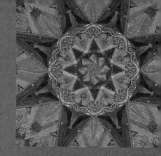

CHAPTER 24
THE FAMILY IN CHILDBIRTH: NEEDS AND CARE

RESOURCE LIBRARY

💿 PRENTICE HALL NURSING MEDIALINK DVD-ROM

Audio Glossary
NCLEX Review
Videos: *First Stage of Labor; First Stage of Labor—Transition; Second Stage of Labor; Third Stage of Labor—Part 1; Third Stage of Labor—Part 2; Third Stage of Labor—Part 3; Newborn Assessment; Delivery of Placenta; Fourth Stage of Labor; Through the Eyes of a Nurse—The Third Trimester*
Animation: *Placental Delivery*

🖥 COMPANION WEBSITE

Additional NCLEX Review
Care Plan Activity: *Presence of Extended Family*
Case Study: *Labor and Birth of Client Who Received No Prenatal Care*
Applications: *Developing a Birth Plan; Positioning Options During Labor and Delivery; Cord Blood Banking*
Critical Thinking

📖 IMAGE LIBRARY

Figure 24.1 Woman and her partner walking in the hospital during labor.
Figure 24.2 The woman's partner provides support and encouragement during labor.
Figure 24.3 The laboring woman is encouraged to choose a position of comfort.
Figure 24.4 A birthing ball is used to promote maternal comfort during labor.
Figure 24.5 The nurse provides encouragement and support during pushing efforts.
Figure 24.6 Using a birthing bar.
Figure 24.7 Birthing positions.

Figure 24.8 A birthing sequence.
Figure 24.9 Hollister cord clamp.
Figure 24.10 Umbilical alarm in place on a newborn infant.
Figure 24.11 A newborn infant being suctioned with a DeLee mucus trap to remove excess secretions from the mouth and nares.
Figure 24.12 Suggested method of palpating the fundus of the uterus during the fourth stage.
Figure 24.13 An adolescent mother receives breastfeeding assistance in the immediate postpartum period.

LEARNING OBJECTIVE 1

Identify nursing diagnoses specific to the first, second, third, and fourth stages of labor.

CONCEPTS FOR LECTURE

1. In the first stage of labor, nursing diagnoses that may apply include the following: fear/anxiety related to discomfort of labor and unknown labor outcome, health-seeking behaviors, and compromised family coping related to labor process.
2. Additional nursing diagnoses for the first stage of labor may include: acute pain related to uterine contractions, cervical dilatation, and fetal descent; deficient knowledge related to lack of information about normal labor process and comfort measures; and fear/anxiety related to unknown birth outcome and anticipated discomfort.
3. Nursing diagnoses for the second and third stages may include the following: acute pain related to uterine contractions, birth process, and/or perineal trauma from birth; deficient knowledge related to lack of information

POWERPOINT LECTURE SLIDES

(NOTE: The number on each PPT Lecture Slide directly corresponds with the Concepts for Lecture.)

1 First Stage Nursing Diagnoses
- Fear/Anxiety related to discomfort of labor and unknown labor outcome
- Health-seeking behaviors
- Compromised family coping related to labor process

2 First Stage Nursing Diagnoses
- Acute pain related to uterine contractions, birth process, and/or perineal trauma from birth
- Deficient knowledge related to lack of information about pushing methods
- Ineffective coping related to birth process
- Fear/Anxiety related to outcome of birth process

about pushing methods; ineffective coping related to birth process; and fear/anxiety related to outcome of birth process.

4. In the fourth stage, possible nursing diagnoses include the following: acute pain related to perineal trauma, deficient knowledge related to lack of information about involutional process and self-care needs, and readiness for enhanced family processes related to incorporation of the newborn into the family.

 Second and Third Stage Nursing Diagnoses
- Acute pain related to uterine contractions, cervical dilatation, and fetal descent
- Deficient knowledge related to lack of information about normal labor process and comfort measures
- Fear/Anxiety related to unknown birth outcome and anticipated discomfort

 Fourth Stage Nursing Diagnoses
- Acute pain related to perineal trauma
- Deficient knowledge related to lack of information about involutional process and self-care needs
- Readiness for enhanced family processes related to incorporation of the newborn into the family

SUGGESTIONS FOR CLASSROOM ACTIVITIES

Discuss nursing interventions that might be appropriate for each of the nursing diagnoses.

SUGGESTIONS FOR CLINICAL ACTIVITIES

Ask students to complete a care plan on a laboring patient that they observed on the unit using one of these nursing diagnoses.

LEARNING OBJECTIVE 2

Describe factors that are assessed in the laboring woman during the admission process.

CONCEPTS FOR LECTURE

1. The labor and birth nurse can obtain essential information regarding the woman and her pregnancy. By doing an admission history, the nurse can initiate any immediate interventions needed and establish individualized priorities. The nurse is then able to make effective nursing decisions regarding intrapartal care. Factors that must be assessed include labor status, fetal and maternal risk factors, need for monitoring, family labor and birth plans, and social support.

2. Physical assessments include: auscultation of fetal heart rate, maternal vital signs, contraction status, cervical dilatation and effacement, and fetal presentation and station. Assessment of laboratory values includes: urine testing for protein, ketones, glucose, and leukocytes; hemoglobin and hematocrit values; serology test for syphilis if one has not been done in the last 3 months or if an antepartal serology result was positive; and HIV screening with consent if the woman has not been screened during pregnancy.

POWERPOINT LECTURE SLIDES

(NOTE: The number on each PPT Lecture Slide directly corresponds with the Concepts for Lecture.)

 Admission Assessment
- Is the woman in labor?
- Are there factors that put the laboring woman or the fetus at risk?
- Should ambulation or bed rest be encouraged?
- Is more frequent monitoring needed?
- What does the woman and/or couple want during labor and birth?
- Who will be with the laboring woman for social support?

 Assessment of the Woman in Labor
- Fetal heart rate
- Maternal vital signs
- Contraction status
- Cervical dilatation and effacement
- Fetal presentation and station
- Urine testing for protein, ketones, glucose, and leukocytes

2a Assessment of the Woman in Labor
- Hemoglobin and hematocrit values
- Serology test for syphilis
- HIV screening with consent

SUGGESTIONS FOR CLINICAL ACTIVITIES

Have students assist a nurse admitting a woman into labor. Ask them to document their observations of the admission process.

LEARNING OBJECTIVE 3

Discuss the components of a social history and its role in caring for the laboring woman.

CONCEPTS FOR LECTURE

1. A social assessment should include: data about the woman's current living situation, availability of resources, preparedness for the infant, community resources, and the woman's social support network.
2. A social assessment should also include the presence of risk factors such as: family violence or sexual assault; use of drugs, alcohol, or tobacco; and presence of sexually transmitted infections. These can influence a woman's labor, birth, and future childrearing choices.

POWERPOINT LECTURE SLIDES

(NOTE: The number on each PPT Lecture Slide directly corresponds with the Concepts for Lecture.)

1. Social Assessment
   - The woman's current living situation
   - Availability of resources
   - Preparedness for the infant
   - Community resources
   - The woman's social support network

2. Risk Factors
   - Family violence
   - Sexual assault
   - Use of drugs, alcohol, or tobacco
   - Presence of sexually transmitted infections

SUGGESTIONS FOR CLASSROOM ACTIVITIES

Ask students to do a mock social assessment of a laboring woman with each other and provide feedback to each other about their interview techniques.

SUGGESTIONS FOR CLINICAL ACTIVITIES

Ask students to assist a nurse admitting a woman in labor doing a social history. Ask them to identify significant findings and the implications for these findings.

LEARNING OBJECTIVE 4

Summarize the importance of incorporating family expectations and cultural beliefs into the nursing care plan.

CONCEPTS FOR LECTURE

1. It is important to understand family expectations regarding labor and birth and to determine whether their expectations are realistic or not. If families have unrealistic expectations, the anxiety level of both the mother and her partner may be affected. Expectations in labor and birth may also be dependent upon social and cultural norms. The nurse should incorporate this information into the care plan for labor and birth.

POWERPOINT LECTURE SLIDES

(NOTE: The number on each PPT Lecture Slide directly corresponds with the Concepts for Lecture.)

1. Family Expectations
   - Unrealistic expectations can increase anxiety
   - Nurse is advocate for the client and her family
   - Experiences in labor are dependent on cultural norms
   - Beliefs and values
   - Variations in issues of modesty and pain

SUGGESTIONS FOR CLASSROOM ACTIVITIES

Ask students to share their cultural beliefs and traditions associated with childbirth in class.

LEARNING OBJECTIVE 5

Discuss nursing interventions to meet the care needs of the laboring woman and her partner during each stage of labor.

CONCEPTS FOR LECTURE

1. During the latent phase of the first stage of labor, most women are responsive to teaching about breathing and other labor-coping techniques as they are not too uncomfortable with the contractions. Additional nursing interventions should include offering clear liquids

POWERPOINT LECTURE SLIDES

(NOTE: The number on each PPT Lecture Slide directly corresponds with the Concepts for Lecture.)

1. Nursing Interventions: Latent Phase
   - Anticipatory guidance
   - Encourage ambulation
   - Offer fluids

and ice chips and encouraging ambulation in the absence of contraindications.

2. Nursing interventions during the active phase of labor include: evaluating contractions, cervical dilatation, effacement, station, and fetal position, encouraging the woman to void, assessing maternal vital signs hourly, and auscultation and evaluation of FHR every 30 minutes. If membranes rupture, immediate auscultation of FHR should be done and the color and odor or the amniotic fluid should be documented. An intravenous electrolyte solution may be required for women experiencing slow progress of labor or the inability to tolerate fluids. Pain management is also an important consideration as the contractions become more frequent and intense.

3. During the transition phase of labor, nursing interventions should include: palpation of contractions at least every 15 minutes, assessment of cervical dilatation, assessment of maternal vital signs every 30 minutes, support with breathing techniques, and helping the woman refrain from pushing until the cervix is completely dilated.

4. During the second stage of labor, nursing interventions include: sterile vaginal examinations to assess fetal descent, assessment of maternal vital signs every 5 minutes, assisting the woman into a comfortable position for pushing, providing information regarding progress and what is happening in labor, and assisting the physician or CNM in preparation for the birth.

5. Nursing care in the third stage focuses on providing initial newborn care and assisting with delivery of the placenta.

6. During the fourth stage of labor, nursing interventions include: uterine palpation every 15 minutes until bleeding is within normal limits, facilitating bonding, assisting with breastfeeding, assessment of maternal vital signs, assessment for bladder distention and assisting the mother to void, catheterization if the mother is unable to void, assessment of the perineum, and the provision of comfort measures for perineal pain and uterine cramping.

2 Nursing Interventions: Active Phase
- Palpate contractions every 15–30 minutes
- Vaginal exams to assess cervical dilatation, effacement, and fetal station and position
- Encourage client to void
- Assess vital signs every hour

2a Nursing Interventions: Active Phase
- Auscultate fetal heart rate every 30 minutes
- Start IV fluid infusion if unable to tolerate fluids
- Assess color and odor of amniotic fluid and fetal heart rate when ruptured

3 Nursing Interventions: Transition Phase
- Palpate contractions every 15 minutes
- Sterile vaginal exams to assess labor progress
- Assess maternal vital signs every 30 minutes
- Assess fetal heart rate every 30 minutes
- Assist with breathing
- Keep woman from pushing until fully dilated

4 Nursing Interventions: Second Stage
- Sterile vaginal exams to assess fetal descent
- Assess maternal vital signs every 5 minutes
- Provide support and information about labor progress
- Assist with pushing
- Assist the physician or CNM with the birth

5 Nursing Interventions: Third Stage
- Provide newborn care
- Assist with delivery of placenta

6 Nursing Interventions: Fourth Stage
- Palpate fundus every 15 minutes for one hour (Figure 24.12)
- Assess vaginal bleeding
- Encourage bonding and breastfeeding
- Assess perineum
- Perineal care

6a See Figure 24.12

SUGGESTIONS FOR CLASSROOM ACTIVITIES

Bring in a cervical dilatation model for students to use to understand assessment of cervical dilatation. Bring an abdominal fundus model to class for student to practice fundal assessments.

SUGGESTIONS FOR CLINICAL ACTIVITIES

Have students assist with the labor and delivery of a client and ask them to discuss their observations in postconference.

Describe nursing interventions for promoting the woman's comfort during each stage of labor.

CONCEPTS FOR LECTURE

1. During the latent phase, frequent position changes (at least every hour) seem to achieve more efficient contractions and contribute to comfort and relaxation. Additional comfort measures may include: allowing the woman to sit up in a rocking chair or other comfortable chair or in the shower, hydrotherapy, perineal care, the provision of clear fluids and ice chips, and the use of birthing balls. To help decrease the anxiety of the mother and her support person, the nurse can give information (which eases fear of the unknown), establish rapport with the couple (which helps them preserve their personal integrity), express confidence in the couple's ability to work with the labor process, and assist with breathing and relaxation techniques. During the active and transition phases of labor, nursing interventions aimed at promoting comfort include: providing information about the nature of the discomfort, encouraging rest between contractions, distraction, effleurage, sacral pressure, visualization, and encouragement and support for controlled breathing techniques.
2. During the second stage of labor, all the comfort measures previously mentioned may be used. Additionally, cool cloths to the face and forehead may cool the woman during the physical exertion of pushing. The woman should be allowed to give birth in a way that will promote her comfort. The nurse should encourage the woman to rest in between contractions and support the woman into a pushing position with each contraction. The nurse should frequently reassure the mother about the progress of the birth.
3. During the fourth stage of labor, a heated bath blanket placed next to the woman and a warm drink may help to alleviate the shivering response. The nurse should also encourage rest and provide nutrition for the couple. Ice packs may be helpful to minimize perineal discomfort.

POWERPOINT LECTURE SLIDES

(NOTE: The number on each PPT Lecture Slide directly corresponds with the Concepts for Lecture.)

1 Comfort Measures: First Stage
- Frequent position changes
- Hydrotherapy
- Perineal care
- Clear fluids and ice chips
- Birthing balls (Figure 24.4)
- Provide information and support

1a See Figure 24.4

1b Comfort Measures: First Stage
- Relaxation between contractions
- Distraction
- Effleurage
- Firm pressure on back or sacrum
- Visualization
- Controlled breathing

2 Comfort Measures: Second Stage
- Same as first stage
- Cool cloths
- Encourage rest between contractions
- Assist into pushing position (Figure 24.7)
- Sips of fluids or ice chips
- Reassurance

2a See Figure 24.7

3 Comfort Measures: Fourth Stage
- Heated blanket
- Provide food
- Encourage rest

SUGGESTIONS FOR CLASSROOM ACTIVITIES

Demonstrate breathing techniques, effleurage, massage, and the use of the birthing ball in class. Have students practice on each other.

SUGGESTIONS FOR CLINICAL ACTIVITIES

Have students utilize comfort measures in assisting with the care of laboring clients. Have them document the interventions and the patient response.

LEARNING OBJECTIVE 7

Summarize immediate nursing care of the newborn following birth.

CONCEPTS FOR LECTURE

1. Immediate care of the newborn following birth includes maintaining respirations by placing the newborn in a modified Trendelenburg position to aid drainage of mucus from the nasopharynx and trachea and suctioning with a bulb syringe or DeLee mucus

POWERPOINT LECTURE SLIDES

(NOTE: The number on each PPT Lecture Slide directly corresponds with the Concepts for Lecture.)

1 Care of the Newborn
- Maintain respirations (Figure 24.11)
- Provide and maintain warmth

trap as needed. The provision and maintenance of warmth is the second priority; therefore, the nurse should dry the newborn immediately and remove the wet blankets to prevent heat loss. The nurse is also responsible for assigning the Apgar score. A physical assessment should be done to detect any abnormalities. The nurse is also responsible for newborn identification which includes braceleting the infant and parents and footprinting the infant. Maternal-infant attachment should also be facilitated.

- Apgar score
- Physical assessment
- Newborn identification
- Facilitate attachment

 See Figure 24.11

SUGGESTIONS FOR CLASSROOM ACTIVITIES

Give students case studies describing newborn status after delivery and ask them to calculate an Apgar score.

SUGGESTIONS FOR CLINICAL ACTIVITIES

Have students assist with the care of newborn immediately following delivery. Ask them to document their assessments.

LEARNING OBJECTIVE 8

Discuss the components of care for the woman during the third stage of labor.

CONCEPTS FOR LECTURE

1. During the third stage of labor, the nurse should gently palpate the uterus to check for ballooning caused by uterine relaxation and subsequent bleeding into the uterine cavity. The physician or CNM will exert gentle traction on the umbilical cord. The nurse should encourage the mother to continue breathing through an open mouth and to relax her abdominal muscles. An oxytocic drug (Pitocin) may be used to stimulate uterine contractions after birth and to reduce the incidence of third-stage hemorrhage.

POWERPOINT LECTURE SLIDES

(NOTE: The number on each PPT Lecture Slide directly corresponds with the Concepts for Lecture.)

 Third Stage of Labor
- Watch for signs of placental separation
- Palpate fundus
- Encourage breathing and abdominal relaxation during delivery of placenta
- Possible administration of Pitocin

LEARNING OBJECTIVE 9

Discuss initial measures to help the woman and family integrate the newborn into family life.

CONCEPTS FOR LECTURE

1. The following measures may help the woman and the family integrate the newborn into their family life: the care providers keep routine investigations to a minimum, delay instillation of ophthalmic antibiotic for the first hour, keep the room slightly darkened, avoid loud noises, talk in quiet tones, and provide privacy. The nurse should encourage both parents to do whatever they feel most comfortable doing in caring for the newborn. They should be encouraged to delay phone calls and visits from friends until after the first hour of birth because it is a time when the baby is the most alert.

POWERPOINT LECTURE SLIDES

(NOTE: The number on each PPT Lecture Slide directly corresponds with the Concepts for Lecture.)

 Facilitating Attachment
- Minimize newborn interventions
- Provide privacy
- Keep lights low
- Facilitate parental wishes

LEARNING OBJECTIVE 10

Explore the nurse's role in providing sensitive care to adolescent parents.

CONCEPTS FOR LECTURE

1. The nurse's role in providing care for adolescent parents includes: close observation during labor, particularly for those adolescents that have not had prenatal care; assessing of fetal well-being; developing a trusting relationship and providing support; and providing encouragement.

POWERPOINT LECTURE SLIDES

(NOTE: The number on each PPT Lecture Slide directly corresponds with the Concepts for Lecture.)

 1 Providing Care to Adolescents
- Assess for complications
- Assess for fetal well-being
- Establish trusting relationship
- Provide emotional support
- Provide positive reinforcement

SUGGESTIONS FOR CLASSROOM ACTIVITIES

Have students form small groups and discuss issues related to adolescent pregnancy and the role of the nurse in assisting the adolescent mother.

SUGGESTIONS FOR CLINICAL ACTIVITIES

Have students attend a class aimed at educating pregnant adolescents about the labor and delivery process. Have students ask the pregnant adolescents to reflect on their fears and concerns.

LEARNING OBJECTIVE 11

Delineate management of a nurse-managed precipitous birth.

CONCEPTS FOR LECTURE

1. There are times when a nurse must manage a precipitous birth. The nurse should keep the woman informed about the progress of labor and assure her that the nurse will stay with her. Auxiliary personnel should be directed to contact a physician or CNM (if they are available) and to retrieve the emergency pack. The nurse should encourage the woman to get into a comfortable position, and then the nurse should scrub (if time permits), put on sterile gloves, and place sterile drapes under the woman's buttocks. The nurse should give clear instructions to the woman, support her, and provide reassurance in a calm and confident manner. The nurse should instruct the woman to blow or pant when the infant's head crowns to decrease her urge to push. If the amniotic sac is intact, the nurse should tear the sac with a clamp. Gentle pressure should be applied against the fetal head with one hand to maintain fetal flexion and prevent it from popping out rapidly. The perineum should be supported with the other hand. Once the head is delivered, the nurse should check to see if the umbilical cord is around the neck and if so, the nurse should pull it over the baby's head, loosen it, or let it slip down over the shoulders. If the cord cannot be slipped over the baby's head, two clamps should be placed on the cord, and the cord cut in between the clamps. The nurse should suction the mouth, throat, and nasal passages after the birth of the head and then place a hand on each side of the head and instruct the woman to push gently to deliver the

POWERPOINT LECTURE SLIDES

(NOTE: The number on each PPT Lecture Slide directly corresponds with the Concepts for Lecture.)

 1 Management of Precipitous Delivery
- Reassure and support mother
- Send auxiliary personnel for help and emergency pack
- Put mother in comfortable position and give clear instructions
- Delivery of infant
- Management of infant after delivery
- Delivery of placenta

rest of the body. The nurse should then provide immediate newborn care and be alert for signs of placental separation. When separation is apparent, the nurse places one hand just above the symphysis pubis to guard the uterus and uses the other hand to maintain gentle downward traction on the cord while instructing the mother to push so that the placenta can be expelled. The placenta should then be inspected to see if it is intact.

SUGGESTIONS FOR CLASSROOM ACTIVITIES

Have students develop a concept map for the assistance of a delivery with a precipitous birth.

CHAPTER 25
PAIN MANAGEMENT DURING LABOR

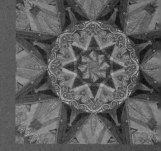

RESOURCE LIBRARY

 PRENTICE HALL NURSING MEDIALINK DVD-ROM

Audio Glossary
NCLEX Review
Videos: *Epidural Placement, Through the Eyes of a Nurse—The Third Trimester*

📖 **IMAGE LIBRARY**

Figure 25.1 Schematic diagram showing pain pathways and sites of interruption.
Figure 25.3 Positioning woman for epidural anesthesia block.
Figure 25.4 Technique for lumbar epidural block.
Figure 25.5 Levels of anesthesia for vaginal and cesarean births.
Figure 25.6 Double-needle technique for spinal injection.

 COMPANION WEBSITE

Additional NCLEX Review
Case Study: *Client Requesting an Epidural*
Care Plan Activity: *Managing Side Effects of an Epidural*
Applications: *Risks and Benefits of Using IV Medications for Pain Relief During Labor; Epidural Analgesia*
Critical Thinking

Figure 25.7 *A*, Pudendal block by the transvaginal approach. *B*, Area of perineum affected by pudendal block.
Figure 25.8 Local infiltration anesthesia.
Figure 25.9 Proper position for fingers in applying cricoid pressure until a cuffed endotracheal tube is placed by the anesthesiologist or certified nurse-anesthetist.

LEARNING OBJECTIVE 1

Discuss the nurse's role in supporting pharmaceutical pain relief measures in labor.

CONCEPTS FOR LECTURE

1. When effective comfort measures during labor and birth do not provide sufficient relief, pharmacologic agents may be used to decrease discomfort, increase relaxation, and reestablish the ability to participate more actively in the labor and birth experience. If a woman decides to use pharmacologic pain management, the nurse should support her decision and explain her options for pain relief in a realistic manner. The nurse should reassure the woman that accepting pain medication is not a failure and should emphasize the goal of a healthy, satisfying outcome for the family.

POWERPOINT LECTURE SLIDES

(NOTE: The number on each PPT Lecture Slide directly corresponds with the Concepts for Lecture.)

🎞 1 Nurse's Role in Pain Relief
- Support decision for pharmaceutical pain relief
- Offer alternative therapies if pharmaceuticals not desired
- Support changes in decision
- Educate about options
- Reassure that accepting medication for pain is not failure

SUGGESTIONS FOR CLASSROOM ACTIVITIES

Have a group discussion about student feelings about pain relief in labor. Discuss cultural influences on pain management in labor.

SUGGESTIONS FOR CLINICAL ACTIVITIES

Have students interview a labor and delivery nurse about his/her role in pain management in labor and discuss their findings.

LEARNING OBJECTIVE 2

Describe the use of systemic analgesics to promote pain relief during labor.

CONCEPTS FOR LECTURE

1. When providing systemic analgesia during labor, the goal is to provide maximal pain relief with minimal risk for the woman and fetus. Effects of the analgesia on the mother can affect the well-being of the fetus because the fetus depends on adequate functioning of the maternal cardiopulmonary system. Pain medication should be administered when the woman is uncomfortable and in a well-established labor pattern with contractions occurring regularly and of significant duration with moderate to strong intensity. If it is administered too early, systemic analgesia may prolong labor and depress the fetus. If systemic analgesia is given too late, it is of no value to the woman and may cause neonatal respiratory depression.

2. The following assessments should be done prior to administering systemic analgesics: the woman is willing to receive medication after being advised about it, vital signs are stable, contraindications are not present, and knowledge of other medications being administered. Fetal assessments include: a fetal heart rate of between 110 and 160 beats per minute, reactive nonstress test (NST), short-term variability is present, long-term variability is average, and periodic late decelerations or nonperiodic (variable) decelerations are absent. An assessment of labor progress should include: the contraction pattern, cervical dilatation, fetal presenting part, and the station of the presenting part.

3. After administration of the medication, the nurse records the drug name, dose, route, site, and the woman's blood pressure and pulse (before and after) on the EFM strip and on the woman's record. Safety precautions should include raising the side rails and assessment of the FHR for possible side effects of the medication.

4. Sedatives may be used in the early latent phase of labor to allow the expectant mother to rest. After rest, either the contractions have ceased or they return and take on a regular pattern. The following are the most common barbiturates used in labor: secobarbital (Seconal) and zolpidem tartrate (Ambien). Benzodiazepines, such as diazepam (Valium), are primarily used to treat anxiety. Some, however, have an amnesic effect which may not be desirable for childbearing women. H1-receptor antagonists can also be used for sedation. These drugs also have anti-Parkinson and antiemetic effects. Common H1-receptor antagonists include promethazine (Phenergan), hydroxyzine (Vistaril), and diphenhydramine (Benadryl).

5. Pain relief agents may include mixed agonist-antagonist narcotic agents such as butorphanol tartrate (Stadol), nalbuphine hydrochloride (Nubain), and meperidine

POWERPOINT LECTURE SLIDES

(NOTE: The number on each PPT Lecture Slide directly corresponds with the Concepts for Lecture.)

1 Systemic Analgesia
- Goal is to provide maximum pain relief with minimal risk
- Alteration in maternal state affects fetus

1a Administration of Systemic Analgesia
- When woman is uncomfortable
- Well-established labor pattern
- Contractions occurring regularly
- Significant duration of contractions
- Moderate to strong intensity

2 Maternal Assessments
- The woman is willing to receive medication
- Vital signs are stable
- Contraindications are not present
- Knowledge of other medications being administered

2a Fetal Assessments
- Fetal heart rate between 110 and 160 bpm
- Reactive nonstress test
- Short-term variability is present
- Long-term variability is average

2b Assessment of Labor Progress
- Contraction pattern
- Cervical dilatation
- Fetal presenting part
- Station of the fetal presenting part

3 Nursing Considerations
- Record the drug name, dose, route, site on EFM strip and chart
- Record the woman's blood pressure and pulse (before and after) on the EFM strip and chart
- Safety precautions
  ○ Raising the side rails
  ○ Assessment of the FHR

4 Sedatives
- Use: early latent phase
- Purpose: relaxation and sleep
- Common medications: Seconal and Ambien

4a H1-receptor antagonists
- Use: Early latent phase
- Purpose: Sedative, antiemetic
- Common medications: Phenergan, Vistaril, Benadryl

(Demerol). The analgesic potency of these medications is greater than that of narcotics such as meperidine and morphine. Naloxone (Narcan) can be used to reverse the mild respiratory depression, sedation, and hypotension following small doses of opiates.

| 5 | Narcotics
- Use: active phase
- Purpose: pain management
- Common medications: Stadol, Nubain, Demerol
- Narcotic antagonist: Narcan

SUGGESTIONS FOR CLASSROOM ACTIVITIES

Ask students to develop medication cards for the systemic medications administered in labor.

SUGGESTIONS FOR CLINICAL ACTIVITIES

Have students do a thorough assessment of a mother and fetus in labor prior to administration of pain medications. Review the assessments to determine whether administration of medication is appropriate at that time.

LEARNING OBJECTIVE 3

Compare the major types of regional analgesia and anesthesia, including area affected, advantages, disadvantages, techniques, and nursing implications.

CONCEPTS FOR LECTURE

1. The temporary and reversible loss of sensation produced by injecting an anesthetic agent into an area that will bring the agent into direct contact with nervous tissue is regional anesthesia. The most commonly used regional anesthetics in childbearing include the epidural, spinal, or combined epidural-spinal.

2. A lumbar epidural is given in the first and second stages of labor and affects the uterus, cervix, vagina, and the perineum. Advantages include: it produces good analgesia, the woman is fully awake during labor and birth, the continuous technique allows different blocking for each stage of labor so that internal rotation of the fetus can be accomplished, and in many cases, the dose of anesthetic agent can be adjusted to preserve the woman's reflex urge to bear down. The primary disadvantage is the risk of maternal hypotension. Also, the onset of analgesia may not occur for up to 30 minutes.

3. A spinal block is given during the first stage of labor and affects the uterus, cervix, vagina, and perineum. Advantages include: the immediate onset of anesthesia, relative ease of administration, a smaller drug volume, and maternal compartmentalization of the drug. The primary disadvantage is that the intense blockade of sympathetic fibers results in a high incidence of hypotension.

4. A combined spinal-epidural (CSE) can be used for labor analgesia and for cesarean birth and affects the uterus, cervix, vagina, and perineum. The spinal analgesia may be given in the latent phase for pain relief and the epidural is given when active labor begins. Advantages include: a faster onset than medications that are injected into the epidural space, it is versatile in that medication can be added to increase the effectiveness, and it preserves motor functioning. Disadvantages include a higher incidence of nausea and pruritus.

POWERPOINT LECTURE SLIDES

(NOTE: The number on each PPT Lecture Slide directly corresponds with the Concepts for Lecture.)

| 1 | Regional Anesthesia
- Temporary and reversible loss of sensation
- Prevents initiation and transmission of nerve impulses
- Types
  - Epidural
  - Spinal
  - Combined epidural-spinal

| 2 | Epidural: Advantages
- Produces good analgesia
- Woman is fully awake during labor and birth
- Continuous technique allows different blocking for each stage of labor
- Dose of anesthetic agent can be adjusted

| 2a | Epidural: Disadvantages
- Maternal hypotension
- Postdural puncture seizures
- Meningitis
- Cardiorespiratory arrest
- Vertigo
- Onset of analgesia may not occur for up to 30 minutes

| 3 | Spinal Block: Advantages
- Immediate onset of anesthesia
- Relative ease of administration
- Smaller drug volume
- Maternal compartmentalization of the drug

| 3a | Spinal Block: Disadvantages
- High incidence of hypotension
- Greater potential for fetal hypoxia

5. A pudendal block technique is given in the second stage of labor for the provision of perineal anesthesia for the second stage of labor, birth, and episiotomy repair. Advantages include: the ease of administration, the small amount of medication that must be used, absence of maternal hypotension, and it allows the use of low forceps or vacuum extraction for birth. The primary disadvantage is that the urge to bear down during the second stage of labor may be decreased.

6. Nursing management prior to the administration of anesthesia includes: an assessment of maternal vital signs and the FHR for baseline information, an assessment of labor progress, explanation of the procedure and expected results to the woman and support person, starting an IV infusion (if one is not already in place), assisting the woman with positioning, and providing physical and emotional support throughout the procedure. Nursing interventions after administration may include: positioning the woman in a semi-reclining position with lateral uterine tilt, assessment of maternal blood pressure and pulse every 5 minutes for at least 30 minutes and then at least every 30 minutes thereafter while the block is present, assessment of respiratory rate every 15 to 30 minutes, and assessment of FHR by continuous electronic fetal monitor. The nurse should assist with corrective measures such as positioning the woman in a left side-lying position, increasing the flow rate of the intravenous infusion, and placing the bed in a 10- to 20-degree Trendelenburg position if hypotension occurs. Ephedrine is given if the maternal blood pressure does not increase within 1 to 2 minutes. Additionally, the nurse should frequently assess the bladder and catheterize the woman if she is unable to void.

- Uterine tone is maintained, making intrauterine manipulation difficult
- Short acting

4 Combined Spinal-Epidural: Advantages
- Spinal agent has a faster onset
- Medication can be added to increase the effectiveness
- Preserves motor functioning
- Most drugs are used in low dose

4a Combined Spinal-Epidural: Disadvantages
- Higher incidence of nausea and pruritus

5 Pudendal (Figure 25.7)
- Perineal anesthesia for the second stage of labor, birth, and episiotomy repair
- Advantages are ease of administration and absence of maternal hypotension
- Urge to bear down may be decreased

5a See Figure 25.7

5b Local
- Used for episiotomy repair
- Advantage is that it involves the least amount of anesthetic agent
- The major disadvantage is that large amounts of solution must be used

6 Nursing Management: Prior to Administration
- Assess maternal and fetal status
- Assess labor progress
- Start an IV and administer preload
- Help woman into position

6a Nursing Management: After Administration
- Monitor maternal and fetal vital signs
- Assess for hypotension
- Tale corrective measures for hypotension
- Administer antiemetics as needed
- Monitor respiratory rate
- Assess bladder and catheterize if unable to void

SUGGESTIONS FOR CLASSROOM ACTIVITIES

Ask students to develop a care plan for a woman who is receiving regional anesthesia.

SUGGESTIONS FOR CLINICAL ACTIVITIES

Have students assist with the administration of regional anesthesia in the clinical setting. Discuss the procedure and the patient response.

LEARNING OBJECTIVE 4

Summarize possible complications of regional anesthesia.

CONCEPTS FOR LECTURE

1. Complications of a lumbar epidural block may include toxic reactions caused by unintentional placement of the drug in the arachnoid or subarachnoid space, excessive amount of the drug in the epidural space (massive epidural), or accidental intravascular injection, and spinal headaches when the dura is accidentally punctured during epidural placement.

2. Spinal anesthesia complications may include hypotension, drug reaction, total spinal neurologic sequelae, and spinal headache. Side effects include nausea, shivering, and urinary retention.

3. Accidental vascular injection can cause a toxic reaction during the administration of a pudendal block. Additional complications may include broad ligament hematoma, perforation of the rectum, and trauma to the sciatic nerve.

POWERPOINT LECTURE SLIDES

(NOTE: The number on each PPT Lecture Slide directly corresponds with the Concepts for Lecture.)

1 Complications of Epidural Anesthesia
- Toxic reactions
  - Unintentional placement of the drug
  - Excessive amount of the drug
  - Accidental intravascular injection
- Spinal headaches

2 Complications of Spinal Anesthesia
- Hypotension
- Drug reaction
- Total spinal neurologic sequelae
- Spinal headache
- Nausea, shivering, and urinary retention
- Ineffective anesthesia

3 Complications of Pudendal Anesthesia
- Systemic toxic reaction
- Broad ligament hematoma
- Perforation of the rectum
- Trauma to the sciatic nerve

SUGGESTIONS FOR CLASSROOM ACTIVITIES

Ask students to identify appropriate nursing interventions for complications related to regional anesthesia administration.

SUGGESTIONS FOR CLINICAL ACTIVITIES

Have students who are caring for women receiving regional anesthesia in labor identify complications that have occurred and the corresponding interventions and client responses.

LEARNING OBJECTIVE 5

Describe the three methods used to provide general anesthesia.

CONCEPTS FOR LECTURE

1. General anesthesia (induced unconsciousness) may be needed for cesarean birth and surgical intervention with some obstetric complications. Anesthesia methods use for cesarean birth include intravenous injection, inhalation of anesthetic agents, or a combination of both methods. Intravenous injection may be done using sodium thiopental (Pentothal) or Ketamine. Ketamine is contraindicated in women with preeclampsia or chronic hypertension. The most commonly used inhaled anesthetic is nitrous oxide as it does not cause significant uterine relaxation. Other low-dose halogenated agents may be used with nitrous oxide to increase maternal inspired oxygen and increase uterine blood flow. Inhalation anesthesia may also be used with spinal or epidural anesthesia where the anesthesia was ineffective or there was a high degree of maternal anxiety.

POWERPOINT LECTURE SLIDES

(NOTE: The number on each PPT Lecture Slide directly corresponds with the Concepts for Lecture.)

1 Methods of General Anesthesia
- Intravenous injection
  - Sodium thiopental (Pentothal)
  - Ketamine
- Inhalation of anesthetic agents
  - Nitrous oxide
  - Low-dose halogenated agents

LEARNING OBJECTIVE 6

Delineate the major complications of general anesthesia.

CONCEPTS FOR LECTURE

1. The major complications of general anesthesia include fetal depression, uterine relaxation, and vomiting and aspiration. Fetal depression is related to the depth and duration of the anesthesia. Due to a decrease in gastrointestinal motility during pregnancy, which is intensified during labor, women often have undigested food remaining in their stomachs during a cesarean birth. This puts the woman at risk for aspiration if vomiting occurs. Even if they have been fasting, the gastric secretions are very acidic and can result in a pneumonitis if aspirated.

POWERPOINT LECTURE SLIDES

(NOTE: The number on each PPT Lecture Slide directly corresponds with the Concepts for Lecture.)

 Complications of General Anesthesia
- Fetal depression
  - Depth and duration
- Uterine relaxation
- Potential for chemical pneumonitis
  - Decrease in gastrointestinal motility
  - Acidic gastric secretions

LEARNING OBJECTIVE 7

Identify contraindications to specific types of analgesia and anesthesia for high-risk mothers.

CONCEPTS FOR LECTURE

1. An immature fetus is more susceptible to depressant drugs and therefore, analgesia should be avoided. The preferred method of pain control for the woman with preeclampsia is regional anesthesia as long as hypotension can be avoided. General anesthesia should be avoided in women with preeclampsia. Regional anesthesia poses complications for the fetus of a mother with diabetes mellitus due to a reduction in placental blood flow and the potential for hypotension. Continuous epidural anesthesia is recommended for women with mitral stenosis and delivery with low forceps birth to avoid cardiovascular changes with pushing. If a woman is actively bleeding, regional blocks are contraindicated because the sympathetic block causes vasodilatation and further reduction of the vascular volume.

POWERPOINT LECTURE SLIDES

(NOTE: The number on each PPT Lecture Slide directly corresponds with the Concepts for Lecture.)

 Contraindications
- Preterm infant
  - Avoid analgesia during labor
- Preeclampsia
  - Regional anesthesia is preferred
  - General anesthesia may aggravate hypertension

 Contraindications
- Diabetes
  - Potential for decreased uteroplacental flow due to hypotension
  - Increased risk of cardiovascular depression with regional
- Cardiac
  - Continuous epidural avoids cardiovascular changes with bearing down

 Contraindications
- Bleeding
  - Regional blocks are contraindication due to reduction in volume

---

SUGGESTIONS FOR CLASSROOM ACTIVITIES

Develop case studies for women with complications and discuss the implications for anesthesia.

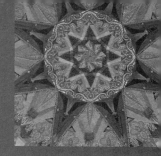

CHAPTER 26
CHILDBIRTH AT RISK
THE INTRAPARTAL PERIOD

RESOURCE LIBRARY

💿 PRENTICE HALL NURSING MEDIALINK DVD-ROM

Audio Glossary
NCLEX Review

COMPANION WEBSITE

Additional NCLEX Review
Case Study: *Client with Placental Problems*
Care Plan Activity: *Prevention of Cord Prolapse*
Applications: *Placenta Pervia; Umblical Cord Prolapse*
Critical Thinking

📖 IMAGE LIBRARY

Figure 26.1 Comparison of labor patterns.
Figure 26.2 Effects of labor on the fetal head.
Figure 26.3 Scanzoni maneuver, anterior rotation.
Figure 26.4 Manual rotation of ROP to OA.
Figure 26.6 Brow presentation.
Figure 26.7 Face presentation.
Figure 26.8 Face presentation.
Figure 26.9 Face presentation.
Figure 26.10 Breech presentation.
Figure 26.11 Transverse lie.

Figure 26.12 McRoberts maneuver.
Figure 26.13 Twins may be in any of these presentations while in utero.
Figure 26.14 Leopold's maneuvers in twin pregnancy.
Figure 26.15 Intrapartal management of nonreassuring fetal status.
Figure 26.16 Abruptio placentae.
Figure 26.17 Placenta previa.
Figure 26.18 Management of placenta previa.
Figure 26.19 Prolapse of the umbilical cord.

LEARNING OBJECTIVE 1

Describe psychologic disorders that may contribute to difficulty in coping during labor and birth.

CONCEPTS FOR LECTURE

1. Women who are depressed may have difficulty coping with labor due to the inability to concentrate or process information, and they may experience fatigue because of the effect of depression on sleeping. This may result in her feeling hopeless or unworthy of motherhood.

2. A manic episode during labor may put a woman and her fetus at risk because of dangerous behaviors such as alcohol or drug use. Women experiencing a manic episode are at an increased risk of suicide and are at greater risk for developing a mood disorder in the postpartum period. They are also at greater risk for postpartum psychosis.

3. Anxiety disorders can cause a wide range of symptoms in laboring women, including intense feelings of terror without warning that result in physical and/or psychologic symptoms. Specific rituals may be used as a means of coping with labor in women with OCD. Labor may trigger flashbacks, avoidance behaviors, or anxiety symptoms in women who have PTSD due to rape. Irrational fears may be exhibited in women with specific phobias.

POWERPOINT LECTURE SLIDES

(NOTE: The number on each PPT Lecture Slide directly corresponds with the Concepts for Lecture.)

1 Psychologic Disorders: Depression
  - Unable to process information
  - Unable to concentrate
  - Fatigue, sleep deprivation
  - Overwhelmed by labor process
  - Unworthy of motherhood
  - Hopelessness

2 Psychologic Disorders: Mania
  - Endangering self or fetus
  - Higher risk of suicide
  - Increased risk for postpartum mood disorder
  - Increased risk for postpartum psychosis

3 Psychologic Disorders: Anxiety
  - Panic attacks
  - Repetition of rituals during labor
  - Flashbacks, avoidance, anxiety
  - Sense of something being wrong during labor
  - Feeling overwhelmed or embarrassed
  - Irrational fears

4. Many medications used to treat schizophrenia are teratogenic; therefore, they cannot be used in pregnancy. Schizophrenic women exhibit exaggerated behaviors during labor. They may need absolute control of everything that happens and refuse to participate until they feel secure. They may not be able to articulate their fears or needs, may not respond to supportive nursing measures, may be unaware of what will happen in labor and birth, and may be unable to understand what is happening. They may be suddenly overwhelmed by terrifying memories.

4 Psychologic Disorders: Schizophrenia
- Exaggerated behaviors during labor
- Demand absolute control over everything
- May not be able to articulate fears or needs
- May not respond to nursing measures
- May be unaware of what is happening

LEARNING OBJECTIVE 2

Discuss dysfunctional labor patterns.

CONCEPTS FOR LECTURE

1. Dysfunctional labor patterns include dystocia, hypertonic contractions, and hypotonic contractions. Dystocia is most often caused by dysfunctional uterine contractions that result in a prolongation of labor. Ineffectual uterine contractions of poor quality that occur in the latent phase of labor and cause an increase in the resting tone of the myometrium are hypertonic contractions. Irregular contractions of low amplitude in which there is commonly less than 1 cm cervical dilatation per hour or there has been no change of cervical dilatation for 2 hours are hypotonic contractions.

POWERPOINT LECTURE SLIDES

(NOTE: The number on each PPT Lecture Slide directly corresponds with the Concepts for Lecture.)

1 Dysfunctional Labor Patterns
- Dystocia
- Hypertonic contractions
- Hypotonic contractions

1a See Figure 26.1A

1b See Figure 26.1B

SUGGESTIONS FOR CLASSROOM ACTIVITIES

Bring electronic fetal monitoring strips to class depicting dysfunctional labor patterns and discuss potential causes.

SUGGESTIONS FOR CLINICAL ACTIVITIES

Ask students to observe women in labor for dysfunctional labor patterns and document observations about the maternal and fetal responses.

LEARNING OBJECTIVE 3

Identify the potential maternal risks of precipitous labor and birth.

CONCEPTS FOR LECTURE

1. Maternal risks from precipitous labor and birth may include abruptio placentae; lacerations of the cervix, vagina, and perineum; and postpartum hemorrhage.

POWERPOINT LECTURE SLIDES

(NOTE: The number on each PPT Lecture Slide directly corresponds with the Concepts for Lecture.)

1 Precipitous Birth: Maternal Risks
- Abruptio placentae
- Cervical, vaginal, or perineal lacerations
- Postpartum hemorrhage

SUGGESTIONS FOR CLASSROOM ACTIVITIES

Discuss in class the implications for nursing in the event of a precipitous labor and birth.

LEARNING OBJECTIVE 4

Describe the impact of postterm pregnancy on the childbearing family.

CONCEPTS FOR LECTURE

1. Women who deliver postterm fetuses are at increased risk for perineal damage (because of the increased size of the fetus), maternal hemorrhage, and cesarean birth. They may also experience anxiety and are emotionally fatigued as their estimated date of birth (EDB) passes.

2. Risks to the fetus are most often associated with placental changes that cause a decrease in the uterine-placental-fetal circulation, which reduces the blood supply, oxygen, and nutrition for the fetus. This puts the fetus at risk for oligohydramnios and small-for-gestational-age (SGA) They may, however, be macrosomic and LGA if uteroplacental-fetal circulation is not compromised. This puts the fetus at increased risk for birth trauma or shoulder dystocia and is also associated with prolonged labor, increased risk of cesarean birth, and cephalopelvic disproportion. Postterm fetuses are also at increased risk for meconium staining of the amniotic fluid, which can lead to nonreassuring fetal status and meconium aspiration at birth.

POWERPOINT LECTURE SLIDES

(NOTE: The number on each PPT Lecture Slide directly corresponds with the Concepts for Lecture.)

1 Impact of Postterm Pregnancy: Maternal
- Perineal damage
- Hemorrhage
- Increased risk of cesarean birth
- Anxiety
- Emotional fatigue
- Persistence of normal discomforts

2 Impact of Postterm Pregnancy: Fetal
- Decreased perfusion
- Oligohydramnios
- Small for Gestational Age (SGA)
- Macrosomia
- Increased risk for meconium staining

SUGGESTIONS FOR CLASSROOM ACTIVITIES

Have a group discussion about the impact of a postterm pregnancy on the emotional status of the mother and her family.

SUGGESTIONS FOR CLINICAL ACTIVITIES

Do a gestational age assessment of a postterm neonate and note variations that can be contributed to the postterm pregnancy.

LEARNING OBJECTIVE 5

Summarize various types of fetal malposition and malpresentation and possible associated problems.

CONCEPTS FOR LECTURE

1. Persistent occiput-posterior (OP) is the most frequent type of fetal malposition. OP occurs when the head remains in the direct occiput posterior position throughout labor. The OP fetal position increases the maternal risks for intense back pain during labor and the possibility of a third- or fourth-degree perineal laceration or extension of a midline episiotomy. A brow presentation is when the forehead of the fetus becomes the presenting part. In the brow presentation, the fetal head is slightly extended instead of flexed, with the result that the fetal head enters the birth canal with the widest diameter of the head foremost. The brow presentation puts the mother at increased risk for a prolonged labor or secondary arrest of labor. There is an increase in risk of fetal mortality due to birth trauma, which, can include cerebral and neck compression and damage to the trachea and larynx. A face presentation is when the face of the fetus is the presenting part. Maternal risks associated with a face presentation include prolonged labor

POWERPOINT LECTURE SLIDES

(NOTE: The number on each PPT Lecture Slide directly corresponds with the Concepts for Lecture.)

1 Malposition/Malpresentation
- Persistent occiput-posterior (OP) position
- Brow presentation
- Face presentation (Figure 26.7A–B)

1a See Figure 26.7A–B

2 Breech Presentation: Types (Figure 26.10A–D)
- Frank
- Single or double footling (incomplete)
- Complete

2a See Figure 26.10 A–D

2b Breech Presentation: Risks
- Head trauma
- Increased risk for infant mortality
- Neonatal complications
- Cord prolapse

and increased chance of infection. Associated fetal risks include facial edema and birth trauma resulting in petechiae and ecchymoses.

2. The most common malpresentation is a breech presentation, and the most common type of breech presentation is a frank breech. In a frank breech, the fetus has flexed hips and extended knees. A single or double footling breech (incomplete breech) is characterized by one or both hips extended and a foot presenting. A final type is a complete breech. There is an increased risk for cord prolapse, infant mortality, and neonatal complications with a breech presentation.

3. In a transverse lie, the infant's long axis lies across the woman's abdomen, and on inspection, the contour of the maternal abdomen appears widest from side to side. Vaginal birth cannot occur with this presentation. When there are two presenting parts, it is a compound presentation. This puts the woman at an increased risk for laceration with a vaginal birth.

 Malpresentation
- Shoulder presentation (Transverse Lie) (Figure 26.11A–B)
- Compound presentation

3a See Figure 26.11A–B

SUGGESTIONS FOR CLASSROOM ACTIVITIES

Bring a model pelvis and fetus to class to demonstrate the malpositions/malpresentations.

SUGGESTIONS FOR CLINICAL ACTIVITIES

Ask students to observe the labor and delivery of births associated with malposition or malpresentation and discuss their observations.

LEARNING OBJECTIVE 6

Discuss the implications of macrosomia and hydrocephalus on the woman and the fetus.

CONCEPTS FOR LECTURE

1. Fetal macrosomia is defined as weight of more than 4500 g. Maternal risks due to macrosomia include: dysfunctional labor, uterine rupture during labor, perineal lacerations, postpartum hemorrhage, and puerperal infection. The most significant fetal complication in macrosomia is shoulder dystocia.

POWERPOINT LECTURE SLIDES

(NOTE: The number on each PPT Lecture Slide directly corresponds with the Concepts for Lecture.)

 Macrosomia Risks
- Dysfunctional labor
- Uterine rupture
- Perineal lacerations
- Postpartum hemorrhage
- Puerperal infection
- Shoulder dystocia

SUGGESTIONS FOR CLINICAL ACTIVITIES

Have students review the charts of women who delivered a macrosomic infant for maternal complications and discuss their findings.

LEARNING OBJECTIVE 7

Identify maternal and fetal risks associated with multiple gestations.

CONCEPTS FOR LECTURE

1. Women with a multiple gestation are more likely to develop the following complications during pregnancy; spontaneous abortions, gestational diabetes, hypertension, acute fatty liver disease, pulmonary embolism, maternal anemia, hydramnios, premature rupture of membranes, incompetent cervix, and intrauterine growth restriction.
2. Complications during labor include: preterm labor, uterine dysfunction due to an overstretched myometrium, abnormal fetal presentations, instrumental or cesarean birth, and postpartum hemorrhage.
3. The woman with a multiple gestation may experience more physical discomfort during her pregnancy, such as shortness of breath, dyspnea on exertion, backaches, round ligament pain, heartburn, pelvic or suprapubic pressure, and pedal edema.

POWERPOINT LECTURE SLIDES

(NOTE: The number on each PPT Lecture Slide directly corresponds with the Concepts for Lecture.)

1 Multiple Gestation: Pregnancy Risks
- Spontaneous abortions
- Gestational diabetes
- Hypertension
- Acute fatty liver disease
- Pulmonary embolism
- Maternal anemia

1a Multiple Gestation: Pregnancy Risks
- Hydramnios
- PROM
- Incompetent cervix
- IUGR

2 Multiple Gestation: Labor Risks
- Preterm labor
- Uterine dysfunction
- Abnormal fetal presentations
- Instrumental or cesarean birth
- Postpartum hemorrhage

3 Multiple Gestation: Physical Discomfort
- Shortness of breath and/or dyspnea on exertion
- Backaches
- Round ligament pain
- Heartburn
- Pelvic or suprapubic pressure
- Pedal edema

LEARNING OBJECTIVE 8

Compare abruptio placentae and placenta previa.

CONCEPTS FOR LECTURE

1. The premature separation of a normally implanted placenta from the uterine wall is an abruptio placentae. It may be caused by maternal hypertension, domestic violence, abdominal trauma, presence of fibroids, uterine overdistension, fetal growth restriction, advanced maternal age, alcohol consumption, cocaine use, a short umbilical cord, and high parity. The three types of placental separation include marginal (where blood passes between the fetal membranes and the uterine wall and escapes vaginally), central (where blood is trapped between the placenta and uterine wall with concealed bleeding), and complete (where there is total separation and massive bleeding).
2. When the placenta is improperly implanted in the lower uterine segment, it is called placenta previa. Dilatation and contraction of the lower uterine segment in the later weeks of pregnancy cause the placental villi to be torn from the uterine wall, thus

POWERPOINT LECTURE SLIDES

(NOTE: The number on each PPT Lecture Slide directly corresponds with the Concepts for Lecture.)

1 Abruptio Placentae: Causes
- Maternal hypertension
- Domestic violence
- Abdominal trauma
- Presence of fibroids
- Uterine overdistension
- Fetal growth restriction

1a Abruptio Placentae: Causes
- Advanced maternal age
- Alcohol consumption
- Cocaine use
- Short umbilical cord
- High parity

1b Abruptio Placentae: Types (Figure 26.16A–C)
- Marginal

exposing the uterine sinuses at the placental site. Associated factors include: multiparity, increasing age, placenta accreta, defective development of blood vessels in the decidua, prior cesarean birth, smoking, a recent spontaneous or induced abortion, and a large placenta. The four degrees of placenta previa include: total placenta previa, partial placenta previa, marginal placenta previa, and low-lying placenta previa.

- Central
- Complete

1c See Figure 26.16A–C

2 Placenta Previa: Causes
- Multiparity
- Increasing age
- Placenta accreta
- Defective development of blood vessels in the decidua
- Prior cesarean birth
- Smoking

2a Placenta Previa: Causes
- Recent spontaneous or induced abortion
- Large placenta

2b Placenta Previa: Types (Figure 26.17A–C)
- Total
- Partial
- Marginal
- Low-lying

2c See Figure 26.17A–C

SUGGESTIONS FOR CLINICAL ACTIVITIES

Have students review maternal charts for placental problems and note the maternal/neonatal outcomes to discuss in post-conference.

LEARNING OBJECTIVE 9

Identify variations that may occur in the umbilical cord and insertion into the placenta.

CONCEPTS FOR LECTURE

1. Succenturiate placenta occurs when one or more accessory lobes of fetal villi have developed on the placenta, with vascular connections of fetal origin. Vessels are only supported by the membranes, which increases the risk of the minor lobes being retained during the third stage of labor. Circumvallate placenta is when the fetal surface of the placenta is exposed through a ring opening around the umbilical cord and the vessels descend from the cord and end at the margin of the ring. Battledore placenta is when the umbilical cord is inserted at or near the placental margin, and, as a result, all fetal vessels transverse the placental surface in the same direction. A prolapsed cord is an umbilical cord that precedes the fetal presenting part. It becomes trapped between the presenting part and the maternal pelvis. The fetus is affected because compression of the umbilical cord occludes blood flow through the umbilical vessels. Umbilical cord abnormalities include: congenital absence of an umbilical artery, insertion variations, cord length variations, and knots and loops of the cord. Insertion variations include velamentous insertion and vasa previa, and cord length problems include long and short cords.

POWERPOINT LECTURE SLIDES

(NOTE: The number on each PPT Lecture Slide directly corresponds with the Concepts for Lecture.)

1 Umbilical Cord Complications
- Succenturiate placenta
- Circumvallate placenta
- Battledore placenta
- Prolapsed umbilical cord (Figure 26.19)
- Velamentous insertion

1a See Figure 26.19

1b Umbilical Cord Complications
- Vasa previa
- Cord length problems

LEARNING OBJECTIVE 10

Discuss the identification, management, and nursing care of women with amniotic fluid embolus, hydramnios, and oligohydramnios.

CONCEPTS FOR LECTURE

1. When a bolus of amniotic fluid enters the maternal circulation and then the maternal lungs, it is called an amniotic fluid embolism. An amniotic fluid level of over 2000 mL is called hydramnios (also called polyhydramnios). Chronic hydramnios occurs in the third trimester, when the fluid volume gradually increases. Acute hydramnios, in contrast, is a rapid increase in volume over a period of a few days and is usually diagnosed between 20 and 24 weeks' gestation. Hydramnios can be due to diabetes, Rh sensitization, and infections such as syphilis, toxoplasmosis, cytomegalovirus, herpes, and rubella. It is managed supportively unless there is maternal or fetal distress. Less than normal amount of amniotic fluid is considered oligohydramnios. While the exact causes are unknown, oligohydramnios is associated with cases of postmaturity, intrauterine growth restriction (IUGR) secondary to placental insufficiency, and with fetal conditions associated with major renal malformations, including renal aplasia with dysplastic kidneys and obstructive lesions of the lower urinary tract. Fetal risks include fetal skin and skeletal abnormalities, because fetal movement is impaired as a result of inadequate amniotic fluid volume, pulmonary hypoplasia, and cord compression.

POWERPOINT LECTURE SLIDES

(NOTE: The number on each PPT Lecture Slide directly corresponds with the Concepts for Lecture.)

 Amniotic Fluid Complications
- Amniotic fluid embolism
- Hydramnios (polyhydramnios)
- Oligohydramnios

LEARNING OBJECTIVE 11

Delineate the effects of pelvic contractures on labor and birth.

CONCEPTS FOR LECTURE

1. Pelvic contractures (narrowing) can result in cephalopelvic disproportion (CPD). This prolongs labor, and premature rupture of the membranes (PROM) can result from the force of the unequally distributed contractions being exerted on the fetal membranes. Additional risks include: uterine rupture, maternal soft tissue damage, cord prolapse, extreme molding of the fetal head, and traumatic forceps-assisted birth.

POWERPOINT LECTURE SLIDES

(NOTE: The number on each PPT Lecture Slide directly corresponds with the Concepts for Lecture.)

 Pelvic Complications
- Cephalopelvic disproportion
  - Uterine rupture
  - Maternal soft tissue damage
  - Cord prolapse
  - Extreme molding
  - Trauma to fetal skull and CNS

SUGGESTIONS FOR CLINICAL ACTIVITIES

Have students observe the labor and delivery of a mother with a pelvic contracture and note the maternal and fetal outcomes.

LEARNING OBJECTIVE 12

Discuss complications of the third and fourth stages of labor.

CONCEPTS FOR LECTURE

1. Common complications of the third and fourth stages of labor include: retained placenta, lacerations, and placenta accreta. Placental adherence complications include placenta accreta (where the chorionic villi attach directly to the myometrium of the uterus), placenta increta (in which the myometrium is invaded), and placenta percreta (in which the myometrium is penetrated). The major complications of placenta accreta include maternal hemorrhage and failure of the placenta to separate following birth of the infant.

POWERPOINT LECTURE SLIDES

(NOTE: The number on each PPT Lecture Slide directly corresponds with the Concepts for Lecture.)

 Third and Fourth Stage Complications
- Retained placenta
- Lacerations
- Placental adherence
  - Accreta
  - Increta
  - Percreta

SUGGESTIONS FOR CLASSROOM ACTIVITIES

Bring in a model of a perineum or illustrations to help students identify the degree of lacerations.

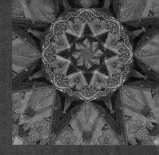

CHAPTER 27
BIRTH-RELATED PROCEDURES

RESOURCE LIBRARY

💿 PRENTICE HALL NURSING MEDIALINK DVD-ROM

Audio Glossary
NCLEX Review
Videos: *Vacuum Extractor*
  Types of Incisions
  Cesarean Birth
    Epidural Placement
    Delivery of Infant
    Assessment of Infant
    Bonding
    Suturing of Uterus
    Scrub Nurse Roles
Through the Eyes of a Nurse—The Third Trimester

🌐 COMPANION WEBSITE

Additional NCLEX Review
Case Study: *Client Undergoing Labor Induction*
Care Plan Activity: *Client with Pitocin for Labor Augmentation*
Applications: *Vacuum Extraction Delivery; Cesarean Birth*
Critical Thinking

📖 IMAGE LIBRARY

Figure 27.1 External (or cephalic) version of the fetus.
Figure 27.2 Use of podalic version and extraction of the fetus to assist in the vaginal birth of the second twin.
Figure 27.3 The two most common types of episiotomies are midline and mediolateral.

Figure 27.4 Forceps are composed of a blade, shank, and handle and may have a cephalic and pelvic curve.
Figure 27.5 Application of forceps in occiput-anterior (OA) position.
Figure 27.6 Vacuum extractor traction.
Figure 27.7 Uterine incisions for a cesarean birth.

LEARNING OBJECTIVE 1

Describe the impact of selected procedures on the childbearing woman and her family or support system.

CONCEPTS FOR LECTURE

1. Obstetric procedures are generally accepted by women and their families during birth based on the belief that the caregiver knows what is necessary for the woman and her fetus. Some women, however, want a natural childbirth without any medical intervention. Their emotional responses to obstetric procedures may include disappointment and/or guilt.

POWERPOINT LECTURE SLIDES

(NOTE: The number on each PPT Lecture Slide directly corresponds with the Concepts for Lecture.)

 Impact of Procedures on Childbearing Woman
- Disappointment
- Guilt
- Conflict between expectation and need for intervention

SUGGESTIONS FOR CLINICAL ACTIVITIES

Have students observe and discuss maternal reactions to different procedures in the clinical setting and identify appropriate nursing interventions.

LEARNING OBJECTIVE 2

Contrast the methods of external cephalic version and internal version and the related nursing management.

CONCEPTS FOR LECTURE

1. External cephalic version (ECV) may be performed if breech or shoulder presentation (transverse lie), oblique lie is detected in the later weeks of pregnancy. Through external manipulation of the maternal abdomen, the position of the fetus may be changed to a cephalic presentation. A podalic version is used only with the second twin during a vaginal birth. An internal version is when the obstetrician places a hand inside the uterus, grabs the fetus's feet, and then turns the fetus from a transverse or non-cephalic presentation to a breech presentation, and then the fetus is then born in a breech presentation. This is used only when the second twin is not in a cephalic position.

2. Nursing management for an external version includes: instructing the woman to fast for 8 hours preceding the version (in case a cesarean birth needs to be performed), assessing maternal vital signs, continuous electronic fetal monitoring, assessment of the presence of uterine contraction, obtaining blood work, and establishing an intravenous line for medication administration and administration of a beta-mimetic agent of intravenous infusion of magnesium sulfate. If epidural analgesia is used, the nurse should assist with that. The nurse should explain the procedure and provide psychological support throughout. After the version, the nurse should monitor the FHR for approximately 1 to 2 hours and assess the maternal-fetal response to the tocolytic agent. Discharge instructions should be given, including monitoring for uterine contractions, being aware of fetal movement (fetal kick counts), and recognizing signs of reversion (excessive movement or a sensation described as the fetus "turning around"). If the woman is Rh negative, RhoGAM should be administered.

POWERPOINT LECTURE SLIDES

(NOTE: The number on each PPT Lecture Slide directly corresponds with the Concepts for Lecture.)

1 Version
- External Cephalic Version (ECV) (Figure 27.1)
- Podalic Version (Internal) (Figure 27.2)

1a See Figure 27.1

1b See Figure 27.2

2 Nursing Management
- Maternal/fetal assessments
- NST
- Lab studies
- Psychologic support
- Education
- Monitor VS

2a Nursing Management
- EFM
- Medication administration—Beta-mimetics, RhoGAM

SUGGESTIONS FOR CLASSROOM ACTIVITIES

Discuss the role of the nurse in cephalic versions and potential risks to the fetus.

SUGGESTIONS FOR CLINICAL ACTIVITIES

Have students observe or assist with a version and document their observations.

LEARNING OBJECTIVE 3

Discuss the use of amniotomy in current maternal-newborn care.

CONCEPTS FOR LECTURE

1. The artificial rupture of the amniotic membranes (AROM) is an amniotomy. It may be used for labor induction or augmentation, to allow access to the fetus in order to apply a fetal heart monitoring electrode, to

POWERPOINT LECTURE SLIDES

(NOTE: The number on each PPT Lecture Slide directly corresponds with the Concepts for Lecture.)

1 Uses of Amniotomy
- Labor induction
- Labor augmentation

insert an intrauterine pressure catheter, or to obtain a fetal scalp blood sample for acid-base determination.

- Allow access to fetus and uterus to
  - Apply an internal fetal heart monitoring scalp electrode
  - Insert an intrauterine pressure catheter
  - Obtain a fetal scalp blood sample

SUGGESTIONS FOR CLASSROOM ACTIVITIES

Bring an amnihook to class and discuss how it is used in an amniotomy.

SUGGESTIONS FOR CLINICAL ACTIVITIES

Have students assist with an amniotomy in labor and delivery and discuss the appropriate nursing interventions.

LEARNING OBJECTIVE 4

Compare methods for inducing labor, explaining their advantages and disadvantages.

CONCEPTS FOR LECTURE

1. Induction of labor may begin by the administration of a prostaglandin E2 (PGE2) gel for cervical ripening. The most common types of gel are Prepidil and Cervidil. Both cause cervical ripening, shorten labor, reduce the rate of cesarean birth, and lower the requirements for oxytocin in labor. Risks include: uterine hyperstimulation, nonreassuring fetal status, a higher incidence of postpartum hemorrhage, and uterine rupture that can occur even in the absence of a previous uterine incision. The advantage of Cervidil is that it can be removed if uterine hyperstimulation occurs. Misoprostol (Cytotec), a synthetic PGE1 analogue, can also be used for this purpose and is a tablet that is inserted into the vagina or taken orally. It is more effective than oxytocin or prostaglandin agents and these women typically deliver within 24 hours of administration.

2. The most frequently used methods of induction or augmentation are stripping the amniotic membranes, amniotomy, and intravenous oxytocin (Pitocin) infusion. Stripping (or sweeping) the amniotic membranes is a nonpharmacologic method of labor induction in which the CNM or physician inserts a gloved finger as far as possible into the internal cervical os and rotates the finger 360 degrees, twice. This causes separation of the amniotic membranes that are lying against the lower uterine segment and internal os from the distal part of the lower uterine segment and is thought to release PGF2oc from the amniotic membranes or PGE2 from the cervix. Discomfort, uterine contractions, cramping, and a bloody discharge can occur. If labor is initiated, it usually begins in 24 to 48 hours.

3. An effective method of initiating uterine contractions to induce labor is the administration of intravenous oxytocin. Risks include hyperstimulation of the uterus resulting in uterine contractions that are too frequent (more often than every 2 minutes), uterine contractions that are too intense, increased uterine resting tone, uterine rupture, water intoxication, and a nonreassuring fetal heart rate pattern.

POWERPOINT LECTURE SLIDES

(NOTE: The number on each PPT Lecture Slide directly corresponds with the Concepts for Lecture.)

1 Cervical Ripening: Prostaglandin E2
- Advantages
  - Cervical ripening
  - Shorter labor
  - Lower requirements for oxytocin during labor induction
  - Vaginal birth is achieved within 24 hours for most women
  - Incidence of cesarean birth is reduced

1a Cervical Ripening: Prostaglandin E2
- Risks
  - Uterine hyperstimulation
  - Nonreassuring fetal status
  - Higher incidence of postpartum hemorrhage
  - Uterine rupture

2 Labor Induction: Stripping Membranes
- Advantages
  - Labor usually occurs in 24–48 hours
- Disadvantages
  - Can be painful
  - Uterine contractions
  - Bloody discharge

3 Labor Induction: Oxytocin
- Risks
  - Hyperstimulation of the uterus
  - Uterine rupture
  - Water intoxication
  - Nonreassuring fetal heart rate patterns

4 Labor Induction: Natural Methods
- Sexual intercourse/lovemaking
- Self or partner stimulation of the woman's nipples and breasts

4. Natural and noninvasive methods that may be suggested to induce labor either at home or in the tertiary care setting include sexual intercourse/lovemaking; self or partner stimulation of the woman's nipples and breasts; the use of herbs, such as blue/black cohosh, evening primrose oil, and red raspberry leaves; the use of homeopathic solutions, such as caulophyllum or pulsatilla; castor oil; enemas; and acupressure/acupuncture. Another method is the use of a Foley catheter with a 25-mL to 80-mL balloon to apply pressure on the internal os of the cervix and acts to ripen the cervix. This may be used alone or in conjunction with other induction methods.

- Use of herbs
  - Blue/black cohosh
  - Evening primrose oil
  - Red raspberry leaves

 Labor Induction: Natural Methods
- Use of homeopathic solutions
  - Caulophyllum or pulsatilla
  - Castor oil, enemas
  - Acupressure/acupuncture
- Mechanical dilatation with balloon catheter

SUGGESTIONS FOR CLASSROOM ACTIVITIES

Bring in samples of some of the herbs and homeopathic solutions used for labor induction.

SUGGESTIONS FOR CLINICAL ACTIVITIES

Have students assist with labor induction in the clinical agency. Document the appropriate assessments and discuss the woman's response to the therapy.

LEARNING OBJECTIVE 5

Discuss the use of transcervical intrapartum amnioinfusion.

CONCEPTS FOR LECTURE

1. An amnioinfusion (AI) can be used intrapartally to increase the volume of fluid when oligohydramnios is present to prevent variable decelerations and to treat variable decelerations. It is also used for meconium dilution in the presence of meconium staining, although its effectiveness for this purpose has been debated. A volume of warmed, sterile, normal saline or Ringer's lactate solution is introduced into the uterus through the use of an intrauterine pressure catheter (IUPC).

POWERPOINT LECTURE SLIDES

(NOTE: The number on each PPT Lecture Slide directly corresponds with the Concepts for Lecture.)

1 Amnioinfusion
- Prevent the possibility of variable decelerations
- Treat nonperiodic decelerations
- Meconium dilution

SUGGESTIONS FOR CLASSROOM ACTIVITIES

Show the students an intrauterine pressure catheter and discuss its use in amnioinfusion.

SUGGESTIONS FOR CLINICAL ACTIVITIES

Have students observe an amnioinfusion in labor and delivery and discuss the indications for the procedure.

LEARNING OBJECTIVE 6

Describe the types of episiotomies performed, the rationale for each, and the associated nursing interventions.

CONCEPTS FOR LECTURE

1. A midline episiotomy extends along the median raphe of the perineum and extends down from the vaginal orifice to the fibers of the rectal sphincter. The advantage of this type of episiotomy is that it avoids muscle fibers and major blood vessels because it divides the insertions of the superficial perineal muscles. Additional advantages of a midline episiotomy include less blood loss, easy repair, and healing with less discomfort for the mother. An episiotomy that begins in the

POWERPOINT LECTURE SLIDES

(NOTE: The number on each PPT Lecture Slide directly corresponds with the Concepts for Lecture.)

1 Episiotomy
- Types (Figure 27.3)
  - Midline
  - Mediolateral

1a See Figure 27.3

midline of the posterior fourchette (to avoid incision into the Bartholin gland) and extends at a 45-degree angle downward to the right or left is a mediolateral episiotomy. In the presence of a short perineum, macrosomia, and instrument-assisted birth (use of forceps or vacuum extractor), a mediolateral episiotomy provides more room and decreases the possibility of a traumatic extension into the rectum.

2. Nursing interventions associated with an episiotomy include: supporting the woman during the procedure, acting as an advocate for the woman in communicating her needs, providing pain medication as needed, documenting the type of episiotomy on the birth record, the provision of pain relief measures, assessment of the perineal tissue, and instructing the woman in perineal hygiene and comfort measures.

2 Nursing Management
- Support
- Assist with communication of woman's needs
- Pain relief measures
- Assessment
- Education

SUGGESTIONS FOR CLASSROOM ACTIVITIES

Bring a perineal model to class to demonstrate the types of episiotomies and discuss the implications of each.

SUGGESTIONS FOR CLINICAL ACTIVITIES

Ask students to assess episiotomies of newly delivered women and to document their assessments, pain relief measures, and the patient response.

LEARNING OBJECTIVE 7

Summarize the indications for forceps-assisted birth, types of forceps that may be used, complications, and related interventions.

CONCEPTS FOR LECTURE

1. Forceps may be used in the presence of any condition that threatens the mother or fetus and that can be relieved by birth. Maternal risk factors include: heart disease, acute pulmonary edema or pulmonary compromise, certain neurological conditions, intrapartal infection, prolonged second stage, or exhaustion. Fetal risk factors include: premature placental separation, prolapsed umbilical cord, and nonreassuring fetal status.
2. Outlet forceps include Elliot, Simpson, and Tucker-McLane forceps. Midforceps include Kielland and Barton forceps. Piper forceps can provide traction and flexion of the head of a fetus in breech presentation.
3. Newborn complications from the use of forceps include: facial ecchymosis and/or edema, caput succedaneum or cephalhematoma, and transient facial paralysis. Additional complications may include: low Apgar scores, retinal hemorrhage, corneal abrasions, ocular trauma, other trauma (Erb's palsy, fractured clavicle), elevated neonatal bilirubin levels, and prolonged infant hospital stay.
4. Maternal complications may include: lacerations of the birth canal, periurethral lacerations, and extensions of a median episiotomy into the anus; this trauma may result in increased bleeding, bruising, hematomas, and pelvic floor injuries.

POWERPOINT LECTURE SLIDES

(NOTE: The number on each PPT Lecture Slide directly corresponds with the Concepts for Lecture.)

1 Forceps-Assisted Birth: Maternal Indications (Figure 27.5A–C)
- Heart disease
- Acute pulmonary edema or pulmonary compromise
- Certain neurological conditions
- Intrapartal infection
- Prolonged second stage
- Exhaustion

1a See Figure 27.5A–C

1b Forceps-Assisted Birth: Fetal Indications
- Premature placental separation
- Prolapsed umbilical cord
- Nonreassuring fetal status

2 Types of Forceps (Figure 27.4)
- Outlet forceps
- Midforceps
- Breech forceps

2a See Figure 27.4

CONCEPTS FOR LECTURE *continued*

5. Nursing interventions include: explanation of the procedure to the woman, monitoring of contractions and advising the physician when one is present, advising the woman not to push when forceps are applied, helping the woman push after the forceps are in place, and supporting the woman. After the birth, the nurse should assess the newborn and the mother, and provide comfort measures for perineal trauma.

POWERPOINT LECTURE SLIDES *continued*

 Fetal Risks
- Ecchymosis, edema, or both along the sides of the face
- Caput succedaneum or cephalhematoma
- Transient facial paralysis
- Low Apgar scores
- Retinal hemorrhage
- Corneal abrasions

 Fetal Risks
- Ocular trauma
- Other trauma (Erb's palsy, fractured clavicle)
- Elevated neonatal bilirubin levels
- Prolonged infant hospital stay

 Maternal Risks
- Lacerations of the birth canal
- Periurethral lacerations
- Extension of a median episiotomy into the anus
- More likely to have a third- or fourth-degree laceration
- Report more perineal pain and sexual problems in the postpartum period
- Postpartum infections

Maternal Risks
- Cervical lacerations
- Prolonged hospital stay
- Urinary and rectal incontinence
- Anal sphincter injury
- Postpartum metritis

 Nursing Management
- Explains procedure to woman
- Monitors contractions
- Informs physician/CNM of contraction
- Encourages woman to avoid pushing during contraction
- Assessment of mother and her newborn
- Reassurance

SUGGESTIONS FOR CLASSROOM ACTIVITIES

Bring different types of forceps to class and discuss the indications for use of each type.

SUGGESTIONS FOR CLINICAL ACTIVITIES

Have students do a newborn assessment of a newly delivered infant born via forceps-assisted birth. Have them note the findings pertaining to trauma related to the use of the forceps.

LEARNING OBJECTIVE 8

Discuss the use of vacuum extraction, including indications, procedure, complications, and related nursing management.

CONCEPTS FOR LECTURE

1. Vacuum extraction is used to assist the birth of a fetus by applying suction to the fetal head. Indications for its use include a prolonged second stage of labor or non-reassuring heart rate pattern.
2. The suction cup is placed against the occiput of the fetal head. The pump is used to create negative pressure (suction) of approximately 50 to 60 mmHg and traction is applied by the physician or CNM in coordination with uterine contractions. Nursing responsibilities include: informing the woman about what is happening, pumping the vacuum to the appropriate level, and assessment of the FHR.
3. Newborn complications may include: scalp lacerations, bruising, subgaleal hematomas, cephalhematomas, intracranial hemorrhages, subconjunctival hemorrhages, neonatal jaundice, fractured clavicle, Erb's palsy, damage to the sixth and seventh cranial nerves, retinal hemorrhage, and fetal death. In addition, there is an increased incidence of shoulder dystocia.
4. Maternal complications may include: perineal trauma, edema, third- and fourth-degree lacerations, postpartum pain, sexual difficulties, and infection.

POWERPOINT LECTURE SLIDES

(NOTE: The number on each PPT Lecture Slide directly corresponds with the Concepts for Lecture.)

1 Indications for Vacuum Extraction
- Prolonged second stage of labor
- Nonreassuring heart rate pattern
- Used to relieve the woman of pushing effort
- When analgesia or fatigue interfere with ability to push effectively
- Borderline CPD

2 Vacuum Extraction Procedure
- Procedure (Figure 27.6A–C)
  ○ Suction cup placed on fetal occiput
  ○ Pump is used to create suction
  ○ Traction is applied
  ○ Fetal head should descend with each contraction

2a See Figure 27.6A–C

2b Nursing Management
- Inform woman about procedure
- Pumps the vacuum
- Supports the woman
- Assesses the mother and neonate for complications

3 Neonatal Risks with Vacuum Extraction
- Scalp lacerations and bruising
- Shoulder dystocia
- Subgaleal hematomas
- Cephalhematomas
- Intracranial hemorrhages
- Subconjunctival hemorrhages

3a Neonatal Risks with Vacuum Extraction
- Neonatal jaundice
- Fractured clavicle
- Erb's palsy
- Damage to the sixth and seventh cranial nerves
- Retinal hemorrhage
- Fetal death

4 Maternal Risks with Vacuum Extraction
- Perineal trauma
- Edema
- Third- and fourth-degree lacerations
- Postpartum pain
- Infection
- More sexual difficulties in the postpartum period

SUGGESTIONS FOR CLASSROOM ACTIVITIES

Show the students the video on the DVD-ROM on vacuum extraction and discuss the procedure.

SUGGESTIONS FOR CLINICAL ACTIVITIES

Have students observe a vacuum extraction birth in labor and delivery and discuss their observations.

Explain the indications for cesarean birth, impact on the family unit, preparation and teaching needs, and associated nursing management.

CONCEPTS FOR LECTURE

1. Indications for cesarean birth include: complete placenta previa, CPD, placental abruption, active genital herpes, umbilical cord prolapse, failure to progress in labor, proven nonreassuring fetal status, and benign and malignant tumors that obstruct the birth canal. Indications that are more controversial include: breech presentation, previous cesarean birth, major congenital anomalies, cervical cerclage, severe Rh isoimmunization, and maternal preference for cesarean birth.

2. The impact of cesarean birth on the family unit may include: stress and anxiety over the surgery and the welfare of the mother and the fetus, loss of the vaginal birth experience, helplessness, loss of control, or relief.

3. Preparation of the couple for a cesarean birth should include preoperative teaching, including: coughing and deep breathing, splinting the incision, and what to expect during and after the surgery.

4. Nursing management before a cesarean birth includes: assisting with the epidural, monitoring maternal vital signs and fetal heart rate, inserting an indwelling urinary catheter, preparing the abdomen and perineum, making sure that all necessary personnel and equipment are present, positioning the woman on the operating table, supporting the couple, and doing an instrument count. Nursing management after the surgery includes: normal newborn post-delivery care, monitoring vital signs, checking the surgical dressing, palpating the fundus and checking lochia, monitoring intake and output, administration of oxytocin as ordered by the physician, and pain management.

POWERPOINT LECTURE SLIDES

(NOTE: The number on each PPT Lecture Slide directly corresponds with the Concepts for Lecture.)

1 Indications of Cesarean Birth
- Complete placenta previa
- CPD
- Placental abruption
- Active genital herpes
- Umbilical cord prolapse
- Failure to progress in labor

1a Indications for Cesarean Birth
- Proven nonreassuring fetal status
- Benign and malignant tumors that obstruct the birth canal
- Breech presentation
- Previous cesarean birth
- Major congenital anomalies
- Cervical cerclage

1b Indications for Cesarean Birth
- Severe Rh isoimmunization
- Maternal preference for cesarean birth

2 Impact on the Family
- Stress and anxiety
- Sense of loss of vaginal birth experience
- Fear
- Relief

3 Preparation for Cesarean Birth
- Preoperative teaching
  - Coughing and deep breathing
  - Splinting
  - What to expect

4 Nursing Management Before Cesarean Birth
- Assisting with the epidural
- Monitoring maternal vital signs and fetal heart rate
- Inserting an indwelling urinary catheter
- Preparing the abdomen and perineum
- Making sure that all necessary personnel and equipment are present
- Positioning the woman on the operating table

4a Nursing Management Before Cesarean Birth
- Supporting the couple
- Instrument count

4b Nursing Management After Cesarean Birth
- Normal newborn postdelivery care
- Monitoring vital signs
- Checking the surgical dressing

- Palpating the fundus and checking lochia
- Monitoring intake and output
- Administration of oxytocin and pain management

SUGGESTIONS FOR CLASSROOM ACTIVITIES

Have students develop a teaching plan to prepare a couple for a cesarean birth.

SUGGESTIONS FOR CLINICAL ACTIVITIES

Have students assist with the preparation of a couple for a cesarean birth in the clinical setting and discuss their observations.

LEARNING OBJECTIVE 10

Discuss vaginal birth following cesarean birth.

CONCEPTS FOR LECTURE

1. While there was an increasing trend in the late 1980s to have a trial of labor and vaginal birth after cesarean (VBAC) birth in cases of nonrecurring indications for a cesarean, recent debate and research have led to a considerable rise in cesarean births and a significant reduction in women attempting VBACs due to the risk of uterine rupture. Success rates, however, have been encouraging. The following conditions must be met for a trial of labor: only one previous cesarean birth and a low transverse uterine incision; an adequate pelvis; no other uterine scars or previous uterine rupture; a physician who is able to do a cesarean needs to be available throughout active labor; and in-house anesthesia personnel are available for emergency cesarean births if warranted.

POWERPOINT LECTURE SLIDES

(NOTE: The number on each PPT Lecture Slide directly corresponds with the Concepts for Lecture.)

 Vaginal Birth After Cesarean (VBAC): Criteria
- One previous cesarean birth and a low transverse uterine incision
- An adequate pelvis
- No other uterine scars or previous uterine rupture
- An available physician who is able to do a cesarean
- In-house anesthesia personnel

 Vaginal Birth After Cesarean (VBAC): Risks
- Uterine rupture
- Stillbirths
- Hypoxia

SUGGESTIONS FOR CLASSROOM ACTIVITIES

Have students discuss the emotional impact of a vaginal birth after cesarean on a couple.

SUGGESTIONS FOR CLINICAL ACTIVITIES

Ask students to assist with the labor of a couple attempting a vaginal birth after cesarean and discuss their observations of labor in post-conference.

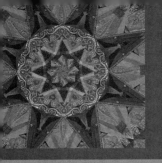

CHAPTER 28
PHYSIOLOGIC RESPONSES OF THE NEWBORN TO BIRTH

RESOURCE LIBRARY

PRENTICE HALL NURSING MEDIALINK DVD-ROM

Audio Glossary
NCLEX Review

 COMPANION WEBSITE

Additional NCLEX Review
Case Study: *Normal Range of Newborn's Vital Signs*
Care Plan Activity: *Physiologic Responses of the Newborn*
Applications: *Newborn Thermoregulation; Physiologic Jaundice*
Critical Thinking

IMAGE LIBRARY

Figure 28.2 Process of absorption of fetal lung fluid during breathing after birth.
Figure 28.3 Fetal oxygen-hemoglobin dissociation curve.
Figure 28.4 Transitional circulation: conversion from fetal to neonatal circulation.
Figure 28.5 Major changes that occur in the newborn's circulatory system.
Figure 28.6 Fetal-neonatal circulation.
Figure 28.7 Response of blood pressure (BP) to changes in neonatal blood volume.

Figure 28.8 Schematic illustration of the mechanisms in placental transfusion (normal term births) through the umbilical vein.
Figure 28.9 Methods of heat loss.
Figure 28.10 The distribution of brown adipose tissue (brown fat) in the newborn.
Figure 28.11 Conjugation of bilirubin in newborns.
Figure 28.12 Newborn stool samples.
Figure 28.13 Mother and baby gaze at each other.
Figure 28.14 Head turning to follow an object.

LEARNING OBJECTIVE 1

Summarize the respiratory and cardiovascular changes that occur during the transition to extrauterine life and during stabilization.

CONCEPTS FOR LECTURE

1. Changes that must take place in the transition to extrauterine life to allow the lungs to function include the following: pulmonary ventilation through lung expansion following birth; and a marked increase in the pulmonary circulation. Lung expansion occurs in response to mechanical, chemical, thermal, and sensory changes at birth; these changes stimulate the neonate to take the first breath, which opens the alveoli. This initial gasp and exhalation begin the removal of lung fluid. A positive intrathoracic pressure is created when the newborn exhales against a partially-closed glottis which distributes the inspired air through the alveoli and establishes a functional residual capacity (FRC).

2. With the onset of respiration, cardiovascular system changes occur. The rise of Po_2 in the alveoli relaxes the pulmonary arteries, which triggers a decrease

POWERPOINT LECTURE SLIDES

(NOTE: The number on each PPT Lecture Slide directly corresponds with the Concepts for Lecture.)

1. Respiratory Adapations
   - Mechanical changes
   - Chemical changes
   - Thermal changes
   - Sensory changes

2. Cardiovascular Adaptations (Figure 28.4, Figure 28.6A–C)
   - Decreased pulmonary vascular resistance and increased blood flow
   - Increased systemic pressure and closure of ductus venosus
   - Increased left atrium and decreased right atrium pressure
     ○ Closure of foramen ovale

in the pumonary vascular resistance and an increase in the vascular flow. As blood returns from the pulmonary veins, pressure in the left atrium increases and pressure in the right atrium drops; this closes the foramen ovale. Systemic vascular resistance increases as umbilical venous flow stops when the cord is clamped and the ductus venosus closes. When the systemic vascular pressure rises above the pulmonary vascular pressure, blood flow reverses through the ductus arteriosus. This, coupled with an increase in the Po_2, causes constriction of the ductus arteriosus.

- Reversal of blood flow through ductus arteriosus and increased Po_2
  - Closure of ductus arteriosus

[2a] See Figure 28.4

[2b] See Figure 28.6A–C

SUGGESTIONS FOR CLASSROOM ACTIVITIES

Have students develop a concept map for the respiratory and cardiovascular changes that occur at birth.

SUGGESTIONS FOR CLINICAL ACTIVITIES

Have students assess a newborn transitioning to extrauterine life and discuss their observations in relation to their knowledge of the processes that are occurring during this time.

LEARNING OBJECTIVE 2

Describe how various factors affect the newborn's blood values.

CONCEPTS FOR LECTURE

1. A relative hypoxia in utero causes increased amounts of erythropoietin to be secreted, which results in active erythropoiesis (an increase in nucleated red blood cells and reticulocytes). As oxygen levels rise after birth, the production of erythropoietin is shut off. Initially, hemoglobin concentration may rise 1 to 2 g/dL above fetal levels as a result of placental transfusion, low oral fluid intake, and diminished extracellular fluid volume but by 1 week after birth, peripheral hemoglobin is comparable to fetal blood counts. It then declines progressively thereafter during the first 2 months after birth, which creates the phenomenon known as physiologic anemia of infancy. Normally, infants have leukocytosis because the stress of birth stimulates increased production of neutrophils during the first few days of life. The leukocyte count then decreases to 35% of the total count by 2 weeks of age.

POWERPOINT LECTURE SLIDES

(NOTE: The number on each PPT Lecture Slide directly corresponds with the Concepts for Lecture.)

[1] Fetal Laboratory Value Changes
- Decreased erythropoietin production
- Rise of hemoglobin concentration
- Physiologic anemia of infancy
- Leukocytosis
- Decreased percentage of neutrophils

SUGGESTIONS FOR CLINICAL ACTIVITIES

Have students review the lab values of a healthy newborn and discuss their findings.

LEARNING OBJECTIVE 3

Correlate the major mechanisms of heat loss in the newborn to the process of thermogenesis in the newborn.

CONCEPTS FOR LECTURE

1. Newborns are more susceptible to heat loss due to a large body surface in relation to mass and a limited amount of insulating subcutaneous fat. Heat loss can occur from convection, radiation, evaporation, and conduction. Convection is the loss of heat from the warm body surface to the cooler air currents. Radiation losses occur when body heat rises to cooler surfaces and objects not in direct contact with the body. Evaporation is the loss of heat incurred when water is converted to a vapor. Conduction is the loss of heat to a cooler surface by direct skin contact.

POWERPOINT LECTURE SLIDES

(NOTE: The number on each PPT Lecture Slide directly corresponds with the Concepts for Lecture.)

| 1 | Thermogenesis in the Newborn
- Large body surface area compared to mass
- Types of heat loss (Figure 28.9A–D)
  - Convection
  - Radiation
  - Evaporation
  - Conduction

| 1a | See Figure 28.9A–D

SUGGESTIONS FOR CLASSROOM ACTIVITIES

Have students demonstrate the types of heat loss using their bodies and items in the classroom. Discuss implications for the newborn.

SUGGESTIONS FOR CLINICAL ACTIVITIES

Have students assess newborns in the clinical area for potential heat loss and identify appropriate nursing interventions.

LEARNING OBJECTIVE 4

Explain the steps involved in conjugation and excretion of bilirubin in the newborn.

CONCEPTS FOR LECTURE

1. The byproduct of hemoglobin that is released from destroyed red blood cells is unconjugated (indirect) bilirubin, which is not excretable and is a potential toxin. Conjugation is the process of transforming the bilirubin into a water-soluble form that can be excreted. Conjugation occurs during the transport of unconjugated bilirubin that is bound to albumin to the hepatocytes where it is bound to intracellular proteins. Unconjugated bilirubin is then attached to glucuronic acid through the activity of the uridine diphosphoglucuronosyl transferase (UDPGT) enzyme, which produces bilirubin glucuronides (conjugated, direct bilirubin). It is then excreted into the tiny bile ducts, then into the common duct and duodenum, progresses down the intestines, where bacteria transform it into urobilinogen (urine bilirubin) and stercobilinogen for excretion.

POWERPOINT LECTURE SLIDES

(NOTE: The number on each PPT Lecture Slide directly corresponds with the Concepts for Lecture.)

| 1 | Types of Bilirubin
- Unconjugated bilirubin
- Conjugated bilirubin
- Total bilirubin

| 1a | Conjugation and Excretion of Bilirubin
- Bilirubin is transported in blood via albumin
- Bilirubin is transferred into the hepatocytes
- Attachment of unconjugated bilirubin to glucuronic acid
- Excreted into bile ducts, then into the common duct and duodenum
- Bacteria transform it into urobilinogen and stercobilinogen
- Bilirubin is excreted in urine and stool

SUGGESTIONS FOR CLASSROOM ACTIVITIES

Have students develop a concept map that illustrates the process of bilirubin conjugation and excretion.

LEARNING OBJECTIVE 5

Discuss the reasons why the newborn may develop jaundice.

CONCEPTS FOR LECTURE

1. Physiologic jaundice is caused by accelerated destruction of fetal RBCs, impaired conjugation of bilirubin, and increased bilirubin reabsorption from the intestinal tract. Any destruction of fetal RBC increases the bilirubin load in the newborn, particularly because a proportionately larger amount of nonerythrocyte bilirubin is formed in the newborn and the newborn liver may not be able to handle the increased load. Neonatal hypoxia decreases oxygen to the liver, which leads to a rise in bilirubin. Additionally, if the newborn does not take in adequate calories, the formation of hepatic intracellular binding proteins diminishes, which results in higher levels of bilirubin. Fatty acids in maternal breast milk compete with bilirubin for albumin binding sites, which impedes bilirubin processing. A delay in intestinal motility for any reason can delay excretion of bilirubin.

POWERPOINT LECTURE SLIDES

(NOTE: The number on each PPT Lecture Slide directly corresponds with the Concepts for Lecture.)

1 Physiologic Jaundice
- Accelerated destruction of fetal RBCs
  ○ Increased amounts of bilirubin delivered to liver
  ○ Inadequate hepatic circulation
- Impaired conjugation of bilirubin
  ○ Defective uptake of bilirubin from the plasma
  ○ Defective conjugation of the bilirubin

1a Physiologic Jaundice
- Increased bilirubin reabsorption
  ○ Defect in bilirubin excretion
  ○ Increased reabsorption of bilirubin from the intestine

SUGGESTIONS FOR CLINICAL ACTIVITIES

Have students assess newborns in the nursery for jaundice and identify potential sources of impaired bilirubin conjugation or excretion.

LEARNING OBJECTIVE 6

Delineate the functional abilities of the newborn's gastrointestinal tract and liver.

CONCEPTS FOR LECTURE

1. The newborn's liver occupies 40% of the abdominal cavity. It plays a significant role in iron storage, carbohydrate metabolism, and coagulation. The iron content of destroyed red blood cells is stored in the liver until it is needed for new red blood cell production. Neonatal carbohydrate reserves are low, with 1/3 of these stores being in the form of liver glycogen. The main source of energy in the first 4 to 6 hours after birth is glucose. After birth, the newborn must begin to conjugate bilirubin and the serum level rises during the first few days of life. Due to a reduction in hepatic activity, a relatively large bilirubin load, and a reduced ability to conjugate bilirubin, the newborn is susceptible to jaundice.

2. There is an absence of normal intestinal flora in the newborn gut which results in low levels of vitamin K and creates a temporary blood coagulation disturbance between days 2 to 5. The coagulation levels rise slowly from a low point at about 2 to 3 days after birth until they reach adult levels at 9 months. The gastrointestinal tract is mature by 36 to 38 weeks of fetal life with the presence of enzymatic activity and the ability to transport nutrients. Amylase, however, is relatively deficient during the first few months of life. The digestion

POWERPOINT LECTURE SLIDES

(NOTE: The number on each PPT Lecture Slide directly corresponds with the Concepts for Lecture.)

1 Liver Adaptations
- Iron content stored in liver
- Low carbohydrate reserves
- Main source of energy is glucose
- Liver begins to conjugate bilirubin
- Lack of intestinal flora results in low levels of vitamin K

2 GI Adaptations
- Sufficient enzymes except for amylase
- Digests and absorbs fats less efficiently
- Salivary glands are immature
- Stomach has capacity of 50–60 mL
- Cardiac sphincter is immature

and absorption of fat is less efficient because of the minimal activity of pancreatic lipase. At birth, the salivary glands are immature, and little saliva is manufactured until the infant is about 3 months old. The newborn's stomach has a capacity of 50 to 60 mL and it empties intermittently, starting within a few minutes of the beginning of a feeding and ending between 2 and 4 hours after feeding. Within the first 30 to 60 minutes of birth, bowel sounds are present. The gastric pH becomes less acidic about a week after birth and remains less acidic than that of adults for the next 2 to 3 months. Regurgitation may occur in the neonatal period because the cardiac sphincter and neural control of the stomach is immature. Caloric intake is often insufficient for weight gain until the newborn is 5 to 10 days old and there may be a weight loss of 5% to 10% in term newborns. Some of the weight loss is due to a shift of intracellular water to the extracellular spaces, as well as insensible water loss.

SUGGESTIONS FOR CLASSROOM ACTIVITIES

Have students discuss the implications of gastrointestinal and liver changes on newborn assessments.

SUGGESTIONS FOR CLINICAL ACTIVITIES

Have students assess the gastrointestinal status of a newborn and discuss their findings in relation to their knowledge about the physiologic changes that are occurring.

LEARNING OBJECTIVE 7

Identify the reasons the newborn's kidneys have difficulty maintaining fluid and electrolyte balance.

CONCEPTS FOR LECTURE

1. Factors that contribute to the newborn's difficulty in maintaining fluid and electrolyte balance include a decreased ability to concentrate urine due to short, narrow tubules, which causes limited tubular reabsorption of water and excretion of solutes in the growing newborn. Because of this, the effect of excessive insensible water loss or restricted fluid intake is unpredictable. The dilutional capabilities of the kidney are also limited.

POWERPOINT LECTURE SLIDES

(NOTE: The number on each PPT Lecture Slide directly corresponds with the Concepts for Lecture.)

1. Fluid and Electrolyte Balance
   - Less able to concentrate urine
   - Limited tubular reabsorption of water
   - Limited excretion of solutes
   - Limited dilutional capabilities

SUGGESTIONS FOR CLINICAL ACTIVITIES

Have students assess the specific gravity of the urine of a newborn.

LEARNING OBJECTIVE 8

List the immunologic responses available to the newborn.

CONCEPTS FOR LECTURE

1. The newborn acquires passive immunity from IgG antibodies that are transferred in utero. This transfer primarily occurs during the third trimester, which puts the

POWERPOINT LECTURE SLIDES

(NOTE: The number on each PPT Lecture Slide directly corresponds with the Concepts for Lecture.)

1. Immunologic Responses in the Newborn
   - IgG—passive acquired immunity via placenta

preterm infant at increased risk for infection. While the newborn does produce antibodies in response to an antigen, the antibodies are not as effective as in an older child. IgM immunoglobulins are produced by the fetus beginning at 10 to 15 weeks' gestation. If elevated levels of IgM are present at birth, it may indicate placental leaks or fetal antigenic stimulation in utero. Infants with high levels of IgM may have been exposed to an intrauterine infection such as syphilis or TORCH syndrome. Newborns begin to produce secretory IgA in their intestinal mucosa at about 4 weeks after birth. The breastfeeding infant receives high levels of IgA through the intake of colostrum.

- IgM—usually not passively transferred
  - Elevated levels may indicate fetal antigenic activity in utero
- IgA—passive acquired immunity via colostrum

LEARNING OBJECTIVE 9

Explain the physiologic and behavioral responses of newborns during the periods of reactivity, and identify possible interventions.

CONCEPTS FOR LECTURE

1. An initial period of reactivity lasts approximately 30 minutes after birth, during which the newborn is awake, active, may appear hungry, and have a strong sucking reflex. Additionally, respirations and heart rate are rapid. There may be retraction of the chest, transient flaring of the nares, grunting, and bowel sounds are usually absent. This phase lasts for approximately 30 minutes, after which the newborn enters a sleep period that may last from a few minutes to 2 to 4 hours. During this time, activity diminishes, the heart rate and respirations decrease, the newborn shows no interest in sucking, and bowel sounds become audible. The second period of reactivity then begins and lasts 4 to 6 hours. During the second period of reactivity, the newborn is again awake and alert. This period is characterized by an increase in heart rate and respiratory rate. The production of respiratory and gastric mucus also increases, and the newborn responds by gagging, choking, and regurgitating. The gastrointestinal tract becomes more active; the newborn often passes the first meconium stool and may also have an initial voiding. At this point, the newborn shows he or she is ready to be fed.

POWERPOINT LECTURE SLIDES

(NOTE: The number on each PPT Lecture Slide directly corresponds with the Concepts for Lecture.)

 1 Periods of Reactivity
- First period of reactivity
- Sleep phase
- Second period of reactivity

SUGGESTIONS FOR CLASSROOM ACTIVITIES

Discuss implications for nursing care with an understanding of the periods of reactivity.

SUGGESTIONS FOR CLINICAL ACTIVITIES

Have students assess a newborn and identify the infant state in relation to reactivity.

LEARNING OBJECTIVE 10

Describe the normal sensory/perceptual abilities and behavioral states present in the newborn period.

CONCEPTS FOR LECTURE

1. The newborn's ability to process and respond to complex stimulation is called habituation. The newborn's ability to be alert to, to follow, and to fixate on complex visual stimuli that have a particular appeal and attraction is called orientation. Newborns have a preference for the human face and eyes and bright shiny objects. The response to auditory stimulation is a definite, organized behavior repertoire that includes a rise in the heart rate and a minimal startle reflex. The newborn will become alert and search for the stimulus if the sound is appealing. The response to taste is varied. The breastfeeding newborn tends to suck in bursts with regular pauses, while the bottle-fed newborn tends to suck at a regular rate with infrequent pauses. Newborns have a sensitivity to being touched, cuddled, and held. If a newborn is settled, he/she is then able to attend to and interact with the environment.

POWERPOINT LECTURE SLIDES

(NOTE: The number on each PPT Lecture Slide directly corresponds with the Concepts for Lecture.)

 Behavioral and Sensory Capabilities
- Habituation
- Orientation (Figure 28.13)
- Auditory
- Olfactory
- Tasting and sucking
- Tactile

1a See Figure 28.13

SUGGESTIONS FOR CLINICAL ACTIVITIES

Have students observe infant behavior and discuss their findings.

CHAPTER 29
NURSING ASSESSMENT OF THE NEWBORN

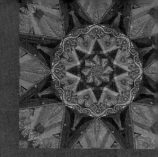

RESOURCE LIBRARY

🔘 PRENTICE HALL NURSING MEDIALINK DVD-ROM

Audio Glossary
NCLEX Review
Videos:
  Assessment of an Infant
  Newborn Reflexes
    Gross and Fine Motor Activity
    Maternal-Newborn Reflexes
    Moro Reflex
    Palmar Grasp
    Rooting
    Sucking
    Babinski
    Trunk Incurvation (Galant Reflex)

📖 IMAGE LIBRARY

Figure 29.1 Newborn maturity rating and classification.
Figure 29.2 Resting posture.
Figure 29.3 Sole creases.
Figure 29.4 Breast tissue.
Figure 29.5 Ear form and cartilage.
Figure 29.6 Male genitals.
Figure 29.7 Female genitals.
Figure 29.8 Square window sign.
Figure 29.9 Scarf sign.
Figure 29.10 Heel-to-ear.
Figure 29.11 Ankle dorsiflexion.
Figure 29.12 Classification of newborns by birth weight and gestational age.
Figure 29.13 Classification of newborns based on maturity and intrauterine growth.
Figure 29.14 Measuring the length of the newborn.
Figure 29.15 *A*, Measuring the head circumference of the newborn. *B*, Measuring the chest circumference of the newborn.
Figure 29.16 Axillary temperature measurement.
Figure 29.17 Temperature monitoring for the newborn.
Figure 29.18 Acrocyanosis.
Figure 29.19 Erythema toxicum.
Figure 29.20 Facial milia.
Figure 29.21 Stork bites.
Figure 29.22 Mongolian spots.
Figure 29.23 Port wine stain.
Figure 29.24 Overlapped cranial bones produce a visible ridge in a small premature infant.

🌐 COMPANION WEBSITE

Additional NCLEX Review
Case Study: *Newborn Maturity Assessment*
Care Plan Activity: *Assessment of the Uncomplicated Newborn*
Applications: *Newborn Gestational Assessment; Newborn Reflexes; Newborn Assessment*
Critical Thinking

Figure 29.25 Cephalhematoma is a collection of blood between the surface of a cranial bone and the periosteal membrane.
Figure 29.26 Caput succedaneum is a collection of fluid (serum) under the scalp.
Figure 29.27 Facial paralysis.
Figure 29.28 Transient strabismus in the newborn may be due to poor neuromuscular control.
Figure 29.29 The nurse inserts the index finger (or "pinky") into the newborn's mouth and feels for any openings along the hard and soft palates.
Figure 29.30 The position of the external ear may be assessed by drawing a line across the inner and outer canthus of the eye to the insertion of the ear.
Figure 29.31 Breast hypertrophy.
Figure 29.32 *A*, Bilaterally palpate the femoral arteries for rate and intensity of the pulses. *B*, Compare the femoral pulses to the brachial pulses by palpating the pulses simultaneously for comparison of rate and intensity.
Figure 29.33 Blood pressure measurement using the Dinemapp and Doppler devices.
Figure 29.34 Umbilical hernia.
Figure 29.35 Right Erb's palsy resulting from injury to the fifth and sixth cervical roots of brachial plexus.
Figure 29.36 *A*, The asymmetry of gluteal and thigh fat folds seen in infant with left developmental of the hip. *B*, Barlow (dislocation) maneuver. *C*, Dislocation is palpable as femoral head slips out of acetabulum. *D*, Ortolani's maneuver puts downward pressure on the hip and then inward rotation.

Figure 29.37 *A*, Unilateral talipes equinovarus (clubfoot). *B*, To determine the presence of clubfoot, the nurse moves the foot to the midline.
Figure 29.38 Tonic neck reflex.
Figure 29.39 Palmar grasping reflex.
Figure 29.40 Moro reflex.

Figure 29.41 Rooting reflex.
Figure 29.42 The Babinski reflex (response).
Figure 29.43 The stepping reflex disappears between 4 and 8 weeks of age.
Figure 29.44 The newborn can bring hand to mouth as a self-soothing activity.

LEARNING OBJECTIVE 1

Explain the various components of the gestational age assessment.

CONCEPTS FOR LECTURE

1. Physical maturity characteristics utilized in gestational age assessment include: resting posture, skin, lanugo, sole creases, breast bud, and male and female genitalia. The preterm newborn's skin appears thin and transparent, with veins prominent over the abdomen early in gestation. The skin of the term infant appears opaque because of increased subcutaneous tissue. Postmature infants usually have skin desquamation due to the disappearance of vernix caseosa. As gestational age increases, lanugo decreases. Sole creases develop at the top portion of the sole and as gestation progresses, continues to the heel. However, the sole creases are only reliable in the first 12 hours of life as superficial creases appear due to drying after that time.

   The breast bud will measure between 0.5 and 1 cm (5 to 10 mm) at term. As the infant is more gestationally mature, the ear will be more formed with a greater amount of cartilage. Prior to 36 weeks, the male infant will have a small scrotum, has few rugae, and the testes are palpable in the inguinal canal. By 40 weeks, the testes are generally in the lower scrotum, which is pendulous and covered with rugae. Female genital appearance is partially dependent upon fat deposition. The clitoris is prominent and the labia majora are smaller than the labia minora in an infant less than 32 weeks. At term, the labia majora completely cover the labia minor and clitoris.

2. Neuromuscular maturity characteristics include: the square window sign recoil, the popliteal angle, the scarf sign, heel-to-ear extension, ankle dorsiflexion, head lag, and ventral suspension.

POWERPOINT LECTURE SLIDES

(NOTE: The number on each PPT Lecture Slide directly corresponds with the Concepts for Lecture.)

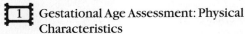 **1** Gestational Age Assessment: Physical Characteristics
- Resting posture
  ○ Preterm: extended
  ○ Term: flexed
- Skin
  ○ Preterm: thin and transparent with veins prominent
  ○ Term: opaque and disappearance of the vernix caseosa

1a Gestational Age Assessment: Physical Characteristics
- Lanugo
  ○ Decreases as gestational age increases
- Sole (plantar) creases
  ○ As gestation progresses, proceeds to the heel
- Breast bud
  ○ Term: the tissue will measure between 0.5 and 1 cm

1b Gestational Age Assessment: Physical Characteristics
- Ear form and cartilage distribution
  ○ Preterm: relatively shapeless and flat, no recoil
  ○ Term: some cartilage and slight incurving of the upper pinna, good recoil
- Male genitals
  ○ Preterm: small scrotum, few rugae, testes are palpable in the inguinal canal
  ○ Term: testes are generally in the lower scrotum, which is pendulous and covered with rugae

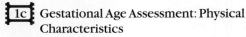 **1c** Gestational Age Assessment: Physical Characteristics
- Female genitals
  ○ Preterm: clitoris is prominent, labia majora are small and widely separated
  ○ Term: labia majora cover the labia minora and clitoris

Assessment of Neuromuscular Characteristics
- Square window
- Recoil
- Popliteal angle
- Scarf sign
- Heel to ear
- Ankle dorsiflexion

 Assessment of Neuromuscular Characteristics
- Head lag
- Ventral suspension

SUGGESTIONS FOR CLASSROOM ACTIVITIES

Bring copies of the Ballard and Dubowitz tools to class for students to view.

SUGGESTIONS FOR CLINICAL ACTIVITIES

Have students complete a gestational age assessment on two infants of different gestational maturity and compare their findings.

LEARNING OBJECTIVE 2

Describe the normal physical and behavioral characteristics of the newborn.

CONCEPTS FOR LECTURE

1. While race, age and size of the parents, the health of the mother, and the interval between pregnancies can influence birth weight, the average weight of the normal full-term Caucasian newborn is 3405 g (7 lb, 8 oz). The average length of the term newborn is 50 cm (20 in). The range of the circumference of the newborn's head is 32 to 37 cm (12.5 to 14.5 in) and is approximately 2 cm greater than the circumference of the chest.

2. Skin color varies with genetic background, although all healthy newborns have a pink tinge to their skin. The head of the newborn is disproportionately large for the body, and two fontanelles may be palpated on the newborn's head; the diamond-shaped anterior fontanelle and the smaller, triangular-shaped posterior fontanelle. The newborn has smooth hair with ethnic texture variations and is usually found high over the eyebrows. Sucking (fat) pads are located in the cheeks, and a labial tubercle (sucking callus) is frequently found in the center of the upper lip, the chin is recessed, and the nose is flattened. The cry is normally tearless because the lacrimal structures are immature at birth and are not usually fully functional until the second month of life. Term newborns have poor oculomotor coordination and absence of accommodation which limits visual abilities. However, they do have peripheral vision and can fixate on near objects in front of their faces for short periods, can accommodate to large objects, and can seek out high-contrast geometric shapes. The nose is small and narrow and they are nose breathers for the first few months of life. Taste buds are developed before birth, and the newborn can easily discriminate between sweet and bitter flavors. The ears are soft and

POWERPOINT LECTURE SLIDES

(NOTE: The number on each PPT Lecture Slide directly corresponds with the Concepts for Lecture.)

 Measurement and Appearance
- Average weight of 3405 g at term
- Average length is 50 cm (20 in.)
- Head circumference is 32–37 cm
- Chest circumference is 30–35 cm
- Skin—pink tinged

 Head
- Proportionally larger than body
- Fontanelles
  ○ Anterior
  ○ Posterior
- Hair
- Face

 Eyes
- Tearless crying
- Peripheral vision
- Can fixate on near objects
- Can perceive faces, shapes, and colors
- Blink in response to bright light
- Pupillary reflex is present

2b Nose and Mouth
- Nose
  ○ Small and narrow
  ○ Must breathe through nose
- Mouth
  ○ Lips pink
  ○ Taste buds present

pliable and should recoil readily when folded and released. In the normal newborn, the top of the ear (pinna) should be parallel to the outer and inner canthus of the eye.

3. Newborns have a short neck creased with skin folds, and because muscle tone is not well developed, the neck cannot support the full weight of the head, which rotates freely. The thorax is cylindrical and symmetric at birth. Frequently newborns have engorged breasts due to maternal hormonal influences. The breasts may also exhibit a whitish secretion from the nipples. The cry should be strong, and normal breathing for a term newborn is 30 to 60 respirations per minute and predominantly diaphragmatic. The normal heart range is 120 to 160 beats per minute.

4. The abdomen is cylindrical, protrudes slightly, and moves with respiration. Bowel sounds should be present by 1 hour after birth. The umbilical cord has two umbilical arteries and one umbilical vein.

5. The labia majora covers the labia minora and the clitoris in the term female infant. The testes are descended, and the scrotum is pendulous with many rugae in the term male infant. Extremities appear short, are generally flexible, and move symmetrically. The nails extend beyond the fingertips, and the legs should be of equal length, with symmetric skin folds.

2c Ears and Neck
- Ears
  - Soft and pliable
  - Ready recoil
  - Pinna parallel with inner and outer canthus
- Neck
  - Short with skin folds

3 Chest
- Chest—cylindrical
- Breasts—engorged, whitish secretion
- Respirations
  - Diaphragmatic
  - 30–60 per minute
- Heart rate 120–160 bpm

4 Abdomen
- Cylindrical and soft
- Bowel sounds present by 1 hour after birth
- Umbilical cord
  - Initially white and gelatinous
  - Two arteries, one vein

5 Genitalia and Extremities
- Genitalia
  - Female—labia majora covers labia minora
  - Male—testes descended, pendulous scrotum
- Extremities
  - Short, flexible, and move symmetrically
  - Legs are equal in length with symmetrical creases

SUGGESTIONS FOR CLINICAL ACTIVITIES

Have students complete a newborn assessment on an infant and summarize their findings.

LEARNING OBJECTIVE 3

Summarize the components of a complete newborn assessment and the significance of normal variations and abnormal findings.

CONCEPTS FOR LECTURE

1. Assessment of the newborn should begin with measurements including: length, weight, head circumference, chest circumference, and abdominal circumference. Assessment of vital signs includes temperature, heart rate, and respiratory rate.

2. Assessment of the skin may include variations such as acrocyanosis (bluish discoloration of the hands and feet) which may be present in the first 2 to 6 hours after birth due to poor peripheral circulation, which results in vasomotor instability and capillary stasis. Mottling is another variation that may be related to chilling, prolonged apnea, sepsis, or hypothyroidism. Occasionally, a Harlequin sign (clown) color change is noted in which a deep color develops over one side of the newborn's body while the other side remains pale.

POWERPOINT LECTURE SLIDES

(NOTE: The number on each PPT Lecture Slide directly corresponds with the Concepts for Lecture.)

1 Measurements
- Weight
- Length
- Head circumference
- Chest circumference
- Abdominal girth
- Temperature

2 Skin Variations
- Acrocyanosis (Figure 29.18)
- Mottling
- Harlequin sign
- Jaundice

This is due to a vasomotor disturbance in which blood vessels on one side dilate while the vessels on the other side constrict, and it usually lasts from 1 to 20 minutes. These are transient and clinically insignificant. A yellowish color (jaundice) may be noted in the baby's skin which is related to elevated bilirubin levels. Erythema toxicum or newborn rash is an eruption in the area surrounding hair follicles of lesions that are firm, vary in size from 1 to 3 mm, and consist of a white or pale yellow papule or pustule with an erythematous base. No treatment is necessary. Exposed sebaceous glands that appear as raised white spots on the face, especially across the nose, are milia. They will clear up spontaneously within the first month. A whitish cheeselike substance that covers the fetus while in utero and lubricates the skin of the newborn is vernix caseosa. The term or postterm newborn has less vernix and frequently is dry. Pale pink or red spots that are frequently found on the eyelids, nose, lower occipital bone, and nape of the neck are telangiectatic nevi (stork bites). They have no clinical significance and usually fade by the second birthday. Macular areas of bluish black or gray-blue pigmentation found on the dorsal area and the buttocks are Mongolian spots. These are common in newborns of Asian, Hispanic, and African descent and other dark-skinned races. They usually fade during the first or second year of life. A capillary angioma directly below the epidermis that is nonelevated, sharply demarcated, and a red to purple area of dense capillaries on the face is a nevus flammeus (port wine stain). It does not fade over time. A capillary hemangioma that consists of newly formed and enlarged capillaries in the dermal and subdermal layers is a nevus vasculosus (strawberry mark). They fade spontaneously after they reach their peak.

3. Asymmetry of the head in a vertex presentation is called molding and is caused by the overriding of the cranial bones during labor and birth. A collection of blood resulting from ruptured blood vessels between the surface of a cranial bone (usually parietal) and the periosteal membrane is a cephalhematoma. They may be unilateral or bilateral and do not cross suture lines. A localized, easily identifiable soft area of the scalp, generally resulting from a long and difficult labor or vacuum extraction, is caput succedaneum. This is due to sustained pressure of the presenting part against the cervix resulting in compression of local blood vessels and a slowing of venous return which causes an increase in tissue fluids, an edematous swelling, and occasional bleeding under the periosteum. The fluid is reabsorbed within 12 hours to a few days after birth.

4. Low set ears may indicate chromosomal abnormalities (especially trisomies 13 and 18), mental retardation, or internal organ abnormalities, especially bilateral renal agenesis as a result of embryologic developmental deviations. During the first few days of life, the eyelids may be edematous because of the pressure associated with birth.

- Erythema toxicum (Figure 29.19)
- Milia (Figure 29.20)

2a See Figure 29.18

2b See Figure 29.19

2c See Figure 29.20

2d Skin Variations
- Vernix Caseosa
- Forceps marks
- Telangiectatic nevi
- Mongolian spots (Figure 29.22)
- Nevus flammeus
- Nevus vasculosus

2e See Figure 29.22

3 Head Variations
- Molding
- Cephalohematoma
- Caput succedaneum

4 Ear and Eye Variations
- Low set ears
- Edema of the eyelids
- Normal variations
- Subconjunctival hemorrhage
- Transient strabismus
- Doll's eye

5 Mouth Variations
- Cleft lip and palate
- Precocious teeth
- Epstein's pearls
- Thrush

6 Neck and Abdomen Variations
- Webbing
- Xiphoid cartilage
- Fractured clavicle

7 Respiratory Variations
- Signs of respiratory distress
  ○ Nasal flaring
  ○ Intercostal or xiphoid retractions
  ○ Expiratory grunting or sighing
  ○ Seesaw respirations
  ○ Tachypnea

8 Cardiac Variations
- Heart is large
- Low pitched murmur
- Decreased strength or absence of femoral pulses (Figure 29.32A–B)

8a See Figure 29.32A–B

9 Female Genitalia Variations
- Vaginal tag
- Pseudomenstruation
- Smegma

Commonly, small subconjunctival hemorrhages caused by changes in vascular tension or ocular pressure during birth are found on the sclera. Transient strabismus (pseudostrabismus) or squinting caused by neuromuscular control of eye muscles that gradually regresses in 3 to 4 months may be seen in the newborn. The "doll's eye" phenomenon is present for about 10 days after birth and can be described as the movement of eyes in the opposite direction when the head is changed to the left and then to the right. This results from underdeveloped integration of head-eye coordination.

5. The mouth should be assessed for a cleft lip and palate. Precocious teeth may be present over the area where the lower central incisor will erupt. They should be removed if they appear loose to prevent aspiration. Epstein's pearls, small glistening white specks (keratin-containing cysts) that feel hard to the touch, may be present on the hard palate and gum margins. They are of no significance and usually disappear in a few weeks. White patches that look like milk curds adhering to the mucous membranes is thrush. It is caused by Candida albicans which is often acquired from an infected vaginal tract during birth, antibiotic use, or poor handwashing when handling the newborn.

6. A lump and a grating sensation (crepitus) during movements may be palpated on the clavicle if a fracture has occurred. The xiphoid cartilage, a protrusion at the lower end of the sternum, is frequently seen. It becomes less apparent after several weeks as the infant accumulates adipose tissue.

7. Signs of respiratory distress include: nasal flaring, intercostal or xiphoid retractions, expiratory grunting or sighing, seesaw respirations, or tachypnea.

8. In the newborn, the heart is relatively large at birth and is located high in the chest, with its apex somewhere between the fourth and fifth intercostal space. A low-pitched, musical murmur heard just to the right of the apex of the heart is fairly common. A decrease in the strength of or absence of femoral pulses may indicate coarctation of the aorta or hypovolemia and require additional investigation.

9. Upon inspection of the female genitalia, a vaginal tag or hymenal tag is often evident and will usually disappear in a few weeks. A vaginal discharge composed of thick whitish mucus may be present during the first week of life. When the discharge is blood-tinged, it is called pseudomenstruation and is caused by the withdrawal of maternal hormones. A white cheeselike substance called smegma is often present between the labia.

10. Upon inspection of the male genitalia, if the urinary meatus is located on the ventral surface of the penis it is called hypospadias. Phimosis occurs when the opening of the foreskin (prepuce) is small, and the foreskin cannot be pulled back over the glans at all. This may interfere with urination, so the adequacy of the urinary stream should be evaluated. Cryptorchidism occurs when the testes fail to descend. In breech births, scrotal

 Male Genitalia Variations
- Hypospadias
- Phimosis
- Hydrocele
- Cryptorchidism

 Variations in Extremities
- **Gross deformities**
- **Extra digits or webbing**
- **Clubfoot**
- **Hip dislocation (Figure 29.36A–D)**

 See Figure 29.36A–D

CONCEPTS FOR LECTURE *continued*

edema and discoloration are common. A hydrocele is a collection of fluid surrounding the testes and is common and resolves without intervention. If the newborn does not pass meconium in the first 24 hours of life, atresia of the gastrointestinal tract or meconium ileus with resultant obstruction must be considered.

11. The presence of extra digits on either the hands or the feet is polydactyly. Fusion (webbing) of fingers or toes is syndactyly. Children with Down syndrome may present with a single palmar crease called a simian line. If a sense of reduction or "clunk" is felt when performing the Ortolani's and Barlow's maneuvers, congenital hip dislocation may be present. Feet should be examined for evidence of a talipes deformity (clubfoot).

SUGGESTIONS FOR CLASSROOM ACTIVITIES	SUGGESTIONS FOR CLINICAL ACTIVITIES
Bring an infant model to class and demonstrate assessment techniques for the students.	Have students perform a physical assessment on a newborn and summarize their findings. Ask them to discuss the variations that they observed and the implications related to those findings.

LEARNING OBJECTIVE 4

Discuss the neurologic and neuromuscular characteristics of the newborn and the reflexes that may be present at birth.

CONCEPTS FOR LECTURE

1. A neurologic examination should include assessment of the following behaviors: the state of alertness, resting posture, cry, and quality of muscle tone and motor activity.

2. The following reflexes should be elicited in the term newborn: tonic neck, Moro, grasping, rooting, sucking, Babinski, and the Trunk incurvation (Galant reflex). Additionally, the newborn has the following protective reflexes: blink, yawn, cough, sneeze, and draw back from pain.

POWERPOINT LECTURE SLIDES

(NOTE: The number on each PPT Lecture Slide directly corresponds with the Concepts for Lecture.)

1 Reflexes
- Tonic neck
- Moro
- Grasping
- Rooting
- Sucking

1a Reflexes
- Babinski (Figure 29.42)
- Trunk incurvation

1b See Figure 29.42

2 Protective reflexes
- Blink
- Yawn
- Cough
- Sneeze

SUGGESTIONS FOR CLASSROOM ACTIVITIES	SUGGESTIONS FOR CLINICAL ACTIVITIES
Bring an infant model to class to demonstrate for students how to elicit reflexes.	Have students attempt to elicit reflexes on an infant and discuss their findings and implications of those findings.

LEARNING OBJECTIVE 5

Describe the categories of the newborn behavioral assessment.

CONCEPTS FOR LECTURE

1. The Brazelton's Neonatal Behavioral Assessment Scale provides guidelines for assessing the newborn's state changes, temperament, and individual behavior patterns. Habituation is the newborn's ability to diminish or shut down innate responses to specific repeated stimuli, such as a rattle, bell, light, or pinprick to heel. The newborn's orientation to inanimate and animate visual and auditory stimuli is assessed by observing how often and where the newborn attends to the stimuli. The motor tone of the newborn is the most characteristic state of responsiveness. Also noted is the frequency of alert states, state changes, color changes, activity, and peaks of excitement. The ability of the newborn to quiet or console themselves is called self-quieting activity. The infant's need for and response to being held is also an important consideration.

POWERPOINT LECTURE SLIDES

(NOTE: The number on each PPT Lecture Slide directly corresponds with the Concepts for Lecture.)

 Brazelton's Neonatal Behavioral Assessment Scale
- Habituation
- Orientation to inanimate and animate visual and auditory assessment stimuli
- Motor activity
- Variations
- Self-quieting activity
- Cuddliness or social behaviors

SUGGESTIONS FOR CLASSROOM ACTIVITIES

Have a group discussion about the benefits of doing a behavioral assessment with the family of an infant.

SUGGESTIONS FOR CLINICAL ACTIVITIES

Have students conduct/observe a behavioral assessment with a family. Ask them to reflect on the experience.

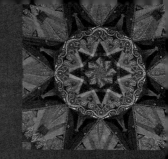

CHAPTER 30

THE NORMAL NEWBORN: NEEDS AND CARE

RESOURCE LIBRARY

 PRENTICE HALL NURSING MEDIALINK DVD-ROM

Audio Glossary
NCLEX Review
Videos: *Newborn Care; Through the Eyes of Nurse—Welcoming the New Arrival at the Postpartal Visit*

COMPANION WEBSITE

Additional NCLEX Review
Case Study: *Newborn Care*
Care Plan Activity: *Infant Care During Transition*
Applications: *Circumcision; Newbon Screening Tests*
Critical Thinking

📖 IMAGE LIBRARY

Figure 30.1 Weighing a newborn.
Figure 30.2 Temperature monitoring for the newborn.
Figure 30.3 Procedure for vitamin K injection.
Figure 30.4 Injection sites.
Figure 30.5 Ophthalmic ointment.
Figure 30.6 The umbilical cord base is carefully cleaned.
Figure 30.7 Circumcision using the Yellen or Gomco clamp.
Figure 30.8 Circumcision using the Plastibel.

Figure 30.9 Following circumcision, petroleum ointment may be applied to the site for the next few diaper changes.
Figure 30.10 A letter from your baby.
Figure 30.11 A father demonstrates competence and confidence in diapering his newborn daughter.
Figure 30.12 Nasal and oral suctioning.
Figure 30.13 Steps in wrapping a baby.
Figure 30.14 Infant car restraint for use from birth to about 12 months of age.
Figure 30.15 An infant teaching checklist is completed by the time of discharge.

LEARNING OBJECTIVE 1

Summarize the essential areas of information to be obtained about a newborn's birth experience and immediate postnatal period.

CONCEPTS FOR LECTURE

1. It is important that information about the condition of the newborn is obtained in the immediate postnatal period. This information will include: the Apgar scores at 1 and 5 minutes, resuscitative measures required in the birthing area, physical examination, vital signs, voidings, and passing of meconium. Additionally, complications that should be noted include: excessive mucus, delayed spontaneous respirations or responsiveness, abnormal number of cord vessels, and obvious physical abnormalities.

2. The duration and course of labor and birth, the status of mother and fetus throughout labor and birth, and any analgesia or anesthesia administered to the mother should be assessed. Complications should be noted, including: prolonged rupture of membranes, abnormal fetal position, meconium-stained amniotic fluid, signs of fetal distress during labor, nuchal cord, precipitous

POWERPOINT LECTURE SLIDES

(NOTE: The number on each PPT Lecture Slide directly corresponds with the Concepts for Lecture.)

1 Assessment Data: Condition of the Infant
- Apgar scores at 1 and 5 minutes
- Resuscitative measures
- Physical examination
- Vital signs
- Voidings
- Passing of meconium

1a Assessment Data: Infant Complications
- Excessive mucus
- Delayed spontaneous respirations or responsiveness
- Abnormal number of cord vessels
- Obvious physical abnormalities

birth, use of forceps or vacuum extraction assisted device, maternal analgesia and anesthesia received within 1 hour of birth, and administration of antibiotics during labor.

3. Maternal complications that may have affected the fetus should be assessed, including: preeclampsia, spotting, illness, recent infections, rubella status, serology results, hepatitis B screen results, exposure to group B streptococci, or a history of maternal substance abuse.

4. Additionally, observations about the parents' interactions with their newborn and their desires regarding care (such as rooming-in, circumcision, and type of feeding) should be documented.

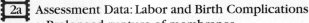 Assessment Data: Labor and Birth
- Duration and course
- Status of mother and fetus
- Analgesia or anesthesia

Assessment Data: Labor and Birth Complications
- Prolonged rupture of membranes
- Meconium-stained amniotic fluid
- Nuchal cord
- Precipitous birth
- Use of forceps or vacuum extraction assisted device
- Fetal distress

Assessment Data: Maternal Complications
- Preeclampsia
- Spotting
- Illness
- Recent infections
- Rubella status
- Serology results

Assessment Data: Maternal Complications
- Hepatitis B screen results
- Exposure to group B streptococci
- History of maternal substance
- Human immunodeficiency virus (HIV) test result

Assessment Data: Family
- Parents' interactions with their newborn
- Their desires regarding infant care
- Information about other children in the home
- Available support systems
- Patterns of interaction within each family unit

SUGGESTIONS FOR CLINICAL ACTIVITIES

Have students review the admission history for a newborn infant. Ask them to identify potential risk factors and the appropriate nursing interventions.

LEARNING OBJECTIVE 2

Relate the physiologic and behavioral responses of newborns to possible interventions needed.

CONCEPTS FOR LECTURE

1. If a newborn exhibits signs of respiratory distress, the airway should be cleared of secretions with a bulb syringe or DeLee wall suction. Additionally, stimulation of the newborn's spine will stimulate respiratory activity. A newborn who is at risk for respiratory or cardiac compromise should be monitored using a cardiorespiratory monitor. If a newborn is noted to have pallor, this may be an early sign of hemorrhage and must be reported to the physician. If a newborn's temperature has decreased, the newborn should be double wrapped with a blanket with a head covering and reassessed. If the temperature does not return to

POWERPOINT LECTURE SLIDES

(NOTE: The number on each PPT Lecture Slide directly corresponds with the Concepts for Lecture.)

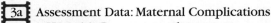 Physiologic Alterations
- Respiratory distress
- Pallor
- Hypothermia
- Alterations in feeding and elimination

normal, the newborn should be placed on a radiant warmer bed and closely monitored. Additionally, infants should be observed for problems with feeding and elimination.

SUGGESTIONS FOR CLASSROOM ACTIVITIES

Use an infant model, bulb syringe, and blanket to demonstrate suctioning and wrapping the infant.

LEARNING OBJECTIVE 3

Discuss the major nursing considerations and activities to be carried out during the first 4 hours after birth (admission and transitional period) and subsequent daily care.

CONCEPTS FOR LECTURE

1. One of the major activities in the first 4 hours after birth is to carry out a preliminary physical examination. Assessment should include: maternal and birth history, airway clearance, vital signs, body temperature, neurologic status, ability to feed, and evidence of complications. This assessment should also include: a review of prenatal and birth information for possible risk factors, a gestational age assessment, and an assessment to ensure that the newborn's adaptation to extrauterine life is proceeding normally. Measurements should include: weight, length, circumference of the head, circumference of the chest, and abdominal girth. Additionally, hematocrit and blood glucose evaluations on at-risk newborns or as clinically indicated should be done. Vital signs for a healthy term newborn should be monitored at least every 30 minutes until the newborn's condition has remained stable for 2 hours.

2. The newborn bath should be done when the newborn's temperature is normal and the condition is stable. After the bath, the temperature should be rechecked and the infant dressed, wrapped, and placed in an open crib. Vitamin K1 (AquaMEPHYTON) is administered intramuscularly to prevent hemorrhage. A prophylactic eye treatment for Neisseria gonorrhea, which may have infected the newborn of an infected mother during the birth process, is also administered. Feeding times will be dependent upon the type of feeding and the newborn's status. Additionally, parent-newborn attachment is facilitated, particularly during the period of first reactivity.

POWERPOINT LECTURE SLIDES

(NOTE: The number on each PPT Lecture Slide directly corresponds with the Concepts for Lecture.)

1 Nursing Care: Assessment
- Airway clearance
- Vital signs
- Body temperature (Figure 30.2)
- Neurologic status
- Ability to feed
- Evidence of complications

1a See Figure 30.2

1b Nursing Care: Assessment
- Review of prenatal and birth information
- Gestational age
- Newborn's adaptation to extrauterine life
- Weight and measurement (Figure 30.1)
- Vital signs every 30 minutes
- Assessment of Hct or blood glucose if warranted

1c See Figure 30.1

2 Admission Procedures
- Newborn bath
- Vitamin K (Figure 30.3)
- Eye prophylaxis (Figure 30.5)
- Observation for distress
- Initiate feeding
- Facilitate parental-infant attachment

2a See Figure 30.3

2b See Figure 30.5

SUGGESTIONS FOR CLASSROOM ACTIVITIES

Use an infant model and materials to simulate Vitamin K administration and eye prophylaxis administration. Demonstrate these procedures to the student and ask them to do a return demonstration.

SUGGESTIONS FOR CLINICAL ACTIVITIES

Have students admit a newborn to the nursery with a preceptor. Have them administer the Vitamin K and eye prophylaxis. Ask them to document their findings and interventions.

LEARNING OBJECTIVE 4

Identify activities that should be included in a daily care plan for a normal newborn.

CONCEPTS FOR LECTURE

1. Daily care of the newborn includes: assessing vital signs, weight, overall color, intake, output, umbilical cord and circumcision, newborn nutrition, parent education, and attachment. Vital signs should be assessed every 6 to 8 hours or more, depending on the newborn's status.

2. Cord care includes keeping the stump clean and dry and performing cord care per agency policy. The cord clamp should be removed within 24–48 hours when it is dry. Skin care includes cleansing the buttock and perianal areas with water and a mild soap with diaper changes and keeping the skin clean and dry. The nurse should monitor the infant's temperature and keep the infant wrapped with the head covered and away from windows and drafts to prevent heat loss. Assessment of infant feeding (either bottle-feeding or breastfeeding) is a primary responsibility of the nurse. The nurse should provide education and support for infant feeding. Nursing care also includes safety measures, such as identification of the newborn and prevention of infection.

POWERPOINT LECTURE SLIDES

(NOTE: The number on each PPT Lecture Slide directly corresponds with the Concepts for Lecture.)

 Daily Assessments
- Vital signs
- Weight
- Overall color
- Intake and output
- Umbilical cord
- Circumcision

 Daily Assessments
- Newborn feeding
- Attachment

 Daily Newborn Care
- Assist with feedings
- Thermoregulation
- Skin care
- Cord care (Figure 30.6)
- Prevention of infection
- Security

 See Figure 30.6

SUGGESTIONS FOR CLINICAL ACTIVITIES

Have students do an assessment of a newborn and document their findings. Ask them to develop a 24-hour care plan for the newborn.

LEARNING OBJECTIVE 5

Determine the common concerns of families regarding their newborns.

CONCEPTS FOR LECTURE

1. Family concerns about their newborns include: how to pick up a newborn, holding and feeding, changing the diaper, interpreting newborn cues, bathing the newborn, cord and circumcision care, and normal voiding and stooling patterns.

POWERPOINT LECTURE SLIDES

(NOTE: The number on each PPT Lecture Slide directly corresponds with the Concepts for Lecture.)

 Common Concerns
- How to pick up a newborn
- Holding and feeding the infant
- Changing the diaper (Figure 30.11)
- Interpreting newborn cues
- Bathing the newborn

See Figure 30.11

Common Concerns
- Cord and circumcision care
- Normal voiding and stooling pattern

LEARNING OBJECTIVE 6

Describe topics and related content to be included in parent teaching on newborn and infant care.

CONCEPTS FOR LECTURE

1. Parent teaching about newborn care should include the following topics: periods of reactivity and expected newborn responses, normal physical characteristics of the newborn, the bonding process, the infant's capabilities for interaction (such as nonverbal communication), the role of touch in facilitating parent-infant interaction, comforting techniques, progression of infant behaviors, and information about available educational pamphlets, videos, and support groups.

POWERPOINT LECTURE SLIDES

(NOTE: The number on each PPT Lecture Slide directly corresponds with the Concepts for Lecture.)

 Parent Education
- Periods of reactivity and expected newborn responses
- Normal physical characteristics of the newborn
- The bonding process
- The infant's capabilities for interaction
- The role of touch in facilitating parent-infant interaction
- Comforting techniques

1a Parent Education
- Progression of infant behaviors
- Information about available educational materials and support

LEARNING OBJECTIVE 7

Identify opportunities to individualize parent teaching and enhance each parent's abilities and confidence while providing infant care in the birthing unit.

CONCEPTS FOR LECTURE

1. Opportunities to teach parents about newborn care include daily newborn care videos or classes and individual instruction. The most effective method is one-to-one teaching while the nurse is in the mother's room. The nurse should observe parental care and feeding while in the hospital and provide feedback and education based upon these observations.

POWERPOINT LECTURE SLIDES

(NOTE: The number on each PPT Lecture Slide directly corresponds with the Concepts for Lecture.)

 Family Education
- Newborn care videos
- Newborn care classes
- Individual instruction
- Observation of parent-infant interaction
- Role modeling

LEARNING OBJECTIVE 8

Delineate the information to be included in discharge planning with the newborn's family.

CONCEPTS FOR LECTURE

1. Discharge information to be provided to the newborn's family includes: immediate safety measures (such as putting the infant back to sleep and demonstrating the use of the bulb syringe to remove excessive mucus), voiding and stool characteristics and patterns, circumcision care and observation for infection, instructions on cleaning the uncircumcised penis, waking and quieting their newborn, car safety, and immunization requirements.

2. Additionally, the nurse should provide information about the signs of illness and the use of a thermometer. The following are signs of illness: temperature above 38C or below 36.6C axillary; continual rise in temperature; forceful or frequent vomiting; refusal of two feedings in a row; difficulty in awakening baby; cyanosis with or without a feeding; absence of breathing longer than 20 seconds; an inconsolable infant or continuous high-pitched cry; discharge or bleeding from umbilical cord, circumcision, or any opening; two consecutive green watery or black stools, or increased frequency of stools; no wet diapers for 18 to 24 hours; fewer than 6 to 8 wet diapers per day after 4 days of age; and development of eye drainage.

POWERPOINT LECTURE SLIDES

(NOTE: The number on each PPT Lecture Slide directly corresponds with the Concepts for Lecture.)

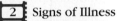

1 Discharge Education
- Safety measures
- Voiding and stool characteristics
- Circumcision care (Figure 30.9)
- Cord care
- Waking and quieting the newborn (Figure 30.13)
- Car safety (Figure 30.14)

1a See Figure 30.9

1b See Figure 30.13

1c See Figure 30.14

1d Discharge Education
- Immunizations
- Signs of illness

2 Signs of Illness
- Temperature above 38C or below 36.6C axillary
- Continual rise in temperature
- Forceful or frequent vomiting
- Refusal of two feedings in a row
- Difficulty in awakening baby
- Cyanosis with or without a feeding

2a Signs of Illness
- Absence of breathing longer than 20 seconds
- Inconsolable infant or continuous high-pitched cry
- Discharge or bleeding from umbilical cord, circumcision, or any opening
- Two consecutive green watery or black stools, or increased frequency of stools
- No wet diapers for 18 to 24 hours
- Fewer than 6 to 8 wet diapers per day after 4 days of age
- Development of eye drainage

SUGGESTIONS FOR CLINICAL ACTIVITIES

Have students develop a discharge education class for new mothers. Have them teach the class on the postpartum unit and provide feedback.

CHAPTER 31
NEWBORN NUTRITION

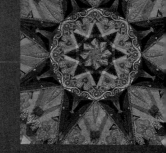

RESOURCE LIBRARY

PRENTICE HALL NURSING MEDIALINK DVD-ROM

Audio Glossary
NCLEX Review
Video: *Breastfeeding; Through the Eyes of a Nurse—Welcoming the New Arrival at the Postpartal Visit*

IMAGE LIBRARY

Figure 31.1 Anatomy of the breast.
Figure 31.2 Modified cradle position.
Figure 31.3 Cradle position.
Figure 31.4 Football hold position.
Figure 31.5 Side-lying position.
Figure 31.6 C-hold hand position.
Figure 31.7 Scissor hold hand position.
Figure 31.8 Nose to nipple.
Figure 31.9 Initial attempt to elicit the rooting reflex.
Figure 31.10 Continued attempt to elicit rooting reflex.

COMPANION WEBSITE

Additional NCLEX Review
Case Study: *Client Undecided on Formula Feeding or Breastfeeding*
Care Plan Activity: *Breastfeeding Concerns*
Applications: *Breastfeeding; Formula Feeding*
Critical Thinking

Figure 31.11 Baby is latched-on.
Figure 31.13 Hand expression.
Figure 31.14 Manual breast pump.
Figure 31.15 Hospital-grade, double electric breast pump.
Figure 31.16 Breastfeeding intake and output expectations.
Figure 31.17 Burping.
Figure 31.18 Bottle feeding.

LEARNING OBJECTIVE 1

Compare the nutritional value and composition of breast milk and formula preparations.

CONCEPTS FOR LECTURE

1. Both breast milk and formula contain almost 90% water, which meets the infant's water needs. Infants that are breastfed exclusively will grow at the same or slightly higher rate than those that are formula-fed in the first 3–4 months. After that, formula-fed infants have a greater weight gain pattern. The fat content is the most variable component in breast milk (ranging from 30–50 grams/liter) and is influenced by maternal parity, duration of pregnancy, and the stage of lactation, and it may vary diurnally or even during a single feeding. The primary carbohydrate in breast milk is lactose, although there are also trace amounts of other carbohydrates such as glucosamines and nitrogen-containing oligosaccharides. Milk-based formulas provide all of their carbohydrate calories from lactose. The carbohydrates in Carnation Good Start® are a blend of 70% lactose and 30% maltodextrin (a table-sugar-like carbohydrate).
2. Whey and casein components in breast milk are not static and change over time to meet the needs of the

POWERPOINT LECTURE SLIDES

(NOTE: The number on each PPT Lecture Slide directly corresponds with the Concepts for Lecture.)

1 Nutritional Comparison: Breast Milk
- 90% water
- Same weight gain or greater during first 3–4 months
- Fat is variable
- Primary carbohydrate is lactose, trace amounts of other carbohydrates

1a Nutritional Comparison: Formula
- 90% water
- Greater weight gain after 3–4 months
- Lactose is only carbohydrate

2 Components of Breast Milk
- Whey/Casein ratio changes according to infant needs
- Whey components include alpha-lactalbumin, serum albumin, lactoferrin, immunoglobulins, and lysozyme

growing infant. There are five major components of whey protein in breast milk: alpha-lactalbumin, serum albumin, lactoferrin, immunoglobulins, and lysozyme. There are many additional kinds of proteins in breast milk, including enzymes, growth modulator, and hormones. Because of its tendency to form curds, milk with high amounts of casein is less easily digested. The whey-casein ratio of cow's milk-based formula is developed to be close to breast milk. The major whey proteins in cow's milk formula are beta-lactoglobulin and alpha-lactalbumin.

3. Breast milk is low in vitamin D (25 IU/L or less). Vitamin B complex and vitamin C readily pass from serum to breast milk. Formula contains adequate amounts of water-soluble vitamins. There are several major and trace minerals in both breast milk and infant formulas. Formula generally contains higher levels of minerals than breast milk to compensate for a lower bioavailability. Breast milk iron is more completely absorbed than the iron in formula.

- Low in vitamin D, adequate vitamin C and B complex
- Mineral content similar
- Iron absorption: 50–60%

 Components of Formula
- Whey/Casein ratio is 60:40
- Whey components are beta-lactoglobulin and alpha-lactalbumin
- Adequate amounts of vitamins
- Mineral content similar

LEARNING OBJECTIVE 2

Discuss the advantages and disadvantages of breastfeeding and formula-feeding for both mother and newborn.

CONCEPTS FOR LECTURE

1. One of the advantages of breast milk is the role that the cholesterol in breast milk may play in myelination and neurologic development. This cholesterol may also stimulate the production of enzymes that lead to more efficient metabolism of cholesterol, thereby reducing its harmful long-term effects on the cardiovascular system. Breast milk composition also varies according to gestational age and stage of lactation. It provides newborns with minerals in more appropriate doses than formulas, and the iron found in breast milk, even though much lower in concentration than that of prepared formulas, is much more readily and fully absorbed.

2. Health advantages that have been supported by research include: a reduced risk of developing type I or type II diabetes mellitus, lymphoma, leukemia, Hodgkin's disease, obesity, hypercholesterolemia, and asthma. There are also immunologic advantages, including varying degrees of protection from respiratory tract and gastrointestinal tract infections, necrotizing enterocolitis, urinary tract infections, otitis media, bacterial meningitis, bacteremia, and allergies.

3. Maternal physical advantages to breastfeeding include: decreased postpartum bleeding and more rapid uterine involution, additional calories burned, a decreased risk of developing breast cancer and ovarian cancer, and a decreased risk of developing postmenopausal osteoporosis. The primary psychosocial advantage of breastfeeding is maternal-infant attachment. Skin-to-skin contact associated with breastfeeding results in the

POWERPOINT LECTURE SLIDES

(NOTE: The number on each PPT Lecture Slide directly corresponds with the Concepts for Lecture.)

1 Advantages of Breastfeeding
- Species specific
- Cholesterol in breast milk plays a role in myelination and neurologic development
- More efficient metabolism of cholesterol
- Composition varies according to gestational age
- Iron is more readily absorbed

2 Infant Benefits
- Reduced risk of
  - Type I or type II diabetes mellitus
  - Lymphoma, leukemia, and Hodgkin's disease
  - Obesity
  - Hypercholesterolemia
  - Asthma

2a Infant Benefits: Immunologic
- Protection from
  - Respiratory tract and gastrointestinal tract infections
  - Necrotizing enterocolitis
  - Urinary tract infections
  - Otitis media
  - Bacterial meningitis

2b Infant Benefits: Immunologic
- Protection from
  - Bacteremia
  - Allergies

newborn having a greater physiologic stability, crying less, sleeping longer, and tending to breastfeed better. Breastfeeding can communicate warmth, closeness, and comfort through tactile stimulation of the newborn and help the newborn and mother learn each other's behavioral cues and needs. Maternal benefits include: a feeling of relaxation and euphoria due to prolactic secretion, a feeling of relaxation and sleepiness, heightened responsiveness and receptivity toward the infant, and increased frequency of nurturing behaviors due to oxytocin secretion. The mother also derives satisfaction from the knowledge that she is providing her infant with the optimal nutritional start in life. Cost savings for the family that chooses breastfeeding may be significant. Societal benefits to breastfeeding may include decreased spending on public assistance programs (e.g., WIC), and environmental benefits in terms of use of natural resources and solid waste disposal.

4. Breastfeeding disadvantages may include: pain due to nipple tenderness, leaking milk when breasts are full, embarrassment about breastfeeding, the stress of finding time to breastfeed and feeling tied down to the demands of breastfeeding, unequal feeding responsibilities/fathers left out, perceptions about diet restrictions, limited birth control options, vaginal dryness, and concerns about the safety of medications and breastfeeding.

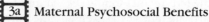

3 Maternal Physical Benefits
- Decreased postpartum bleeding
- More rapid uterine involution
- Burns additional calories
- Decreased risk of developing
  - Breast and ovarian cancer
  - Postmenopausal osteoporosis

3a Maternal Psychosocial Benefits
- Improved maternal-infant attachment
- Skin-to-skin contact
- Tactile communication
- Learn behavioral cues and needs
- Prolactin increases feelings of relaxation and euphoria
- Oxytocin heightens responsiveness and receptivity toward infant

4 Disadvantages to Breastfeeding
- Pain due to nipple tenderness
- Leaking milk when breasts are full
- Embarrassment about breastfeeding
- Feeling tied down to the demands of breastfeeding
- Unequal feeding responsibilities/fathers left out
- Perceptions about diet restrictions

4a Disadvantages to Breastfeeding
- Limited birth control options
- Vaginal dryness
- Concerns about the safety of medications and breastfeeding

SUGGESTIONS FOR CLASSROOM ACTIVITIES

Ask students to interview women who have breastfed and assess their reasons for breastfeeding. Ask them to share their findings in class.

SUGGESTIONS FOR CLINICAL ACTIVITIES

Have students develop and teach a breastfeeding class on the postpartum unit, focusing on the advantages of breastfeeding.

LEARNING OBJECTIVE 3

Develop guidelines for helping both breastfeeding and formula-feeding mothers to feed their infants successfully.

CONCEPTS FOR LECTURE

1. In assisting the mother with feeding her infant, the nurse should assess for readiness to feed, including: active bowel sounds, absence of abdominal distention, and a lusty cry that quiets and is replaced with rooting and sucking behaviors when a stimulus is placed near the lips. Skin-to-skin contact can begin immediately after birth. The nurse can assist the mother with breastfeeding in the birthing room. Formula-fed infants are fed according to hospital policy and when they demonstrate feeding cues. The nurse should teach the mother how to feed and hold the infant and observe the feeding to ensure the mother's understanding of

POWERPOINT LECTURE SLIDES

(NOTE: The number on each PPT Lecture Slide directly corresponds with the Concepts for Lecture.)

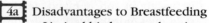

1 Feeding Interventions: Birthing Room
- Assess for signs of readiness to feed
- Place newborn on mother's chest
- Breastfeeding may begin in birthing room
- Assess infant physiologic status during feeding

2 Feeding Interventions
- Monitor progress
- Education
- Anticipatory guidance
- Evaluate the need for follow-up after discharge

the information and ability of the infant to tolerate the feeding.

2. Breastfeeding progress should be monitored throughout the birthing unit stay. This provides the opportunity to teach the new mother about lactation and the breastfeeding process, provide anticipatory guidance, and evaluate the need for follow-up care after discharge. The bottle-fed infant should be monitored throughout the birthing unit stay as well, and the nurse should educate parents about formula preparation and bottlefeeding techniques.

SUGGESTIONS FOR CLASSROOM ACTIVITIES

Have students role play teaching a new mother how to breastfeed and formula feed. Have students provide feedback.

SUGGESTIONS FOR CLINICAL ACTIVITIES

Have students teach new mothers about breastfeeding and formula feeding on the postpartum unit. Ask them to share their observations of client responses.

LEARNING OBJECTIVE 4

Delineate nursing responsibilities for client teaching regarding infant feeding issues.

CONCEPTS FOR LECTURE

1. Nurses need to educate both breastfeeding and formula-feeding parents about "on demand" feeding patterns, infant feeding cues, normal feeding/sleeping patterns, satiety behaviors, and growth patterns.

2. Breastfeeding parents should be taught about positioning, latching, and breast milk pumping, storage, and supplementation.

3. Formula feeding parents need to learn about the feeding pattern for a formula-fed infant. They need to know intake and output expectations, the recommended type of formula for their infant, how to prepare and store formula, what equipment they will need, feeding technique, and safety precautions.

POWERPOINT LECTURE SLIDES

(NOTE: The number on each PPT Lecture Slide directly corresponds with the Concepts for Lecture.)

1 Infant Feeding Education
- "On Demand" feeding pattern
- Infant feeding cues
- Normal feeding/sleeping patterns
- Satiety behaviors (Figure 31.16)
- Growth patterns

1a See Figure 31.16

2 Breastfeeding Education
- Positioning
- Latching
- Breast milk pumping and storage (Figure 31.15)
- Supplementation

2a See Figure 31.15

3 Formula Feeding Education
- Intake and output expectations
- Preparation and storage of formula
- Feeding technique
- Equipment
- Safety precautions

SUGGESTIONS FOR CLASSROOM ACTIVITIES

Use an infant model to demonstrate correct breastfeeding and formula feeding positions.

SUGGESTIONS FOR CLINICAL ACTIVITIES

Have students develop an educational plan for infant feeding for their clients on the postpartum unit.

LEARNING OBJECTIVE 5

Incorporate knowledge of newborn nutrition and normal growth patterns into parent education and infant assessment.

CONCEPTS FOR LECTURE

1. The nurse should teach the mother that both breastfed and formula-fed infants will experience growth spurts at certain times and require increased feeding. A mother who breastfeeds can meet these increased demands by nursing more frequently to increase her milk supply, and she should be aware that it takes about 72 hours for the milk supply to increase adequately to meet the new demand. The mother who uses formula can slightly increase the amount of feedings to meet the infant's growth demands.

POWERPOINT LECTURE SLIDES

(NOTE: The number on each PPT Lecture Slide directly corresponds with the Concepts for Lecture.)

 Growth Rates
- Both breastfed and formula-fed infants experience growth spurts requiring increased feedings
- Breastfeeding mother should nurse more frequently
- Formula feeding mother should slightly increase amount of feeding

LEARNING OBJECTIVE 6

Recognize the influence of cultural values on infant care, especially feeding practices.

CONCEPTS FOR LECTURE

1. Cultural values can influence feeding practices. For example, breast exposure is often viewed in a sexual context, leading to disapproval of the mother attempting to breastfeed in public. Hispanics, Navajo Indians, Filipinos, and Vietnamese believe that colostrum is "unclean" and do not offer it to their newborns. The language used in infant feeding may also be culturally related, such as the African-Americans referring to their infant as "greedy," a term that is often used as an expression of approval of the infant's vigorous feeding.

POWERPOINT LECTURE SLIDES

(NOTE: The number on each PPT Lecture Slide directly corresponds with the Concepts for Lecture.)

 Influence of Culture on Infant Feeding
- Perception of breasts as sexual organ
- Perceptions of colostrum
- Language

SUGGESTIONS FOR CLASSROOM ACTIVITIES

Ask students to share their own cultural beliefs about infant feeding in the classroom.

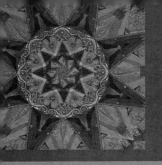

CHAPTER 32
THE NEWBORN AT RISK: CONDITIONS PRESENT AT BIRTH

RESOURCE LIBRARY

 PRENTICE HALL NURSING MEDIALINK DVD-ROM

Audio Glossary
NCLEX Review
Video: *Through the Eyes of a Nurse—Welcoming the New Arrival at the Postpartal Visit*

COMPANION WEBSITE

Additional NCLEX Review
Case Study: *Infant with Postmaturity Syndrome*
Care Plan Activity: *Infant of a Diabetic Mother*
Applications: *Care of the Preterm Infant; Congenital Defects*
Critical Thinking

 IMAGE LIBRARY

Figure 32.1 Newborn classification and neonatal mortality risk chart.

Figure 32.2 Neonatal morbidity by birth weight and gestational age.

Figure 32.3 Thirty-five-week gestational age twins.

Figure 32.4 Macrosomic infant of a Class B insulin-dependent diabetic mother born at 38 weeks' gestation weighing 3402 grams.

Figure 32.5 The skin of the postterm infant exhibits deep cracking and peeling.

Figure 32.6 A 6-day-old, 28 weeks' gestational age, 960-g preterm infant.

Figure 32.7 Mother breastfeeding her premature infant.

Figure 32.8 Measuring gavage tube length.

Figure 32.9 Auscultation for placement of gavage tube.

Figure 32.10 Father participates in feeding experience with his premature infant.

Figure 32.11 Kangaroo (skin-to-skin) care facilitates a closeness and attachment between parents and their premature infant.

Figure 32.12 Family bonding occurs when parents have opportunities to spend time with their infant.

Figure 32.13 An 8-day-old, 30 weeks' gestational age, 860-gram IUGR infant is "nested."

Figure 32.14 Nonnutritive suckling on a pacifier has a calming effect on newborn.

LEARNING OBJECTIVE 1

Identify factors present at birth that help identify an at-risk newborn.

CONCEPTS FOR LECTURE

1. Factors present at birth that may help identify an at-risk newborn include maternal factors such as a low socioeconomic status and limited or no prenatal care; exposure to environmental dangers; preexisting maternal conditions, such as heart disease, diabetes, hypertension, hyperthyroidism, and renal disease; age, parity, and medical conditions related to pregnancy; and pregnancy complications such as abruptio placentae, oligohydramnios, preterm labor, premature rupture of membranes, and preeclampsia.

POWERPOINT LECTURE SLIDES

(NOTE: The number on each PPT Lecture Slide directly corresponds with the Concepts for Lecture.)

 1 Identification of At-Risk Newborn
- Low socioeconomic level of the mother
- Limited or no prenatal care
- Exposure to environmental dangers
- Preexisting maternal conditions

 1a Identification of At-Risk Newborn
- Maternal factors such as age or parity
- Medical conditions related to pregnancy
- Pregnancy complications

SUGGESTIONS FOR CLASSROOM ACTIVITIES

Discuss the identification of risk factors for newborn conditions and the associated nursing assessments.

LEARNING OBJECTIVE 2

Compare the underlying etiologies of the physiologic complications of small-for-gestational-age (SGA) newborns and preterm appropriate-for-gestational-age (Pr AGA) newborns.

CONCEPTS FOR LECTURE

1. The underlying physiologic complications of small-for-gestational-age (SGA) newborns may include maternal factors such as: primiparity or grand multiparity, multiple-gestation pregnancy, poor or lack of prenatal care, age under 16 or over 40, and low socioeconomic status. Additionally, maternal diseases that affect blood flow to the uterus (such as preeclampsia, hypertension, and diabetes) can affect fetal growth. Heart disease, substance abuse, sickle cell anemia, PKU, and pyelonephritis have also been associated with SGA. Environmental factors may also play a role in growth restriction, including: high altitude, exposure to x-rays, excessive exercise, work-related exposure to toxins, and hyperthermia. Placental factors causing decreased blood flow (such as a small placenta, placental infarcts, abnormal cord insertions, placenta previa, or thrombosis) may also cause SGA. Fetal factors such as congenital infection, congenital malformations, discordant twins, sex of the fetus, chromosomal abnormalities, and inborn errors of metabolism can also affect fetal growth.

POWERPOINT LECTURE SLIDES

(NOTE: The number on each PPT Lecture Slide directly corresponds with the Concepts for Lecture.)

1 Small-for-Gestational-Age
- Maternal factors
- Maternal disease
- Environmental factors
- Placental factors
- Fetal factors

SUGGESTIONS FOR CLINICAL ACTIVITIES

Have students do a gestational assessment of an SGA infant and a preterm infant and compare their results.

LEARNING OBJECTIVE 3

Describe the impact of maternal diabetes mellitus on the newborn.

CONCEPTS FOR LECTURE

1. Newborns born to mothers with diabetes mellitus (DM) are typically LGA due to exposure to high levels of maternal glucose via the placenta and the subsequent production of increased amounts of insulin. Mothers who have vascular complications associated with diabetes may have SGA infants due to the vascular compromise to the fetus. Complications may include hypoglycemia, hypocalcemia, hyperbilirubinemia, birth trauma, polycythemia, RDS, and congenital malformations.

POWERPOINT LECTURE SLIDES

(NOTE: The number on each PPT Lecture Slide directly corresponds with the Concepts for Lecture.)

1 Impact of Maternal Diabetes Mellitus (DM) on the Newborn
- LGA
- SGA
- Hypoglycemia
- Hypocalcemia
- Hyperbilirubinemia

 1a Impact of Maternal Diabetes Mellitus (DM) on the Newborn
- Birth trauma
- Polycythemia
- RDS
- Congenital malformations

SUGGESTIONS FOR CLASSROOM ACTIVITIES

Discuss the mechanisms of maternal diabetes that contribute to the development of neonatal complications and potential strategies for preventing these complications.

SUGGESTIONS FOR CLINICAL ACTIVITIES

Have students do an assessment of an infant born to a diabetic mother and identify any complications and the appropriate nursing interventions.

LEARNING OBJECTIVE 4

Compare the characteristics and underlying etiologies of potential complications of the postterm newborn and the newborn with postmaturity syndrome.

CONCEPTS FOR LECTURE

1. Newborns who are born postterm are generally normal in size and health, while some can continue growing to over 4000 g at birth. Potential complications for these newborns include cephalopelvic disproportion (CPD) and shoulder dystocia. Newborns born with postmaturity syndrome may suffer from the following effects of decreased placental function: hypoglycemia, meconium aspiration, oligohydramnios, polycythemia, congenital anomalies, seizures, and cold stress.

POWERPOINT LECTURE SLIDES

(NOTE: The number on each PPT Lecture Slide directly corresponds with the Concepts for Lecture.)

1. Postmaturity Syndrome
   - Hypoglycemia
   - Meconium aspiration and oligohydramnios
   - Polycythemia
   - Congenital anomalies
   - Seizures
   - Cold stress

SUGGESTIONS FOR CLASSROOM ACTIVITIES

Discuss the mechanism of the development of fetal postmaturity syndrome.

SUGGESTIONS FOR CLINICAL ACTIVITIES

Have students do an assessment of a postterm infant of normal size and one with postmaturity syndrome and compare their results.

LEARNING OBJECTIVE 5

Discuss the physiologic characteristics of the preterm newborn that predispose each body system to various complications and are used in development of a plan of care.

CONCEPTS FOR LECTURE

1. Preterm newborns face many potential complications due to the immaturity of their systems. The preterm newborn is at significant risk for problems with respiration because they do not produce adequate amounts of surfactant, the muscular coat of the pulmonary blood vessels is not completely developed, and they are at greater risk for the ductus arteriosis to remain open due to a higher susceptibility to hypoxia.

2. The preterm infant is also susceptible to risks due to the effects of their immaturity on thermogenesis. As both glycogen and brown fat do not appear until the third trimester, they do not have those mechanisms available for heat production. Additionally, a hypoxic newborn cannot increase oxygen consumption in response to cold stress and becomes progressively colder. Preterm infants have a high ratio of body surface area to body weight, increasing their exposure to the cold. As preterm infants are extended (rather than flexed, like the term newborn) they also increase their exposed body surface area. These newborns also have a decreased ability to vasoconstrict superficial blood vessels to conserve core body heat.

POWERPOINT LECTURE SLIDES

(NOTE: The number on each PPT Lecture Slide directly corresponds with the Concepts for Lecture.)

1. Preterm Infant: Respiratory Alterations
   - Inadequate surfactant production
   - Muscular coat of pulmonary blood vessels is not completely developed
   - Greater risk for the ductus arteriosis to remain open

2. Preterm Infant: Alterations in Thermogenesis
   - Unavailability of glycogen and brown fat
   - Inability to increase oxygen consumption
   - High ratio of body surface area to body weight
   - Extended position increases body surface area
   - Decreased ability to vasoconstrict superficial blood vessels

3. Preterm Infant: GI Alterations
   - Poorly developed gag reflex
   - Incompetent esophageal cardiac sphincter
   - Poor sucking and swallowing reflexes
   - Difficulty meeting caloric needs for growth

3. Another issue of concern for preterm infants is GI immaturity, including: a danger of aspiration due to a poorly developed gag reflex, an incompetent esophageal cardiac sphincter, and poor sucking and swallowing reflexes; a difficulty in meeting caloric needs for growth due to small stomach capacity; the inability to handle the increased osmolarity of formula protein due to kidney immaturity; a difficulty with absorbing saturated fats due to decreased bile salts and pancreatic lipase; a difficulty with lactose digestion; a deficiency of calcium and phosphorous (as 2/3 of these minerals are deposited in the third trimester); an increased basal metabolic rate and increased oxygen requirements (due to fatigue associated with sucking); and feeding intolerance and potential for the development of necrotizing enterocolitis (NEC).

4. Preterm infants have a lower glomerular filtration rate (GFR) due to decreased renal blood flow. They also have a limited ability to concentrate urine or excrete large amounts of fluid. These newborns begin excreting glucose at a lower serum glucose level than the term infant, and the kidney's buffering capacity is reduced, which predisposes them to metabolic acidosis. The immaturity of the preterm newborn's renal system also affects their ability to excrete drugs because the excretion time is longer.

5. Glycogen stores in the liver are used rapidly for energy after birth. These stores are further affected by asphyxia and cold stress. This puts the preterm infant at risk for hypoglycemia. As iron is also stored in the liver during the third trimester, the preterm infant is born with low iron stores. Conjugation is also impaired, causing bilirubin levels to rise more rapidly than in the term infant.

6. Preterm newborns are also at greater risk for infection than the term infant due to the fact that passive immunity from maternal IgG immunoglobulins generally occurs in the third trimester. Breast milk can provide protection through the passive transfer of IgA. The skin of the preterm newborn is also easily excoriated, placing them at risk for nosocomial infections.

7. The most rapid period of brain growth and development occurs in the third trimester. This puts the preterm newborn at risk for intraventricular hemorrhage (IVH) and intracranial hemorrhage (ICH). Additionally, the newborn's periods of reactivity are delayed due to their immaturity.

- Inability to handle the increased osmolarity of formula protein
- Difficulty with absorbing saturated fats

3a Preterm Infant: GI Alterations
- Difficulty with lactose digestion
- Deficiency of calcium and phosphorous
- Increased basal metabolic rate and increased oxygen requirements
- Feeding intolerance
- Potential for the development of necrotizing enterocolitis (NEC)

4 Preterm Infant: Kidney Alterations
- Lower glomerular filtration rate (GFR)
- Limited ability to concentrate urine or excrete large amounts of fluid
- Excrete glucose at a lower serum glucose level
- Buffering capacity is reduced
- Excretion time of drugs is longer

5 Preterm Infants: Liver Alterations
- Glycogen stores are used rapidly
- Glycogen stores are affected by asphyxia and cold stress
- Low iron stores
- Conjugation is impaired

6 Preterm Infants: Other Alterations
- Immunologic
  - Lack of passive IgG antibodies
  - Skin is easily excoriated

7 Preterm Infants: Other Alterations
- Neurologic
  - Increased risk for IVH and ICH
  - Delayed or absent reactivity

SUGGESTIONS FOR CLASSROOM ACTIVITIES

Have students view the animation "Early Premature Labor" on the DVD-ROM. Discuss the risk factors for the premature infant.

SUGGESTIONS FOR CLINICAL ACTIVITIES

Have students review the clinical charts of premature infants being cared for in the NICU and identify complications related to prematurity.

LEARNING OBJECTIVE 6

Identify the information used in developing the nursing diagnoses required to plan interventions for the care of the preterm AGA newborn.

CONCEPTS FOR LECTURE

1. Information needed for the development of nursing diagnoses to plan interventions for the care of the preterm AGA newborn includes: an assessment of physical characteristics and gestational age, maternal prenatal risk factors, delivery risk factors, a thorough physical assessment noting abnormal findings, and a family assessment.

POWERPOINT LECTURE SLIDES

(NOTE: The number on each PPT Lecture Slide directly corresponds with the Concepts for Lecture.)

1 Assessment of the Preterm Newborn
- Physical characteristics
- Gestational age
- Maternal prenatal risk factors
- Delivery risk factors
- Physical assessment
- Family assessment

LEARNING OBJECTIVE 7

Summarize the nursing assessments of and initial interventions for a newborn born with selected congenital anomalies.

CONCEPTS FOR LECTURE

1. The following assessments should be done on an infant with congenital hydrocephalus: occipital-frontal baseline measurements and then daily head circumferences, skin integrity, signs and symptoms of infection, and signs of widening of suture lines. Nursing interventions include: assisting with head ultrasounds and transillumination, maintaining skin integrity by changing position frequently, cleaning skin creases, and keeping a sheepskin under the head. Postoperatively the head should be positioned off the operative site.

2. Assessment of the infant with choanal atresia should include a thorough respiratory assessment, observing for cyanosis and retractions at rest, noisy respiration, difficulty breathing during feeding, thick mucous, and the patency of the nares. A feeding tube should be passed to confirm the diagnosis. Nursing interventions include assisting with taping the airway in the mouth to prevent respiratory distress and elevating the head to improve air exchange.

3. Infants with a cleft lip and/or palate should be assessed for the extent of the cleft, difficulty in sucking, and expulsion of formula through the nose. Nursing interventions include: providing nutrition through feedings with a special nipple and frequent burping, monitoring weight gain, cleaning the cleft with sterile water, supporting parent coping, and providing role modeling. Infants should also be placed prone or in a side-lying position to facilitate drainage, and the nasopharyngeal cavity should be suctioned to prevent aspiration.

4. Infants with a tracheoesophageal fistula with esophageal atresia should be assessed for: excessive oral secretions, constant drooling, abdominal distention, periodic choking and cyanosis, immediate regurgitation of feeding, clinical symptoms of aspiration pneumonia,

POWERPOINT LECTURE SLIDES

(NOTE: The number on each PPT Lecture Slide directly corresponds with the Concepts for Lecture.)

1 Hydrocephalus: Nursing Assessments
- Occipital-frontal baseline measurements
- Daily head circumferences
- Skin integrity
- Signs and symptoms of infection
- Signs of widening of suture lines

1a Hydrocephalus: Nursing Interventions
- Assist with head ultrasounds and transillumination
- Change position frequently
- Clean skin creases
- Keeping a sheepskin under the head
- Postoperatively position head off the operative site

2 Choanal Atresia: Nursing Assessment
- Cyanosis and retractions at rest
- Noisy respirations
- Difficulty breathing during feeding
- Thick mucous
- Patency of the nares
- Pass feeding tube to confirm the diagnosis

2a Choanal Atresia: Nursing Interventions
- Assist with taping the airway in the mouth
- Elevate the head to improve air exchange

3 Cleft Lip and/or Palate: Nursing Assessment
- The extent of the cleft
- Difficulty in sucking
- Expulsion of formula through the nose

and the inability to pass a nasogastric tube. Nursing interventions include: maintenance of respiratory status and prevention of aspiration, withholding feedings until esophageal patency is determined, place on low intermittent suction to control saliva and mucus, and maintaining fluid and electrolyte balance. The nurse should try to keep the infant quiet and comfortable, placing him in a warmed, humidified incubator and elevating the head of the bed 20–40 degrees. The nurse should also provide parent education and information.

5. Infants born with a diaphragmatic hernia should be assessed for: adequate respiratory status, barrel chest and scaphoid abdomen, asymmetric chest expansion, absent breath sounds, displacement of heart sounds to the right, spasmodic attacks of cyanosis and difficulty feeding, and bowel sounds heard in thoracic cavity. Nursing interventions should include: maintenance of adequate respiratory status, gastric decompression, involve parents in care, place infant in high semi-Fowler's position, and turn to affected side to allow unaffected lung expansion.

3a Cleft Lip and/or Palate: Nursing Interventions
- Provide nutrition through feedings with a special nipple
- Monitor weight gain
- Clean the cleft with sterile water
- Supporting parent coping
- Provide role modeling
- Position infant prone or side-lying

4 Tracheoesophageal Fistula: Nursing Assessments
- Excessive oral secretions
- Constant drooling
- Abdominal distention
- Periodic choking and cyanosis
- Immediate regurgitation of feeding
- Inability to pass a nasogastric tube

4a Tracheoesophageal Fistula: Nursing Interventions
- Withholding feedings until esophageal patency is determined
- Place on low intermittent suction to control saliva and mucus
- Place in a warmed, humidified incubator
- Keep infant quiet and elevate head of bed 20–40 degrees
- Maintain fluid and electrolyte balance
- Provide parent education and information

5 Diaphragmatic Hernia: Nursing Assessments
- Barrel chest and scaphoid abdomen
- Asymmetric chest expansion
- Absent breath sounds
- Displacement of heart sounds to the right
- Spasmodic attacks of cyanosis and difficulty feeding
- Bowel sounds heard in thoracic cavity

5a Diaphragmatic Hernia: Nursing Interventions
- Maintenance of adequate respiratory status
- Gastric decompression
- Involve parents in care
- Place infant in high semi-Fowler's position
- Turn to affected side to allow unaffected lung expansion

SUGGESTIONS FOR CLASSROOM ACTIVITIES

Use illustrations of the congenital anomalies to discuss the implications for the newborn. Bring in a feeding device used for infants with a cleft lip/palate and demonstrate use with a mannequin.

LEARNING OBJECTIVE 8

Explain the special care needed by drug-exposed newborn.

CONCEPTS FOR LECTURE

1. Nursing care of the drug-exposed newborn includes: neonatal abstinence scoring as per hospital protocol, monitoring temperature for hyperthermia, monitoring of pulse, respirations every 15 minutes and pulse oximetry until stable, stimulation of the infant if apnea

POWERPOINT LECTURE SLIDES

(NOTE: The number on each PPT Lecture Slide directly corresponds with the Concepts for Lecture.)

1 Nursing Care of the Drug-Exposed Newborn
- Neonatal abstinence scoring
- Monitoring VS and pulse oximetry until stable

occurs, small frequent feedings, IV therapy if needed, positioning on the right side-lying or semi-Fowler's to avoid possible aspiration, monitoring frequency of diarrhea and vomiting and weigh infant every 8 hours during withdrawal, swaddle infant, protect face and extremities from excoriation by using mittens and soft sheets or sheepskin, and place infant in quiet, dimly lighted area of the nursery. Medications that may be administered include oral morphine, phenobarbital, and tincture of opium.

- Small frequent feedings
- IV therapy if needed
- Positioning on the right side-lying or semi-Fowler's
- Monitoring frequency of diarrhea and vomiting

 Nursing Care of the Drug-Exposed Newborn
- Weigh infant every 8 hours during withdrawal
- Swaddle infant
- Protect face and extremities from excoriation
- Place infant in quiet, dimly lighted area of the nursery
- Administration of medications

SUGGESTIONS FOR CLASSROOM ACTIVITIES

Discuss implications of intrauterine drug exposure and have a group discussion about possible ways to prevent maternal drug abuse.

SUGGESTIONS FOR CLINICAL ACTIVITIES

Have students observe an infant that is going through withdrawal due to drug exposure. Have them complete neonatal abstinence scoring and discuss their results.

LEARNING OBJECTIVE 9

Relate the consequences of maternal HIV/AIDS to the management of the infant in the neonatal period.

CONCEPTS FOR LECTURE

1. Newborns who have been exposed to maternal HIV/AIDS are generally premature, SGA, and show failure to thrive. They may exhibit signs of an enlarged spleen and liver, swollen glands, recurrent respiratory infections, rhinorrhea, interstitial pneumonia, recurrent gastrointestinal problems such as diarrhea and weight loss, urinary infections, persistent or recurrent oral and genital candidiasis infection, and loss of developmental milestones. Nursing care should include: providing comfort, keeping the newborn well nourished, keeping the infant protected from infections, and facilitating growth, development, and attachment.

POWERPOINT LECTURE SLIDES

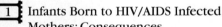

(NOTE: The number on each PPT Lecture Slide directly corresponds with the Concepts for Lecture.)

 Infants Born to HIV/AIDS Infected Mothers: Consequences
- Prematurity
- SGA
- Failure to thrive
- Enlarged spleen and liver
- Swollen glands

 Infants Born to HIV/AIDS Infected Mothers: Consequences
- Recurrent respiratory infection
- Rhinorrhea
- Recurrent GI problems
- Persistent or recurrent candidiasis

Nursing Care of the Infant Born to HIV/AIDS Infected Mothers
- Provide comfort
- Keep the newborn well nourished
- Keep the infant protected from infections
- Facilitate growth, development, and attachment

SUGGESTIONS FOR CLASSROOM ACTIVITIES

Have students develop a care plan for an infant born to a mother with HIV/AIDS.

SUGGESTIONS FOR CLINICAL ACTIVITIES

Have students observe the care for an infant in the intensive care nursery that has been born to a mother with HIV/AIDS. Have them discuss their observations in post-conference.

LEARNING OBJECTIVE 10

Identify physical examination findings suggestive of a congenital cardiac defect.

CONCEPTS FOR LECTURE

1. The most common cardiac defects seen in the early newborn period include: left ventricular outflow obstructions, hypoplastic left heart, coarctation or the aorta, patent ductus, ventricular septal defect, or atrial septal defects. The most common symptoms of a cardiac defect are cyanosis, detectable heart murmur, and signs of congestive heart failure such as tachycardia and tachypnea.

POWERPOINT LECTURE SLIDES

(NOTE: The number on each PPT Lecture Slide directly corresponds with the Concepts for Lecture.)

 Congenital Cardiac Disease: Symptoms
- Cyanosis
- Heart murmur
- Signs of congestive heart failure

SUGGESTIONS FOR CLASSROOM ACTIVITIES

Use illustrations of common congenital cardiac anomalies to show the students how the anomalies affect the infant.

SUGGESTIONS FOR CLINICAL ACTIVITIES

Have students do an assessment on an infant with a cardiac anomaly in the intensive care nursery and discuss their observations.

LEARNING OBJECTIVE 11

Explain the special care needed by a newborn with an inborn error of metabolism.

CONCEPTS FOR LECTURE

1. Nursing care for the newborn with an inborn error of metabolism is focused on assessment of the signs of the disorder, carrying out state-mandated newborn testing, referral of parents to support groups and centers to provide them with information about the genetics, and dietary management.

POWERPOINT LECTURE SLIDES

(NOTE: The number on each PPT Lecture Slide directly corresponds with the Concepts for Lecture.)

 Nursing Care of the Newborn with Inborn Errors of Metabolism
- Assessment of signs of the disorder
- State-mandated newborn testing
- Referral of parents to support groups
- Referral of parents to centers for education
- Dietary management

SUGGESTIONS FOR CLASSROOM ACTIVITIES

Review the screening tests that are included for newborn screening in your state.

SUGGESTIONS FOR CLINICAL ACTIVITIES

Review the hospital policy for newborn screening and the mechanisms in place for reporting abnormal results.

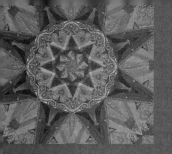

CHAPTER 33
THE NEWBORN AT RISK: BIRTH-RELATED STRESSORS

RESOURCE LIBRARY

 PRENTICE HALL NURSING MEDIALINK DVD-ROM

Audio Glossary
NCLEX Review
Video: *Infant Receiving Phototherapy*

COMPANION WEBSITE

Additional NCLEX Review
Case Study: *Newborn with Jaundice*
Care Plan Activity: *Infection in a Newborn*
Applications: *Infant with Respiratory Distress Syndrome; Meconium Aspiration Syndrome*
Critical Thinking

📖 IMAGE LIBRARY

Figure 33.1 Demonstration of resuscitation of an infant with bag and mask.

Figure 33.2 Endotracheal intubation is accomplished with the infant's head in the "sniffing" position.

Figure 33.3 External cardiac massage.

Figure 33.4 Cycle of events of RDS leading to eventual respiratory failure.

Figure 33.5 RDS chest x-ray.

Figure 33.6 One-day-old, 29 weeks' gestational age, 1450-g baby on respirator and in isolette.

Figure 33.7 Evaluating respiratory status using the Silverman-Andersen index.

Figure 33.8 This baby born at 36 weeks' gestational age had severe RDS.

Figure 33.9 Premature infant under oxygen hood.

Figure 33.10 Chest x-ray of a left-sided pneumothorax.

Figure 33.11 The baby with BPD has ongoing oxygen and nutritional needs as well as the need for gentle individualized care.

Figure 33.12 A baby requiring oxygen at greater than 36 weeks' gestational age.

Figure 33.13 Cold stress chain of events.

Figure 33.14 Potential sites for heel sticks.

Figure 33.15 Heel stick.

Figure 33.16 Guidelines for phototherapy in hospitalized infants or 35 or more weeks' gestation.

Figure 33.17 Transfusion level nomogram.

Figure 33.18 Infant receiving phototherapy.

Figure 33.19 Newborn on fiberoptic "bili" mattress and under phototherapy lights.

Figure 33.20 Mother of a 26 weeks' gestational age infant with respiratory distress syndrome on a ventilator is getting acquainted with her baby.

Figure 33.22 This 25 weeks' gestational age infant with respiratory distress syndrome may be frightening for her parents to see for the first time because of the technology that is attached to her.

Figure 33.23 Mother of this 26 weeks' gestational age 600-g baby begins attachment through fingertip touch.

Figure 33.24 This mother of a 31 weeks' gestational age infant with respiratory distress syndrome is spending time with her newborn and meeting the baby's need for cuddling.

Figure 33.25 Cobedding of twins facilitates delivery of care and parent interaction with healthcare members.

Figure 33.26 Twins from Figure 33.25 on the happy day of discharge, being held by staff in the NICU.

LEARNING OBJECTIVE 1

Discuss how to identify infants in need of resuscitation and the appropriate method of resuscitation based on the antepartal/labor record and physiologic indicators apparent at birth.

CONCEPTS FOR LECTURE

1. The nurse should anticipate neonatal resuscitation if the mother has antepartal and intrapartal risk factors as mentioned in previous chapters. Additionally, the following fetal/neonatal factors may also alert the nurse to anticipate a possible neonatal resuscitation: nonreassuring

POWERPOINT LECTURE SLIDES

(NOTE: The number on each PPT Lecture Slide directly corresponds with the Concepts for Lecture.)

 1 Fetal/Neonatal Risk Factors for Resuscitation
- Nonreassuring fetal heart rate pattern
- Difficult birth

© 2008 Pearson Education, Inc.

fetal heart rate pattern, difficult birth or prolonged bradycardia, fetal scalp/capillary blood sample-acidosis pH < 7.20, meconium in amniotic fluid, prematurity, macrosomia, male infant SGA, significant intrapartum bleeding, structural lung abnormality, oligohydramnios, congenital heart disease, maternal infection, narcotic use in labor, an infant of a diabetic mother, arrhythmias, cardiomyopathy, and fetal anemia.

- Fetal scalp/capillary blood sample-acidosis pH < 7.20
- Meconium in amniotic fluid
- Prematurity
- Macrosomia or SGA

1a Fetal/Neonatal Risk Factors for Resuscitation
- Male infant
- Significant intrapartum bleeding
- Structural lung abnormality or oligohydramnios
- Congenital heart disease
- Maternal infection
- Narcotic use in labor

1b Fetal/Neonatal Risk Factors for Resuscitation
- An infant of a diabetic mother
- Arrhythmias
- Cardiomyopathy
- Fetal anemia

SUGGESTIONS FOR CLINICAL ACTIVITIES

Have students review the charts of newborns in the NICU and review the documentation of the resuscitative efforts at birth. Have students identify risk factors that predisposed the newborn to distress.

LEARNING OBJECTIVE 2

Based on clinical manifestation, differentiate among the various types of respiratory distress (respiratory distress syndrome, transient tachypnea of the newborn, meconium aspiration syndrome, and persistent pulmonary hypertension) in the newborn and the nursing care related to each type.

CONCEPTS FOR LECTURE

1. Respiratory distress syndrome (RDS) is due to the absence, deficiency, or alteration in the production of surfactant, which is required to maintain alveolar stability. Instability of the alveoli causes atelectasis upon expiration. This can then further inhibit the production of surfactant and causes pulmonary vasoconstriction. This causes hypoxemia, hypercarbia, and acidemia. RDS is due to either prematurity or surfactant deficiency disease. Nursing care of infants with RDS should focus on maintaining an adequate respiratory status by observing for signs of distress, providing oxygen and suction as needed, and assessing vital signs and oxygenation status. Another goal of nursing care is to maintain adequate neonatal nutrition by assessing ability to feed orally or via gavage safely, providing enteral feedings as tolerated, providing TPN as indicated, and monitoring intake, output, and weight gain. It is also important for the nurse to maintain adequate hydration by assessing hydration status, providing enteral feedings or IV fluids as ordered, and monitoring intake and output.

2. Respiratory distress manifested primarily by LGA and near-term infants that resembles RDS is called transient tachypnea (TTN) of the newborn. It is due to failure to clear the lungs of fluid, mucus, and debris, or an excess

POWERPOINT LECTURE SLIDES

(NOTE: The number on each PPT Lecture Slide directly corresponds with the Concepts for Lecture.)

1 Respiratory Distress Syndrome (RDS)
- Deficiency or absence of surfactant
- Atelectasis (Figure 33.5)
- Hypoxemia, hypercarbia, academia
- May be due to prematurity or surfactant deficiency

1a See Figure 33.5

1b RDS: Nursing Care
- Maintain adequate respiratory status (Figure 33.9)
- Maintain adequate nutritional status
- Maintain adequate hydration
- Education and support of family

1c See Figure 33.9

2 Transient Tachypnea of the Newborn (TTN)
- Failure to clear lung fluid, mucus, debris
- Exhibit signs of distress shortly after birth
- Symptoms
  ○ Expiratory grunting and nasal flaring
  ○ Subcostal retractions
  ○ Slight cyanosis

of lung fluid due to aspiration of amniotic or tracheal fluid. These infants usually do not exhibit signs of respiratory distress immediately after birth, but shortly thereafter they will develop expiratory grunting, nasal flaring, subcostal retractions, and mild cyanosis. They will usually develop tachypnea by 6 hours of age and may have a mild respiratory and metabolic acidosis. Symptoms usually disappear by 24 hours of age but may last up to 72 hours. Nursing care should include: monitoring of respiratory status; provision of oxygen as needed and monitoring oxygenation status; assessing the infant's ability to receive enteral feedings safely; assessing intake, output, and weight; and assessing hydration status.

3. Increased intestinal peristalsis and relaxation of the anal sphincter is often a physiologic response to fetal asphyxia. The fetus then releases meconium, which is then mixed in with the amniotic fluid, creating the potential for aspiration in the tracheobronchial tree in utero or during the infant's first breaths. Meconium in the lungs may produce a mechanical obstruction of the airways, a chemical pneumonitis, vasoconstriction of the pulmonary vessels, and inactivation of natural surfactant. The infant may demonstrate signs of distress at birth, including: pallor, cyanosis, apnea, and slow heartbeat; continued respiratory distress requiring mechanical ventilation; an overdistended, barrel-shaped chest; decreased air movement with rales and rhonchi; a displaced liver; and yellowish/pale green staining of the skin, nails, and umbilical cord. Nursing interventions should include an ongoing assessment of the respiratory status, observing for complications, as well as normal nursing care for an infant with respiratory distress.

4. Persistent pulmonary hypertension (PPHN) is a condition in which blood is shunted away from the lungs (R-L) through the patent ductus arteriosus and foramen ovale. Primary PPHN results from pulmonary vascular changes before birth, which cause abnormally high pulmonary vascular resistance (PVR). Secondary PPHN occurs when events after birth result in an increase in the PVR. Nursing interventions include assessing for the onset of symptoms, which generally occurs within 12–24 hours after birth, signs of respiratory distress, and cyanosis. Minimal stimulation is very important because agitation can lead to hypoxemia, which further increases the PVR. Provision of oxygen and frequently mechanical ventilation is required, and the nurse should continually assess the infant's oxygenation status and monitor for excess secretions. Vital signs should be monitored frequently and good skin care should be provided. The nurse should also assess for signs of a pneumothorax, which is a potential side effect of mechanical ventilation. The nurse also plays an important role in educating the parents about their infant's condition and subsequent changes and supporting the family.

 TTN: Nursing Care
- Maintain adequate respiratory status
- Maintain adequate nutritional status
- Maintain adequate hydration
- Support and educate family

 Meconium Aspiration Syndrome (MAS)
- Mechanical obstruction of the airways
- Chemical pneumonitis
- Vasoconstriction of the pulmonary vessels
- Inactivation of natural surfactant

 MAS: Nursing Care
- Assess for complications related to MAS
- Maintain adequate respiratory status
- Maintain adequate nutritional status
- Maintain adequate hydration

 Persistent Pulmonary Hypertension (PPHN)
- Blood shunted away from lungs
- Increased pulmonary vascular resistance (PVR)
- Primary
  - Pulmonary vascular changes before birth resulting in PVR
- Secondary
  - Pulmonary vascular changes after birth resulting in PVR

 PPHN: Nursing Care
- Minimize stimulation
- Maintain adequate respiratory status
- Observe for signs of pneumothorax (Figure 33.10)
- Maintain adequate nutritional status
- Maintain adequate hydration status
- Support and educate family

4b See Figure 33.10

SUGGESTIONS FOR CLASSROOM ACTIVITIES

Have students compare and contrast the different types of respiratory disorders and the nursing interventions.

SUGGESTIONS FOR CLINICAL ACTIVITIES

Have students participate in the care of a newborn with respiratory distress and discuss their assessments and interventions.

LEARNING OBJECTIVE 3

Discuss selected metabolic abnormalities (including cold stress and hypoglycemia), their effects on the newborn, and their nursing implications.

CONCEPTS FOR LECTURE

1. Cold stress in the newborn is excessive heat loss which results in increased respirations and nonshivering thermogenesis to maintain body temperature. The ability of the infant to compensate for cold stress is impaired due to hypoxemia, CNS abnormalities, and hypoglycemia. Several metabolic consequences can occur as a result of cold stress, including an increase in oxygen requirements, an increase in utilization of glucose, acids are released in the bloodstream, and surfactant production decreases. Prevention is the key nursing intervention, along with observation for signs of cold stress, including increased movements and respirations, decreased skin temperature and peripheral perfusion, development of hypoglycemia, and possibly development of metabolic acidosis. Nursing interventions should include maintaining a neutral thermal environment (NTE), warming the baby slowly, frequent monitoring of skin temperature, warming IV fluids before infusion, prevent further heat loss, and treat the accompanying hypoglycemia or respiratory distress.

2. Hypoglycemia is defined as a glucose oxidase reagent strip value of 40–50 mg/dL and a plasma serum glucose of less than 20–25 mg/dL. Infants at risk for developing hypoglycemia include preterm infants who have not had sufficient time to store glucose and fat and therefore have a decreased ability to carry out gluconeogenesis, the infant of a diabetic mother who develops hyperinsulinemia in response to maternal glucose, and a small-for-gestation-age infant who has used up glycogen and fat stores. Symptoms of hypoglycemia include: lethargy, jitteriness, poor feeding and sucking, vomiting, hypothermia, pallor, hypotonia, tremors, seizure activity, high pitched cry, and an exaggerated mororeflex. Nursing care should include routine screening for all at-risk newborns for the first 4 hours of life, treatment with parenteral D10W for hypoglycemia, and prevention of hypoglycemia through early feedings.

POWERPOINT LECTURE SLIDES

(NOTE: The number on each PPT Lecture Slide directly corresponds with the Concepts for Lecture.)

1 Cold Stress (Figure 33.13)
- Increase in oxygen requirements
- Increase in utilization of glucose
- Acids are released in the bloodstream
- Surfactant production decreases

1a See Figure 33.13

1b Cold Stress: Nursing Care
- Observe for signs of cold stress
- Maintain NTE
- Warm baby slowly
- Frequent monitoring of skin temperature
- Warming IV fluids
- Treat accompanying hypoglycemia

2 Hypoglycemia Symptoms
- Lethargy or jitteriness
- Poor feeding and sucking
- Vomiting
- Hypothermia and pallor
- Hypotonia, tremors
- Seizure activity, high pitched cry, exaggerated moro reflex

2a Hypoglycemia: Nursing Care
- Routine screening for all at risk infants (Figures 33.14 and 33.15)
- Early feedings
- D10W infusion

2b See Figure 33.14

2c See Figure 33.15

SUGGESTIONS FOR CLASSROOM ACTIVITIES

Use a newborn model to demonstrate the appropriate method of doing a heel stick to obtain a capillary blood sample for glucose analysis.

SUGGESTIONS FOR CLINICAL ACTIVITIES

Have students do an assessment of a newborn experiencing cold stress and hypoglycemia and document their findings.

LEARNING OBJECTIVE 4

Differentiate between physiologic and pathologic jaundice according to timing of onset (in hours), cause, possible sequelae, and specific management.

CONCEPTS FOR LECTURE

1. Physiologic jaundice generally appears after the first 24 hours of life and disappears within 14 days. The cause is due to an increase in red cell mass due to a shorter red cell lifespan, a slower uptake of bilirubin by the liver, a lack of intestinal bacteria, and/or poorly established hydration from initial breastfeeding.

2. Pathologic jaundice is due to a decrease in the number or quality of available serum albumin-binding sites available for conjugation. It appears within the first 24 hours of life, the serum bilirubin concentration rises by more than 0.2 mg/dL per hour, the total serum bilirubin concentrations exceed the 95th percentile on the nomogram, the conjugated bilirubin concentrations are greater than 2 mg/dL or more than 20% of the total serum bilirubin concentration, and clinical jaundice persists for more than 2 weeks in a term newborn. Causes of pathologic hyperbilirubinemia include: hemolytic disease of the newborn, erythroblastosis fetalis, hydrops fetalis, ABO incompatibility, polycythemia (central hematocrit 65% or more), pyloric stenosis, obstruction or atresia of the biliary duct or of the lower bowel, low-grade urinary tract infection, sepsis, hypothyroidism, enclosed hemorrhage (cephalhematoma, extensive bruising), asphyxia neonatorum, hypothermia, acidemia, and hypoglycemia. Maternal conditions predisposing the infant to hyperbilirubinemia include: hereditary spherocytosis, diabetes, intrauterine infections, gram-negative bacilli infections that stimulate production of maternal alloimmune antibodies, drug ingestion (such as sulfas, salicylates, novobiocin, and diazepam), and oxytocin administration.

3. The resulting outcome of an infant with hyperbilirubinemia is dependent upon the extent of the hemolytic process and cause. Potential sequelae may include: fetal or early neonatal death, kernicterus that may result in mental retardation, death, hearing loss, perceptual impairment, delayed speech development, hyperactivity, muscle incoordination, or learning difficulties. Treatment is directed toward resolving anemia, removing maternal antibodies and sensitized erythrocytes, increasing serum albumin levels, reducing serum bilirubin levels, and minimizing the consequences of hyperbilirubinemia. Phototherapy, exchange transfusions, and drug therapy may be used to treat hemolytic disease.

POWERPOINT LECTURE SLIDES

(NOTE: The number on each PPT Lecture Slide directly corresponds with the Concepts for Lecture.)

1 Physiologic Hyperbilirubinemia
- Appears after first 24 hours of life
- Disappears within 14 days
- Due to an increase in red cell mass

2 Pathologic Hyperbilirubinemia
- Appears within first 24 hours of life
- Serum bilirubin concentration rises by more than 0.2 mg/dL per hour
- Bilirubin concentrations exceed the 95th percentile
- Conjugated bilirubin concentrations are greater than 2 mg/dL
- Clinical jaundice persists for more than 2 weeks in a term newborn

2a Causes of Pathologic Hyperbilirubinemia
- Hemolytic disease of the newborn
- Erythroblastosis fetalis
- Hydrops fetalis
- ABO incompatibility

3 Treatment of Pathologic Hyperbilirubinemia
- Resolving anemia
- Removing maternal antibodies and sensitized erythrocytes
- Increasing serum albumin levels
- Reducing serum bilirubin levels
- Minimizing the consequences of hyperbilirubinemia

SUGGESTIONS FOR CLINICAL ACTIVITIES

Have students review the charts of newborns with hyperbilirubinemia and identify the cause and treatment.

Explain how Rh incompatibility or ABO incompatibility can lead to the development of hyperbilirubinemia.

CONCEPTS FOR LECTURE

1. Rh incompatibility when an Rh-negative mother is pregnant with an Rh-positive fetus and maternal antibodies cross the placenta. They attach to and destroy fetal red blood cells. ABO incompatibility occurs when a mother who is type O has a fetus that is type A or B. Antibodies from both of these maternal-fetal antibodies causes destruction of the fetal red blood cells. This causes an increase in bilirubin load, which the newborn may not be able to conjugate and excrete effectively.

POWERPOINT LECTURE SLIDES

(NOTE: The number on each PPT Lecture Slide directly corresponds with the Concepts for Lecture.)

 Maternal-Fetal Blood Incompatibility
- Rh incompatibility
  - Rh-negative mother
  - Rh-positive fetus
- ABO incompatibility
  - O mother
  - A or B fetus

SUGGESTIONS FOR CLASSROOM ACTIVITIES

Discuss strategies to prevent Rh incompatibility in women and their newborns.

SUGGESTIONS FOR CLINICAL ACTIVITIES

Have students review the charts of infants with hyperbilirubinemia related to maternal-infant blood incompatibility and discuss predisposing factors that contributed to the development of hyperbilirubinemia.

Identify the nursing responsibilities in caring for the newborn receiving phototherapy.

CONCEPTS FOR LECTURE

1. Nursing responsibilities in caring for a newborn receiving phototherapy include: maximizing exposure of the skin surface to the light, periodic assessment of serum bilirubin levels, protecting the newborn's eyes with patches, measuring irradiance levels with a photometer, good skin care, reposition infant at least every 2 hours, maintaining an NTE, and maintenance of adequate hydration and nutrition.

POWERPOINT LECTURE SLIDES

(NOTE: The number on each PPT Lecture Slide directly corresponds with the Concepts for Lecture.)

 Phototherapy: Nursing Care (Figure 33.18)
- Maximize exposure of the skin surface to the light
- Periodic assessment of serum bilirubin levels
- Protect the newborn's eyes with patches
- Measure irradiance levels with a photometer
- Good skin care and reposition infant at least every 2 hours
- Maintain an NTE and adequate hydration and nutrition

 See Figure 33.18

SUGGESTIONS FOR CLASSROOM ACTIVITIES

Show students pictures of a newborn receiving phototherapy and discuss the nursing management.

SUGGESTIONS FOR CLINICAL ACTIVITIES

Have students assist in the care of a newborn receiving phototherapy and discuss the rationale for their interventions.

LEARNING OBJECTIVE 7

Discuss selected hematologic problems such as anemia and polycythemia and the nursing implications associated with each.

CONCEPTS FOR LECTURE

1. Infants with a hemoglobin value of less than 14 mg/dL and 13 mg/dL are anemic. Anemia in the newborn may be due to blood loss, hemolysis, and impaired red blood cell production. Nursing management includes: assessment of the newborn for pallor, shock, poor weight gain, tachycardia, tachypnea, and apnea. The anemia is confirmed by laboratory testing. If signs of shock are demonstrated, the nurse should initiate interventions to treat the shock.

2. Polycythemia is defined as an increase in blood volume and hematocrit values. It often occurs in intrauterine growth restricted (IUGR); full-term, or close-to-full-term infants; newborns with placental transfusion caused by delayed cord clamping or cord stripping; infants receiving maternal-fetal or twin-to-twin transfusions; babies who have been exposed to intrauterine hypoxia; and babies of mothers who smoke, suffer from asphyxia, diabetes (DM), or hypertension, or take propranolol during pregnancy. Nursing interventions include screening of the newborn hematocrit, observing for signs of distress. If the newborn receives an exchange transfusion, the nurse observes for distress or change in vital signs and monitors for potential complications.

POWERPOINT LECTURE SLIDES

(NOTE: The number on each PPT Lecture Slide directly corresponds with the Concepts for Lecture.)

1 Anemia
- Hemoglobin of less than 14 mg/dL (term)
- Hemoglobin of less than 13 mg/dL (preterm)
- Nursing management
  - Observe for symptoms
  - Initiate interventions for shock

2 Polycythemia
- Increase in blood volume and hematocrit
- Nursing management:
  - Assessment of hematocrit
  - Monitor for signs of distress
  - Assist with exchange transfusion

SUGGESTIONS FOR CLASSROOM ACTIVITIES

Discuss the signs and symptoms of anemia and polycythemia.

LEARNING OBJECTIVE 8

Describe the nursing assessment that would lead the nurse to suspect newborn sepsis.

CONCEPTS FOR LECTURE

1. The following nursing assessments may lead the nurse to suspect newborn sepsis: lethargy or irritability, hypotonia, hypotension, pallor, duskiness, cyanosis, cool and clammy skin, temperature instability, feeding intolerance, hyperbilirubinemia, and tachycardia followed by apnea/bradycardia.

POWERPOINT LECTURE SLIDES

(NOTE: The number on each PPT Lecture Slide directly corresponds with the Concepts for Lecture.)

1 Signs and Symptoms of Sepsis
- Lethargy or irritability
- Hypotonia
- Hypotension
- Pallor, duskiness, or cyanosis
- Cool and clammy skin

1a Signs and Symptoms of Sepsis
- Temperature instability
- Feeding intolerance
- Hyperbilirubinemia
- Tachycardia followed by apnea/bradycardia

LEARNING OBJECTIVE 9

Relate the consequences of selected maternally transmitted infections, such as maternal syphilis, gonorrhea, herpesviridae family (HSV or CMV), and chlamydia, to the management of the infant in the neonatal period.

CONCEPTS FOR LECTURE

1. Infants born to mothers infected with syphilis may demonstrate: rhinitis, fissures on mouth corners and excoriated upper lip, a red rash around the mouth and anus, irritability, generalized edema, hepatosplenomegaly, congenital cataracts, SGA, and failure to thrive. Nursing interventions include: initiating isolation until the infant has been treated with antibiotics for 48 hours, administering penicillin, and providing emotional support for the family.

2. Infants born to mothers affected by gonorrhea may exhibit: conjunctivitis, purulent discharge and corneal ulcerations, and neonatal sepsis. Nursing interventions include administration of ophthalmic antibiotic ointment and initiation of follow-up referral.

3. Infants born to mothers infected with herpes may exhibit: small cluster vesicular skin lesions over the entire body, DIC, pneumonia, hepatitis, hepatosplenomegaly, and neurologic abnormalities. Nursing interventions include: careful hand washing and gown and glove isolation with linen precautions, administration of IV vidarabine or acyclovir, initiation of follow-up referral, and support and education of parents.

4. Infants born to mothers infected with chlamydia may demonstrate pneumonia and conjunctivitis. Nursing interventions include installation of ophthalmic erythromycin and follow-up referral.

POWERPOINT LECTURE SLIDES

(NOTE: The number on each PPT Lecture Slide directly corresponds with the Concepts for Lecture.)

1 Symptoms of Syphilis
- Rhinitis
- Red rash around the mouth and anus
- Irritability
- Generalized edema and hepatosplenomegaly
- Congenital cataracts
- SGA and failure to thrive

1a Syphilis: Nursing Management
- Initiate isolation
- Administer penicillin
- Provide emotional support for the family

2 Gonorrhea
- Symptoms
  - Conjunctivitis
  - Corneal ulcerations
- Nursing management
  - Administration of ophthalmic antibiotic ointment
  - Referral for follow-up

3 Symptoms of Herpes
- Small cluster vesicular skin lesions over the entire body
- DIC
- Pneumonia
- Hepatitis
- Hepatosplenomegaly
- Neurologic abnormalities

3a Herpes: Nursing Management
- Careful hand washing and gown and glove isolation
- Administration of IV vidarabine or acyclovir
- Initiation of follow-up referral
- Support and education of parents

4 Chlamydia
- Symptoms
  - Pneumonia
  - Conjunctivitis
- Nursing management
  - Administration of ophthalmic antibiotic ointment
  - Referral for follow-up

LEARNING OBJECTIVE 10

Describe interventions to facilitate parental attachment with the at-risk newborn.

CONCEPTS FOR LECTURE

1. Nursing interventions that facilitate parental attachment with the at-risk newborn include: facilitating family visits, allowing the family to hold and touch the baby, giving the family a picture of the baby to take home, liberal visiting hours, and encouraging the family to get involved in the care of the newborn.

POWERPOINT LECTURE SLIDES

(NOTE: The number on each PPT Lecture Slide directly corresponds with the Concepts for Lecture.)

1. Facilitating Parental Attachment
   - Facilitating family visits (Figure 33.20)
   - Allowing the family to hold and touch the baby
   - Giving the family a picture of the baby
   - Liberal visiting hours
   - Encouraging the family to get involved in the care

1a. See Figure 33.20

SUGGESTIONS FOR CLASSROOM ACTIVITIES

Have students form small groups and discuss their perception of what a parent must experience after having an at-risk newborn.

SUGGESTIONS FOR CLINICAL ACTIVITIES

Have students interview NICU nurses about strategies that they use to facilitate parental attachments and share their findings in post conference.

LEARNING OBJECTIVE 11

Identify the special initial and long-term needs of parents of at-risk infants.

CONCEPTS FOR LECTURE

1. Initial and long-term needs of the parents of at-risk infants include: realistically perceiving the infant's medical condition and needs, adapting to the infant's hospital environment, assuming primary caretaking role, assuming total responsibility for the infant upon discharge, and possibly coping with the death of the infant if it occurs.

POWERPOINT LECTURE SLIDES

(NOTE: The number on each PPT Lecture Slide directly corresponds with the Concepts for Lecture.)

1. Needs of Parents of At-Risk Infants
   - Realistically perceiving the infant's medical condition and needs
   - Adapting to the infant's hospital environment
   - Assuming primary caretaking role
   - Assuming total responsibility for the infant upon discharge
   - Possibly coping with the death of the infant if it occurs

SUGGESTIONS FOR CLASSROOM ACTIVITIES

Discuss potential interventions for meeting family needs after having an at-risk newborn.

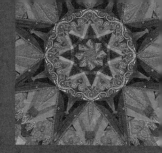

CHAPTER 34
POSTPARTAL: ADAPTATION AND NURSING ASSESSMENT

RESOURCE LIBRARY

 PRENTICE HALL NURSING MEDIALINK DVD-ROM

Audio Glossary
NCLEX Review
Videos: *Postpartum Assessment; Through the Eyes of a Nurse—Welcoming the New Arrival at the Postpartal Visit*

COMPANION WEBSITE

Additional NCLEX Review
Case Study: *Mother-Infant Bonding*
Care Plan Activity: *Postpartum Client Requesting Relief*
Applications: *Identifying Strategies to Enhance Father-Infant Interactions; Exploring Cultural Differences Regarding Postpartum Care*
Critical Thinking

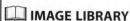 **IMAGE LIBRARY**

Figure 34.1 Involution of the uterus.
Figure 34.2 The uterus becomes displaced and deviated to the right when the bladder is full.
Figure 34.3 Diastasis recti abdominis, a separation of the musculature, commonly occurs after pregnancy.
Figure 34.4 The mother has direct face-to-face and eye-to-eye contact in the *en face* position.

Figure 34.5 The father experiences strong feelings of attraction during engrossment.
Figure 34.6 Measuring the descent of the fundus for the woman having a vaginal birth.
Figure 34.8 Intact perineum with hemorrhoids.
Figure 34.9 Homans' sign: With the woman's knees flexed, the nurse dorsiflexes the foot.

LEARNING OBJECTIVE 1

Describe the basic physiologic changes that occur in the postpartum period as a woman's body returns to its prepregnant state.

CONCEPTS FOR LECTURE

1. Changes in the uterus include a decrease in weight from 1000 g in the immediate postpartal period to 100 g at the completion of involution. The spongy layer of the decidua is sloughed off and the basal layer differentiates into two layers within the first 72 hours. The outer layer sloughs off and the inner layer begins the foundation for the new endometrium. The placental site heals by exfoliation with the superficial tissue becoming necrotic and sloughing off. The uterine cells will atrophy with the decreased levels of estrogen and progesterone. Within 6 to 12 hours postpartum, the fundus rises to the level of the umbilicus. On the first postpartum day, the fundus is located about 1 cm below the level of the umbilicus and descends about 1 cm per day until it is in the pelvis on the 10th day. The uterus will reach its prepregnant size by 5 to 6 weeks postpartum. The debris in the uterus is discharged through lochia. Lochia rubra is red and is present for the first 2–3 days postpartum; lochia serosa

POWERPOINT LECTURE SLIDES

(NOTE: The number on each PPT Lecture Slide directly corresponds with the Concepts for Lecture.)

1 Postpartum Uterine Changes (Figure 34.1)
- Decrease in weight 100 g
- Spongy layer of the decidua is sloughed off
- Basal layer differentiates into two layers
  - Outer layer sloughs off
  - Inner layer begins the foundation for the new endometrium
- Placental site heals by exfoliation

1a Postpartum Uterine Changes
- Uterine cells will atrophy
- Uterine debris in the uterus is discharged through lochia
  - Lochia rubra is red (first 2–3 days)
  - Lochia serosa is pink (day 3 to day 10)
  - Lochia alba is white (continues until the cervix is closed)

is pink and is present from day 3 to day 10; lochia alba is white and continues until the cervix is closed.

2. After birth, the cervix is spongy, flabby, and may appear bruised. The external os may have lacerations that occurred during birth, be irregular, and close slowly. The shape of the external os is permanently changed after birth. The dimpled os changes to a lateral slit. After birth, the vagina may be edematous and bruised with small superficial lacerations, and the rugae have been obliterated. The size decreases and rugae reappear within 3–4 weeks. By 6 weeks, it is back to its prepregnant state.

3. The perineum may be edematous, with bruising and lacerations or an episiotomy in the early postpartal period. The woman may experience some discomfort. Menstruation will return at varying times for each woman; however for nonbreastfeeding women, it generally returns between 6 and 10 weeks after birth with 50% of the first cycles being anovulatory. The return is due to increasing levels of serum progesterone.

4. The abdomen will continue to appear loose and flabby but will respond to exercise. The uterine ligaments will gradually return to their prepregnant state. A diastasis recti abdominus, which is a separation of the rectus abdominus muscles, may occur in some pregnancies. This may result in a pendulous abdomen and maternal backache; however, it usually responds to exercise. Striae will take on different colors based on the mother's skin color. In Caucasian mothers, striae fade to silver or white where striae of mothers with darker skin will be darker than the surrounding skin. Under the influence of estrogen and progesterone during pregnancy, breasts will be prepared for lactation. Through the secretion of maternal hormones, milk production is established.

5. After birth, women often experience hunger and thirst. The bowels will be sluggish due to the effects of progesterone, decreased abdominal muscle tone, and bowel evacuation during labor and delivery. The presence of an episiotomy, lacerations, or hemorrhoids may further delay elimination due to the fear of pain.

6. In the postpartum period, the woman has an increased bladder capacity, a swelling and bruising of tissues around the urethra, a decrease in sensitivity to fluid pressure, and a decrease in sensation of bladder filling. This puts the woman at risk for overdistention, incomplete emptying, and a buildup of residual urine. Urinary output is greater in the early postpartal period because of puerperal diuresis as the kidneys must eliminate between 2000–3000 mL of extracellular fluid. Due to dilated ureters and renal pelves, urinary stasis may increase the chances for infection. These structures return to the prepregnant level by 6 weeks after birth. Hematuria may occur resulting from bladder or urethral trauma.

7. The maternal temperature may be elevated to 38C for up to 24 hours after birth because of exertion and

1b See Figure 34.1

2 Postpartum Cervical and Vaginal Changes
- Cervix is spongy, flabby, and may appeared bruised
- External os may have lacerations and is irregular and closes slowly
- Shape of the external os changes to a lateral slit
- Vagina may be edematous, bruised with small superficial lacerations
- Size decreases and rugae reappear within 3–4 weeks
- Returns to prepregnant state by 6 weeks

3 Perineal Changes and Return of Menstruation
- Perineum may be edematous, with bruising
- Lacerations or an episiotomy may be present
- Menstruation generally returns between 6 and 10 weeks (nonbreastfeeding)

4 Postpartum Abdominal and Breast Changes
- Loose and flabby but will respond to exercise
- Uterine ligaments will gradually return to their prepregnant state
- Diastasis recti abdominis (Figure 34.3)
- Striae will take on different colors based on the mother's skin color
- Breasts are ready for lactation

4a See Figure 34.3

5 Postpartum Bowel Changes
- Bowels will be sluggish
- Episiotomy, lacerations, or hemorrhoids may delay elimination

6 Postpartum Bladder Changes
- Increased bladder capacity
- Swelling and bruising of tissues around the urethra
- Decrease in sensitivity to fluid pressure
- Decrease in sensation of bladder filling
- Urinary output is greater due to puerperal diuresis
- Increased chance of infection due to dilated ureters and renal pelves

7 Postpartum Changes in Vital Signs
- Temperature may be elevated to 38C for up to 24 hours after birth
- Temperature may be increased for 24 hours after the milk comes in
- BP rises early and then returns to normal
- Bradycardia occurs during first 6–10 days

8 Postpartum Changes in Lab Values
- Nonpathologic leukocytosis occurs in the early postpartum period
- Blood loss averages 200–500 mL (vaginal), 700–1000 mL (cesarean)
- Plasma levels reach the prepregnant state by 4–6 weeks postpartum

dehydration during labor. The temperature may also be increased for 24 hours after the milk comes in. In the early postpartal period, there is a brief rise in the systolic and diastolic blood pressure, which returns to normal over the first few days. Orthostatic hypotension may develop within the first 48 hours due to abdominal engorgement that occurs after birth. Bradycardia normally occurs during the first 6–10 days postpartum, which may be related to decreased cardiac strain, decreased blood volume, contraction of the uterus, and increased stroke volume.

8. Blood values will normally return to their normal prepregnant state by the end of the postpartal period. In the immediate postpartum period, nonpathologic leukocytosis occurs with white blood cell (WBC) counts up to 25,000 to 30,000/mm³. These values will return to normal at the end of the first postpartum week. Blood loss averages 200–500 mL with a vaginal birth and 700 to 1000 mL with a cesarean birth. Because of changing blood volumes, hemoglobin and hematocrit levels are difficult to interpret. Plasma levels reach the prepregnant state by 4–6 weeks postpartum. Platelet levels will initially decrease due to placental separation and then begin to increase by the third to fourth postpartum day, returning to normal by the sixth postpartum week. The entire hemostatic system reaches the prepregnant state by 3–4 weeks. Initially, maternal hypervolemia occurs because of the expulsion of the placental circulation. This is a protective effect against excess blood loss. Cardiac output will reach normal levels by 6 to 12 weeks. Diuresis in the early postpartum period helps to decrease the extracellular fluid.

9. The most common neurologic symptom in the postpartum woman is headache. Women experience an initial weight loss of 10–12 lbs due to the birth of the infant, placenta, and amniotic fluid. Postpartum diuresis causes an additional loss of 5 lb. Women may return to their prepregnant weight by the 6th to 8th week postpartum if they gained an average of 35 to 30 lb.

- Platelet levels will return to normal by the 6th week
- Diuresis
- Cardiac output returns to normal by 6–12 weeks

 9 Postpartum Weight Changes
- Initial weight loss of 10–12 lb
- Postpartum diuresis causes a loss of 5 lb
- Return to their prepregnant weight by the 6th to 8th week

SUGGESTIONS FOR CLASSROOM ACTIVITIES

Have students develop a teaching plan for a postpartum discharge class to instruct new mothers about the postpartum changes they can expect.

SUGGESTIONS FOR CLINICAL ACTIVITIES

Have students do a postpartum assessment on a woman and note any physical changes that have occurred since delivery.

LEARNING OBJECTIVE 2

Discuss the psychological adjustments that normally occur during the postpartum period.

CONCEPTS FOR LECTURE

1. A new mother enters the "taking-in" phase during the first day or two following birth. She tends to be preoccupied with her own needs and wants to talk about the labor and birth. The "taking-hold" phase occurs by

POWERPOINT LECTURE SLIDES

(NOTE: The number on each PPT Lecture Slide directly corresponds with the Concepts for Lecture.)

1 Maternal Psychological Adjustment (Figure 34.4)

the second or third day after birth when the mother is ready to resume control of her body, her mothering, and her life.

2. The process by which a woman learns mothering behaviors is called maternal role attainment. There are four stages: the anticipatory stage (where she looks to role models), the formal stage (when the child is born and the woman is influenced by the guidance of others), the informal stage (when the mother begins to make her own choices about mothering), and the personal stage (in which the mother is comfortable with her identity as a mother).

3. Postpartum blues is a transient period of depression that sometimes occurs during the first few days postpartum. Women may experience mood swings, anger, weepiness, anorexia, difficulty sleeping, and a feeling of letdown. Causes of postpartum blues may include changing hormones and a lack of a supportive environment.

- "Taking in"
- "Taking hold"

1a See Figure 34.4

2 Maternal Role Attainment
- Anticipatory stage
- Formal stage
- Informal stage
- Personal stage

3 Postpartum Blues
- Transient period of depression; sometimes occurs during the first few days postpartum
  - Mood swings
  - Anger
  - Weepiness
  - Anorexia
  - Difficulty sleeping
  - Feeling of let down

3a Causes of Postpartum Blues
- Changing hormones
- Lack of a supportive environment

SUGGESTIONS FOR CLASSROOM ACTIVITIES

Discuss which observations may indicate that a woman is in one of the stages of maternal role attainment.

SUGGESTIONS FOR CLINICAL ACTIVITIES

Have students assess a postpartum woman and identify the stage of psychological adaptation that she is in.

LEARNING OBJECTIVE 3

Discuss the impact of cultural influence upon the postpartum period.

CONCEPTS FOR LECTURE

1. Many non-Western cultures emphasize the postpartum period over the birth. New mothers and their infants are expected to stay in the home of her husband's family after birth, with only limited visits (primarily from women from her own family). Women of European background may expect to eat a full meal and drink large amounts of iced liquids after the birth based upon the belief that food restores energy and fluids help replace liquids. Islamic women must be completely covered, with only hands and feet exposed, and no man other than her husband or a family member may be alone with her. Women of Hispanic, African, and Asian cultures avoid cold after birth, while traditional Mexican women avoid eating hot foods to restore the hot-cold balance. Often the grandmother plays a primary role in assisting the new mother and her newborn. It is important that the nurse respects the mother's culture and facilitates her wishes.

POWERPOINT LECTURE SLIDES

(NOTE: The number on each PPT Lecture Slide directly corresponds with the Concepts for Lecture.)

1 Cultural Influence in the Postpartum Period
- Non-Western cultures emphasize postpartum period
- Food and liquids after birth
- Hot-cold balance
- Role of grandmother

SUGGESTIONS FOR CLASSROOM ACTIVITIES

Ask students to share any particular cultural issues in their family that may be significant for the postpartum period.

SUGGESTIONS FOR CLINICAL ACTIVITIES

Have students observe cultural behaviors of new mothers on the postpartum unit and discuss their findings.

LEARNING OBJECTIVE 4

Delineate the physiologic and psychosocial components of a normal postpartum assessment.

CONCEPTS FOR LECTURE

1. Principles for completing an assessment of the postpartum woman include: selecting the time that will provide the most accurate data, providing an explanation of the purpose of the assessment, ensuring that the woman is relaxed before starting and performing the procedures as gently as possible, recording and reporting the results clearly, and taking appropriate precautions to prevent exposure to body fluids.

2. Physical assessment should be guided using the acronym BUBBLEHE: breast, uterus, bladder, bowel, lochia, episiotomy/laceration, Homans'/hemorrhoids, and emotional.

3. The breasts are assessed for size and shape, any abnormalities, reddened areas, or engorgement. The presence of breast fullness due to milk presence should be assessed by palpation. Visual inspection of the nipples should be done to assess for cracks, fissures, soreness, or inversion.

4. Prior to assessment of the abdomen, the woman should void. The fundus of the uterus should be palpated and evaluated for position in relation to the umbilicus, the midline of the body, and firmness. If a woman has had a cesarean section, the incision should also be assessed for bleeding, approximation, and signs of infection.

5. The lochia should be assessed for amount, color, and odor. The nurse should also document the presence of any clots. After asking the woman to lie in the Sim's position, the buttocks are lifted to examine the perineum and anus. If the woman has had a laceration or an episiotomy, the wound is assessed for approximation, redness, edema, ecchymosis, and discharge. The nurse should also assess for the presence of hemorrhoids. Level of comfort/discomfort should also be assessed along with the efficacy of any comfort measures that the woman is using.

6. The lower extremities should be assessed for the presence of thrombophlebitis by performing an assessment for a Homan's sign. If a positive Homan's sign is present, the woman's calf should be assessed for redness and warmth and the findings reported to her practitioner. The nurse should assess the adequacy of urinary elimination, bladder distention, and pain during urination. Intestinal elimination should also be assessed as well as maternal concerns regarding bowel movements.

7. The psychological adaptation to motherhood should also be assessed at varying times to determine the mother's progress with this task. Rest should be

POWERPOINT LECTURE SLIDES

(NOTE: The number on each PPT Lecture Slide directly corresponds with the Concepts for Lecture.)

1 Principles of Conducting a Postpartum Assessment
- Selecting the time that will provide the most accurate data
- Providing an explanation of the purpose of the assessment
- Ensuring that the woman is relaxed before starting
- Recording and reporting the results clearly
- Body fluid precautions

2 Postpartum Assessment
- B – Breasts
- U – Uterus
- B – Bowel
- B – Bladder
- L – Lochia
- E – Episiotomy/Lacerations

2a Postpartum Assessment
- H – Homans'/Hemorrhoids
- E – Emotions

3 Breast Assessment
- Size and shape
- Abnormalities, reddened areas, or engorgement
- Presence of breast fullness due to milk presence
- Assess nipples for cracks, fissures, soreness, or inversion

4 Abdominal Assessment
- Position of fundus related to umbilicus (Figure 34.6)
- Position of fundus to midline (Figure 34.2)
- Firmness
- Assess incision for bleeding, approximation, and signs of infection

4a See Figure 34.6

4b See Figure 34.2

5 Assessment of Lochia and Perineum
- Assess lochia for amount, color, and odor
- Presence of any clots
- Wound is assessed for approximation, redness, edema, ecchymosis, and discharge
- Presence of hemorrhoids (Figure 34.8)
- Level of comfort/discomfort
- Efficacy of any comfort measures

encouraged to prevent difficulty with this due to fatigue. The nutritional status of the mother should also be noted. Particular attention should be paid to the nutritional status of women who have had a cesarean birth, assessing for the return of bowel function and tolerance of dietary progression.

5a See Figure 34.8

6 Assessment of Extremities, Bowel, and Bladder
- Homan's sign
- Assess calf for redness and warmth
- Adequacy of urinary elimination
- Bladder distention and pain during urination
- Intestinal elimination
- Maternal concerns regarding bowel movements

7 Assessment of Psychological Adaptation and Nutrition
- Adaptation to motherhood
- Fatigue
- Nutritional status
- Cesarean birth
  - Return of bowel function
  - Tolerance of dietary progression

SUGGESTIONS FOR CLASSROOM ACTIVITIES

Use breast and uterine models to have students practice doing a breast and fundal postpartum assessment.

SUGGESTIONS FOR CLINICAL ACTIVITIES

Have students do a thorough BUBBLEHE assessment and document their findings. Have them identify any variations from normal findings.

LEARNING OBJECTIVE 5

Summarize the physical and developmental tasks that the mother must accomplish during the postpartum period.

CONCEPTS FOR LECTURE

1. In the postpartum period, the woman must gain competence in caregiving and confidence in her role as a parent. Physically, all of the woman's systems must return to their prepregnant state.

POWERPOINT LECTURE SLIDES

(NOTE: The number on each PPT Lecture Slide directly corresponds with the Concepts for Lecture.)

1 Physical and Developmental Tasks
- Gain competence in caregiving
- Confidence in role as parent
- Return of all physical systems to prepregnant state

SUGGESTIONS FOR CLASSROOM ACTIVITIES

Conduct a group discussion on possible issues that may interfere with maternal completion of these tasks.

LEARNING OBJECTIVE 6

Summarize the factors that influence the development of parent-infant attachment.

CONCEPTS FOR LECTURE

1. Factors that may influence the development of parent-infant attachment include: family of origin, relationships, stability of the home environment, communication patterns, and the degree of nurturing the parents received as children.

POWERPOINT LECTURE SLIDES

(NOTE: The number on each PPT Lecture Slide directly corresponds with the Concepts for Lecture.)

1 Factors that Influence Parent-Infant Attachment
- Family of origin
- Relationships
- Stability of the home environment
- Communication patterns
- The degree of nurturing the parents received as children

Have students observe parental attachment of the families they are caring for on the postpartum unit. Ask students to identify any issues that may be interfering with the family's attachment and potential nursing interventions to help them resolve those issues.

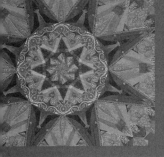

CHAPTER 35
THE POSTPARTAL FAMILY: NEEDS AND CARE

RESOURCE LIBRARY

PRENTICE HALL NURSING MEDIALINK DVD-ROM

Audio Glossary
NCLEX Review
Video: *Through the Eyes of a Nurse—Welcoming the New Arrival at the Postpartal Visit*

COMPANION WEBSITE

Additional NCLEX Review
Case Studies: *Perineal Discomfort; Postpartum Client*
Care Plan Activity: *Postpartal Care Following Cesarean Birth*
Applications: *Perineal Discomfort; Clinical Pathway to Promote Family Wellness; Caring for the Postpartum Adolescent; Discharge Planning*
Critical Thinking

IMAGE LIBRARY

Figure 35.1 Postpartal exercises.
Figure 35.2 The sister of this newborn becomes acquainted with the new family member.

Figure 35.3 The nurse provides discharge instructions to the mother and father before discharge.

LEARNING OBJECTIVE 1

Delineate nursing responsibilities for client teaching during the early postpartal period.

CONCEPTS FOR LECTURE

1. Nursing responsibilities for client teaching in the early postpartal period include assessing educational needs through observation, sensitivity to nonverbal clues, and questions. The nurse should then develop a teaching plan that provides education in a logical, nonthreatening way with respect for family culture, values, and beliefs. After implementing the teaching plan, the nurse must evaluate client learning and revise the teaching plan as needed.

POWERPOINT LECTURE SLIDES

(NOTE: The number on each PPT Lecture Slide directly corresponds with the Concepts for Lecture.)

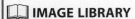 Nursing Responsibilities for Client Teaching
- Assess educational needs
- Develop and implement a teaching plan
- Evaluate client learning
- Revise plan as needed

SUGGESTIONS FOR CLASSROOM ACTIVITIES

Have students develop a teaching plan for a postpartal family.

SUGGESTIONS FOR CLINICAL ACTIVITIES

Have students assess the learning needs of their postpartal client, develop and implement a teaching plan, and evaluate client learning.

LEARNING OBJECTIVE 2

Discuss appropriate nursing interventions to promote maternal comfort and well-being.

CONCEPTS FOR LECTURE

1. In order to assess maternal well-being, the nurse should complete an assessment of the uterus, noting the position in relation to the umbilicus and midline

POWERPOINT LECTURE SLIDES

(NOTE: The number on each PPT Lecture Slide directly corresponds with the Concepts for Lecture.)

1 Uterine Well-Being and Comfort Measures
- Assess uterus

and firmness. Additionally, the lochia should be assessed for color, amount, odor, and the presence of clots. Woman may experience pain due to intermittent uterine contractions as the uterus returns to the prepregnant state. This more commonly occurs in multiparous women. The woman can lie prone with a small pillow under the lower abdomen to help alleviate the discomfort. This applies pressure to the uterus and maintains a constant contraction after which the afterpains will stop. Ambulation and administration of analgesia, including ibuprofen (Motrin), acetaminophen (Tylenol), acetaminophen with codeine (Tylenol #3), or acetaminophen with oxycodone (Percocet) may be effective in reducing pain.

2. After childbirth, women often experience perineal discomfort. Prior to selecting a method, the nurse should assess the perineum and any particular concerns or wishes regarding preferred interventions. It is of primary importance that the woman use good hygiene when caring for the perineum. Perineal care should be done after each elimination to clean the perineum and promote comfort. This can be done using peri-bottles, a Surgigator®, moist antiseptic towelettes, or toilet paper in a blotting motion. Additionally, perineal pads should be changed frequently to prevent infection. An ice pack is helpful if the woman has an episiotomy or laceration to reduce edema and promote comfort. These are used for the first 24 hours and should be applied for 20 minutes at a time, with a 10-minute rest period between applications. Sitz baths may also provide comfort, decrease pain, and increase circulation to the tissues, which promotes healing and reduces the incidence of infection. The woman should soak in the sitz bath for 20 minutes at a time. Topical anesthetics may also be effective for relieving discomfort. These should be applied after a sitz bath or perineal care. They include anesthetic sprays, foams, ointments, or Tucks® pads and may be used to relieve perineal or hemorrhoid pain.

3. New mothers often experience discomfort related to postpartal diaphoresis. The nurse can encourage fluids, frequent showers, and provide dry gowns and linens to promote comfort. Suppression of lactation is important in women who choose not to breastfeed. Engorgement will peak by day 4 and spontaneously resolve by day 10. Comfort measures included minimizing symptoms by having the woman wear a supportive bra as soon as possible after birth, application of cold compresses or cabbage leaves, and anti-inflammatory medications.

4. Administration of the rubella vaccine is important for women who are not rubella-immune. This is administered prior to discharge. Rh-negative women with Rh-positive babies must receive Rh immune globulin (RhoGAM) within 72 hours after childbirth to prevent sensitization.

- Assess lochia
- Afterpains
  - Positioning
  - Ambulation
  - Analgesics

2 Perineal Well-Being and Comfort Measures
- Assess perineum
- Perineal care
- Ice packs
- Surgigator®
- Topical Anesthetics

3 Comfort Measures
- Diaphoresis
- Suppression of lactation
  - Well-fitting bra
  - Cold compresses or cabbage leaves
  - Anti-inflammatory medication

4 Pharmacologic Interventions
- Rubella vaccine
- RhoGAM

5 Emotional Stress Interventions
- Encourage mothers to tell birth stories
- Maternal role attainment

5. New mothers often experience emotional stress due to the physiologic changes that are occurring and her adjustment to her new role as a mother. It is important to encourage mothers to tell their birth stories; this allows them to discuss fears, concerns, and disappointments. Additionally, it is important to help her to understand her strengths and to feel connected. Maternal-infant attachment should be assessed and the nurse must facilitate maternal role attainment through education and positive reinforcement.

SUGGESTIONS FOR CLASSROOM ACTIVITIES

Bring perineal products, a sitz bath, a peri-bottle, and so on to demonstrate use to students.

SUGGESTIONS FOR CLINICAL ACTIVITIES

Have students develop a care plan for a postpartum client and assess client response to nursing interventions.

LEARNING OBJECTIVE 3

Describe the nurse's role in promoting maternal rest and helping the mother to resume gradually an appropriate level of activity.

CONCEPTS FOR LECTURE

1. The nurse's role in promotion of maternal rest is to evaluate individual needs in order to provide opportunities for rest. Limiting family visits and providing a space for rest of the partner may be helpful in accomplishing this. Fatigue affects the physical and psychological adaptations of the mother. Encouraging frequent rest periods helps to facilitate these adaptations. Activity will gradually increase after discharge; however, the new mother should avoid heavy lifting, frequent stair climbing, and strenuous activity during the first few weeks at home. Resumption of full activity can usually occur after 4–5 weeks when the lochia ceases.

POWERPOINT LECTURE SLIDES

(NOTE: The number on each PPT Lecture Slide directly corresponds with the Concepts for Lecture.)

 Rest and Activity
- Provide opportunities for rest
- Encourage frequent rest periods
- Resumption of activity
  - Avoid heavy lifting
  - Avoid frequent stair climbing
  - Avoid strenuous activity

SUGGESTIONS FOR CLASSROOM ACTIVITIES

Have a group discussion to brainstorm ideas to facilitate maternal rest in the hospital and at home.

SUGGESTIONS FOR CLINICAL ACTIVITIES

Have students conduct discharge teaching with their postpartum clients about rest and activity and evaluate client learning.

LEARNING OBJECTIVE 4

Identify client teaching topics for promoting postpartal family wellness.

CONCEPTS FOR LECTURE

1. Family-centered care, which focuses on keeping the mother and baby together as much as the mother desires, is an important component of postpartal family wellness. Family wellness is dependent upon receiving appropriate information, adequate time for interaction with the infant, and a supportive environment. Sibling visitation provides an opportunity to meet the needs of the siblings and the mother through contact with the mother and the new baby.

POWERPOINT LECTURE SLIDES

(NOTE: The number on each PPT Lecture Slide directly corresponds with the Concepts for Lecture.)

 Postpartal Family Wellness
- Family-centered care (Figure 35.3)
- Information
- Time for interaction
- Supportive environment

2. Resumption of sexual activity is advised after episiotomy is healed and lochia has stopped. Couples should be encouraged to express their affection in other ways until this time. Postpartum women may experience vaginal dryness, therefore lubrication may be recommended. Maternal fatigue and infant demands may limit sexual activity. Information about contraception should be provided prior to discharge as sexual activity is usually resumed prior to the postpartal exam. Couples should be educated about their options and implications of the different types of contraception so that they can make an informed choice.

3. In order to facilitate parent-infant attachment, the following nursing interventions should be considered: determine the childbearing and childrearing goals of the family and incorporate them in the plan of care, postpone eye prophylaxis for 1 hour after delivery to facilitate eye contact, provide private time in the first hour after birth for the family to become acquainted, encourage skin-to-skin contact between the baby and the mother/father, encourage the mother to tell her birth story, encourage involvement of the siblings, use anticipatory guidance to prepare parents for potential problems with adjustment, include parents in developing a plan of care, initiate and support measures to minimize fatigue of parents, and help parents identify, understand, and accept feelings related to the birth, the newborn, and parenting.

1a See Figure 35.3

2 Resumption of Sexual Activity
- Resume after episiotomy healed and lochia stopped
- Lubrication may be required
- Contraception
- Potential limiting factors
  - Fatigue
  - Demands of the infant

3 Parent-Infant Attachment
- Incorporate family goals in care plan
- Postpone eye prophylaxis for 1 hour after delivery
- Provide private time for the family to become acquainted
- Encourage skin-to-skin contact
- Encourage mother to tell her birth story

3a Parent-Infant Attachment
- Encourage involvement of the sibling (Figure 35.2)
- Prepare parents for potential problems with adjustment
- Initiate and support measures to minimize fatigue
- Help parents identify, understand, and accept feelings

3b See Figure 35.2

SUGGESTIONS FOR CLINICAL ACTIVITIES

Have students assess family interactions on the postpartum unit and identify strategies to encourage family well-being.

LEARNING OBJECTIVE 5

Compare the nursing needs of a woman who experienced a cesarean birth with the needs of a woman who gave birth vaginally.

CONCEPTS FOR LECTURE

1. Promotion of the well-being of mothers after cesarean birth includes minimizing complications related to the surgery including pulmonary infection, abdominal distention and discomfort, blood clots, deep vein thrombosis, and pulmonary embolus. Deep breathing, incentive spirometry, ambulation, and pain management are effective nursing interventions. Pain may be due to the incision, gas, uterine contractions, or pain from voiding, defecation, or constipation. Frequent rest should also be encouraged. Effective methods of pain management may include epidural analgesia immediately after the surgery and patient-controlled analgesia (PCA). Interventions to minimize gas pains may include leg exercises, abdominal tightening, lying on her left side, and avoiding carbonated or very hot or cold beverages, and the use of straws. Antiflatulents,

POWERPOINT LECTURE SLIDES

(NOTE: The number on each PPT Lecture Slide directly corresponds with the Concepts for Lecture.)

1 Care of the Mother After Cesarean Birth
- Minimize complications
  - Deep breathing and incentive spirometry
  - Ambulation
  - Pain management
- Rest
- Minimize gas pains

1a Pharmacologic Management of Pain
- Epidural analgesia
- PCA

1b Needs After Discharge
- Increased need for rest and sleep
- Incisional care

suppositories, and enemas may also be helpful. Women who have had a cesarean birth have the following particular needs after discharge: increased need for rest and sleep, incisional care, assistance with household chores, infant and self-care, and relief of pain and discomfort.

2. Promotion of parent-infant interaction after cesarean birth may be hindered by the physical condition of the mother and the newborn, maternal reactions to stress, anesthesia, and medications. Newborn safety after birth is a concern because of maternal fatigue and an altered level of consciousness due to medications. These mothers will require constant support and observation when they are with their newborn to ensure maternal and infant safety.

- Assistance with household chores
- Infant and self-care
- Relief of pain and discomfort

 Parent-Infant Attachment
- Factors that hinder attachment
  - Physical condition of the mother and the newborn
  - Maternal reactions to stress
  - Anesthesia
  - Medications
- Newborn safety

SUGGESTIONS FOR CLASSROOM ACTIVITIES

Have students develop a care plan for mothers who have had a cesarean birth.

SUGGESTIONS FOR CLINICAL ACTIVITIES

Have students observe maternal responses to nursing interventions following a cesarean birth and discuss their observations in postconference.

LEARNING OBJECTIVE 6

Summarize the nursing needs of the childbearing adolescent during the postpartal period.

CONCEPTS FOR LECTURE

1. Adolescent mothers may require additional assistance with postpartum hygiene and care due to a lack of knowledge about their own body. The nurse should give clear directions and assess the understanding of the new mother. It is necessary to provide contraceptive counseling prior to discharge to ensure that the teen has a plan in place and knows how to properly use the type of contraceptive she chooses. The nurse should use role modeling to teach the adolescent mother how to care for her newborn, ensuring that the mother has the knowledge and skills to care for her newborn before discharge. The nurse should include the family in teaching to ensure a supportive home environment. Positive feedback is instrumental in developing adolescent confidence and self-esteem. After discharge, special needs may include: child care so that she can attend work or school; assistance with transportation to school, work, and health care appointments; financial support; nonjudgmental emotional support; education regarding newborn care and illness; and education regarding self-care.

POWERPOINT LECTURE SLIDES

(NOTE: The number on each PPT Lecture Slide directly corresponds with the Concepts for Lecture.)

 Nursing Care of the Adolescent
- Postpartum hygiene
- Contraceptive counseling
- Newborn care
- Include family in teaching
- Positive feedback

 Post-Discharge Adolescent Needs
- Child care
- Transportation
- Financial support
- Nonjudgmental emotional support
- Education regarding newborn care and illness
- Education regarding self-care

SUGGESTIONS FOR CLASSROOM ACTIVITIES

Have students bring to class resources for adolescent mothers in the area and compile a comprehensive list for use in a teen pregnancy class.

SUGGESTIONS FOR CLINICAL ACTIVITIES

Have students care for adolescent mothers on the postpartum unit and note differences in client needs when compared with an older mother.

LEARNING OBJECTIVE 7

Describe possible approaches to sensitive, holistic nursing care for the woman who relinquishes her newborn.

CONCEPTS FOR LECTURE

1. Mothers who relinquish their infants for adoption have particular needs in the postpartum period. Nurses who care for these mothers must use active listening, provide nonjudgmental support, show concern and compassion, and personalize care for the mother. Staff should be informed about her decision and special requests should be respected. The woman should be encouraged to express her emotions. The nurse should also provide support to family members. Privacy requests should also be respected. If the intended adoptive parents have an established relationship with the mother and are present for the delivery, the nurse should take cues from the birth mother as to how to provide support for everyone; however, the birth mother is the primary responsibility. Referral for grief counseling may be an important nursing intervention for mothers who view this as a loss.

POWERPOINT LECTURE SLIDES

(NOTE: The number on each PPT Lecture Slide directly corresponds with the Concepts for Lecture.)

1 Care of the Mother Who Relinquishes Her Infant
- Active listening
- Provide nonjudgmental support
- Show concern and compassion
- Personalize care for the mother

SUGGESTIONS FOR CLASSROOM ACTIVITIES

Have a group discussion about personal biases regarding mothers who relinquish their infants.

LEARNING OBJECTIVE 8

Determine the nurse's responsibilities related to early postpartum discharge.

CONCEPTS FOR LECTURE

1. Early postpartum discharge may make discharge teaching difficult for the nurse. However, the nurse should ensure that the following information is included in discharge teaching: signs of possible complications, rest and activity, resumption of sexual activity, referral numbers for questions, contact information about local agencies or support groups, bottle or breastfeeding information, a scheduled postpartal examination visit and newborn well-baby visit, procedure for obtaining the birth certificate, newborn care, and signs and symptoms of infant complications.

POWERPOINT LECTURE SLIDES

(NOTE: The number on each PPT Lecture Slide directly corresponds with the Concepts for Lecture.)

1 Early Discharge
- Signs of possible complications
- Rest and activity
- Resumption of sexual activity
- Referral numbers for questions
- Contact information about local agencies or support groups
- Bottle or breastfeeding information

1a Early Discharge
- A scheduled postpartal and newborn well-baby visit
- Procedure for obtaining the birth certificate
- Newborn care
- Signs and symptoms of infant complications

SUGGESTIONS FOR CLASSROOM ACTIVITIES

Have students develop a teaching plan for early discharge.

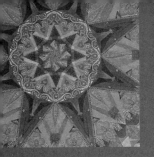

CHAPTER 36
HOME CARE OF THE POSTPARTAL FAMILY

RESOURCE LIBRARY

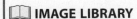 **PRENTICE HALL NURSING MEDIALINK DVD-ROM**

Audio Glossary
NCLEX Review
Video: *Through the Eyes of a Nurse—Welcoming the New Arrival at the Postpartal Visit*

 COMPANION WEBSITE

Additional NCLEX Review
Case Study: *Follow-Up with the Client at Home*
Care Plan Activity: *Breastfeeding Pain*
Applications: *Positioning and Handling the Newborn; Maintaining Lactation after Returning to Work*
Critical Thinking

IMAGE LIBRARY

Figure 36.1 Nurse arriving for a home visit.
Figure 36.2 Various positions for holding an infant.
Figure 36.3 When bathing the newborn, the caregiver must support the head.

Figure 36.4 Infants should be placed on their backs when sleeping.
Figure 36.5 Air-drying the nipples can help prevent cracking and fissures.

LEARNING OBJECTIVE 1

Explain the history of the controversy surrounding length of stay.

CONCEPTS FOR LECTURE

1. In the 1980s, consumers often requested early discharge. In the 1990s, length of stay (LOS) was decreased to only 24 hours after an uncomplicated vaginal delivery to reduce healthcare costs. The safety of this practice was questioned by professional organizations, and in the mid-1990s, Congress responded by enacting the Newborns' and Mothers' Health Protection Act (NMHPA). This act guarantees a minimum stay of up to 48 hours following vaginal birth and 96 hours following an uncomplicated cesarean birth. The American Academy of Pediatrics (AAP) and the American College of Obstetricians and Gynecologists (ACOG) developed LOS guidelines along with follow-up care for mothers and their newborns. This recommends that a home visit or a follow-up telephone call by a healthcare provider be done within 48 hours of discharge of a mother who had a shortened LOS. An examination of the newborn by a healthcare provider is recommended for newborns who are discharged prior to 48 hours of age. The American Nurses Association (ANA) also advocates for a home visit.

POWERPOINT LECTURE SLIDES

(NOTE: The number on each PPT Lecture Slide directly corresponds with the Concepts for Lecture.)

 Controversy over Length of Stay (LOS)
- Consumer request for early discharge (1980s)
- Healthcare payer decreased LOS to 24 hours (1990s)
- NMHPA enacted 1996
- ACOG, AAP, ANA recommend home visit after early discharge

SUGGESTIONS FOR CLASSROOM ACTIVITIES

Discuss the possible ramifications of early discharge for mothers and their newborns and how they can be prevented through home visits.

LEARNING OBJECTIVE 2

Discuss the components of postpartal home care.

CONCEPTS FOR LECTURE

1. Components of a postpartal home care visit include assessment of the mother and her newborn, teaching about care of the newborn and the new mother, and counseling. If the mother is breastfeeding, the progress of the breastfeeding process should be assessed and teaching about breastfeeding should be continued. Opportunities should be given to the new family to ask questions and the nurse should ensure family understanding of the information. Additionally, any necessary referrals for maternal or newborn care should be made at this time.

POWERPOINT LECTURE SLIDES

(NOTE: The number on each PPT Lecture Slide directly corresponds with the Concepts for Lecture.)

1 Components of Postpartal Home Care
- Assessment of mother and her newborn
- Teaching about care of the newborn and mother
- Assessment of breastfeeding and reinforcement of teaching
- Answer family questions
- Make appropriate referrals

SUGGESTIONS FOR CLASSROOM ACTIVITIES

Have students develop a plan of care for a home visit with a new mother and her newborn.

SUGGESTIONS FOR CLINICAL ACTIVITIES

Have students conduct a home visit of a new mother and her newborn with an experienced nurse. Have them discuss their observations of the interactions in the home environment.

LEARNING OBJECTIVE 3

Identify the main purposes of home visits during the postpartum period.

CONCEPTS FOR LECTURE

1. The purpose of postpartal home care includes an opportunity to expand upon and reinforce information about self and infant care techniques that were presented in the hospital. This allows the nurse an opportunity to interact with the family in a more relaxed environment in which the family has control of the setting. The nurse also has the opportunity to assess home safety.

POWERPOINT LECTURE SLIDES

(NOTE: The number on each PPT Lecture Slide directly corresponds with the Concepts for Lecture.)

1 Purpose of Postpartal Home Care (Figure 36.1)
- Expand upon and reinforce information
- Interact with the family in a more relaxed setting
- Family has control of the setting
- Opportunity to assess home safety

1a See Figure 36.1

SUGGESTIONS FOR CLINICAL ACTIVITIES

After completing a home visit with a new mother and her newborn, have students discuss their evaluation of the achievement of the proposed goals of the home visit.

LEARNING OBJECTIVE 4

Summarize actions the nurse should take to ensure personal safety during a home visit.

CONCEPTS FOR LECTURE

1. Safety rules for conducting a home safety include: confirm the address and directions, trace the route to the client's home, provide a daily schedule of visits and contact information to the supervisor, notify the supervisor when leaving for a visit and check in when the visit is completed, carry a cell phone with a charged battery, carry a phone card, make sure the vehicle used

POWERPOINT LECTURE SLIDES

(NOTE: The number on each PPT Lecture Slide directly corresponds with the Concepts for Lecture.)

1 Safety Rules for a Home Visit
- Confirm the address and directions
- Trace the route to the client's home
- Provide a daily schedule of visits and contact information

for visits is in good condition and has enough fuel, wear a name tag and carry identification, carry a flashlight and food and water, avoid wearing expensive jewelry, lock personal belongings in the trunk of the car, call clients when you are on your way to confirm they are home and expecting you, pay attention to the body language of anyone present during the visit, request that threatening or sexually inappropriate behavior stop immediately, be aware of personal body language, leave the home immediately if a weapon is visible and the person refuses to put it away, ask clients to keep threatening pets in a secured area, request that clients and family members avoid the use of illegal substances during the visit, have car keys in your hand prior to returning to the vehicle, and lock doors and drive away upon return to the vehicle.

- Notify the supervisor when leaving for a visit
- Check in when the visit is completed
- Carry a cell phone with a charged battery

 Safety Rules for a Home Visit
- Carry a phone card
- Make sure the vehicle is in good condition and has enough fuel
- Wear a name tag and carry identification
- Carry a flashlight and food and water
- Avoid wearing expensive jewelry
- Lock personal belongings in the trunk of the car

 Safety Rules for a Home Visit
- Call clients when you are on your way
- Pay attention to the body language of anyone present
- Request that threatening or sexually inappropriate behavior stop
- Be aware of personal body language
- Leave the home immediately if a weapon is visible
- Ask clients to keep threatening pets in a secured area

 Safety Rules for a Home Visit
- Request that clients and family members avoid the use of illegal substances
- Have car keys in your hand
- Lock doors and drive away upon return to the vehicle

SUGGESTIONS FOR CLASSROOM ACTIVITIES

Have students role-play scenarios that they might encounter where their personal safety may be compromised during a home visit. Strategize ways to deal with the situations.

LEARNING OBJECTIVE 5

Delineate aspects of fostering a caring relationship in the home.

CONCEPTS FOR LECTURE

1. One of the aspects of nursing care that foster a caring relationship in the home is regard. The nurse should introduce himself/herself to the family and call the members by their surnames unless asked to use a less formal name. The nurse should ask to be introduced to other present family members, use active listening, and maintain objectiveness. A second aspect is genuineness. The nurse should mean what he/she says, and ensure that communication is nonjudgmental and the verbal and nonverbal messages are congruent. Caring behaviors should be demonstrated and questions should be answered honestly. A nurse should develop empathy by listening to the family without judgment and being attentive to what the birth experience means to them. A final aspect is developing trust and rapport. The nurse should do what he/she says he/she will do, be prepared for the visit, and be on time.

POWERPOINT LECTURE SLIDES

(NOTE: The number on each PPT Lecture Slide directly corresponds with the Concepts for Lecture.)

 Fostering a Caring Relationship in the Home
- Regard
- Genuineness
- Empathy
- Trust and Rapport

LEARNING OBJECTIVE 6

Describe assessment, care of the newborn, and reinforcement of parent teaching in the home.

CONCEPTS FOR LECTURE

1. Physical assessment of the newborn at home should include an assessment of vital signs, plus the skin, respiratory, cardiovascular, gastrointestinal, genitourinary, musculoskeletal, and neurologic body systems. An assessment of the infant's behavioral state along with parent-infant interaction should also be assessed. The presence of jaundice, the condition of the umbilical cord and circumcision, reflexes, hydration, nutritional status, feeding history, elimination of urine and stool, sleep-wake cycles, activity, and weight should also be noted. The nurse should ensure that the screening exams have been completed and any required follow-up is scheduled.

2. Assessment and reinforcement of knowledge about the following newborn care issues should also be done: positioning and handling, skin care and bathing, cord care, nail care, dressing the newborn, temperature assessment, fever and illness, stools and urine, sleeping, sleep-wake states, and injury prevention.

POWERPOINT LECTURE SLIDES

(NOTE: The number on each PPT Lecture Slide directly corresponds with the Concepts for Lecture.)

1 Physical Assessment of the Newborn
- Vital signs
- Assessment of systems
- Infant's behavioral state
- Parent-infant interaction
- Presence of jaundice
- Condition of the umbilical cord and circumcision

1a Physical Assessment of the Newborn
- Reflexes and activity
- Hydration, nutritional status, and feeding history
- Elimination of urine and stool
- Sleep-wake cycles
- Weight
- Ensure that the screening exams have been completed

2 Newborn Care
- Positioning and handling
- Skin care and bathing (Figure 36.3)
- Cord and nail care
- Dressing the newborn
- Temperature assessment

2a See Figure 36.3

2b Newborn Care
- Fever and illness
- Stools and urine
- Sleeping, sleep-wake states (Figure 36.4)
- Injury prevention

2c See Figure 36.4

LEARNING OBJECTIVE 7

Discuss maternal and family assessment and anticipated progress after birth.

CONCEPTS FOR LECTURE

1. The initial goal of the postpartum visit is to assess the woman's perceptions of her current home circumstances; her recovery from childbirth; her adjustment, and that of her partner, to parenthood; the newborn's condition; family-newborn bonding; and any concerns of the woman. Specifically, the nurse should assess the progression of lochia; the presence of fever or malaise; the presence of dysuria or difficulty voiding; the presence of pain in the pelvis or perineum; the presence of painful, reddened hot spots or shooting pain in the breasts; and the presence of areas of redness, edema, tenderness, or warmth in the legs. An assessment of the mother's diet, level of fatigue, ability to rest and sleep, pain management, signs of postpartal complications, activity level, sexuality issues, self-care ability, social support system, and any cultural or religious practices related to postpartum or newborn care should be done.

2. An assessment of maternal attachment, adjustment to the parental role, maternal emotions, sibling adjustment, and educational needs should be done. The nurse should provide information about community resources available to the family. Family interaction should be observed if possible and any questions that the family might have should be answered. Concerns or questions regarding family planning should also be addressed.

POWERPOINT LECTURE SLIDES

(NOTE: The number on each PPT Lecture Slide directly corresponds with the Concepts for Lecture.)

1 Assessment of Maternal Perceptions
- Current home circumstances
- Recovery from childbirth
- Mother's adjustment, and that of her partner, to parenthood
- The newborn's condition
- Family-newborn bonding
- Concerns of the woman

1a Physical Assessment of the Mother
- Progression of lochia
- Presence of fever or malaise
- Presence of dysuria or difficulty voiding
- Presence of pain of the pelvis or perineum
- Presence of painful, reddened hot spots or shooting pain in the breasts
- Presence of areas of redness, edema, tenderness, or warmth in the legs

1b Maternal Assessment
- Diet
- Level of fatigue
- Ability to rest and sleep
- Pain management
- Signs of postpartal complications
- Activity level

1c Maternal Assessment
- Sexuality issues
- Self-care ability
- Social support system
- Cultural or religious practices

2 Maternal Assessment
- Maternal attachment
- Adjustment to parental role
- Maternal emotions
- Sibling adjustment
- Educational needs

2a Maternal Assessment
- Provide information about community resources
- Observe family interaction
- Address concerns or questions regarding family planning

SUGGESTIONS FOR CLASSROOM ACTIVITIES

Discuss findings during a maternal exam during a home visit that would require follow-up by the nurse and the appropriate nursing intervention.

SUGGESTIONS FOR CLINICAL ACTIVITIES

Have students conduct a maternal exam during a home visit and document their findings.

4 Behavioral Responses
- Withdrawal
- Dependence
- Fear of being alone
- Memorializing the loss
- Disorientation
- Sleep and appetite disturbances

4a Behavioral Responses
- Absent-minded behavior
- Dreams of the deceased
- Crying and sighing
- Restlessness
- Avoiding of behaviors
- Treasuring of mementos

5 Spiritual Responses
- Blaming God (or spiritual equivalent)
- Hostility toward God (or spiritual equivalent)
- Lack of meaning or direction
- Wishing to join the deceased
- Isolation
- Feelings of betrayal

5a Spiritual Responses
- Hopelessness
- Destruction or strengthening of beliefs
- Feelings of being punished
- Acceptance as "Divine Will"
- Assigning of deceased infant as an "angel" in heaven

SUGGESTIONS FOR CLINICAL ACTIVITIES

Have students observe families in the clinical setting that are experiencing a perinatal loss and identify any of the responses mentioned above. Discuss in postconference.

LEARNING OBJECTIVE 3

Explore the personal and societal issues that may complicate responses to perinatal loss.

CONCEPTS FOR LECTURE

1. Personal issues that may complicate responses to perinatal loss include age, family dynamics, and gender. Age plays a big role in grief responses. For example, couples in their thirties may feel anxiety from the loss because they feel that they are running out of time while couples in their twenties feel that they still have time to have more children. Adolescents are at the greatest risk because although they have a mature concept of death, they have a sense that "it can't happen to me." Mistrust of authority figures may further complicate the care of these women. Family dynamics play a big role in parental responses to grief. Parents with supportive, cohesive families will be able to deal with the grief more effectively than those who have poor

POWERPOINT LECTURE SLIDES

(NOTE: The number on each PPT Lecture Slide directly corresponds with the Concepts for Lecture.)

1 Personal Issues Complicating Grief
- Age
- Family dynamics
- Gender

2 Other Complicating Factors
- Insecurity
- Anxiety or low self-esteem
- Psychiatric history
- Excessive anger and guilt

---

communication, lack trust and cohesiveness, and those that deny that the event even happened. Gender issues also play a role in grief response. Women are primarily "intuitive" grievers. They feel their way through the loss, and rely on emotional and psychosocial support. Men are primarily "instrumental" grievers. They use cognitive skills to deal with the loss and they value acceptance, acknowledgement of their pain, information about the loss, what to expect in the aftermath, and tasks that are connected to the loss. They appreciate problem-solving support.

2. Individuals who are insecure, or who have anxiety or low self-esteem, a psychiatric history, excessive anger and guilt, a physical disability or illness, previous unresolved losses, an inability to express emotion, and concurrent problems of living have additional risks for dealing with their grief.

3. In crisis, spirituality may provide comfort to some while others may question their spirituality because of the crisis. The spiritual needs of parents experiencing a perinatal loss may include honest exchange of information, empathy and presence, continuing bonds, spiritual rites, attachment with others, and grief support.

 Other Complicating Factors
- Physical disability or illness
- Previous unresolved losses
- Inability to express emotion
- Concurrent problems of living

 Spirituality
- Honest exchange of information
- Empathy and presence
- Continuing bonds
- Spiritual rites
- Attachment with others
- Grief support

SUGGESTIONS FOR CLASSROOM ACTIVITIES

Discuss strategies to assist the adolescent with perinatal grief.

LEARNING OBJECTIVE 4

Identify nursing diagnoses and interventions to meet the special needs of parents and their families related to perinatal loss and grief.

CONCEPTS FOR LECTURE

1. The following nursing diagnoses are applicable to meeting the needs of families experiencing a perinatal loss:
   - *Anticipatory Grieving* related to the imminent loss of a child
   - *Powerlessness* related to lack of control in current situational crisis
   - *Compromised Family Coping* related to death of a child/unresolved feelings regarding perinatal loss
   - *Interrupted Family Processes* related to fetal demise
   - *Hopelessness* related to sudden, unexpected fetal loss
   - *Risk for Spiritual Distress* related to intense suffering secondary to unexpected fetal loss

2. Nursing interventions will include preparing the family for the birth and the death, supporting the family in decision making, providing postpartum care, supporting siblings and family members, actualizing the loss, providing discharge care, and making referrals to community services.

POWERPOINT LECTURE SLIDES

(NOTE: The number on each PPT Lecture Slide directly corresponds with the Concepts for Lecture.)

 Nursing Diagnoses
- *Anticipatory Grieving* related to the imminent loss of a child
- *Powerlessness* related to lack of control in current situational crisis
- *Compromised Family Coping* related to death of a child/unresolved feelings regarding perinatal loss
- *Interrupted Family Processes* related to fetal demise
- *Hopelessness* related to sudden, unexpected fetal loss
- *Risk for Spiritual Distress* related to intense suffering secondary to unexpected fetal loss

 Nursing Interventions
- Preparing the family for the birth and the death
- Supporting the family in decision making

POWERPOINT LECTURE SLIDES *continued*

- Providing postpartum care
- Supporting siblings and family members

 2a Nursing Interventions
- Actualizing the loss
- Providing discharge care
- Making referrals to community services

SUGGESTIONS FOR CLASSROOM ACTIVITIES

Have students develop a plan of care for a family experiencing a perinatal loss.

LEARNING OBJECTIVE 5

Differentiate between helpful and nonhelpful responses in caring for families experiencing perinatal loss and grief.

CONCEPTS FOR LECTURE

1. Minimizing the pain of the loss by saying that a couple can try to have another child is not helpful. It is more helpful to acknowledge that the deceased infant is unique and validate the loss. A sentence should never be started with the words "at least" as it diminishes whatever follows. It is helpful to acknowledge the future plans that the couple had for the infant that will never be realized. Statements that attempt to explain the outcome of the pregnancy such as, "It's a blessing in disguise" are incorrect and not helpful. It is better to acknowledge that you do not know why the tragedy happened and offer reassurance that they will not be alone. Nurses should not impose their own belief systems on families. It is better to address their pain and reassure them of the nurse's caring presence.

POWERPOINT LECTURE SLIDES

(NOTE: The number on each PPT Lecture Slide directly corresponds with the Concepts for Lecture.)

1 Nonhelpful Responses
- Minimizing the pain
- "At least ..."
- Offering explanation for loss
- Imposing belief system

1a Helpful Responses
- Acknowledging that the infant is unique
- Validate the loss
- Acknowledge that future plans will not be realized
- Offer reassurance that they are not alone
- Address pain
- Reassure them of the caring presence of nurses

SUGGESTIONS FOR CLASSROOM ACTIVITIES

Have students role-play caring for a family with a perinatal loss. Provide feedback on their communication.

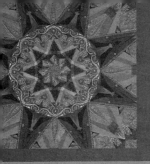

CHAPTER 38
THE POSTPARTAL FAMILY AT RISK

RESOURCE LIBRARY

 PRENTICE HALL NURSING MEDIALINK DVD-ROM

Audio Glossary
NCLEX Review

COMPANION WEBSITE

Additional NCLEX Review
Case Study: *Postpartal Thromboembolic Disease*
Care Plan Activity: *Postpartal Perineal Pain*
Applications: *Postpartum Hemorrhage; Caring for the Client with Mastitis*
Critical Thinking

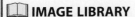 **IMAGE LIBRARY**

Figure 38.1 *A*, Manual compression of the uterus and massage with the abdominal hand usually will effectively control hemorrhage from uterine atony. *B*, Manual removal of placenta.

Figure 38.2 Mastitis.
Figure 38.3 Homans' sign.

LEARNING OBJECTIVE 1

Describe assessment of the woman for predisposing factors, onset, signs, and symptoms of various postpartum complications to facilitate early and effective management of complications.

CONCEPTS FOR LECTURE

1. Assessment of the woman with postpartal hemorrhage includes frequent assessment of fundal height and tone. Monitoring of vaginal bleeding is essential through pad counts or by weighing perineal pads. In the presence of bleeding, women should be monitored for signs of hypovolemic shock and the development of coagulation problems. The nurse should evaluate the woman for signs of anemia, and review the hematocrit.

2. Assessment of the woman with infection should include inspection of the woman's perineum every 8 to 12 hours for signs of infection using the REEDA scale: *r*edness, *e*dema, *e*cchymosis, *d*ischarge, and *a*pproximation. Woman should also be assessed for the following signs of infection: fever, malaise, abdominal pain, foul-smelling lochia, larger than expected uterus, tachycardia, and other signs of infection. A 30% increase in the WBC level in a 6-hour period may be indicative of infection.

3. Nursing assessment of a woman for an overdistended bladder includes assessment of the abdomen for a large mass, which reaches sometimes to the umbilicus and displaces the uterine fundus upward. Additionally, the woman will have increased vaginal bleeding, a boggy fundus, and cramping. Women may also complain of backache and restlessness.

4. A nursing assessment for cystitis should include observation for symptoms which often appear 2 to 3 days after birth. They include frequency, urgency, dysuria, and

POWERPOINT LECTURE SLIDES

(NOTE: The number on each PPT Lecture Slide directly corresponds with the Concepts for Lecture.)

1 Assessment of Postpartum Hemorrhage
- Fundal height and tone
- Vaginal bleeding
- Signs of hypovolemic shock
- Development of coagulation problems
- Signs of anemia

2 Assessment of Infection: REEDA Scale
- R: redness
- E: edema
- E: ecchymosis
- D: discharge
- A: approximation

2a Assessment of Infection
- Fever
- Malaise
- Abdominal pain
- Foul-smelling lochia
- Larger than expected uterus
- Tachycardia

3 Assessment of Overdistention of the Bladder
- Large mass in abdomen
- Increased vaginal bleeding
- Boggy fundus

nocturia. Additionally, hematuria, suprapubic pain, and a slightly elevated temperature may also be present. Progression to pyelonephritis is a possibility so the woman should be observed for systemic symptoms including chills, high fever, flank pain (unilateral or bilateral), nausea, and vomiting. A urine culture and sensitivity specimen should be obtained by the nurse to confirm the diagnosis.

5. Assessment of the woman with mastitis includes a daily assessment of breast consistency, skin color, surface temperature, nipple condition, and presence of pain is essential to detect early signs of problems that may predispose to mastitis. When an infection is present, the woman should be assessed for contributing factors including: cracked nipples, poor hygiene, engorgement, supplemental feedings, change in routine or infant feeding pattern, abrupt weaning, or lack of proper breast support.

6. Assessment of the postpartal woman for thrombosis or thrombophlebitis includes: assessment for Homan's sign; pain in the leg, inguinal area, or lower abdomen; edema; temperature change; or pain with palpation.

7. Assessment of the woman for postpartum psychiatric disorders should begin prenatally. Depression scales such as the Edinburgh Postnatal Depression Scale may be used to screen for postpartum depression. The nurse should observe for signs of depression including anxiety, irritability, poor concentration, forgetfulness, sleeping difficulties, appetite change, fatigue, and tearfulness.

- Cramping
- Backache
- Restlessness

4 Assessment of Cystitis
- Frequency and urgency
- Dysuria
- Nocturia
- Hematuria
- Suprapubic pain
- Slightly elevated temperature

5 Assessment of Mastitis (Figure 38.2)
- Breast consistency
- Skin color
- Surface temperature
- Nipple condition
- Presence of pain

5a See Figure 38.2

6 Assessment of Thrombophlebitis
- Homan's sign (Figure 38.3)
- Pain in the leg, inguinal area, or lower abdomen
- Edema
- Temperature change
- Pain with palpation

6a See Figure 38.3

7 Assessment of Postpartum Psychiatric Disorders
- Depression scales
- Anxiety and irritability
- Poor concentration and forgetfulness
- Sleeping difficulties
- Appetite change
- Fatigue and tearfulness

SUGGESTIONS FOR CLASSROOM ACTIVITIES

Discuss signs and symptoms of postpartum complications and how to incorporate these assessments in normal postpartal care.

SUGGESTIONS FOR CLINICAL ACTIVITIES

Have students care for a new mother with a postpartum complication and identify symptoms of that complication.

LEARNING OBJECTIVE 2

Incorporate preventive measures for various complications of the postpartal period into nursing care of the postpartum woman.

CONCEPTS FOR LECTURE

1. Postpartal hemorrhage may be prevented by adequate prenatal care, good nutrition, avoidance of traumatic procedures, risk assessment, early recognition, and management of complications.

2. Measures to prevent infection include good perineal care, hygiene practices to prevent contamination of the perineum, and thorough handwashing. Sitz baths,

POWERPOINT LECTURE SLIDES

(NOTE: The number on each PPT Lecture Slide directly corresponds with the Concepts for Lecture.)

1 Prevention of Postpartum Hemorrhage
- Adequate prenatal care
- Good nutrition
- Avoidance of traumatic procedures
- Risk assessment

adequate fluid intake, and a diet high in protein and vitamin C may also be helpful in preventing infection.

3. Frequent monitoring of the bladder in the early postpartum period can prevent overdistension of the bladder. The nurse should encourage the mother to void spontaneously and should assist the woman to a normal voiding position. Providing medication for pain may decrease the reflex spasm of the urethra and perineal ice packs will minimize edema.

4. Prevention of a UTI may include good perineal hygiene, good fluid intake, and frequent emptying of the bladder. After intercourse is resumed, the woman should be encouraged to void before and after intercourse. Cotton underwear may also reduce the risk of developing a UTI. The nurse should advise the woman to avoid carbonated beverages, which increase the alkalinity of urine, and to drink juices, which increase the acidity of the urine.

5. Women should be instructed about proper feeding techniques. Women should also be instructed to wear a supportive bra at all times to avoid milk stasis in order to prevent mastitis. Additionally, the mother should use good handwashing. Prompt attention should be given to women who have blocked milk ducts.

6. The nurse should teach the woman to avoid prolonged standing or sitting to prevent thrombophlebitis. She should also be instructed to avoid crossing her legs and take frequent breaks while taking car trips or if she sits for most of the day while she is working.

7. Postpartum psychiatric disorders can be prevented by helping prospective parents understand the lifestyle changes and role demands of parenthood. The nurse should provide realistic information, anticipatory guidance, and dispel myths about the perfect mother or the perfect newborn to prevent postpartum depression. The family of the mother should be made aware of the possibility of postpartum blues in the early days after birth. Mother should be made aware of the symptoms of postpartum depression and should be encouraged to call her healthcare provider if symptoms occur.

- Early recognition and management of complications

2 Prevention of Infection
- Good perineal care
- Hygiene practices to prevent contamination of the perineum
- Thorough handwashing
- Sitz baths
- Adequate fluid intake
- Diet high in protein and vitamin C

3 Prevention of Bladder Overdistension
- Frequent monitoring of the bladder
- Encourage spontaneously voiding
- Assist the woman to a normal voiding position
- Provide medication for pain
- Perineal ice packs

4 Prevention of a UTI
- Good perineal hygiene
- Good fluid intake
- Frequent emptying of the bladder
- Void before and after intercourse
- Cotton underwear
- Increase acidity of the urine

5 Prevention of Mastitis
- Proper feeding techniques
- Supportive bra worn at all times to avoid milk stasis
- Good handwashing
- Prompt attention to blocked milk ducts

6 Prevention of Thrombophlebitis
- Avoid prolonged standing or sitting
- Avoid crossing her legs
- Take frequent breaks while taking car trips

7 Prevention of Postpartum Psychiatric Disorders
- Help parents understand the lifestyle changes and role demands
- Provide realistic information
- Anticipatory guidance
- Dispel myths about the perfect mother or the perfect newborn
- Educate about the possibility of postpartum blues
- Educate about the symptoms of postpartum depression

SUGGESTIONS FOR CLASSROOM ACTIVITIES

Divide students into groups and have them develop a teaching plan for prevention of one of the postpartal complications.

SUGGESTIONS FOR CLINICAL ACTIVITIES

Have students teach clients on the postpartum unit about prevention of these complications prior to discharge.

LEARNING OBJECTIVE 3

List the causes of and appropriate nursing interventions for hemorrhage during the postpartal period.

CONCEPTS FOR LECTURE

1. Postpartum hemorrhage may be caused by uterine atony; lacerations of the genital tract; episiotomy; retained placental fragments; vulvar, vaginal, or subperitoneal hematomas; uterine inversion; uterine rupture; problems of placental implantation; and coagulation disorders.

2. Nursing interventions for postpartum hemorrhage should include uterine massage if a soft, boggy uterus is detected. Clots may be expressed during fundal massage. The nurse should encourage frequent voiding or catheterize the woman if she is unable to void. Vascular access should be initiated in labor and maintained until the uterus is well-contracted. The nurse should review the hemoglobin and hematocrit levels and notify the physician of any abnormalities. Urinary output should be assessed to assess renal perfusion. The woman should be encouraged to rest as much as possible and the nurse should take safety precautions to ensure that the woman does not injure herself due to dizziness or fatigue. The woman may also need assistance in caring for the infant.

POWERPOINT LECTURE SLIDES

(NOTE: The number on each PPT Lecture Slide directly corresponds with the Concepts for Lecture.)

1. Causes of Postpartum Hemorrhage
   - Uterine atony
   - Lacerations of the genital tract
   - Episiotomy
   - Retained placental fragments
   - Vulvar, vaginal, or subperitoneal hematomas

1a. Causes of Postpartum Hemorrhage
   - Uterine inversion
   - Uterine rupture
   - Problems of placental implantation
   - Coagulation disorders

2. Nursing Interventions
   - Uterine massage if a soft, boggy uterus is detected
   - Encourage frequent voiding or catheterize the woman
   - Vascular access
   - Assess abnormalities in hematocrit levels
   - Assess urinary output
   - Encourage rest and take safety precautions

SUGGESTIONS FOR CLASSROOM ACTIVITIES

Bring a fundal model into class and discuss the assessment of the uterus and techniques for uterine massage. Have students practice on the model.

SUGGESTIONS FOR CLINICAL ACTIVITIES

Have students develop a care plan for a woman with postpartum hemorrhage.

LEARNING OBJECTIVE 4

Develop a nursing care plan that reflects knowledge of etiology, pathophysiology, and current clinical management for the woman experiencing postpartal hemorrhage, reproductive tract infection, urinary tract infection, mastitis, thromboembolic disease, or a postpartal psychiatric disorder.

CONCEPTS FOR LECTURE

1. Nursing diagnoses for women with postpartum hemorrhage may include: *Health Seeking Behaviors* related to lack of information about signs of delayed postpartal hemorrhage, and *Fluid Volume Deficit* related to blood loss secondary to uterine atony, lacerations, hematomas, coagulation disorders, or retained placental fragments.

2. Nursing diagnoses for women with a puerperal infection may include: *Risk for Injury* related to the spread of infection, *Pain* related to the presence of infection, *Deficient Knowledge* related to lack of information about condition and its treatment, and *Risk for Altered Parenting* related to delayed parent-infant attachment secondary to woman's pain and other symptoms of infection.

POWERPOINT LECTURE SLIDES

(NOTE: The number on each PPT Lecture Slide directly corresponds with the Concepts for Lecture.)

1. Nursing Diagnoses: Postpartum Hemorrhage
   - *Health-seeking Behaviors* related to lack of information about signs of delayed postpartal hemorrhage
   - *Fluid Volume Deficit* related to blood loss secondary to uterine atony, lacerations, hematomas, coagulation disorders, or retained placental fragments

2. Nursing Diagnoses: Puerperal Infection
   - *Risk for Injury* related to the spread of infection
   - *Pain* related to the presence of infection

3. Nursing diagnoses for a woman with bladder overdistension may include: **Risk for Infection** related to urinary stasis secondary to overdistension, **Urinary Retention** related to decreased bladder sensitivity and normal postpartal diuresis.

4. Nursing diagnoses for a woman with a UTI may include: **Pain** with voiding related to dysuria secondary to infection, and **Health-seeking Behaviors** related to need for information about self-care measures to prevent UTI.

5. Nursing diagnoses for a woman with mastitis may include: **Health-seeking Behaviors** related to lack of information about appropriate breastfeeding practices, and **Ineffective Breastfeeding** related to pain secondary to development of mastitis.

6. Nursing diagnoses for a woman with thromboembolic disease may include **Altered Tissue Perfusion** in **periphery** related to obstructed venous return, **Pain** related to tissue hypoxia and edema secondary to vascular obstruction, **Risk for Altered Parenting** related to decreased maternal-infant interaction secondary to bed rest and intravenous lines, **Altered Family Processes** related to illness of family member, and **Deficient Knowledge** related to self-care after discharge on anticoagulant therapy.

7. Nursing diagnoses for a woman with a psychiatric disorder may include: **Ineffective Individual Coping** related to postpartum depression, **Risk for Altered Parenting** related to postpartal mental illness, and **Risk for Violence** against self (suicide), newborn, and other children related to depression.

- **Deficient Knowledge** related to lack of information about condition and its treatment
- **Risk for Altered Parenting** related to delayed parent-infant attachment secondary to woman's pain and other symptoms of infection

3 Nursing Diagnoses: Bladder Distention
- **Risk for Infection** related to urinary stasis secondary to overdistention
- **Urinary Retention** related to decreased bladder sensitivity and normal postpartal diuresis

4 Nursing Diagnoses: UTI
- **Pain** with voiding related to dysuria secondary to infection
- **Health-seeking Behaviors** related to need for information about self-care measures to prevent UTI

5 Nursing Diagnoses: Mastitis
- **Health-seeking Behaviors** related to lack of information about appropriate breastfeeding practices
- **Ineffective Breastfeeding** related to pain secondary to development of mastitis

6 Nursing Diagnoses: Thromboembolic Disease
- **Pain** related to tissue hypoxia and edema secondary to vascular obstruction
- **Risk for Altered Parenting** related to decreased maternal-infant interaction secondary to bed rest and intravenous lines
- **Altered Family Processes** related to illness of family member
- **Deficient Knowledge** related to self-care after discharge on anticoagulant therapy

7 Nursing Diagnoses: Postpartum Psychiatric Disorder
- **Ineffective Individual Coping** related to postpartum depression
- **Risk for Altered Parenting** related to postpartal mental illness
- **Risk for Violence** against self (suicide), newborn, and other children related to depression

SUGGESTIONS FOR CLASSROOM ACTIVITIES

Have students choose one of the postpartum complications and a corresponding nursing diagnosis and develop a care plan for that diagnosis.

LEARNING OBJECTIVE 5

Evaluate the mother's knowledge of self-care measures, signs of complications to be reported to the primary care provider, and measures to prevent recurrence of complications.

CONCEPTS FOR LECTURE

1. The woman with postpartum hemorrhage should be taught about normal changes in lochia and fundus and signs of abnormal bleeding. Strategies to prevent bleeding should include fundal massage, ways to assess fundal height and consistency, and inspection of the episiotomy and lacerations if present. The woman should be advised to contact her healthcare provider if she has excessive or bright red bleeding, a boggy fundus that does not respond to massage, abnormal clots, leukorrhea, high temperature, or any unusual pelvic or rectal discomfort or backache.

2. A woman with a puerperal infection should be instructed about activity, rest, medications, diet, and signs and symptoms of complications. Completion of antibiotic therapy should also be emphasized.

3. Postpartal women with a UTI should be instructed to continue good perineal hygiene following discharge. She should also be instructed to maintain adequate fluid intake, and to empty her bladder when she feels the urge to void or at least every 2–4 hours while awake.

4. A woman who is breastfeeding and develops mastitis should be made aware of the importance of regular, complete emptying of the breasts, good infant positioning and latch-on, and the principles of supply and demand. If she is taking antibiotics, she should be made aware of the importance of taking the full course. The nurse should tell the woman that all flu-like symptoms should be considered a sign of mastitis and if these symptoms develop, she should notify her healthcare provider.

5. The woman with thromboembolic disease should be instructed about her condition and treatment, the importance of compliance, and safety factors. She should be given contact information for concerns/follow-up. She should be instructed about ways of avoiding circulatory stasis, and precautions while taking anticoagulants.

6. The woman with a psychiatric disorder after childbirth should be instructed about the signs and symptoms of postpartum depression and told to contact her healthcare provider if the symptoms do not go away or if she has any concerns. She should be given contact information for any questions or concerns that she might have.

POWERPOINT LECTURE SLIDES

(NOTE: The number on each PPT Lecture Slide directly corresponds with the Concepts for Lecture.)

1 Self-Care Measures: Postpartum Hemorrhage
- Fundal massage, assessment of fundal height and consistency
- Inspection of the episiotomy and lacerations if present
- Report:
  ○ Excessive or bright red bleeding, abnormal clots
  ○ Boggy fundus that does not respond to massage
  ○ Leukorrhea, high temperature, or any unusual pelvic or rectal discomfort or backache

2 Self-Care Measures: Puerperal Infection
- Activity and rest
- Medications
- Diet
- Signs and symptoms of complications
- Importance of completion of antibiotic therapy

3 Self-Care Measures: UTI
- Good perineal hygiene
- Maintain adequate fluid intake
- Empty bladder when she feels the urge to void or at least every 2–4 hours while awake

4 Self-Care Measures: Mastitis
- Importance of regular, complete emptying of the breasts
- Good infant positioning and latch-on
- Principles of supply and demand
- Importance of taking a full course of antibiotics
- Report flu-like symptoms

5 Self-Care: Thromboembolic Disease
- Condition and treatment
- Importance of compliance and safety factors
- Ways of avoiding circulatory stasis
- Precautions while taking anticoagulants

6 Self-Care: Postpartum Psychiatric Disorders
- Signs and symptoms of postpartum depression
- Contact information for any questions or concerns

SUGGESTIONS FOR CLINICAL ACTIVITIES

Have students teach women on the postpartum unit who have been diagnosed with postpartum complications appropriate self-care techniques prior to discharge. Have them document the woman's response to teaching.

LEARNING OBJECTIVE 6

Identify ways to provide continuity of nursing care for women with postpartum complications in the community setting.

CONCEPTS FOR LECTURE

1. Considerations for caring for a woman with postpartum hemorrhage in the community includes clear explanations given to the family about the woman's condition and need for recovery. Women should be advised to rise slowly to minimize orthostatic hypotension and should be seated while holding the newborn. She should be encouraged to eat foods high in iron. She should be instructed to continue to observe for signs of hemorrhage or infection.

2. The woman with a puerperal infection may need assistance when she is discharged from the hospital and may need a referral for home care services. The family needs instruction about care of the newborn and the mother should be instructed about breast pumping to maintain lactation if she is unable to breastfeed.

3. The home care nurse may be the first to suspect mastitis because it often does not occur until after discharge. The nurse may obtain a sample of milk for culture and sensitivity analysis. If the mother is too ill to breastfeed, the nurse can teach the mother how to pump and help her obtain the appropriate supplies. She should assist her with dealing with feelings about being unable to breastfeed. She should be referred to a lactation consultant or La Leche League for support.

4. The woman with thromboembolic disease will be dependent on others for her initial home care. The nurse should provide instructions to family members. If there are no family members available, and may need to make a referral for home care. The family should be provided with resources for follow-up or questions and concerns. Since thrombophlebitis may not develop until after discharge, all families should be taught to observe for the signs and symptoms.

5. For women with psychiatric disorders, home visits are valuable to foster positive adjustments in the new family. Telephone follow-up should continue after a few weeks to assess the mother's adaptation. A brief assessment of maternal depression can also be done at well-child visits. Families should be taught that the presence of 3 symptoms on one day or one symptom on 3 days may indicate postpartum depression and she should contact a health professional immediately. If the infant is rejected or threatened, immediate referral should also be made. The nurse should assist family members by identifying community resources and making referrals as needed.

POWERPOINT LECTURE SLIDES

(NOTE: The number on each PPT Lecture Slide directly corresponds with the Concepts for Lecture.)

1 Community Based Care: Postpartum Hemorrhage
- Clear explanations about condition and the woman's need for recovery
- Rise slowly to minimize orthostatic hypotension
- Woman should be seated while holding the newborn
- Encourage to eat foods high in iron
- Continue to observe for signs of hemorrhage or infection

2 Community Based Care: Puerperal Infection
- May need assistance when discharged from the hospital
- May need a referral for home care services
- Instruct family on care of the newborn
- Instruct mother about breast pumping to maintain lactation if she is unable to breastfeed

3 Community Based Care: Mastitis
- Home care nurse may be the first to suspect mastitis
- Obtain a sample of milk for culture and sensitivity analysis
- Teach mother how to pump if necessary
- Assist with feelings about being unable to breastfeed
- Referral to lactation consultant or La Leche League

4 Community Based Care: Thromboembolic Disease
- Instruct family members on care of mother and newborn
- Referral for home care if necessary
- Provide resources for follow-up or questions
- Teach all families to observe for signs and symptoms

5 Community Based Care: Postpartum Psychiatric Disorders
- Foster positive adjustments in the new family
- Assessment of maternal depression
- Teach families symptoms of depression
- Give contact information for community resources
- Make referrals as needed

SUGGESTIONS FOR CLINICAL ACTIVITIES

Have students do a home visit with a professional nurse on a family with a postpartum complication. Have them discuss their assessment and the nursing interventions.

1.1 An experienced nurse is working with a new graduate. The experienced nurse suspects that the multiparous client is going to deliver precipitously, while the new graduate is unaware that the labor is proceeding rapidly. One reason for this difference in interpretation of the client situation is because experienced nurses are able to view situations more holistically because they

1. are more aware of subtle cues that indicate client changes.
2. need less supervision in managing complex clinical situations.
3. spend less time providing direct client care.
4. know more about the pathophysiology of diseases.

Answer: 1
Rationale: Experienced nurses have internalized knowledge and judgment that they draw on to understand a situation and the possibilities of the situation. Experienced nurses often provide more direct client care because of their knowledge base, which may include, but is not limited to, the pathophysiology of disease processes. Although expert nurses require less supervision during complex client situations, this does not lead to a holistic view of the client.
Assessment
Safe, Effective Care Environment
Application
Learning Objective 1.1

1.2 Self-care has gained wide acceptance with clients, the healthcare community, and third-party payors due to research findings that suggest that it has

1. shortened newborn length of stay.
2. decreased use of home health agencies.
3. reduced healthcare costs.
4. decreased the number of emergency room visits.

Answer: 3
Rationale: The self-care movement began in the late 1960s, as clients began to see themselves as consumers of health care and assumed responsibility for their health. Because maternal-newborn nursing care is generally health focused, active participation (self-care) is encouraged. Research indicates self-care significantly reduces healthcare costs. Length of stay is often determined by third party payor (insurance company) policies as well as physiologic stability of the mother and newborn. Home healthcare agencies often are involved in client care to decrease hospital stay time. Acute emergencies are addressed by emergency departments, and are not delayed by those practicing self-care.
Planning
Health Promotion and Maintenance
Application
Learning Objective 1.2

1.3 The new graduate is learning about advanced practice nursing. Which of the following situations best illustrates an advanced practice nursing role? (Select all that apply.)

1. an experienced registered nurse who is the manager of a large obstetrical unit
2. a registered nurse who is the circulating nurse at surgical (cesarean) deliveries
3. a clinical nurse specialist who is working as a staff nurse on a mother-baby unit
4. a nurse practitioner who is consulting with a physician in the newborn nursery
5. a nurse-midwife attending vaginal deliveries of uncomplicated pregnancies.

Answer: 4, 5
Rationale: Advanced practice nurses have received additional specialized education beyond registered nursing, and tend to have a clinical focus. Nurse practitioners make clinical judgment and begin treatment, and consult a physician as needed. Management roles are often held by professional nurses. Unit-specific skills such as circulating during cesarean births do not require additional formal education. An advanced practice nurse working as a staff nurse is not working in the role of advanced practice. It is within the scope of practice for Certified Nurse-Midwives to attend deliveries of essentially normal patients with essentially normal pregnancies.
Planning
Health Promotion and Maintenance
Analysis
Learning Objective 1.3

1.4 The nurse at an elementary school is performing TB screenings on all of the students. Permission slips were returned for all children except for the Nguyen children. When the nurse phones to obtain permission, the mother states in clearly understandable English that she is unable to give permission at this time because her grandmother is out of town for two more weeks. Which of the following elements of culture is contributing to the dilemma that faces the nurse?

1. permissible physical contact with strangers
2. belief and understanding about the concepts of health and illness
3. religion and social beliefs
4. presence and influence of the extended family

Answer: 4

Rationale: Many elements of the cultural background of the childbearing family will impact their values. The role of a family elder in healthcare decision making is a common example of the influence of extended family. This is not an example of permissible contact with strangers, nor beliefs and understanding about the concepts of health and illness, nor religion and social beliefs.

Planning
Health Promotion and Maintenance
Application
Learning Objective 1.4

1.5 The insurance company is demanding that a client who is experiencing complications be discharged in two days, because her benefits will run out. The physician and nurses who are involved in this client's care all feel that, because there is no one at home to provide assistance, it is an ethical breach of duty to send this client home when she cannot care for herself. Which of the six components of ethical decision making is the nurse considering when evaluating the driving and restraining forces and assessing the likelihood of a successful outcome?

1. data gathering
2. conflict resolution
3. plan formulation
4. action and implementation

Answer: 2

Rationale: Using an ethical decision-making model helps the nurse to confront conflicts systematically. Data gathering is the first step, and involves determining who is involved in the dilemma, the decision, and the outcome. A plan is formulated to outline all potential options and their consequences. Conflict resolution is accomplished by reviewing driving and restraining forces, assessing risks and benefits, and assessing the likelihood of success of each option. A plan is selected and then implemented after determining who is most impacted by the outcome.

Planning
Safe, Effective Care Environment
Application
Learning Objective 1.5

1.6 The nurse is reviewing care of clients on a mother-baby unit. Which of the following situations should be reported to the supervisor?

1. A 2-day-old infant has breastfed every three hours and voided four times.
2. An infant was placed in the wrong crib after examination by the physician.
3. The client who delivered by cesarean delivery yesterday received oral narcotics.
4. A primiparous client who delivered today is requesting discharge within 24 hours.

Answer: 2

Rationale: Placing an infant in the wrong crib is negligence. Negligence is omitting information or committing an act that a reasonable person would not omit or commit under the same circumstances. Negligence has four elements: a duty to provide care, breach of that duty, injury, and the breach of duty that caused the injury. The other answer choices are normal findings, and not examples of negligence.

Evaluation
Safe, Effective Care Environment
Analysis
Learning Objective 1.5

1.7 The nurse manager is planning a presentation on ethical issues in caring for the childbearing families. Which of the following should the nurse manager include as an example of maternal-fetal conflict?

1. A client chooses an abortion after her fetus is diagnosed with a genetic anomaly.
2. A 39-year-old nulliparous client undergoes therapeutic insemination.
3. A family of a child with leukemia requests cord blood banking at this birth.
4. A cesarean delivery of a breech fetus is court-ordered after the client refuses.

Answer: 4

Rationale: Maternal-fetal conflict is a special ethical situation where the rights of the fetus and the rights of the mother are considered separately. Coercion by court order to undergo operative delivery is one example of a maternal-fetal conflict, which infringes on the autonomy of the mother. Abortion is a different type of ethical situation, as are cord blood banking, and achieving pregnancy through the use of therapeutic insemination as a form of reproductive assistance.

Planning

Safe, Effective Care Environment

Application

Learning Objective 1.6

1.8 The nurse is working at a community clinic. For which of the following clients must the nurse seek parental permission to obtain informed consent?

1. a 16-year-old who is seeking information on contraceptive use
2. an emancipated minor who is requesting treatment for a urinary tract infection
3. a married 17-year-old who is recommended for a planned cesarean birth
4. a 12-year-old with an ectopic (tubal) pregnancy who requires surgery

Answer: 4

Rationale: Depending on state law, minors can seek information and treatment on sexually transmitted infections and contraceptive methods. A 12-year-old who requires surgery is a situation in which parental consent must be obtained. An emancipated minor is a self-supporting adolescent who is not subject to parental control. Married teens are considered legal adults in most states.

Planning

Safe, Effective Care Environment

Analysis

Learning Objective 1.5

1.9 In explaining descriptive statistics to the student nurse, the experienced nurse should include which of the following examples?

1. comparison of maternal mortality rates across racial groups
2. determining why the infant mortality is declining in the United States
3. assessment of maternal nutrition with age and birth weight
4. understanding the behavioral variations within a cultural group

Answer: 1

Rationale: Descriptive statistics summarize data in a concise manner. Birth and mortality rates are two examples of descriptive statistics. Determining cause and effect requires inferential statistics, as does analysis of multiple variables such as race, maternal nutrition, age, and birth weight. The variations within a cultural group are rarely examined statistically.

Planning

Physiologic Integrity

Application

Learning Objective 1.7

1.10 The nurse knows the birth rate by age group in the state. Which research question could be developed for further study from this data?

1. What is the average number of children per family in the United States?
2. How does educational level affect the incidence of unplanned pregnancy?
3. What is the overall nutritional status of adolescents?
4. Which high schools provide day care for student parents?

Answer: 2

Rationale: Research questions often come from a nurse's desire to further understand an issue. How educational level affects the incidence of unplanned pregnancy is a question that flows from the known data of birth rate by age group. Determining the average number of children nationally will not yield additional information about this state, nor will studying the nutritional status of adolescents. Schools that provide student parent day care may indicate the incidence of teen pregnancy in the population served by the school, but not pregnancy rates of those who are not in high school.

Planning

Health Promotion and Maintenance

Analysis

Learning Objective 1.8

1.11 The nurse manager is leading an in-service educational session about evidence-based nursing practice. Which participant statement indicates the need for additional information? "Evidence-based nursing practice

1. incorporates research findings into clinical practice."
2. is unnecessary on a unit with established policies."
3. is supported by current, valid research."
4. is a lifelong learning approach to client care."

Answer: 2
Rationale: An unfortunate reality is that some nurses and units still operate on an "old-school" system, which can lead to conflict between those nurses who seek to practice in a more responsible, evidence-based manner. Evidence-based nursing practice is using only those interventions that are supported by current, valid research evidence, and provides a client-centered approach to problem solving. This self-directed approach involves lifelong learning, building on the actions needed to transform research findings into clinical practice. Evidence-based practice also considers other forms of evidence, such as statistical data and risk management measures when making clinical practice decisions.
Evaluation
Safe, Effective Care Environment
Analysis
Learning Objective 1.9

1.12 State nurse practice acts define the legal scope of nursing practice. How can the policies of an institution or organization such as a hospital influence nursing practice? The institution (Select all that apply.)

1. can restrict nurses from doing some things that are allowed by the state nurse practice act.
2. can permit nurses to do some things that are forbidden by the state practice act.
3. cannot redefine in any way the limits set by the practice act.
4. can either restrict or expand the limits of the practice act.
5. should remain aware of changes or updates as they are enacted.

Answer: 1, 5
Rationale: Hospitals can restrict nurses from doing some things allowed by the state nurse practice act, because the states have the legal right to limit the scope of practice. Nurse practice acts are subject to change and hospitals should keep abreast of the changes and modify policies and procedures accordingly. Hospitals cannot permit nurses to do some things forbidden by the state practice act, nor can they redefine in any way the limits set by the practice act, or restrict or expand the limits of the practice act.
Planning
Safe, Effective Care Environment
Application
Learning Objective 1.5

1.13 The maternity nurse has been named in a negligence malpractice suit. The best defense against the accusation of negligence is if the nurse

1. followed the physician's written orders.
2. met the Association of Women's Health, Obstetric and Neonatal Nurses (AWHONN) standards of practice.
3. is a certified nurse midwife or nurse practitioner.
4. was acting on the advice of the nurse manager.

Answer: 2
Rationale: Meeting the AWHONN standards of practice would cover the maternity nurse against an accusation of malpractice or negligence, because the standards are rigorous and cover all bases of excellent nursing practice. Following the physician's written orders or acting on the advice of the nurse manager are not enough to defend the nurse from accusations, because the orders and/or advice may be wrong or unethical. Being a certified nurse midwife or nurse practitioner does not defend the nurse against these accusations if they do not follow the AWHONN standards of practice.
Assessment
Health Promotion and Maintenance
Application
Learning Objective 1.5

1.14 The nurse is planning care in a labor and delivery unit. Which of the following families is most likely to request cord blood banking?

1. a family with a history of leukemia
2. a family with a history of infertility
3. a family who wishes to select the sex of a future child
4. a family who wishes to avoid a future intrauterine fetal surgery

Answer: 1
Rationale: Families with a history of leukemia might find cord blood banking useful because cord blood, like bone marrow and embryonic tissue, contains regenerative stem cells, which can replace diseased cells in the affected individual. Cord blood banking would not help a family with a history of infertility, or one who wishes to select the sex of a future child or avoid a future intrauterine surgery.
Planning
Physiologic Integrity
Application
Learning Objective 1.6

1.15 A nurse has attended a cesarean birth. Without first consulting the parents the nurse goes to the waiting room and tells family members the sex of a newborn baby. In this situation, the nurse would be considered to have committed

1. a breach of privacy.
2. negligence.
3. malpractice.
4. a breach of ethics.

Answer: 1

Rationale: A breach of privacy would have been committed in this situation, because it violates the right to privacy of this family. The right to privacy is the right of a person to keep his or her person and property free from public scrutiny (even other family members). Negligence and malpractice are punishable legal offenses and are more serious. A breach of ethics does not apply to this situation.

Implementation

Safe, Effective Care Environment

Learning Objective 1.5

CHAPTER 2

2.1 Which examples of a pregnant client's culture may influence her decision making? (Select all that apply.)

1. The client's grandfather makes the family's major healthcare decisions.
2. The client follows the nutrition advice of the certified nurse-midwife.
3. The client's husband comes to a prenatal visit to hear the fetal heartbeat.
4. The client plans to return to work full-time at six weeks postpartum.
5. The client includes specific foods in her diet every day during pregnancy.

Answers: 1, 5

Rationale: Cultural influences on decision making during pregnancy include weighing the opinions of family more heavily over healthcare team member opinions. In many cultures, the oldest male relative (for example, the client's grandfather) holds a great deal of power in the decision making process, even making the healthcare decisions for the extended family. The wisdom of the elders is honored and revered in many cultures, and sought out for advice and assistance in making decisions. Following the nurse-midwife's nutritional counseling is not a cultural issue. The role of the father of the baby during pregnancy, labor, and birth will vary from one culture to another and within cultures. Returning to work at six weeks postpartum is a common practice in the United States, based more on today's economic realities than culture. Eating specific foods each day of pregnancy is a cultural practice that is believed to facilitate the physical and/or emotional development of the fetus.

Assessment

Safe, Effective Care Environment

Application

Learning Objective 2.1

2.2 At 38 weeks' gestation, the client reports to the nurse that she will return to work when her child is 2 weeks old, and her grandmother will care for the infant. This is an example of

1. a developmental task.
2. a spiritual belief.
3. an economic employment trend.
4. a family development stage.

Answer: 3

Rationale: One of the biggest changes in society since the 1950s is the number of families in which both parents work outside the home. When the client's place of employment does not offer paid maternity leave, it is often an economic necessity for the client to return to work early after delivery. Family members often provide child care for each other, which eliminates the cost of day care. A developmental task is a specific task to be achieved in a development stage, the changes and adaptations that a family goes through over time. Spiritual beliefs relate to concerns about the spirit or soul.

Assessment

Health Promotion and Maintenance

Application

Learning Objective 2.2

2.3 The public health nurse is working with a student nurse. The student nurse asks which of the six groups of people seen today are families. How should the nurse respond? "The clients we visited today that are families are the (Select all that apply.)

1. married heterosexual couple without children."
2. gay couple with two adopted children."
3. unmarried heterosexual couple with two biological children."

Answer: 1, 2, 3, 5

Rationale: Families take many forms in today's society. The basis of a family is a commitment to each other, with sharing of responsibilities, chores, and expenses. A couple without children is still a family. A family may be formed without a legal marriage. However, if a couple without children together does not live together, they are considered dating and not yet a family. Gay and lesbian families are increasingly more common, although laws vary from state to state regarding adoption by gay or lesbian parents. Lesbians often seek artificial insemination to achieve pregnancy. Extended family members, including parents or grandparents, will often live with their adult children or grandchildren, creating intergenerational families.

Assessment

Health Promotion and Maintenance

Application

Learning Objective 2.3

4. lesbian couple not living together that have no children"
5. married heterosexual couple with three children, living with grandparents."

2.4 The nurse is preparing a community presentation on family development. Which of the following statements should the nurse include? 1. The youngest child's age determines the family's current stage. 2. A family does not experience overlapping of stages. 3. Family development ends when the youngest child leaves home. 4. The stages describe the family's progression over time.	Answer: 4 Rationale: Family development stages describe the changes and adaptations that a family goes through over time as children are added to the family. The oldest child's age is the marker for which stage the family is in, except for the two last stages, which occur after the children have left home. Families with more than one child may experience multiple stages simultaneously. Assessment Health Promotion and Maintenance Application Learning Objective 2.4
2.5 The family the nurse is caring for in the community has a 2-month-old child. The infant is breastfed, and the father helps care for the child by changing diapers, and dressing and bathing the baby. The mother will be returning to work when the baby is three months old, and a day care provider has been arranged. Although the mother occasionally feels fatigued, the couple has resumed having sexual relations, although not as frequently as before the pregnancy. Which family model best describes this family? 1. Model of the Childbearing Family 2. Model Incorporating the Unattached Young Adult 3. Model of the Nuclear Family 4. Model of the Breastfeeding Mother	Answer: 1 Rationale: The Model of the Childbearing Family describes the transitions that the family undertakes in their home and their lives with the birth of the first child. The nurse's role is to assist the family in identifying possible safety issues, facilitating communication among family members. The Model of Incorporating the Unattached Young Adult encompasses the time from the young adult leaving home and becoming financially independent until marriage. Neither a Model of the Nuclear Family nor a Model of the Breastfeeding Mother exists. Assessment Health Promotion and Maintenance Analysis Learning Objective 2.3
2.6 The pregnant client reports to the nurse that she is eating dirt on a weekly basis, and was told to do this by her grandmother to have a healthy pregnancy. How should the nurse respond? 1. "The soil may contain contaminants that could harm your baby." 2. "This practice is completely unhealthy and should be stopped." 3. "Your grandmother gave you bad advice. Stop at once." 4. "There is no problem with this practice. Feel free to continue."	Answer: 1 Rationale: It is a common practice for African Americans, especially those with familial roots in the South, to eat a specific type of clay dirt during pregnancy. However, the soil may have bacterial, viral, or chemical contaminants, and this practice should be discouraged to prevent maternal or fetal harm. Therapeutic communication must be used at all times with clients, thus the nurse should not tell a client that familial advice or practices are bad. Therapeutic communication requires explaining the rationale for not eating dirt, not just telling the client to stop. Planning Physiologic Integrity Analysis Learning Objective 2.6
2.7 The nurse is performing a cultural assessment using the Transcultural Assessment Model. What aspect of communication should the nurse keep in mind when planning the assessment? 1. Personal space does not vary from one culture to another.	Answer: 4 Rationale: The Transcultural Assessment Model views each client as a culturally unique individual. In planning an assessment using this model, the nurse must remember that the use of silence will differ among groups. Personal space and nonverbal communication will vary from one culture to another. Although the United States norm is a future orientation, not all cultural groups will adhere to this norm.

2. Cultural groups living in America are future-oriented. 3. Nonverbal communication is consistent across cultures. 4. The use of silence may differ among different groups.	Planning Health Promotion and Maintenance Application Learning Objective 2.9
2.8 A family is said to be acculturating to U.S. norms when the parent makes which of the following statements? 1. "The children are much less well-behaved than they used to be." 2. "Our diet now includes hamburgers and French fries." 3. "We celebrate the same holidays that we used to at home." 4. "When the children leave the house, I worry about them."	Answer: 2 Rationale: Acculturation is the process an immigrant or refugee undergoes in adopting the values and beliefs of the new culture. Unfortunately, many health outcomes decrease as a result of acculturation. Inclusion of fast food in the diet is an indication of acculturation, as it indicates a belief in the nutritional value of these foods and an acceptance of purchasing fast food as equivalent in value to home-cooked meals. The holidays that are celebrated may or may not change as a part of acculturation. Concern about behavior of the children is nearly universal, and is not an indicator of a family's acculturation. Assessment Psychosocial Integrity Analysis Learning Objective 2.6
2.9 The nurse is working with an immigrant group in the community that has been in the state for several years. Which of the following findings would indicate that the immigrant group is acculturating? 1. increased rates of cervical cancer screening exams 2. decreased incidence of obesity in adults and children 3. fewer screening mammograms 4. lowered cholesterol levels and insulin resistance	Answer: 1 Rationale: Acculturation is the process an immigrant or refugee undergoes in adopting values and beliefs of the new culture lived in. Health outcomes often change as a result of acculturation of recent immigrants and refugees to the United States, including improved or decreased outcomes. Acculturation also improves some health outcomes, specifically vaccinations and screening tests such as pap smears and mammograms. Nutrition-related issues including obesity, increased cholesterol levels, increased insulin resistance, and poorly balanced diets are among the most commonly encountered issues. Assessment Health Promotion and Maintenance Application Learning Objective 2.6
2.10 The nurse manager in a hospital with a large immigrant population is planning an inservice. The nurse manager is aware of how ethnocentrism affects nursing care. Which statement should the nurse manager include? "The belief that one's own values and beliefs are the only or the best 1. means that newcomers to the United States should adopt U.S. norms and values." 2. can create barriers to communication through misunderstanding." 3. leads to an expectation that all clients will exhibit pain the same way." 4. improves the quality of care provided to culturally diverse clients."	Answer: 2 Rationale: Ethnocentrism is the conviction that one's own values and beliefs either are the only that exist, or they are the best. When the nurse assumes that a client has the same values and beliefs as the nurse, misunderstanding will frequently occur, which in turn may negatively impact nurse-client communication. Expression of pain is one area that varies greatly from one culture to another. Although acculturation involves adoption of some of the majority culture's practices and beliefs, each cultural group will continue to hold and express their own set of values and beliefs. Planning Psychosocial Integrity Application Learning Objective 2.8
2.11 When planning care of childbearing families, the nurse encounters different spiritual and religious beliefs and practices. Which of the following is a spiritual practice that could impact the nurse's care of the childbearing family? 1. a strong belief in reincarnation, and thus refusal of an autopsy	Answer: 1 Rationale: Spirituality relates to issues of the soul or spirit. Many people believe that the body will be reincarnated after death, and that procedures like autopsy and organ donation or transplantation will affect the form of the reincarnated body. Thus the nurse must assess the family's preferences and not assume that an autopsy will be performed. Candles are often used in religious and spiritual ceremonies; however, the nurse's role in an acute care setting is to inform the family that candles are a fire hazard, and the smoke can set off the fire alarm

2. the desire to light candles at home during a naming ceremony
3. request by the family to speak to a Roman Catholic priest
4. refusing consent for a blood transfusion by a Jehovah's Witness

system, and thus may not be able to be used. Roman Catholic and Jehovah's Witness are two formal religions, not spiritual or religious beliefs.
Planning
Psychosocial Integrity
Application
Learning Objective 2.10

2.12 When preparing to teach a group of culturally diverse childbearing families about hospital birthing options, in order to be culturally competent, the nurse should:
1. understand that the family has the same values as the nurse.
2. teach the family how childbearing takes place in the United States.
3. insist that the client answer questions instead of her husband.
4. learn about the cultural groups that are likely to attend the class.

Answer: 4
Rationale: Cultural competence is the development of skills and knowledge necessary to appreciate, understand, and work with individuals from other cultures than the culture of the nurse. Through gaining knowledge of the cultures that are likely to be encountered professionally, the nurse is able to understand the aspects of the client's culture that may impact how care should best be given to be accepted by the client. Assuming that the family has the same values is ethnocentrism. The husband answering questions may be a cultural norm, and insisting that the client answer may decrease the family's trust in the healthcare system. Although it is important to explain health care during pregnancy and childbearing, this is not the top priority.
Planning
Health Promotion and Maintenance
Application
Learning Objective 2.8

2.13 The laboring client is being tended by her mother, older sisters, and aunts. The husband of the client is not at the hospital. The most likely explanation for this, based on an understanding of the client's culture, is
1. the husband is angry at his wife.
2. the client and her husband are not legally married.
3. this is the indirect communication of this culture.
4. labor support is to be provided by adult women, not men.

Answer: 4
Rationale: The people who are appropriate to provide labor support and be present during birth can vary from the husband to only women who have given birth themselves. It is important to not make assumptions about the relationship of the husband and wife, or about communication patterns. Politely inquiring who will be present during the birth will yield the information the nurse needs.
Assessment
Health Promotion and Maintenance
Analysis
Learning Objective 2.7

2.14 The nurse in the community should use a family assessment tool to obtain what type of information?
1. how long the family has lived at their current address
2. what other health insurance the family has had in the past
3. how they meet their nutritional needs and obtain food
4. what eye color they desire in their unborn child

Answer: 3
Rationale: The family assessment tool is used by the community nurse to more fully understand a family through the tool's focus on meeting the needs of the family members; childrearing practices; communication; support and security; growth-producing relationships; community relationships; hopes for children; unity and loyalty of family members; and acceptance of outside help in time of crisis. The length of time at this residence, what health care coverage they have had in the past, and the desired eye color are less important.
Assessment
Health Promotion and Maintenance
Application
Learning Objective 2.5

2.15 The laboring client the nurse is caring for speaks English well, and has identified her race as Asian. She has requested only warm water to drink, and has refused ice chips and cold liquids throughout the labor. The nurse understands that this is most likely related to
1. the client's belief in the role of hot and cold in health.
2. the fact that the client has not yet become thirsty.

Answer: 1
Rationale: Humeral theory, or hot-cold theory, includes prescriptions on foods that possess either hot or cold properties, as well as the optimal temperature for foods, beverages, and the environment. Humeral theory is commonly practiced by Asian and Latin American cultures. The labor process involves muscle activity, and therefore thirst will occur. Control of the environment would likely include such aspects of the room as sound and lighting. Folk beliefs regarding a desired gender usually center on conception, not labor.
Assessment
Physiologic Integrity
Application
Learning Objective 2.7

---

3. a desire to have complete control of the environment.
4. folklore concerning the desired sex of the unborn child.

CHAPTER 3

3.1 The client states "I am using homeopathic remedies to help with my morning sickness." The nurse understands that the client is utilizing
1. a complementary therapy.
2. an alternative therapy.
3. traditional Chinese medicine.
4. naturopathy.

Answer: 1
Rationale: A complementary therapy is that which is an adjunct to traditional medical treatment, and has been shown through rigorous scientific testing to be reliable. Alternative therapies are those that have not undergone rigorous scientific testing. Traditional Chinese medicine includes acupuncture and herbology. Naturopathy is an eclectic combination of nutrition, botanical medicine, homeopathy, acupuncture, hydrotherapy, and physiotherapy.
Assessment
Physiologic Integrity
Analysis
Learning Objective 3.1

3.2 Complementary and alternative therapies are becoming more commonly used in the United States. Based on an understanding of how clients learn about these therapies, which client is most likely to use either a complementary or an alternative therapy?
1. an elderly couple on a fixed income without a computer at home
2. a middle-aged woman who travels internationally for her job
3. an adolescent male who plays many sports through school
4. a young mother of three preschoolers who works part-time

Answer: 2
Rationale: Increased awareness of the limitations and drawbacks of traditional medicine, increased international travel, increased media attention, and advent of the internet are the greatest factors that contribute to the rise in the use of complementary and alternative therapies. Participation in sports would not directly increase knowledge or use of complementary or alternative therapies, although many sports trainers are incorporating them into their repertoire. Neither the age of one's children nor working part-time are predictive of the use of complementary or alternative therapies.
Planning
Physiologic Integrity
Analysis
Learning Objective 3.2

3.3 The National Center for Complementary and Alternative Medicine (NCCAM) is responsible for
1. ensuring the safety of complementary and alternative therapies.
2. endorsing products for further approval by the FDA.
3. performing testing on new therapies and products.
4. disseminating information to consumers.

Answer: 4
Rationale: The NCCAM was mandated by Congress in 1998 to promote research into complementary and alternative therapies, and to disseminate those research findings to consumers. The research that NCCAM sponsors looks for evidence of both safety and efficacy of complementary and alternative therapies, not to disseminate consumer information. Most complementary and alternative therapies are not regulated by the FDA.
Assessment
Physiologic Integrity
Application
Learning Objective 3.3

3.4 The nurse is planning a community education program on the role of complementary and alternative therapies during pregnancy. Which statement should the nurse include? "Alternative and complementary therapies
1. bring about cures for illnesses and diseases."
2. are invasive but effective for achieving health."
3. emphasize prevention and wellness."
4. prevent pregnancy complications."

Answer: 3
Rationale: Complementary and alternative therapies have many benefits during pregnancy. The use of these therapies emphasizes prevention and wellness, aiming for holistic health rather than cure or treatment. They are noninvasive. No method of treatment can prevent all pregnancy complications.
Planning
Physiologic Integrity
Application
Learning Objective 3.4

3.5 The pregnant client asks the nurse about the safety and risks of using complementary and alternative therapies. How should the nurse respond? "The use of complementary and alternative therapies is

1. completely safe and therefore not a problem during pregnancy."
2. not regulated by the FDA and little has been proven about some methods."
3. very inexpensive and can easily be tried to see if they help your health."
4. safe as long as you see a certified and registered practitioner of the therapy."

Answer: 2
Rationale: Some complementary and alternative therapies (such as homeopathy) are FDA approved, but not all are regulated by the FDA. Similarly, some states and municipalities require the practitioner of complementary and alternative therapies to be certified, but not all require formal training, testing, and certification. Research into many of the therapies is lacking and unscientific, with claims of health based on "testimonials" of clients who have benefited from the therapy. Some therapies are known to be unsafe during pregnancy. As an example, the herbs blue and black cohosh are contraindicated during pregnancy due to the potential for spontaneous abortion or preterm labor. Unfortunately, most health insurance plans do not cover the use of complementary and alternative therapies, and thus the cost can be quite high for the client.
Implementation
Physiologic Integrity
Application
Learning Objective 3.5

3.6 The nurse is teaching a community education class on complementary and alternative therapies. To assess learning, the nurse asks this question about traditional Chinese medicine: "What is the invisible flow of energy in the body that maintains health and assures physiologic functioning?" Which answer indicates teaching was successful?
1. Meridians
2. Chi
3. Yin
4. Yang

Answer: 2
Rationale: Chi is the energy that flows through the body along meridians, or pathways, to maintain health; a blockage of chi can result in illness or pain. Yin and yang are opposites: yin is the female force, passive, cool, wet, and close to the earth; while yang is the masculine force: Aggressive, hot, dry, and celestial. Yin and yang cannot exist independently because they are complementary and both are essential.
Evaluation
Physiologic Integrity
Application
Learning Objective 3.6

3.7 The client reports to the nurse that she is utilizing Ayurvedic medicine. Which statements would the nurse expect this client to make? "Ayurvedic medicine (Select all that apply.)
1. is knowledge of how to live a vital, healthful life."
2. combines heat and cold with spinal manipulation."
3. uses both traditional means with current modern medicine."
4. cures an illness with a like substance."
5. seeks balance to achieve harmony in my life."

Answer: 1, 5
Rationale: Aryurveda is knowledge of how to live a vital, healthful life. The five elements (ether, wind, fire, water, and earth) take form in the body as three tendencies, called *doshas*: vata, pitta, and kapha. The ayurvedic physician seeks to balance the doshas to achieve harmony and holism. Spinal manipulation is chiropractic treatment. Like cures like is the basis for homeopathy. Naturopathy combines traditional treatment and prevention with the most current advances in modern medicine.
Assessment
Physiologic Integrity
Application
Learning Objective 3.6

3.8 The nurse is seeing clients at the wellness clinic. Which client is most likely to be using a form of chromotherapy?
1. a baby with spina bifida
2. a client with cancer
3. a client with severe burns
4. a client with a seasonal mood disorder

Answer: 4
Rationale: Chromotherapy is the use of color to treat a condition. When sunlight is decreased during winter months, some people develop a seasonal mood disorder. The use of a light box can replace sunlight, improving mood. Spina bifida, cancer, and burns are not treated with chromotherapy.
Assessment
Psychosocial Integrity
Application
Learning Objective 3.12

3.9 The nurse is teaching a class to the community on mind-body therapies. A class participant gives an example of a friend with leukemia who was taught by her complementary therapist to

Answer: 1
Rationale: Guided imagery involves picturing a desired outcome, such as making antibodies to fight cancer cells. Qigong involves the use of breathing, meditation, self-massage, and movement. Biofeedback is learning to control physiologic

concentrate on making antibodies that will fight and kill the cancer cells in the blood stream. The nurse would describe this technique as
1. guided imagery.
2. qigong.
3. biofeedback.
4. homeopathy.

responses to stimuli or thoughts. Homeopathy is not a mind-body therapy, but uses the concept of like curing like.
Assessment
Physiologic Integrity
Analysis
Learning Objective 3.7

3.10 The client reports using an alternative therapy that involves the manipulation of soft tissues. This therapy has reduced the client's stress, diminished pain, and increased circulation. This therapy is most likely
1. guided imagery.
2. homeopathy.
3. massage therapy.
4. reflexology.

Answer: 3
Rationale: Massage therapy involves the manipulation of soft tissues. Guided imagery involves picturing a desired outcome. Reflexology is the application of pressure to designated points or reflexes on the client's feet, hands, or ears using the thumb and fingers. Homeopathy uses the concept of like curing like.
Assessment
Physiologic Integrity
Application
Learning Objective 3.8

3.11 The client asks why she should not use a sauna or sweat bath in the first trimester of pregnancy. The best explanation by the nurse is that saunas and sweat baths have been associated with fetal
1. craniofacial defects.
2. neural tube defects.
3. gastroschisis.
4. patent ductus arteriosus.

Answer: 2
Rationale: High temperatures in the first trimester have been associated with neural tube defects, thus saunas and sweat baths should be avoided. Saunas and sweat baths are not associated with craniofacial defects, gastroschisis, or patent ductus arteriosus.
Implementation
Health Promotion and Integrity
Application
Learning Objective 3.9

3.12 The client reports relief from headaches when she rubs the temples on each side of the head. The nurse understands that this is a form of
1. acupressure.
2. acupuncture.
3. the Feldenkrais method.
4. the Alexander technique.

Answer: 1
Rationale: Acupressure uses pressure from the fingers and thumbs to stimulate pressure points to relieve symptoms. Acupuncture uses six to twelve very fine stainless steel needles placed to stimulate specific points depending on the client's medical assessment and condition. The Feldenkrais method uses verbal instruction and hands-on assistance to help clients become aware of their movements and to develop alternate ways of moving. The Alexander technique focuses on movement to achieve proper alignment of the head, neck, and trunk.
Assessment
Physiologic Integrity
Analysis
Learning Objective 3.10

3.13 The nurse is reviewing charts. A client seen in the clinic yesterday reported seeing a practitioner that placed his hands above a painful abdomen in order to transfer energy. This resulted in a decrease in pain simultaneously with an improved overall sense of well-being. The nurse understands this therapy to be:
1. Reiki.
2. Therapeutic touch.
3. Homeopathy.
4. Chiropractic.

Answer: 1
Rationale: Reiki practitioners place their hands on or above specific problem areas and transfer energy from themselves to their clients to restore the balance of the client's energy fields. Therapeutic touch practitioners balance the energy flow of clients. Homeopathy is giving a substance to a client based on the concept of like healing like. Chiropractic treatments involve manipulation of the spine.
Evaluation
Physiologic Integrity
Analysis
Learning Objective 3.11

3.14 The nurse is preparing a class on complementary and alternative medicine (CAM). One fact that could be included in this presentation is

Answer: 2
Rationale: Thirty-six percent of Americans use CAM, but when prayer regarding health and megavitamin therapy is included in the definition, the number increases to 62%. Women and people of higher educational levels are most likely to use CAM.

---

1. men are more likely to use CAM than women.	Planning
2. 36% of Americans use some form of CAM.	Physiologic Integrity
3. people of lower educational levels use more CAM.	Application
4. prayer and megavitamin therapy are not considered CAM	Learning Objective 3.12

3.15 The pregnant client has brought an herbal remedy to the clinic to learn about the safety of the remedy. The nurse should include which statements about herbal therapies? "Herbal remedies (Select all that apply.) 1. are subject to FDA approval." 2. are used to eliminate certain diseases." 3. cannot be sold over the counter." 4. are different from homeopathic remedies." 5. are not subject to safety and effectiveness testing."	Answer: 4, 5 Rationale: Homeopathic remedies are not the same as herbal remedies, and are FDA approved. Much of the information on effectiveness is based on hearsay, not scientific studies. Although herbal therapies have been used since ancient times, they are not subject to Food and Drug Administration (FDA) premarket testing for safety and effectiveness. Herbal therapies are sold over the counter. Planning Physiologic Integrity Application Learning Objective 3.9

CHAPTER 4

4.1 A client asks her nurse "Is it okay for me to take a tub bath during the heavy part of my menstruation?" The best response by the nurse is 1. "tub baths are contraindicated during menstruation." 2. "you should shower and douche daily instead." 3. "either a bath or a shower is fine at that time." 4. "you should bathe and use a feminine deodorant spray during menstruation."	Answer: 3 Rationale: Bathing, whether it is a tub bath or shower, is as important (if not more so) during menses as at any other time. Douching and feminine deodorant sprays are unnecessary, and may cause irritation or increase the incidence of vaginal infections. Implementation Health Promotion and Maintenance Application Learning Objective 4.2

4.2 An adolescent client is asking the nurse about using tampons during heavy menstrual flow. Which answer is best for the nurse to provide? 1. Tampons should be avoided when the menstrual flow is heavy. 2. Super tampons with added deodorants are recommended for the day, while regular tampons may be worn at night. 3. Tampons should be used during the day; change to napkins at night when flow is lighter to decrease the risk of toxic shock syndrome. 4. Tampons are recommended for use at the end of the menstrual period rather than at the beginning.	Answer: 3 Rationale: The use of super absorbent tampons has been linked to toxic shock syndrome. Women should be taught to change either their pad or tampon every three to six hours while awake to decrease this risk. Tampons and pads with deodorant can cause vulvar or vaginal irritation, and should be avoided. Implementation Health Promotion and Maintenance Application Learning Objective 4.2

4.3 The nurse is beginning to take a sexual history from the client. List the answer choices in chronological order of how the nurse should proceed. Your answer should be a four digit number.

1. Ask specific questions about the client's current sexual practices.
2. Ask the client mostly open-ended questions.
3. Have the client fill out a comprehensive questionnaire.
4. Explain that the history is obtained from all clients and will be confidential.

Answer: 4321
Rationale: Introducing the sexual history as a confidential aspect of the client health record, and explaining that it is obtained from all clients will allay fears the client may have about why the information is being obtained. Having the client fill out a questionnaire is helpful prior to the interview. Open-ended questions are the most therapeutic and useful in eliciting information. The sexual history interview should proceed from general questions to more specific and personal questions.
Assessment
Health Promotion and Maintenance
Application
Learning Objective 4.1

4.4 The nurse has successfully completed a client's sexual and gynecologic history. Which of the following questions is the nurse most likely to have included?

1. When was the last time you had intercourse?
2. Have you ever had any type of surgery?
3. Have you had any elective abortions?
4. Have you had a sexually-transmitted infection?

Answer: 2
Rationale: To facilitate a therapeutic relationship and successfully obtain the needed information, the sexual history should begin with less intimate information and work toward more intimate information. Asking about surgery is the least intimate question listed. Asking about intercourse, abortions, and sexually-transmitted diseases are more intimate.
Implementation
Psychosocial Integrity
Analysis
Learning Objective 4.1

4.5 A 19-year-old woman comes to the gynecologist's office. When the nurse asks the reason for this visit, the woman explains that she has never had a menstrual period and that she is concerned there may be something wrong. The diagnosis that the physician is most likely to make based on this information is:

1. primary dysmenorrhea.
2. secondary infertility.
3. primary amenorrhea.
4. secondary amenorrhea.

Answer: 3
Rationale: Primary amenorrhea is the term for never having had a mense while secondary amenorrhea develops after menses have occurred. Primary dysmenorrhea is when menses have always been painful, and secondary dysmenorrhea means menses later became painful.
Assessment
Health Promotion and Maintenance
Application
Learning Objective 4.3

4.6 The nurse is interviewing an adolescent client. The client reports a weight loss of 50 pounds over the last four months, and reports running at least five miles per day. The client asserts that her menarche was five years ago. Her menses are usually every 28 days, but her last menstrual period was four months ago. The client denies any sexual activity. Which of the following statements is best for the nurse to make?

1. "Your lack of menses may be related to your rapid weight loss."
2. "It is common and normal for runners to stop having any menses."
3. "Increase your intake of iron-rich foods to reestablish menses."
4. "Adolescents rarely have regular menses, even if they used to be regular."

Answer: 1
Rationale: Secondary amenorrhea can be caused by rapid weight loss, including the development of the eating disorders anorexia and bulimia. Runners with low body fat may have irregular menses, but amenorrhea is not a normal condition. Iron deficiency does not impact menstrual regularity. Although the first year or two after menarche may be characterized by irregular menses, once menses are established and regular, the lack of menses is secondary amenorrhea.
Implementation
Health Promotion and Maintenance
Analysis
Learning Objective 4.3

4.7 A client comes to the clinic complaining of severe menstrual cramps. She has never been pregnant, has been diagnosed with ovarian cysts, and has had an intrauterine device (IUD) for two years. The most likely cause for the client's complaint is

1. primary dysmenorrhea.
2. secondary dysmenorrhea.
3. menorrhagia.
4. hypermenorrhea.

Answer: 2
Rationale: Secondary dysmenorrhea is associated with pathology of the reproductive tract, and usually appears after menstruation has been established. Conditions that most frequently cause secondary dysmenorrhea include ovarian cysts and the presence of an intrauterine device. Primary dysmenorrhea is defined as cramps without underlying disease. Menorrhagia is excessive, profuse flow. Hypermenorrhea is an abnormally long menstrual flow.
Assessment
Health Promotion and Maintenance
Analysis
Learning Objective 4.4

4.8 A teaching plan for a client with premenstrual syndrome (PMS) should include a recommendation to restrict her intake of

1. high-starch foods such as potatoes and spaghetti.
2. chicken, eggs, and fish.
3. whole grain breads and cereals, and beans.
4. coffee, colas, and chocolate cake.

Answer: 4
Rationale: A client with PMS is advised to restrict her intake caffeine, as contained in foods such as chocolate, cola, and coffee. She should increase her intake of complex carbohydrates and proteins.
Planning
Health Promotion and Maintenance
Application
Learning Objective 4.4

4.9 A 49-year-old client comes to the clinic with complaints of severe perimenopausal symptoms including hot flashes, night sweats, urinary urgency, and vaginal dryness. The physician has prescribed a combination hormone replacement therapy of estrogen and progestin. When the client asks the nurse why she must take both hormones, the best reply is

1. "Hot flashes respond better when replacement includes both hormones."
2. "You are having very severe symptoms, so you need more hormones replaced."
3. "There is an increased risk of tissue abnormality inside the uterus if only one is given."
4. "Your blood pressure may become elevated if only one hormone is used."

Answer: 3
Rationale: Uterine endometrial cancer risks increase if only estrogen therapy is given to menopausal women with an intact uterus. Estrogen, not progestin, improves hot flashes and most other perimenopausal symptoms. The severity of symptoms will be considered by the physician in determining the appropriate dose for the client. Estrogen therapy does not cause hypertension.
Implementation
Physiologic Integrity
Analysis
Learning Objective 4.5

4.10 The nurse is answering the perimenopausal client's questions about hormone replacement therapy. Which client statement indicates a need for additional teaching? "The Women's Health Initiative of 2002 reported that long-term hormone replacement therapy caused decreased

1. hip fractures."
2. risk of heart attack."
3. risk of gallbladder disease."
4. risk of blood clots to the lungs."

Answer: 1
Rationale: The development of osteoporosis can be prevented or delayed when postmenopausal women take estrogen therapy. Estrogen therapy was shown to increase the risk of heart attack, stroke, gallbladder disease, and emboli of the legs when taken for more than four years.
Evaluation
Physiologic Integrity
Analysis
Learning Objective 4.5

4.11 Rank the following clients in order from highest to lowest risk for developing osteoporosis. Your answer should be a four-digit number.

Answer: 3124
Rationale: Smoking, thin build, non-white race, high caffeine intake, post-menopause, family history, and female gender are risk factors for developing

---

1. small-boned, underweight 40-year-old woman 2. overweight 55-year-old with type II diabetes 3. 60-year-old African American woman who smokes 4. 75-year-old male who plays tennis three times per week	osteoporosis. Diabetes does not increase the risk of osteoporosis. Weight-bearing exercise helps maintain bone density. Assessment Health Promotion and Maintenance Analysis Learning Objective 4.6
4.12 The client is given a prescription for hormone replacement therapy (HRT). She asks the nurse, "What type of side effects or consequences should I expect from taking this medicine?" The nurse's best response would be "You may 1. notice chest pains initially that will subside." 2. experience irregular, heavy menstrual bleeding." 3. notice some intermittent abdominal cramping." 4. have a decrease in vaginal dryness."	Answer: 4 Rationale: The client's symptoms such as hot flashes and vaginal dryness should improve when HRT is started. Hormone replacement therapy (HRT) increases the risk of myocardial infarction, therefore clients should be taught to report the onset of chest pain immediately. Irregular heavy bleeding can be a symptom of uterine cancer. No abdominal cramping occurs with HRT. Implementation Physiologic Integrity Application Learning Objective 4.7
4.13 A menopausal woman tells her nurse that she experiences discomfort from vaginal dryness during sexual intercourse and asks, "What should I use as a lubricant?" The nurse should recommend 1. petroleum jelly. 2. a water-soluble lubricant. 3. body cream or body lotion. 4. less frequent intercourse.	Answer: 2 Rationale: A water-soluble jelly should be used. Petroleum jelly, body creams, and body lotions are not water-soluble. Less frequent intercourse is an inappropriate response. Planning Health Promotion and Maintenance Application Learning Objective 4.7
4.14 The client is experiencing symptoms of menopause, and states that she would prefer to use herbs rather than medication. Which statement indicates that no further teaching is indicated? 1. "Black cohosh will reduce the frequency of my hot flashes and mood swings." 2. "Studies have shown significant improvement of menopausal symptoms." 3. "Soy protein may be helpful, but should not be taken over a long time period." 4. "Dong quai decreases hot flashes, and does not interfere with medications."	Answer: 3 Rationale: Long term use of soy protein may thicken the uterine lining, which precedes the development of uterine cancer. No studies on botanicals have shown significant improvement of symptoms of menopause. Dong quai will increase the activity of warfarin (Coumadin), leading to bleeding problems. Evaluation Physiologic Integrity Analysis Learning Objective 4.7
4.15 The nurse is conducting health screening at a community clinic. The client has asked if there are any risks with body piercing and tattooing, or if these activities would impact sexual activity. How should the nurse respond? 1. "You should avoid piercing your genitalia and your nipples." 2. "There are no problems that occur with either body piercing or tattooing."	Answer: 3 Rationale: Body piercing and tattooing involve puncturing the skin, creating a possible entry point of bacteria that can cause infection of the site. If the ink, needles, or other equipment have not been sterilized between use, hepatitis B and C can be spread from one client to another. Genitalia and nipple piercing may cause problems during childbearing and breastfeeding, but the practice is undertaken by some people. The physiologic risk of infection outweighs the psychologic benefit of beautification. Implementation Physiologic Integrity

3. "Both piercing and tattooing carry risks of infection, including hepatitis."
4. "The benefit of body art outweighs any risk of infection of a tattoo or piercing."

Application
Learning Objective 4.1

CHAPTER 5

5.1 The nurse is discussing the use of contraception with a client. Which factors should the nurse include when educating the client on contraceptive methods? (Select all that apply.)
1. contraindications in the client's health history
2. religious or moral beliefs
3. partner's belief in the effectiveness of the choice
4. personal motivation to use method
5. future pregnancy plans

Answer: 1, 2, 4, 5
Rationale: Decisions about contraception should take into consideration any contraindications to the client's health. For example, women over the age of 35 who smoke should not take oral contraceptives. Religious or moral beliefs often impact which choices are acceptable. Personal motivation also needs to be considered. Plans for future pregnancy contradict sterilization as an alternative. The cost, and therefore ability, to obtain the method reliably will impact the actual use of the method. The partner's belief in the effectiveness has no bearing on the actual effectiveness.
Planning
Health Promotion and Maintenance
Application
Learning Objective 5.1

5.2 The client asks the nurse how the cervical mucus method of contraception differs from the calendar (rhythm) method. The nurse's best response is, "The cervical mucus method
1. is more effective for women with irregular cycles."
2. is free, safe, and acceptable to women of many religions."
3. provides an increased awareness of the body."
4. requires no artificial substances or devices."

Answer: 1
Rationale: The cervical mucus method can be used by women with irregular cycles. The other choices apply to both methods.
Planning
Health Promotion and Maintenance
Application
Learning Objective 5.2

5.3 The nurse is planning an educational session about contraception. What is the most significant factor in choosing a specific method of contraception in order to avoid pregnancy?
1. absolute reliability
2. ease of use
3. consistency of use
4. cost

Answer: 3
Rationale: No method of contraception is reliable if not used consistently. Ease of use can impact consistency of use, as can cost. Absolute reliability is based on statistics, not the consistency of one person's use.
Planning
Health Promotion and Maintenance
Application
Learning Objective 5.1

5.4 A client asks, "Can you explain to us how to use the basal body temperature method to detect ovulation and prevent pregnancy?" What would be the best reply by the nurse?
1. "Take your temperature every evening at the same time and keep a record for a period of several weeks. A noticeable drop in temperature indicates that ovulation has occurred."
2. "Take your temperature every day at the same time and keep a record of the findings. A noticeable rise in temperature indicates ovulation."

Answer: 3
Rationale: Basal body temperatures should be taken and recorded every day prior to rising from bed. A drop in temperature occurs prior to ovulation, and indicates when intercourse should be avoided for three days. A rise in temperature indicates that ovulation has occurred. This method is quite successful when intercourse is avoided on the appropriate days.
Planning
Health Promotion and Maintenance
Application
Learning Objective 5.2

3. "Take your temperature each day, immediately upon awakening, and keep a record of each finding. A noticeable drop in temperature indicates that ovulation is about to occur."

4. "This is an unscientific and unproven method of determining ovulation and is not recognized as a means of birth control."

5.5 A client wants to use the vaginal sponge as a method of contraception. Which of the following statements indicate that she will need further instruction? "I need to (Select all that apply.) " 1. use a lubricant prior to insertion." 2. add spermicidal cream prior to intercourse." 3. moisten it with water prior to use." 4. leave it in no longer than six hours." 5. use the sponge on my most fertile days."	Answer: 1, 2, 4, 5 Rationale: To activate the spermicide in the vaginal sponge, the sponge must be moistened thoroughly with water. Neither lubricant nor spermicidal creams are needed. The sponge can remain in place for 24 hours. Consistent use is important to the success rate of all methods. Evaluation Health Promotion and Maintenance Analysis Learning Objective 5.3
5.6 When teaching a woman about use of the diaphragm, it is important to instruct her that the diaphragm should be rechecked for correct size 1. every five years routinely. 2. when weight gain or loss beyond five pounds has occurred. 3. after each pregnancy. 4. only after significant weight loss.	Answer: 3 Rationale: The diaphragm should be rechecked for correct size after each childbirth or abortion and whenever a woman has gained or lost ten pounds or more. Routine checking for size is not recommended. Planning Health Promotion and Maintenance Application Learning Objective 5.4
5.7 Instructions concerning the use of a diaphragm should include that it is an excellent method of contraception, provided that the woman 1. does not use any spermicidal creams or jellies with it. 2. removes it promptly following intercourse and then douches. 3. leaves it in place for six hours following intercourse. 4. inserts it at least two hours prior to intercourse.	Answer: 3 Rationale: The diaphragm can be inserted anytime prior to intercourse, must always be used with contraceptive cream or jelly, and should be left in place for six hours after the last episode of intercourse. Additional cream or jelly should be inserted into the vagina if intercourse occurs while the diaphragm is in place. Douching is not recommended, because it disrupts the natural vaginal flora. Planning Health Promotion and Maintenance Application Learning Objective 5.4
5.8 The nurse at the family planning clinic has done some teaching on oral contraceptives in the waiting room. The nurse knows that the teaching has been effective when one of the clients responds 1. "I can't take 'the pill' if I'm over 30." 2. "I can take 'the pill,' even though I smoke heavily." 3. "My periods will become slightly heavier when I take 'the pill'." 4. "I can't take 'the pill' if I have gallbladder disease."	Answer: 4 Rationale: Combination oral contraceptive use is contraindicated in women with gallbladder disease and those who are heavy smokers. There is not an age limit to use. Menstrual flow is decreased with the use of oral contraceptives. Evaluation Health Promotion and Maintenance Analysis Learning Objective 5.5

5.9 The nurse has taught a client about combined oral contraceptive use. Additional teaching is required if the client makes which statement? "Taking combined oral contraceptives will give me a
1. lower risk for breast cancer."
2. higher risk for cervical cancer."
3. lower risk for ovarian cancer."
4. higher risk for uterine cancer."

Answer: 3
Rationale: The use of combined oral contraceptives decreases the risk of developing both ovarian and endometrial cancer. No change occurs in the risk of breast cancer. Multiple sexual partners and contracting human papilloma virus increase the risk for cervical cancer.
Evaluation
Health Promotion and Maintenance
Analysis
Learning Objective 5.5

5.10 The client is 36 years old, weighs 250 pounds, is monogamous, does not smoke, and desires birth control. In preparing an educational session for this client, the nurse understands that which of the following methods is inappropriate for this client?
1. intrauterine device
2. vaginal sponge
3. combined oral contraceptives
4. transdermal hormonal contraception

Answer: 4
Rationale: Transdermal hormonal contraception is contraindicated due to the client's obesity. This client may use an intrauterine device, the vaginal sponge, or combined oral contraceptives.
Planning
Health Promotion and Maintenance
Application
Learning Objective 5.6

5.11 The nurse is preparing educational materials at a family planning clinic. The client who is an appropriate candidate for using emergency contraception would be one who reports
1. forgetting to start her pill pack yesterday.
2. unprotected intercourse during her menses.
3. that a condom broke yesterday in the middle of her cycle.
4. increased dysmenorrhea since IUD insertion.

Answer: 3
Rationale: Emergency contraception (EC) is taken to prevent pregnancy when unprotected intercourse occurs during the midcycle within the past 72 hours. Intercourse during menses does not lead to pregnancy. A client who forgets to start a new pill pack on time should be instructed to use a barrier method for the cycle. An IUD in place prevents conception, and mild dysmenorrhea is common after IUD insertion.
Assessment
Health Promotion and Maintenance
Application
Learning Objective 5.7

5.12 The nurse is planning a group education session on the IUD. The nurse understands that the IUD is contraindicated for a woman
1. with three children and who is monogamous.
2. desiring another child in four years.
3. without children and has two sex partners.
4. who has smoked heavily for several years.

Answer: 3
Rationale: The IUD is contraindicated for clients who have never had a child, and who are not in a mutually monogamous relationship. Neither desire for a future pregnancy nor smoking are contraindications for IUD use.
Planning
Health Promotion and Maintenance
Analysis
Learning Objective 5.8

5.13 A couple asks the nurse what would be the safest method of sterilization. The nurse should reply, "Generally, the safest surgical method of permanent sterilization would be a
1. laparotomy tubal ligation."
2. laparoscopy tubal ligation."
3. minilaparotomy."
4. vasectomy."

Answer: 4
Rationale: Vasectomy is a relatively minor procedure. Female sterilization procedures involve more risks due to the need for general anesthesia.
Planning
Health Promotion and Maintenance
Application
Learning Objective 5.9

5.14 The client is using oral contraceptives. She tells the nurse that her family is complete, and that she now desires permanent contraception. Which statement should the nurse include in teaching this client about sterilization options?
1. "Essure becomes effective three months after insertion."
2. "Vasectomy is effective immediately after the procedure."
3. "Tubal ligation is not advised until the client is age 35."
4. "Oral contraception should be taken until menopause."

Answer: 1
Rationale: Essure involves insertion of stainless steel inserts into the fallopian tubes via hysteroscopy. The inserts create a tissue response that results in tubal occlusion in about three months. Vasectomy requires several ejaculations to clear the remaining sperm from the vas deferens before sterility occurs. Tubal ligation can be performed at any age. Oral contraceptives are effective, but the client desires a permanent method.
Planning
Health Promotion and Maintenance
Application
Learning Objective 5.9

5.15 The client reports that she was raped three weeks ago, and now her menses is a week late. The client is extremely upset when a pregnancy test confirms that she is pregnant, and requests information regarding pregnancy termination. Which statement is best for the nurse to include?
1. "Abortion is morally wrong and should not be undertaken."
2. "You are too late to have a medical abortion."
3. "Surgical abortion can result in uterine perforation."
4. "Both medical and surgical abortions are 100% effective."

Answer: 3
Rationale: Surgical abortion approaches 100% effectiveness, and the risks include uterine perforation and infection (although the risk is very small). Although many nurses have strong moral objections against abortion, in order to be effective in a therapeutic relationship the nurse must avoid being judgmental. Medical abortion is 96% effective, and is undertaken within the first seven weeks of pregnancy.
Planning
Health Promotion and Maintenance
Application
Learning Objective 5.10

CHAPTER 6

6.1 A nonpregnant client reports a fishy smelling, thin, white, watery vaginal discharge. She is diagnosed with bacterial vaginosis (BV). The client reports an allergy to sulfa. The nurse would expect to administer
1. penicillin G (Bicillin) 2 million units IM one time.
2. zithromax (Azithromycin) 1 mg po bid for two weeks.
3. doxycycline (Vibramycin) 100 mg po bid for a week.
4. metronidazole (Flagyl) 500 mg po bid for a week.

Answer: 4
Rationale: The nonpregnant woman who is diagnosed with bacterial vaginosis (BV) is treated with metronidazole (Flagyl) 500 mg orally twice a day for seven days. Penicillin, zithromax, and doxycycline are not used to treat BV. An allergy to sulfa is not contraindicated in the use of metronidizole.
Planning
Physiologic Integrity
Application
Learning Objective 6.1

6.2 The client being given discharge instructions with a diagnosis of vulvo-vaginal candidiasis (VVC) demonstrates understanding when she states, "I need to (Select all that apply.)
1. apply the miconazole (Monistat) for 10 days."
2. douche daily."
3. add yogurt to my diet."
4. wear nylon panties."
5. have the rash on my husband's penis checked.

Answer: 3, 5
Rationale: Eating yogurt with active cultures helps prevent candidiasis recurrence. A genital rash on a male can be candidiasis, and should be checked and treated as appropriate. Douching daily and wearing nylon panties predispose clients to developing vulvovaginal candidiasis. Miconazole is used for seven days.
Evaluation
Physiologic Integrity
Analysis
Learning Objective 6.1

6.3 The physician has prescribed metronidazole (Flagyl) for a woman diagnosed with trichomoniasis. The nurse's instructions to the woman should include

1. "Both partners must be treated with the medication."
2. "Alcohol does not need to be avoided while taking this medication."
3. "It will turn your urine orange."
4. "This medication may produce drowsiness."

Answer: 1
Rationale: Both partners should be treated with the medication. Alcohol should be avoided. Metronidazole does not turn the urine orange or cause drowsiness.
Planning
Physiologic Integrity
Application
Learning Objective 6.2

6.4 The couple demonstrates understanding of the consequences of not treating chlamydia when they state (Select all that apply.)

1. "She could become pregnant."
2. "She could have severe vaginal itching."
3. "He could get an infection in the tube that carries the urine out."
4. "It could cause us to develop a rash."
5. "She could develop a worse infection of the uterus and tubes."

Answer: 3, 5
Rationale: Chlamydia is a major cause of nongonococcal urethritis (NGU) in men. Chlamydia cervicitis can ascend and become pelvic inflammatory disease, or infection of the uterus, fallopian tubes, and sometimes ovaries. It does not cause a woman to become pregnant, vaginal itching, or a rash.
Evaluation
Physiologic Integrity
Application
Learning Objective 6.2

6.5 Which of the following clients should be treated with ceftriaxone (Rocephin) IM and doxycycline (Vibramycin) orally?

1. a pregnant client with gonorrhea and a yeast infection
2. a nonpregnant client with gonorrhea and chlamydia
3. a pregnant client with syphilis
4. a nonpregnant client with chlamydia and trichomoniasis

Answer: 2
Rationale: This combined treatment provides dual treatment for gonorrhea and chlamydia because the two infections frequently occur together. Doxycycline is contraindicated during pregnancy. Syphilis is treated with penicillin. Trichomoniasis is treated with metronidizole.
Planning
Physiologic Integrity
Application
Learning Objective 6.2

6.6 Which of the following statements by the client verifies correct knowledge about vaginal herpes?

1. "I should douche daily to prevent infection."
2. "I may have another breakout during my period."
3. "I am more likely to develop cancer of the cervix."
4. "I should use sodium bicarbonate on the lesions to relieve discomfort."

Answer: 2
Rationale: Menstruation seems to trigger recurrences of herpes. Douches do not prevent infection. There is no relationship between herpes and cancer of the cervix. Burow's (aluminum acetate) solution relieves discomfort, not sodium bicarbonate.
Evaluation
Physiologic Integrity
Analysis
Learning Objective 6.3

6.7 A client is hospitalized for pelvic inflammatory disease (PID). Which of the following orders should the nurse implement first?

1. encourage oral fluids
2. administer cefotetan IV
3. enforce bed rest
4. instruct the client to discontinue use of her diaphragm

Answer: 2
Rationale: Administration of medications to treat the disease is priority. Bed rest and encouraging oral fluids are not a priority. Diaphragm use is not associated with increased risk of PID.
Planning
Physiologic Integrity
Analysis
Learning Objective 6.4

6.8 Which of the following diagnostic tests would the nurse question when ordered for a client diagnosed with pelvic inflammatory disease (PID)?
1. CBC (complete blood count) with differential
2. vaginal culture for *Neisseria gonorrhea*
3. throat culture for *Streptococcus A*
4. RPR (rapid plasma reagin)

Answer: 3
Rationale: Streptococcus of the throat is not associated with PID. CBC with differential will give an indication of the severity of the infection. Gonorrhea is a common cause of PID, and the client should be tested for this. RPR is a test for syphilis, another cause of PID.
Implementation
Physiologic Integrity
Analysis
Learning Objective 6.4.

6.9 A nurse is assessing a pregnant client for right-sided flank pain. The nurse explains to the client that this type of pain is a common symptom of pyelonephritis in the pregnant client because of:
1. displacement of the urinary bladder.
2. nausea and vomiting.
3. the position of the uterus in the abdomen.
4. a colicky large intestine.

Answer: 3
Rationale: The right side is almost always involved if the woman is pregnant because the large bulk of intestines to the left pushes the uterus to the right. Nausea and vomiting are symptoms from the pyelonephritis. A colicky large intestine and displacement of the urinary bladder do not cause right-sided flank pain in pregnancy.
Implementation
Physiologic Integrity
Application
Learning Objective 6.5

6.10 The client gives correct information regarding ways to prevent a recurrence of her urinary tract infection when she states, "I should
1. wipe from back to front after urination."
2. urinate when I feel the urge."
3. try to restrict my intake of fruits."
4. use a diaphragm."

Answer: 2
Rationale: Retention over-distends the bladder and can lead to infection. Wiping from back to front after urination may transfer bacteria from the anorectal area to the urethra. Organic acids from fruits inhibit bacterial growth. The use of a diaphragm may cause recurrent urinary tract infections.
Evaluation
Physiologic Integrity
Analysis
Learning Objective 6.5

6.11 A client comes to the clinic complaining of difficulty urinating, flu-like symptoms, genital tingling, and blisterlike vesicles on the upper thigh and vagina. She denies having ever had these symptoms before. The most likely medication for the physician to order would be:
1. oral acyclovir.
2. ceftriaxone IM.
3. azithromycin po.
4. penicillin G 2.4 million units IM.

Answer: 1
Rationale: Malaise, dysuria, and tingling or painful vesicles are indicative of a primary herpes simplex outbreak. Acyclovir treats herpes. Neither ceftriaxone IM, azithromycin, nor penicillin G treat herpes.
Implementation
Physiologic Integrity
Application
Learning Objective 6.2

6.12 The client has been diagnosed with hepatitis B. Which statement indicates a need for further education?
1. "This infection could be sexually transmitted."
2. "I might get jaundiced from this illness."
3. "An immunization exists to prevent getting hepatitis B."
4. "I may have gotten this infection from food."

Answer: 4
Rationale: Hepatitis A and E are foodborne, and transmitted via fecal-oral contamination. Hepatitis is found in blood and body fluids, and therefore can be sexually transmitted. Hepatitis can cause jaundice. An immunization is available for both hepatitis A and B.
Evaluation
Physiologic Integrity
Application
Learning Objective 6.6

6.13 The client who is in the first trimester of pregnancy has been diagnosed with syphilis. Which statement about congenital syphilis indicates that further education is necessary? "Syphilis infection during pregnancy could cause my baby to have

1. intrauterine growth restriction."
2. preterm birth."
3. stillbirth."
4. vesicular rash."

Answer: 4
Rationale: Congenital syphilis can cause intrauterine growth restriction, preterm birth, or stillbirth. Vesicular rash is not associated with congenital syphilis.
Evaluation
Physiologic Integrity
Analysis
Learning Objective 6.3

6.14 The nurse is planning a community education presentation about hepatitis. Which statement should be included?

1. Hepatitis A is the most common viral infection in the world.
2. Hepatitis C is the most common bloodborne illness in the United States.
3. Hepatitis A will develop into a chronic condition.
4. Hepatitis B can be prevented with use of the birth control pill.

Answer: 2
Rationale: Hepatitis C is the most common bloodborne illness in the United States today, and like hepatitis B and D, can become a chronic infection. Hepatitis A is not the most common viral illness, and does not become chronic. Condoms are the only method of birth control that will decrease the risk of hepatitis B transmission.
Planning
Physiologic Integrity
Application
Learning Objective 6.6

6.15 A client comes in complaining of wart-like lesions on the vulva, painful wrist and finger joints, and a chronic and hoarse sore throat. The appropriate treatment would be

1. penicillin G (Bicillin) IM
2. acyclovir (Zovirax) po
3. ceftriaxone (Rocephin) IM
4. metronidizole (Flagyl) po

Answer: 1
Rationale: The symptoms are the result of syphilis. Syphilis is treated with penicillin G administered intramuscularly. Acyclovir, ceftriaxone, and metronidizole are not used to treat syphilis.
Implementation
Physiologic Integrity
Application
Learning Objective 6.3

CHAPTER 7

7.1 The nurse is planning a community health presentation about screening examinations that are recommended for women. The nurse should include the American Cancer Society's current recommendation that a woman should begin annual mammograms at the age of

1. 30.
2. 35.
3. 40.
4. 45.

Answer: 3
Rationale: The American Cancer Society recommends annual mammogram screening for women beginning at age 40. The National Cancer Institute recommends a mammogram every one to two years, beginning at the same age. The ages of 30 and 35 are too young, and 45 is later than American Cancer Society recommendations.
Planning
Health Promotion and Maintenance
Application
Learning Objective 7.1

7.2 A client is concerned about her risk for breast cancer. Following the initial history, the nurse identifies which of the following as a high risk factor for breast cancer?

1. history of late menarche and early menopause
2. sister with premenopausal breast cancer
3. mother with fibrocystic breast disease
4. multiparity

Answer: 2
Rationale: Nulliparity and age over 30 at first childbearing are associated with increased risk of breast cancer, as is premenopausal breast cancer in a first degree relative.
Early menarche combined with late menopause is a breast cancer risk. Neither fibrocystic breast disease nor multiparity are breast cancer risk factors.
Assessment
Health Promotion and Maintenance
Analysis
Learning Objective 7.1

7.3 The nurse is working with a woman who is undergoing chemotherapy for breast cancer. The client states, "First, the cancer seemed unreal. Now I feel like I can cope." The best response of the nurse would be, "Women with breast cancer often

1. go through several stages of adjustment."
2. cope better than their partners cope."
3. seek multiple opinions before starting treatment."
4. usually become angry after treatment begins."

Answer: 1
Rationale: Psychological adjustment to breast cancer involves four stages: shock, reaction, recovery, and reorientation. The client's statement indicates shock followed by reaction. Partners are often the primary support person during treatment, but may also have difficulty adapting to the diagnosis. Some clients seek multiple opinions, some do not. Anger is not a stage of adjustment.
Assessment
Psychosocial Integrity
Analysis
Learning Objective 7.2

7.4 The nurse interviews a 28-year-old client with a new medical diagnosis of endometriosis. Which of the following questions are most appropriate? (Select all that apply.)

1. "Are you having hot flashes?"
2. "Are you experiencing pain during intercourse?"
3. "Is a vaginal discharge present?"
4. "Are you having pain during your period?"
5. "Have you noticed any skin rashes?"

Answer: 2, 4
Rationale: The primary symptoms of endometriosis include dysmenorrhea, dyspareunia, and infertility. Hot flashes, vaginal discharge, and skin rashes are not symptoms of endometriosis.
Assessment
Physiologic Integrity
Analysis
Learning Objective 7.3

7.5 The client has been diagnosed with endometriosis. She asks the nurse if there are any long-term health risks associated with this condition. The nurse should include which statement in the client teaching about endometriosis?

1. "There are no other health risks associated with endometriosis."
2. "Pain with intercourse rarely occurs as a long-term problem."
3. "You are at increased risk for ovarian and breast cancer."
4. "Most women with this condition develop fibromyalgia."

Answer: 3
Rationale: Dyspareunia is a common symptom of endometriosis. There are long-term health risks associated with endometriosis, including an increased risk for cancer of the ovary and breast, melanoma, non-Hodgkins lymphoma, and an increased incidence of fibromyalgia.
Planning
Physiologic Integrity
Analysis
Learning Objective 7.3

7.6 The client is undergoing lab work and ultrasound for a possible diagnosis of polycystic ovarian syndrome (PCOS). Which problem does the nurse expect to find in the client's history?

1. multiple first trimester fetal losses
2. dyspareunia
3. vulvitis
4. oligomenorrhea

Answer: 4
Rationale: PCOS causes 85–90% of oligomenorrhea. Dyspareunia is associated with endometriosis. Neither first trimester fetal loss nor vulvitis are associated with polycystic ovarian syndrome (PCOS).
Assessment
Physiologic Integrity
Application
Learning Objective 7.4

7.7 The client with polycystic ovarian syndrome (PCOS) has been prescribed metformin (Glucophage). Education about this medication should include: "This medication will (Select all that apply.)

1. decrease your excessive hair growth."

Answer: 1, 2, 4
Rationale: Polycystic ovarian syndrome (PCOS) treatment with metformin decreases hirsuitism, improves weight loss success, decreases acne, increases ovulation and therefore menstrual regularity and fertility, and treats type II diabetes by decreasing glucose production in the liver and improves glucose uptake by cells.
Planning
Physiologic Integrity

2. make it easier to lose weight." 3. increase your acne." 4. improve your chances of pregnancy." 5. make your menstrual periods irregular."	Application Learning Objective 7.4
7.8 The 12-year-old client reports that menarche occurred five months ago. She has had bleeding every day this month, and is very worried. The nurse should explain that the most common cause of this bleeding is 1. anovulation. 2. diabetes mellitus. 3. pregnancy. 4. Von Willebrand disease.	Answer: 1 Rationale: Chronic anovulation is very common in the first year after menarche. Although Von Willebrand disease can cause irregular uterine bleeding, it is quite rare. Uterine bleeding is not a symptom of either diabetes mellitus nor pregnancy. Implementation Physiologic Integrity Application Learning Objective 7.5
7.9 The nurse is scheduling an ultrasound for a 45-year old woman with a suspected uterine tumor. The nurse includes in the client's teaching that the most common benign uterine tumor seen in women in their forties is a 1. fibroid tumor. 2. fibroadenoma. 3. fibrocystic tumor. 4. lymphoma.	Answer: 1 Rationale: Fibroid tumors frequently occur in perimenopausal women. Fibroadenoma is a benign tumor of the breast, and are sometimes referred to as a fibrocystic tumor. Lymphoma is cancer of the lymphatic system. Planning Physiologic Integrity Application Learning Objective 7.5
7.10 The client has been found to have vitiligo on her vulva. Which statement indicates that the client requires additional teaching on this condition? 1. "This may occur in other places on my body." 2. "Vitiligo is only a decrease of pigmentation." 3. "Other serious health conditions are common with vitiligo." 4. "There usually are no other symptoms of this condition."	Answer: 3 Rationale: Vitiligo is an absence of melanin, which results in white patches that are especially noticeable on dark-skinned individuals. It can occur in multiple areas on the body, and has no associated symptoms nor health conditions. Evaluation Physiologic Integrity Analysis Learning Objective 7.6
7.11 The client has been diagnosed with vulvitis. The nurse is performing teaching on this condition. Which statement by the client indicates that additional information is required? 1. "I should stop having sexual intercourse." 2. "Deodorized tampons may make this condition recur." 3. "Wearing pantyhose daily will improve the problem." 4. "A different brand of soap might eliminate the irritation."	Answer: 3 Rationale: Vulvitis is inflammation of the vulva. Tight clothing, especially if made of synthetic fibers, can predispose women to the condition. Pantyhose are one example. Use of deodorized and heavily scented products that come in contact with the vulva (toilet paper, soap, bubble bath, pads and tampons, etc.) can cause the inflammation. Abstaining from intercourse until the vulva are healed is helpful, but long-term abstinence is not required. Evaluation Health Promotion and Maintenance Analysis Learning Objective 7.7
7.12 The nurse has presented a community education class on recommended health screenings for women. Which statement by a class member indicates that additional teaching is necessary? "The Pap smear 1. is recommended every year." 2. diagnoses cervical cancer."	Answer: 2 Rationale: The Pap smear is a screening tool, and detects abnormal cervical cells that may indicate precancerous or cancerous conditions. The Pap does not diagnose cervical cancer. The American College of Obstetrics and Gynecology (ACOG) recommends the procedure every year; the American Cancer Society (ACS) recommends every three years after having three consecutive exams with normal findings. Evaluation

3. can be done every three years in some women." 4. detects abnormal cells."	Health Promotion and Maintenance Analysis Learning Objective 7.8
7.13 The nurse obtains a health history from the following clients. To which one should she give priority for teaching about cervical cancer prevention? 1. age 30, treated for human papilloma virus (HPV) 2. age 25, monogamous 3. age 20, pregnant 4. age 27, uses a diaphragm	Answer: 1 Rationale: Exposure to sexually transmitted infections indicates that one or both partners is not monogamous, and the client is not using condoms. Exposure to sexually transmitted infections includes possible exposure to human papilloma virus (HPV). Contracting HPV increases risk of abnormal cervical cell changes and cervical cancer. Pregnancy, use of a diaphragm, and practicing monogamy do not increase risks of cervical cancer. Planning Health Promotion and Maintenance Analysis Learning Objective 7.9
7.14 The 22-year-old client is scheduled for her first gynecologic examination. What can the nurse do to make the client more comfortable during this exam? (Select all that apply.) 1. have a female physician perform the exam 2. show the client what the speculum looks like 3. reduce her fear by not telling the client what the exam involves 4. ask the client why she has delayed her first Pap this long 5. provide a mirror for the client	Answer: 1, 2, 5 Rationale: The first pelvic examination can be a frightening experience. To reduce fear and improve the client's sense of control, schedule the exam with a female provider, show the client all of the equipment to be used, provide a mirror to increase learning about anatomy, and create a trusting atmosphere. Avoid being judgmental. Implementation Health Promotion and Maintenance Application Learning Objective 7.10
7.15 The client's Pap smear result is ASC-US. The best way for the nurse to explain this result is: "ASC-US means (Select all that apply.) 1. abnormal squamous cells of undetermined significance." 2. cancer has invaded the upper cervix." 3. a sexually transmitted infection is present." 4. the Pap should be repeated in four months." 5. the cervical cells are abnormal, but the reason why is unknown."	Answer: 1, 3, 5 Rationale: ASC-US stands for abnormal squamous cells of undetermined significance. This result is equivocal, and requires follow-up either through repeating the Pap every four to six months, or with a colposcopic examination for more detailed information. A large number of women with cervical intraepithelial neoplasia (CIN) initially present with ASC-US Pap results. Cervicitis caused by human papilloma virus (HPV) or another sexually transmitted infection can lead to an ASC-US result, but the results can also be caused by recent sexual intercourse. ASC-US does not indicate cancer. Planning Health Promotion and Maintenance Analysis Learning Objective 7.8

CHAPTER 8

8.1 The nurse is planning a community educational presentation for people living below poverty level. The nurse knows that the highest population in this socioeconomic category is 1. adults in communal living situations. 2. young married couples under the age of 20. 3. single women with children. 4. single adults.	Answer: 3 Rationale: Single women with children, regardless of previous marital status, are the group most likely to be living below the poverty level. Unmarried couples who live together, young married couples, and single adults are not the most likely to encounter poverty. Planning Health Promotion and Maintenance Application Learning Objective 8.1
8.2 The nurse manager is examining a complaint about wage discrimination. To resolve this complaint the nurse manager	Answer: 1 Rationale: Comparable worth means equal pay for work that is of comparable value and requires comparable skills, responsibility, education, and experience.

must understand that the basic premise of "comparable worth" means that
1. men and women doing the same job should receive the same pay.
2. a person's pay should be based more on the number of hours worked rather than on the type of work performed.
3. women are especially well-suited for some kinds of jobs, as are men for others.
4. unemployment compensation should be based on the salary the person was making while employed.

Number of hours worked is not a factor. Assuming that one gender is more suited to a particular type of work than the other gender is sex discrimination. Unemployment compensation is a different issue than comparable worth.
Planning
Safe, Effective Care Environment
Application
Learning Objective 8.2

8.3 The community clinic nurse manager is working on a long-term budget. The manager understands that in the next few years, Medicaid is expected to pay for fewer births. This is, in part, because
1. the U.S. economy is becoming stronger.
2. more women are able to pay for private insurance.
3. new public policies are providing other forms of payment.
4. eligibility rules for Medicaid have been changed.

Answer: 4
Rationale: Eligibility for Medicaid has decreased eligibility for pregnant women. The strength of the economy is not a factor in Medicaid regulations. Private insurance is expensive, and not affordable to poor women who would be Medicaid-eligible. Although some states are implementing affordable healthcare options, not all states have chosen to do so.
Planning
Health Promotion and Maintenance
Analysis
Learning Objective 8.3

8.4 The nurse is working with a client who is seeking a family and medical leave. Which of the following is an eligibility requirement of the Family and Medical Leave Act of 1993? The employee must
1. work at least 40 hours per week.
2. have been employed for at least one month.
3. work for a company with less than 50 employees.
4. furnish a physician's statement that verifies the need.

Answer: 4
Rationale: The Family and Medical Leave Act (FMLA) of 1993 permits employees to take up to 12 weeks of unpaid leave from work following the birth or adoption of a child or the placement of a foster child, if faced with serious illness, or the illness of a spouse, child, or parent. A physician's statement must verify the need. Only companies with 50 or more employees are covered by FMLA, and coverage is not mandated for employees who work fewer than 25 hours per week, or who have been employed less than one year.
Assessment
Safe, Effective Care Environment
Application
Learning Objective 8.4

8.5 The pregnant client is employed at a factory. The client asks the nurse if exposure to chemicals can cause harm to her fetus. The nurse should advise that exposure to which substance can lead to neurological damage?
1. lead
2. latex
3. formaldehyde
4. benzene

Answer: 1
Rationale: Lead exposure during pregnancy, as well as during childhood, can cause neurological damage. Exposure to latex, formaldehyde, or benzene is not known to cause neurological damage.
Assessment
Health Promotion and Maintenance
Application
Learning Objective 8.5

8.6 The community nurse has presented an educational presentation at a low-income assisted living facility with residents from several races and ethnic groups. Which statement made by an older African American woman

Answer: 3
Rationale: African-American women have higher rates of chronic disease and death from chronic disease than white women. The poor elderly often face barriers when obtaining health care, leading to poor outcomes. Generic medications have the same pharmacologic effect as trade name medications.
Evaluation

indicates that teaching has been effective?

1. "I have a lower risk of dying from diabetes than my white friend."
2. "Income doesn't affect our health risks as compared to rich people."
3. "I am twice as likely to have coronary heart disease as my white neighbor."
4. "Generic medications might not work as well as the trade name pills."

Health Promotion and Maintenance
Application
Learning Objective 8.8

8.7 The nurse manager is preparing an educational in-service for staff nurses about elder abuse. The nurse manager develops a hypothetical situation: A wheelchair-bound client who lives with her daughter has experienced hunger because she cannot reach the cupboards to make lunch. Which category of elder abuse does this example describe?

1. Psychologic abuse
2. Physical abuse
3. Neglect
4. Financial abuse

Answer: 3
Rationale: Neglect can either be by a caretaker or neglecting oneself. Psychologic abuse is usually verbal. Physical abuse involves some degree of violence. Financial abuse involves money.
Planning
Health Promotion and Maintenance
Application
Learning Objective 8.7

8.8 The community health nurse manager is reviewing the charts of elderly clients. Which issue are these clients most likely to experience?

1. adequate financial resources to purchase medications
2. senior services that provide transportation to healthcare appointments
3. multiple medications prescribed by different physicians
4. medicare that covers healthcare costs so no out of pocket expenses occur

Answer: 3
Rationale: Polypharmacy, or medication prescriptions from different providers that results in the client taking multiple medications, has the potential to cause problems with side effects and medication interactions. The elderly are more likely to encounter poverty, and too often forgo medications to buy food. Not all elderly have adequate access to transportation for health care. Medicare rarely covers all healthcare expenses, and if a client does not have co-insurance, out of pocket expenses can be substantial.
Assessment
Health Promotion and Maintenance
Application
Learning Objective 8.8

8.9 The nurse is planning care at a retirement community. The nurse understands that, compared to a male of the same age, a 75-year-old woman is more likely to have a

1. living spouse.
2. pension.
3. disability.
4. better education.

Answer: 3
Rationale: More elderly women experience disabilities, in part because of their longer life spans. Men tend to have shorter life spans than women. Elderly women are less likely to have held jobs that provided a pension. Most families believed that education of girls was less important than education of boys when the elderly were of school-age.
Assessment
Health Promotion and Maintenance
Application
Learning Objective 8.6

8.10 The nurse at a women's clinic is reviewing a new client health information questionnaire. Which question would be found insulting and discriminatory by lesbian clients?

1. Who should be contacted in case of emergency?
2. What method of birth control do you use?

Answer: 2
Rationale: Assuming that a client uses birth control assumes that the client is heterosexual, creating a heterosexist atmosphere. Emergency contact information is important for all clients. Lesbians should be assessed for chemical dependency and domestic abuse.
Assessment
Health Promotion and Maintenance
Analysis
Learning Objective 8.12

---

3. How often do you drink alcohol?
4. Do you feel safe in your relationship?

8.11 The nurse is reviewing charts. Documentation would be accurate if a client with severe hearing loss is categorized as having what type of disability?
1. sensory
2. developmental
3. neurological
4. psychiatric

Answer: 1
Rationale: Loss of hearing is a sensory disability. Developmental, neurologic, and psychiatric disabilities do not involve sensory loss.
Assessment
Safe, Effective Care Environment
Application
Learning Objective 8.9

8.12 The student nurse is beginning a clinical experience in an assisted living facility that serves a disabled population. Which statement indicates that the student understands the healthcare implications of disability?
1. "More of the clients are female than male because men with disabilities are more likely to be employed."
2. "These disabled women will receive the same healthcare services that able-bodied people have."
3. "Statistics indicate that women with disabilities earn the same as women without disabilities."
4. "Disabled women are just as likely to face poverty as are men who have a disability."

Answer: 1
Rationale: Disabled women are less likely to be gainfully employed than men with disabilities, and those who are employed earn significantly less than either men with disabilities or women without disabilities. Disabled women are also more likely to live in poverty than disabled men. Access to health care is impacted by disability through architectural obstructions, poverty leading to inability to pay for services and medications, and inability to obtain transportation to a healthcare facility.
Evaluation
Safe, Effective Care Environment
Analysis
Learning Objective 8.10

8.13 The nurse has presented an educational session to local politicians about the health impact of discrimination based on sexual orientation. Which statements indicate that further education is needed? (Select all that apply.)
1. "Lesbians who stay at home to raise children receive healthcare benefits through their partner's employer."
2. "A lesbian will receive her partner's retirement funds if the partner dies unexpectedly."
3. "Lesbian couples can be homeless because of eviction based solely on their sexual orientation."
4. "A veteran discharged from the Army because she is lesbian cannot receive care at the Veteran's Administration."
5. "A parent with children can be fired in most states if it becomes known that she is a lesbian."

Answer: 1, 2
Rationale: Gay couples experience many sources of economic discrimination based on sexual orientation, including not receiving pensions or retirement funds after the death of a partner, and not being offered healthcare benefits that a legally-married spouse is entitled to receive. Discharge from the armed forces based on sexual orientation prevents access to Veterans Administration benefits. Most states allow overt discrimination, including on the job discrimination and housing discrimination, based on sexual orientation.
Evaluation
Health Promotion and Maintenance
Analysis
Learning Objective 8.11

8.14 The nurse working at a homeless shelter is studying case statistics. Of the total homeless population served at the

Answer: 1
Rationale: Homelessness among families with children, especially single-parent families with a female head of household, is rising faster than any other group.

---

shelter, which group would the nurse's statistics likely uncover as the fastest-growing group?
1. unemployed women
2. families with children
3. the mentally ill
4. the elderly

Unemployment is one aspect of this trend, but it is not the group with the fastest increase in homelessness, nor are the mentally ill or the elderly.
Assessment
Health Promotion and Maintenance
Application
Learning Objective 8.2

8.15 The nurse is working with a group of recent immigrants from a country that practices female genital mutilation (FGM). In order to be effective in teaching about gynecologic care in the United States, the nurse must keep which issues in mind? (Select all that apply.)
1. Women may undergo FGM willingly to support the status quo of society.
2. Women may undergo the procedure to be considered for marriage.
3. Societies that practice FGM view women as having equal rights with men.
4. FGM is usually done during infancy so women have no memory of the procedure.
5. Women will view the term *female genital mutilation* as culturally appropriate.

Answer: 1, 2
Rationale: Societies that practice FGM are strongly patriarchal, and value females based on the labor they can perform and childbearing. However, if FGM is the norm, and only those females who have had the procedure can be married, women seeking the security of marriage will willingly submit to the practice. FGM is rarely performed during infancy, and is usually done during adolescence. Many find the term female genital mutilation disrespectful and inappropriate because it implies that women have been mutilated, are not whole, and that these people are cruel mutilators.
Planning
Health Promotion and Maintenance
Application
Learning Objective 8.13

CHAPTER 9

9.1 The nurse has been talking to a woman about the reorganization phase following a rape. Which of the following responses would indicate that the client understands this phase?
1. "By using denial and suppression in this phase, I will eventually be able to accept what has happened to me."
2. "During this time I won't talk much about the rape because I am examining my inward feelings regarding the rape."
3. "During this time I will repeatedly replay the role of the victim until I come to terms with the experience."
4. "My perception of a normal sexual relationship will be similar to my perception prior to the rape."

Answer: 3
Rationale: During reorganization, a victim adjusts her self-concept to include the rape. Flash backs of being a rape victim may indicate post-traumatic stress disorder. Denial and suppression indicate the client is experiencing the outward adjustment phase of rape trauma syndrome. During the outward adjustment phase, the victim will not talk about the rape, but because the experience is being pushed deeper into the subconscious. Sexual relationships often develop dysfunction after rape.
Evaluation
Psychosocial Integrity
Analysis
Learning Objective 9.13

9.2 A man has brought his wife to the emergency room. Because of her visible injuries and demeanor, the nurse suspects partner abuse. The man is doing most of the talking, and the wife sits quietly with her head down. In preparing to examine the woman, the nurse should
1. ask her if she would like her husband to wait in the waiting room.

Answer: 4
Rationale: One way that abusers maintain control is by preventing the person being abused from freely talking to healthcare providers or the police. The client must be alone to be in a confidential and safe environment that will promote trust before she will divulge her history of battering to the nurse.
Assessment
Psychosocial Integrity
Application
Learning Objective 9.2

---

2. find a chair so that the husband can sit by her during the examination.
3. ask the husband if he would like to be present during the examination.
4. tell the husband to wait in the waiting room while his wife is being examined.

9.3 The nurse is planning a community education presentation on battering. Which statements about battering should the nurse include?
1. Battering occurs in a small percentage of the population.
2. Battering is mainly a lower-class, blue-collar problem.
3. Battered women are at greatest risk for severe violence when they leave the batterer.
4. If the batterer stops drinking, the violence usually stops.

Answer: 3
Rationale: The greatest risk for severe violence is when victims of abuse attempt to leave the abuser. Battering occurs in one out of four women, across all socioeconomic and cultural groups. Although alcoholism can be a contributing factor, if the batterer abstains from alcohol, it does not ensure that violent behavior will stop.
Planning
Psychosocial Integrity
Application
Learning Objective 9.4

9.4 The nurse is interviewing a client that has admitted to being a victim of spousal abuse. Which of the following is the most typical description of how the spousal violence developed in her relationship?
1. "He changed overnight. Everything was fine, and all of a sudden he flipped out and beat me up; he nearly killed me."
2. "It was severe from the beginning. As soon as we got married, he began hitting me and threatening to kill me."
3. "We've both always dated other people. I thought that was understood. He was as emotionally abusive in the beginning as he is now."
4. "I don't know when it started, really. It was gradual. First, just yelling and shoving. Then the beatings started; and now they're more frequent."

Answer: 3
Rationale: Spousal violence usually begins slowly and subtly after a form of commitment such as engagement. Escalation occurs after the commitment, progressing from minor verbal battering to increasingly more violent physical abuse. Domestic violence does not begin suddenly, and will always escalate.
Assessment
Psychosocial Integrity
Analysis
Learning Objective 9.1

9.5 A 35-year-old client in the women's health clinic has just told the nurse about being abused by her husband for the past ten years. The nurse's most appropriate intervention, initially, is to
1. offer to call the police and help her to file charges.
2. ask her to tell you the details surrounding the abuse.
3. reassure her that many women experience the same problem.
4. listen to her account of the situation and offer support.

Answer: 4
Rationale: The initial step in caring for women who have disclosed abuse is to establish trust and ensure confidentiality. Once trust is established, only the detail on what type of violence has occurred is necessary to collect. And although reassuring the client that she is not alone, this is not the most important step. Filing charges will come later.
Implementation
Psychosocial Integrity
Application
Learning Objective 9.7

9.6 Which of the following is most important when screening a woman for partner abuse?

1. ensuring privacy and confidentiality
2. conveying warmth and empathy
3. asking specific, direct questions about abuse
4. clarifying her myths about battering

Answer: 1

Rationale: All women should be screened for partner abuse. Ensuring privacy and confidentiality is critical to gain the trust of the abused woman. Warmth and empathy are helpful, but confidentiality is more important. Clarifying myths is not essential during screening. General questions about possible abuse will both facilitate trust building and is more likely to obtain accurate information.

Implementation
Psychosocial Integrity
Application
Learning Objective 9.8

9.7 A woman has come to the emergency room with multiple bruises over her body and a small laceration over her upper lip. She says she fell down the stairs while doing her housework. Which of the following observations would most likely cause you to suspect that she has been a victim of battering? The client

1. is hesitant to provide details about how the injuries occurred.
2. was accompanied to the ER by her mother instead of her partner.
3. seems eager to go back home.
4. does not seem to be in pain.

Answer: 1

Rationale: Hesitation to provide details about how the injury occurred is a common sign of abuse. Who accompanies the client is not significant for abuse. Abused women often are anxious to get back home quickly to avoid escalation of violence into another attack. Pain level is not indicative of abuse.

Assessment
Psychosocial Integrity
Analysis
Learning Objective 9.9

9.8 The client with limited English language skills has a black eye, and bruises across her face and arms. The client's husband has been acting as an interpreter for the client, and answers all of the questions the nurse asks, often without talking to his wife first. The nurse suspects the client has been a victim of domestic abuse. What should the nurse do next?

1. Ask the husband if he has beaten his wife.
2. Ask the husband to have a female friend come in with his wife.
3. Provide written materials in English for the client to read at home.
4. Ask the husband to step out of the room and obtain a professional interpreter.

Answer: 4

Rationale: Asking an abuser if he has abused his spouse is useless, as most abusers see their behavior as appropriate. A friend may not understand the legal or medical terminology, or may protect the husband by filtering the nurse's words, which may lead to inaccurate interpretation. Written proficiency develops after verbal fluency; therefore, written materials in English are inappropriate for this client. A professional medical interpreter, preferably the same gender as the client, will provide the most accurate translation of the nurse's words as well as the client's.

Implementation
Psychosocial Integrity
Application
Learning Objective 9.10

9.9 The client reports being beaten by her spouse two weeks ago. The client tells the nurse "my husband was so apologetic after he hit me, and brought me flowers." The nurse understands that the husband's behavior indicates which phase of the cycle of violence?

1. tension building
2. acute battering
3. honeymoon period
4. end of violence

Answer: 3

Rationale: Apologies and gifts characterize the tranquil phase or honeymoon period, when the abuser has feelings of guilt. The tension building phase follows the honeymoon period, and extends into the next episode of acute battering. Only behavioral therapy will end the violence.

Assessment
Psychosocial Integrity
Application
Learning Objective 9.5

9.10 The client has been a victim of a violent sadistic rape. She is crying, and asks the nurse, "Why would someone do something like that?" The nurse should explain that the primary purpose of sadistic rape is to
1. take pleasure from the victim's struggle and pain.
2. express feelings of rage.
3. feel a sense of power or mastery.
4. relieve intolerable anxiety.

Answer: 1
Rationale: Sadistic rapists inflict pain on victims; this torture and suffering creates pleasure for the rapist. Anger rape involves brutality and degradation of the victim, and expresses the rapist's sense of rage and unexpressed anger. Power rape provides a sense of dominance and mastery over the victim for the rapist, who often believes the victim enjoys the assault. Anxiety is not associated with a type of rape.
Planning
Psychosocial Integrity
Application
Learning Objective 9.12

9.11 Which woman would you expect to experience the most intense post-traumatic stress disorder as a result of being raped?
1. a woman who fought back during the rape
2. a woman who had a psychiatric disorder prior to being assaulted
3. a woman who was afraid to fight back during the rape
4. a woman who had no visible physical injuries from the assault

Answer: 2
Rationale: Post-traumatic stress disorder is often greatest for women who had a psychiatric disorder prior to the assault. Fighting back, not fighting back, and lack of visible injuries are not factors that will increase the intensity of post-traumatic stress disorder.
Planning
Psychosocial Integrity
Application
Learning Objective 9.13

9.12 A client comes to the reproductive health clinic and reports that she woke up in a strange room this morning, that her perineal area is sore, and she can't clearly remember what happened the previous evening. The client says that she is afraid that she was a victim of a drug-facilitated sexual assault. Which statement should the nurse include when discussing this possibility with the client?
1. "Drinking alcohol can lead to uninhibited sexual behavior, which is not the same as rape."
2. "Some men use drugs mixed into a drink to subdue a potential victim prior to a rape."
3. "It is rare that a woman doesn't remember what happened if she were actually raped."
4. "We need to check for forensic evidence of rape before we can be sure what happened."

Answer: 2
Rationale: Drug-facilitated sexual assault occurs when a drug such as Rohypnol, which dissolves easily and is odorless, is slipped into the drink of an unsuspecting woman, which creates amnesia of the attack. Although an effect of alcohol is decreased inhibition which can lead to less cautious sexual behavior, if a woman is drugged, the sexual act is nonconsensual and, therefore, rape. Forensic evidence is collected for possible legal prosecution of the attacker, but the absence of collectable evidence does not eliminate the possibility of rape.
Implementation
Psychosocial Integrity
Analysis
Learning Objective 9.14

9.13 The nurse is teaching an in-service educational presentation about working with battered women. The nurse should discuss that it is often frustrating for nurses to work with battered women because (Select all that apply.)
1. there is little the nurse can really do to help.
2. the woman is looking for a temporary solution to the problem.
3. both husband and wife must agree to therapy.

Answer: 1, 4, 5
Rationale: Working with victims of domestic abuse can be extremely frustrating because the nurse is seeing the problem from a more detached clinical perspective, while the victim experiences the violence emotionally. The abuser must seek behavior change therapy to accomplish permanent change. Nurses can offer suggestions for leaving the abuser, but cannot force the client to leave. Even if women have experienced nonviolent relationships, they often return to an abusive situation because they lack alternatives or fear reprisal. Women are often convinced by the abusers that it is their own behavior that causes the violence.
Implementation
Psychosocial Integrity
Analysis
Learning Objective 9.15

4. these women may return to the abusive situation.
5. women often accept that they are the cause of the violence.

9.14 A woman comes to the crisis prevention center anxious and upset. She tells the volunteer nurse who is working as a client advocate that she has been raped. The client says, "I think it is my fault this happened. I should never have worn that tight skirt." Which response by the nurse would be most appropriate?
1. "You should not dwell on why it happened. Now you need to deal with the complications that may occur because of the rape."
2. "Your reaction represents a myth. Women do not have to provoke the assailant to be raped."
3. "You need to stop blaming yourself."
4. "Even if you did provoke the assailant by wearing a tight skirt, he is responsible for his behavior."

Answer: 2
Rationale: Many women believe that their behavior has provoked their rapist's behavior, but this belief is a myth. And although rapists are responsible for their behavior, it is important to emphasize that nothing the victim did provoked the rape. Therapeutic communication prohibits telling clients what to think. It is important for women to not blame themselves, but it is critical for the nurse to use therapeutic communication techniques.
Implementation
Psychosocial Integrity
Analysis
Learning Objective 9.16

9.15 The emergency room nurse is admitting a client who has been sexually assaulted. The nurse is explaining how the physical evidence will be collected. Which statement made by the client indicates that teaching has been effective?
1. "All the evidence will be kept in a cupboard until the police arrive."
2. "You have to collect evidence to prove I wasn't sexually active."
3. "The evidence you collect may be able to identify the rapist."
4. "I will find out if the rapist has HIV from the evidence."

Answer: 3
Rationale: The evidence must remain in the hands of the nurse until handed directly to the police. One function of collecting evidence is to corroborate that sexual activity has taken place. DNA can be obtained from collected evidence to identify the rapist. Because diagnosis of infection cannot be made from evidence, rape victims are given preventative therapy against sexually transmitted infections (including gonorrhea, syphilis, and HIV) at the time of assault.
Evaluation
Psychosocial Integrity
Analysis
Learning Objective 9.17

CHAPTER 10

10.1 The pregnant client asks the nurse when the male and female reproductive organs begin to differentiate. The best answer would be, "This happens at
1. 4 weeks."
2. 8 weeks."
3. 14 weeks."
4. 20 weeks."

Answer: 2
Rationale: Reproductive organs begin differentiation at 8 weeks, and by 14 weeks the differences are apparent to the naked eye. Four weeks is too early and 20 weeks is too late.
Implementation
Health Promotion and Maintenance
Application
Learning Objective 10.1

10.2 The nurse is teaching a middle school class about embryonic reproductive organ development. Which statement indicates that the student understands this process?
1. "Boys are born with all the sperm they will ever have."
2. "Girls are born with all the ova they will ever have."

Answer: 2
Rationale: All the oocytes are present at birth; none develop later in life. Spermatogenesis (the development of sperm) does not occur until puberty, and continues throughout life for all males.
Evaluation
Health Promotion and Maintenance
Analysis
Learning Objective 10.1

---

3. "Girls develop additional ova as they mature." 4. "Some boys develop more sperm as they mature."	
10.3 A school nurse, teaching a health class to adolescent males, explains that spermatozoa become motile and fertile during the two to ten days they are stored in the 1. epididymis. 2. vas deferens. 3. prostate gland. 4. urethra.	Answer: 1 Rationale: The epididymis provides a reservoir where maturing spermatozoa become both motile and fertile. The spermatozoa remain in the epididymis for two to ten days. The vas deferens connects the epididymis to the prostate. The prostate gland secretes a fluid that protects the sperm from the acidic environment of the vagina. The urethra is the passageway for both urine and semen. Planning Health Promotion and Maintenance Application Learning Objective 10.2
10.4 The nurse is reviewing documentation by a student nurse. The student nurse encountered a 15-year-old girl who reported that she has no pubic or axillary hair and has not yet experienced growth of her breasts. The student nurse asks about the physiology of this occurrence. The nurse should explain to the student that this indicates the client probably lacks which hormone? 1. estrogen 2. progesterone 3. testosterone 4. prolactin	Answer: 1 Rationale: Estrogen is the primary hormone responsible for the development of secondary sex characteristics in females. Progesterone and prolactin do not accomplish this change. Testosterone is the primary hormone responsible for the development of secondary sex characteristics in males. Implementation Health Promotion and Maintenance Application Learning Objective 10.2
10.5 The nurse is teaching a class on erectile dysfunction. Based on the anatomy of the male external genitalia, which of the following is the most logical cause of the inability to achieve erection? 1. weakness or atrophy of the penile muscles 2. poor circulation to the penis 3. an undescended testicle 4. decreased functioning of the seminiferous tubules	Answer: 2 Rationale: Poor circulation to the penis is the most logical cause because the penis becomes erect as a result of innervation from the pudendal nerve, which causes its blood vessels to become engorged. Weakness or atrophy of the penile muscle, an undescended testicle, and decreased function of the seminiferous tubules do not play a primary role in the inability to achieve erection. Assessment Health Promotion and Maintenance Application Learning Objective 10.3
10.6 The nurse is preparing a handout on sterilization methods. The handout should explain that a man who has had a vasectomy becomes functionally sterile because the sperm 1. are no longer being produced. 2. are no longer motile and fertile. 3. cannot reach the outside of the body. 4. cannot penetrate an ovum.	Answer: 3 Rationale: Sperm cannot reach the outside of the body in a man who has a vasectomy. The main function of the vas deferens, which is ligated in a vasectomy, is to squeeze the sperm from their storage site into the urethra. Sperm continue to be produced in the seminiferous tubules in the testes and are not affected by a vasectomy. It is true that sperm cannot penetrate an ovum, but only because they cannot reach the outside of the body due to the ligation. A vasectomy does not affect motility or fertility of sperm. Planning Health Promotion and Maintenance Application Learning Objective 10.3
10.7 The client shows an understanding of the pelvic cavity divisions by stating: 1. "The true pelvis is made up of the sacrum, coccyx, and the innominate bones."	Answer: 1 Rationale: The true pelvis is made up of the sacrum, coccyx, and innominate bones and represents the bony limits of the birth canal. The true pelvis consists of the inlet, the pelvic cavity, and the outlet. The false pelvis is the portion above the pelvic brim. It is, therefore, the relationship between the true pelvis (not the false) and the fetal head that is of paramount importance.

2. "The false pelvis consists of the inlet, the pelvic cavity, and the outlet." 3. "The true pelvis is the portion above the pelvic brim." 4. "The relationship between the false pelvis and the fetal head is of paramount importance."	Evaluation Health Promotion and Maintenance Analysis Learning Objective 10.4
10.8 A pregnant adolescent asks the nurse, "Why does the physician call measuring my uterus 'a fundal height'?" The nurse's answer is based on the fact that the fundus of the uterus is located 1. in the elongated portion where the fallopian tubes enter. 2. in the lower third area. 3. at the uppermost (dome-shaped top) portion. 4. between the internal cervical os and the endometrial cavity.	Answer: 3 Rationale: The rounded uppermost (dome-shaped top) portion of the uterus that extends above the points of attachment of the fallopian tubes is called the fundus. The elongated portion where the fallopian tubes enter the uterus is called the cornua, and the lower third of the uterus is called the cervix or neck. The isthmus is the portion of the uterus between the internal cervical os and the endometrial cavity. Implementation Health Promotion and Maintenance Application Learning Objective 10.4
10.9 A nurse teaches newly pregnant clients that if an ovum is fertilized and implants in the endometrium, the hormone the fertilized egg begins to secrete is 1. estrogen. 2. human chorionic gonadotropin (hCG). 3. progesterone. 4. luteinizing hormone.	Answer: 2 Rationale: When the ovum is fertilized and implants in the endometrium, the fertilized egg begins to secrete human chorionic gonadotropin (hCG) hormone to maintain the corpus luteum. Estrogen and progesterone are ovarian hormones and luteinizing hormone is excreted by the anterior pituitary. Implementation Health Promotion and Maintenance Application Learning Objective 10.5
10.10 A school nurse is teaching a health class to middle school children. The nurse explains that the follicle-stimulating hormone (FSH) and luteinizing hormone (LH) are secreted by the 1. hypothalamus. 2. ovaries and testes. 3. posterior pituitary. 4. anterior pituitary.	Answer: 4 Rationale: The anterior pituitary secretes FSH and LH, which are primarily responsible for maturation of the ovarian follicle. The hypothalamus secretes gonadotropin-releasing hormone to the pituitary gland in response to signals from the central nervous system. The ovaries secrete the female hormones estrogen and progesterone, and the testes secrete testosterone. The posterior pituitary gland secretes oxytocin and anti-diuretic hormone. Implementation Health Promotion and Maintenance Analysis Learning Objective 10.5
10.11 The nurse is explaining the menstrual cycle to a group of women. The teaching on phases of the menstrual cycle should include the fact that the corpus luteum begins to degenerate, estrogen and progesterone levels fall, and the blood supply to the endometrium is reduced in which phase? 1. menstrual phase 2. proliferative phase 3. secretory phase 4. ischemic phase	Answer: 4 Rationale: The ischemic phase is characterized by ischemia of the endometrium. The menstrual phase is the mense. The proliferative phase is characterized by proliferation of the endometrium, while the secretory phase involves glycogen secretion by the endometrium after ovulation. Implementation Health Promotion and Maintenance Application Learning Objective 10.6
10.12 Which statement best indicates that the client understands the differences in the follicular and luteal phases of the ovarian cycle?	Answer: 2 Rationale: For a female with a 28-day cycle, the follicular phase comprises days 1–14 of the menstrual cycle, and the luteal phase comprises days 15–28. The

1. "My period will be every 28 days." 2. "The first part of my period may vary in length, but not the second." 3. "The follicular phase is the second half of my cycle." 4. "The follicular phase is when the egg is fertilized."	follicular phase may vary, resulting in cycle length other than 28 days, but the luteal phase does not vary. Evaluation Health Promotion and Maintenance Analysis Learning Objective 10.6
10.13 The nurse is preparing a handout for female adolescents on the menstrual cycle. The nurse is including information on the phases of the menstrual cycle. What term should be used for the phase in which the vascularity of the uterus increases and the endometrium becomes prepared for a fertilized ovum? 1. menstrual 2. proliferative 3. secretory 4. ischemic	Answer: 2 Rationale: The proliferative phase refers to the buildup of the endometrium as blood supply and uterine size is increased. The menstrual phase refers to the cyclic uterine bleeding in response to hormonal changes. The secretory phase occurs after ovulation and the ischemic phase occurs if fertilization does not occur. Planning Health Promotion and Maintenance Application Learning Objective 10.7
10.14 A woman is experiencing mittelschmerz and increased vaginal discharge. Her temperature has increased by 0.6°C (1.0° F) for the past 36 hours. This most likely indicates that 1. menstruation is about to begin. 2. ovulation will occur soon. 3. ovulation has occurred. 4. she is pregnant and will not menstruate.	Answer: 3 Rationale: Signs that ovulation has occurred include: pain associated with rupture of the ovum (mittelschmerz), increased vaginal discharge, and a temperature increase of 0.6°C for the past 36 hours. A temperature increase does not occur when menstruation is about to begin or before ovulation has occurred. Pregnancy can only be detected through testing the urine or serum for the presence of human chorionic gonadotropin hormone. Assessment Health Promotion and Maintenance Application Learning Objective 10.7
10.15 The nurse has presented a class on reproduction at a college. The nurse knows that teaching has been effective if a student states, "Once the ovum has entered the fallopian tube, movement of the ovum through the fallopian tube and toward the uterus is facilitated by 1. estrogen-induced tubal peristalsis." 2. progesterone-induced cervical mucus changes." 3. motions of the fallopian fimbriae." 4. movements of the corona radiata of the ovum."	Answer: 1 Rationale: Estrogen-induced tubal peristalsis helps move the ovum through the tube, as the ovum has no inherent power of movement. Progesterone-induced cervical changes also can aid in ovum transport but are not the primary mover. Motions of the fallopian fimbriae occur as the ovum is released at ovulation but do not facilitate the movement through the fallopian tube. Movements of the corona radiata of the ovum surround the zona pellucida, and since the ovum has no inherent power of movement, it does not facilitate movement through the fallopian tube. Evaluation Health Promotion and Maintenance Analysis Learning Objective 10.3

CHAPTER 11

11.1 The nurse is preparing a class on reproduction. The cell division process that results in two identical cells, each with the same number of chromosomes as the original cell, should be termed 1. meiosis. 2. mitosis. 3. oogenesis. 4. gametogenesis.	Answer: 2 Rationale: Mitosis is the process of cell division that was described. Meiosis is a process of cell division that leads to the development of eggs and sperm. Oogenesis is the process by which female gametes, or ova, are produced. Gametogenesis is the process by which germ cells are produced. Planning Health Promotion and Maintenance Application Learning Objective 11.1
11.2 The nurse is present for the delivery of a preterm fetus. The fetus is wrinkled, covered with vernix, opens	Answer: 2 Rationale: The fetus in the description is at 25 weeks gestation. At 23 weeks, the fetal skin is reddish and wrinkled, and the eyes are still closed. At 34 weeks, the

and closes its eyelids, and has physiologically immature lungs that cannot sufficiently provide gas exchange. What gestational age is this fetus?
1. 23 weeks
2. 25 weeks
3. 34 weeks
4. 36 weeks

fetus has less wrinkled skin and lanugo begins to disappear. At 36 weeks, lung maturity has occurred to provide for gas exchange.
Assessment
Health Promotion and Maintenance
Analysis
Learning Objective 11.5

11.3 The nurse is presenting a class to pregnant clients. The nurse asks, "The fetal brain is developing rapidly and the nervous system is complete enough to provide some regulation of body function on its own at which fetal development stage?" It is clear that education has been effective when a participant responds
1. "the 17th to 20th week."
2. "the 25th to 28th week."
3. "the 29th to 32nd week."
4. "the 33rd to 36th week."

Answer: 2
Rationale: Nervous system function that is complex enough to provide body function regulation occurs around the 25th to 28th week, which is when a fetus has a good chance of survival if born. The other dates are either too early or too late in gestation.
Evaluation
Health Promotion and Maintenance
Analysis
Learning Objective 11.5

11.4 The nurse is presenting a class on conception to a group of middle school students. Which answer to this question indicates that learning has occurred? "In order for fertilization to occur, what portion of the sperm must enter the ovum?"
1. the entire sperm
2. only the head
3. only the tail
4. either the head or the tail

Answer: 2
Rationale: Only the head of the sperm is required to enter the ovum for fertilization to occur. For this reason, none of the other answers (the entire sperm, only the tail, and either the head or the tail) are correct.
Evaluation
Health Promotion and Maintenance
Application
Learning Objective 11.3

11.5 A pregnant woman tells the midwife, "I've heard that if I eat certain foods during my pregnancy, the baby will be a boy." The nurse midwife's response should explain that this is a myth, and that the sex of the baby is determined at the time of
1. ejaculation.
2. fertilization.
3. implantation.
4. differentiation.

Answer: 2
Rationale: Fertilization is the time when the sex of the zygote is determined. Ejaculation is the release of sperm from the male. Implantation is when the fertilized ovum is implanted in the uterine endometrium. Differentiation refers to a cell division process.
Implementation
Health Promotion and Maintenance
Application
Learning Objective 11.3

11.6 A client tells you that her mother was a twin, two of her sisters have twins, and several cousins either are twins or gave birth to twins. The client, too, is expecting twins. Because there is a genetic predisposition to twins in her family, there is a good chance that the client will have
1. dizygotic twins.
2. monozygotic twins.
3. identical twins.
4. nonzygotic twins.

Answer: 1
Rationale: A familial history of twins usually results in dizygotic (fraternal) twins, or twins that result from two separate ova. Monozygotic twins, also known as identical twins, are not familial. Nonzygotic twins do not exist.
Assessment
Health Promotion and Maintenance
Analysis
Learning Objective 11.4

11.7 Which statement by a pregnant client would indicate that additional teaching was necessary?
1. "Because of their birth relationship, fraternal twins are more similar to each other than if they had been born singly."
2. "Identical twins may be the same or different sex."
3. "Congenital abnormalities are more prevalent in identical twins."
4. "Identical twins occur more frequently than fraternal twins."

Answer: 3
Rationale: Due to variations in the timing of the splitting of the embryo, congenital abnormalities such as conjoining are more common in monozygotic twins. Identical or monozygotic twins have identical chromosomal structures, and therefore are always the same sex. Dizygotic, or fraternal twins, occur more frequently than monozygotic twins.
Evaluation
Health Promotion and Maintenance
Analysis
Learning Objective 11.4

11.8 The nurse is evaluating information that was taught about conception and fetal development. When the client verbalizes her understanding about transportation time of the zygote through the fallopian tube and into the cavity of the uterus, which statement shows correct understanding?
1. "It will take at least three days for the egg to reach the uterus."
2. "It will take eight days for the egg to reach the uterus."
3. "It will only take 12 hours for the egg to go through the fallopian tube."
4. "It will take 18 hours for the fertilized egg to implant in the uterus."

Answer: 1
Rationale: It takes at least three days for fertilized egg to reach the uterus. The other statements do not accurately describe the transportation time of the zygote through the fallopian tube and into the cavity of the uterus.
Evaluation
Health Promotion and Maintenance
Application
Learning Objective 11.3

11.9 The pregnant client who is at 14 weeks' gestation asks the nurse why the doctor used to call her baby an embryo, and now calls it a fetus. What is the best answer to this question?
1. "A fetus is the term used from the ninth week of gestation and onward."
2. "We call a baby a fetus when it is larger than an embryo."
3. "An embryo is a baby from conception until the eighth week."
4. "The official term for a baby in utero is really *zygote*."

Answer: 1
Rationale: The fetal stage begins in the ninth week. The pre-embryonic stage is from conception until day 15. The embryonic stage ends with the eighth week. A zygote is a fertilized ovum.
Implementation
Health Promotion and Maintenance
Application
Learning Objective 11.5

11.10 During a prenatal examination, an adolescent client asks, "How does my baby get air?" The nurse would give correct information by saying:
1. "The lungs of the fetus carry out respiratory gas exchange in utero similar to what an adult experiences."
2. "The placenta assumes the function of the fetal lungs by supplying oxygen and allowing the excretion of carbon dioxide into your bloodstream."
3. "The blood from the placenta is carried through the umbilical artery,

Answer: 2
Rationale: The placenta assumes the function of the fetal lungs by supplying oxygen and allowing the excretion of carbon dioxide into the maternal bloodstream. Most of the blood supply bypasses the fetal lungs, since they do not carry out respiratory gas exchange. The blood from the placenta is carried through the umbilical vein, not the umbilical artery. The fetus has a hemoglobin concentration that is 50% greater prior to birth.
Implementation
Health Promotion and Maintenance
Application
Learning Objective 11.6

which penetrates the abdominal wall of the fetus."

4. "The fetus is able to obtain sufficient oxygen due to the fact that your hemoglobin concentration is 50% greater during pregnancy."

11.11 The client has read that the placenta produces hormones that are vital to the function of the fetus. It is evident that the client understands the function of the placenta if she states which hormone is primarily responsible for the maintenance of pregnancy past the eleventh week?

1. human chorionic gonadotropin (hCG)
2. human placental lactogen (hPL)
3. estrogen
4. progesterone

Answer: 4
Rationale: Progesterone is primarily responsible for maintenance of pregnancy past the eleventh week because it decreases the contractility of the uterus, thus preventing uterine contractions from causing spontaneous abortion. Human chorionic gonadotropin (HCG) begins to decrease as placental hormone production increases. Human placental lactogen (hPL) stimulates certain changes in the mother's metabolic processes and can be detected by four weeks after conception. Estrogen that is secreted by the placenta is in the form of estriol and cannot be synthesized by the placenta alone.
Evaluation
Health Promotion and Maintenance
Analysis
Learning Objective 11.6

11.12 The client is at 20 weeks' gestation, and asks the nurse what would be typical of a fetus at 20 weeks? How should the nurse reply? (Select all that apply.)

1. "The fetus has a body weight of 435 to 465 g."
2. "The fetus actively sucks and swallows amniotic fluid."
3. "The kidneys begin to produce urine."
4. "Nipples appear over the mammary glands."
5. "Activity and movement happens about once per day."

Answer: 1, 2, 4
Rationale: A fetus at 20 weeks has a body weight of 435 to 465 g, can actively suck and swallow amniotic fluid, has nipples that appear over the mammary glands, and has lanugo that covers the entire body. Kidneys begin to produce urine between nine and twelve weeks' gestation. Fetal activity develops earlier.
Implementation
Health Promotion and Maintenance
Analysis
Learning Objective 11.7

11.13 At her first prenatal visit, a woman and the nurse are discussing fetal development. The client asks, "When will my baby actually have a heartbeat?" The nurse should reply, "The heartbeat of an embryo is distinguishable by week number _____ of development."

1. four
2. six
3. eight
4. twelve

Answer: 1
Rationale: The tubular heart beats at a regular rhythm and pushing its own primitive blood cells through the main blood vessels in the fourth week of fetal development. The other answers are stages that are too late.
Implementation
Health Promotion and Maintenance
Application
Learning Objective 11.7

11.14 The nurse is preparing a preconception information class. Information about causes of fetal organ malformation in the first trimester will be presented. What prenatal influences on the intrauterine environment should be included in the instruction? (Select all that apply.)

1. the use of saunas or hot tubs
2. the use of drugs
3. the quality of the sperm or ovum
4. maternal nutrition
5. age of the mother at conception

Answer: 1, 2, 4
Rationale: The use of saunas or hot tubs is associated with maternal hyperthermia, and is associated with neural tube defects. Many drugs can have teratogenic effects. Maternal nutrition, if deficient, can cause damage to the fetus. Vitamins and folic acid taken prior to and during the pregnancy can have beneficial effects. The quality of the sperm or ovum can affect fertility, but not organ formation. A maternal age of 35 or older is associated with genetic defects that occur at conception, not later in the first trimester.
Implementation
Health Promotion and Maintenance
Application
Learning Objective 11.8

11.15 The nurse is presenting information on pregnancy and fetal development. In order to evaluate learning, the nurse asks the following question. "When a female reaches adolescence, the ova continue to divide by the process of meiosis. How many chromosomes do the resulting cells then have?"
1. 46 double-structured chromosomes
2. 46 single chromosomes
3. 23 double-structured chromosomes
4. 23 single chromosomes

Answer: 3
Rationale: Meiosis is the process of cells splitting their genetic material during replication. The first meiotic division of ova results in half the original number of chromosomes. The second meiotic division occurs after adolescence and creates 23 double-structured chromosomes.
Evaluation
Health Promotion and Maintenance
Application
Learning Objective 11.2

CHAPTER 12

12.1 The nurse is planning a class to teach couples about factors that influence fertility. What should be included in the teaching plan?
1. sexual intercourse should occur one to three times a week
2. get up to urinate immediately after intercourse
3. douche at least twice per week
4. use stress reduction techniques

Answer: 1
Rationale: Intercourse should occur one to three times per week at intervals of no less than 48 hours. Women should be instructed to wait to urinate for one hour after intercourse, and to avoid douching. Stress reduction techniques should be included in the teaching plan.
Planning
Health Promotion and Maintenance
Application
Learning Objective 12.1

12.2 The nurse obtains a health history from the following client. Which piece of data should alert the nurse to include infertility teaching in her discussion?
1. circumcision as a newborn
2. history of premature ejaculation
3. history of measles at age 12
4. employment as an engineer

Answer: 2
Rationale: Premature ejaculation is a possible cause of infertility. Circumcision, having the measles, and being an engineer do not affect fertility.
Assessment
Health Promotion and Maintenance
Application
Learning Objective 12.2

12.3 A nurse is reviewing the basal body temperature method with a couple. Which of the following statements would indicate that the teaching has been successful?
1. "I have to go buy a special type of thermometer."
2. "I need to wait five minutes after smoking a cigarette before I take my temperature."
3. "I need to take my temperature before I get out of the bed in the morning."
4. "I need to take my temperature for at least two minutes every day."

Answer: 3
Rationale: In the basal body temperature method, the woman takes her temperature for five minutes every day before arising, and before starting any activity, including smoking. The temperature can be taken with a standard oral or rectal thermometer.
Evaluation
Health Promotion and Maintenance
Analysis
Learning Objective 12.3

12.4 A client calls the urologist's office to receive instructions about semen analysis. The nurse should instruct the client to
1. avoid sexual intercourse 24 hours prior to obtaining specimen.
2. use a latex condom to collect the specimen.
3. expect that a repeat test may be required.
4. expect a small sample.

Answer: 3
Rationale: A repeat semen analysis may be required to adequately assess the man's fertility potential. The specimen is collected after two to three days of abstinence, usually by masturbation. Regular condoms should not be used, because of the spermicidal agents that they contain. Instructing the client to expect a small sample is not appropriate.
Implementation
Health Promotion and Maintenance
Application
Learning Objective 12.3

12.5 The nurse in a fertility clinic is working with a woman who has been undergoing infertility treatment with clomiphene citrate (Clomid) and menotropin (Repronex). Which statement would the nurse expect the woman to make?

1. "I feel moody so much of the time."
2. "If this doesn't work, I think my husband will leave me."
3. "This combination of medications will guarantee a pregnancy."
4. "My risk of twins or triplets is the same as the general population."

Answer: 1
Rationale: Moodiness is a common side effect when menotropins are used for infertility treatment. Although infertility can be stressful on a marriage relationship, the nurse does not expect a marriage to end if pregnancy is not achieved. There is no guarantee for any medication. Multifetal pregnancies are more likely when any medication is used to stimulate fertility.
Assessment
Health Promotion and Maintenance
Application
Learning Objective 12.4

12.6 An infertile couple confides in the nurse at the infertility clinic that they feel overwhelmed with the decisions that face them. Which of the following nursing strategies would be most appropriate?

1. Refer them to a marriage counselor in the same building.
2. Provide them with information throughout the diagnostic process.
3. Express concern and provide counseling to the couple.
4. Inquire about the names they have chosen for their baby.

Answer: 2
Rationale: The nurse can provide comfort to couples by offering a sympathetic ear, a nonjudgmental approach, and appropriate information and instruction throughout the diagnostic and therapeutic process. Expressing concern, inquiring about names, and referring the couple to a counselor are not appropriate.
Implementation
Health Promotion and Maintenance
Application
Learning Objective 12.5

12.7 The nurse is planning a group session for parents who are beginning infertility evaluation. Which statement should be included in this session? (Select all that apply.)

1. "Infertility can be stressful for a marriage."
2. "The doctor will be able to tell why you have not conceived."
3. "Your insurance will pay for the infertility treatments."
4. "Keep communicating with one another through this process."
5. "Taking a vacation usually results in pregnancy."

Answer: 1, 4
Rationale: Infertility is often stressful on a marriage, as a result of the need to schedule intercourse, pay for treatments, and the societal expectation to have children. Communication is important to help cope with stress. A nurse should always encourage clients to ask questions. Some infertility cannot be explained despite extensive treatments. Insurance often does not pay for infertility treatment. A common myth is that taking a vacation or just relaxing will result in conception.
Planning
Health Promotion and Maintenance
Application
Learning Objective 12.5

12.8 The nurse is reviewing preconception questionnaires in charts. Which couple is the most likely candidate for preconceptual genetic counseling?

1. wife is 30 years old, husband is 31 years old
2. wife and husband are both 29 years old, first baby for husband, wife has a normal 4-year-old
3. wife's family has a history of hemophilia
4. single 32-year-old woman, using donor sperm

Answer: 3
Rationale: Hemophilia is a sex-linked disorder; therefore, the couple with hemophilia in the wife's family is at risk for hemophilia in male offspring. An age of less than 35 is not a risk factor for genetic abnormalities. Sperm donors are screened for genetic disorders, and men with a possible genetic problem are not accepted for sperm donation.
Planning
Health Promotion and Maintenance
Application
Learning Objective 12.6

12.9 A couple is at the clinic for preconceptual counseling. Both parents are 40 years old. The nurse knows that the education session has been successful when the wife states (Select all that apply.)

1. "We are at low risk for having a baby with Down syndrome."
2. "Our children are more likely to have genetic defects."
3. "Children born to parents this age have sex-linked disorders."
4. "The tests for genetic defects can be done early in pregnancy."
5. "It will be almost impossible for us to conceive a child."

Answer: 2, 4

Rationale: When a mother will be 35 years or older at the time of delivery, there is an increased risk of genetic defects like trisomy 21 (Down syndrome.) Genetic testing such as amniocentesis and chorionic villus sampling are done in the first trimester. Sex-linked disorders are not related to the age of either parent. Parents undergo genetic testing if there is a known or suspected family history of a genetic disorder, not based on their age. Fertility decreases somewhat after age 35, but age over 35 does not mean that conception is impossible.

Evaluation

Health Promotion and Maintenance

Application

Learning Objective 12.6

12.10 A 45-year-old mother gave birth to a baby boy two days ago. The nurse assesses a single palmar crease, poor muscle tone, and low-set ears on the newborn. The nurse understands that these signs most likely indicate the infant has which autosomal abnormalities?

1. trisomy 13
2. trisomy 18
3. trisomy 21
4. trisomy 26

Answer: 3

Rationale: A single palmar crease and low-set ears are characteristics of trisomy 21 (Down syndrome). They are not characteristics of trisomy 13 or trisomy 18. Trisomy 26 is not an autosomal abnormality.

Assessment

Health Promotion and Maintenance

Application

Learning Objective 12.7

12.11 A nurse counsels a couple who have concerns about a sex-linked disorder. Both parents are carriers of the disorder. They ask the nurse how this disorder will affect any children they may have. What is the nurse's best response?

1. "If you have a daughter, she will not be affected."
2. "If you have a son, he will not be affected."
3. "There is a 25% chance that a daughter will have the disorder."
4. "There is a 50% chance that a son will be a carrier."

Answer: 4

Rationale: If both parents carry a sex-linked disorder, they each have one normal sex chromosome and one abnormal female sex chromosome. There is a 50% chance of male offspring being carriers and a 50% chance of males being normal. With female offspring, there is a 50% of being a carrier, and a 50% chance of having the disorder.

Implementation

Health Promotion and Maintenance

Analysis

Learning Objective 12.7

12.12 The couple has had an ultrasound at 19 weeks' gestation, and their fetus was found to have anencephaly. The nurse is completing counseling for the couple on the ultrasound findings. Which statement indicates that additional teaching is needed?

1. "We won't know if something is wrong until the baby's chromosomes are tested."
2. "This problem is not caused by one of us having a genetic problem."
3. "Our baby has an incomplete brain, and may not be born alive."
4. "Waiting until our 30s did not cause this problem to develop."

Answer: 1

Rationale: Anencephaly is a condition in which the skull does not cover the brain completely, and the brain consists mostly of brain stem with little other brain development. This condition is clearly visualized with ultrasound, and does not require genetic testing to verify a diagnosis. Folic acid deficiency is a contributing factor, but neither age nor genetic abnormalities in either parent are related to anencephaly.

Evaluation

Health Promotion and Maintenance

Analysis

Learning Objective 12.8

12.13 A male infant was born two days ago, and the nurse assessed the infant as having single palmar crease, poor muscle tone, and low-set ears. Genetic testing of the infant has been ordered by the physician. Which statement should the nurse include when explaining this plan to the parents?

1. "We will draw blood from both of you to check for abnormal genes."
2. "Your son will have his chromosomes sampled and then studied."
3. "When your son is two years old, he will need a blood test."
4. "After your breast milk is in, we will draw blood from your son."

Answer: 2

Rationale: A single palmar crease, poor muscle tone, and low-set ears may indicate trisomy 18. This diagnosis is confirmed by chromosomal analysis of the infant, using either a buchal smear or a blood specimen. The chromosome studies will be undertaken as soon as possible. The parents' chromosomes do not need to be assessed in order to diagnose the infant. It is not necessary to wait until the breast milk has come in.

Planning

Health Promotion and Maintenance

Application

Learning Objective 12.8

12.14 The couple at 12 weeks' gestation has been told that their fetus has sickle cell disease. Which statement by the couple indicates that they are adequately coping?

1. "We knew we were both carriers of sickle cell. We shouldn't have tried to have a baby."
2. "If we had been healthier when we conceived, our baby wouldn't have this disease now."
3. "Taking vitamins before we got pregnant would have prevented this from happening."
4. "The doctor told us there was a 25% chance that our baby would have sickle disease."

Answer: 4

Rationale: A true statement indicates coping. When both the mother and father are carriers of an autosomal recessive disease like sickle cell, there is a 25% chance of a normal child, a 25% chance of a child with sickle cell disease, and a 50% chance of a child with sickle cell trait. Preconception health and nutrition do not affect transmission of an autosomal recessive trait. Self-blame and judgment do not indicate coping.

Assessment

Health Promotion and Maintenance

Application

Learning Objective 12.9

12.15 The 28-year-old husband and wife have just been told their child has trisomy 21. Their 3-year-old child has no health problems. What statement should the nurse include in counseling this family?

1. "Don't worry. Everything will turn out for the best."
2. "It can be very difficult to understand why God chose you for this problem."
3. "Your child's disorder was not predictable, and not the fault of either of you."
4. "Your 3-year-old will need extra attention given a sibling with special needs."

Answer: 3

Rationale: Therapeutic communication avoids clichés and philosophical answers involving God. The needs of the 3-year-old are less important right now than reassuring the couple that neither of them caused the genetic abnormality of their newborn.

Planning

Health Promotion and Maintenance

Analysis

Learning Objective 12.9

CHAPTER 13

13.1 A primigravida is admitted to the labor unit with contractions every seven to eight minutes. She is 3 cm dilated, 70% effaced, and at 0 station. She is very anxious, is having difficulty coping with

Answer: 1

Rationale: Abdominal breathing and progressive relaxation assist the client in relaxing and allow the uterine muscles to work more efficiently. Patterned paced breathing and touch relaxation are exercises that are taught in childbirth

---

contractions, and states that she did not attend prenatal classes. Which of the following would be the most effective nursing intervention?
1. Instruct the client in abdominal breathing and progressive relaxation.
2. Instruct the client in patterned paced breathing and touch relaxation.
3. Instruct the client in pelvic tilt and pelvic rock exercises.
4. Call the physician and request a sedative.

preparation classes and involve the use of a partner. Pelvic tilt and rock exercises are body-conditioning exercises. Providing sedatives would not allow the client to participate actively in the process.
Implementation
Health Promotion and Maintenance
Application
Learning Objective 13.1

13.2 The nurse is assisting an expectant couple in developing a birth plan. Which of the following instructions would the nurse include in the teaching plan?
1. The birth plan includes only client choices and does not take into account standard choices of the healthcare provider.
2. The birth plan allows the client to make choices about the birth process; however, these choices cannot be altered.
3. The birth plan is a legally-binding contract between the client and the healthcare provider.
4. The birth plan is a communication tool between the client and the healthcare provider.

Answer: 4
Rationale: The birth plan is used as a tool for communication among the expectant parents, the healthcare provider, and the healthcare professionals at the birth setting. It is not a legal document. The written plan identifies options that are available; thus, it can be altered.
Planning
Health Promotion and Maintenance
Application
Learning Objective 13.1

13.3 A couple would like their 5-year-old to attend the birth. Which statement by the nurse would assist in the family's plan to include their 5-year-old in the birth?
1. "You should let your child stay home because you will be focusing on the birth."
2. "Children under 12 are not allowed to be present at the birth."
3. "You should bring someone who can tend only to any specific needs of your child."
4. "Bring some toys to keep your child occupied."

Answer: 3
Rationale: A sibling should have his or her own support person whose primary responsibility is to take care of the child's needs so that the child will have support if anxiety develops over the birth process, and the mother can concentrate on the labor and birth. Children are allowed to be present at births. Preparing the child on what to expect is beneficial. Toys will not sustain a 5-year-old's attention for an extended time period.
Implementation
Health Promotion and Maintenance
Application
Learning Objective 13.1

13.4 While teaching a preconception class, the nurse should include which of the following recommendations to decrease the risk of neural tube defects?
1. 500 mg vitamin C every day
2. 0.4 mg folate every day
3. 1500 mg calcium every day
4. 600 mg vitamin A every day

Answer: 2
Rationale: Folic acid supplementation prior to conception is recommended since this decreases the risk of neural tube defects. The other nutrients do not decrease the risk of neural tube defects.
Planning
Health Promotion and Maintenance
Application
Learning Objective 13.2

13.5 An expectant couple desires to determine compatibility with a care provider. They ask the nurse for assistance. Which of the following

Answer: 3
Rationale: A thorough understanding of the provider's philosophy is essential to determining compatibility. Children's attendance, a husband's presence for a cesarean birth, and episiotomy percentages are complements to the provider's philosophy.

---

questions should the nurse encourage the couple to ask first? 1. "Can my children attend the birth?" 2. "If I have a cesarean birth, can my husband attend?" 3. "What is your philosophy of birth?" 4. "What percentage of your clients has episiotomies?"	Implementation Health Promotion and Maintenance Analysis Learning Objective 13.2
13.6 Regardless of the method of childbirth preparation, most childbirth classes 1. present ways of alleviating fear. 2. teach imagery for relaxation. 3. use patterned paced breathing techniques. 4. present the benefits of epidural anesthesia.	Answer: 1 Rationale: The overall goal of prenatal classes is to decrease fear through increasing knowledge and teaching participants skills to help cope with labor. These skills include various relaxation methods and breathing techniques. Not all classes teach imagery, nor do all use patterned paced breathing. Many couples will be able to avoid an epidural by using the techniques they learned in classes. Planning Health Promotion and Maintenance Application Learning Objective 13.6
13.7 An expectant mother asks a nurse, "Why do I need to learn breathing patterns for use during labor?" The nurse relates to the client that the primary reason for using controlled breathing patterns during labor is to 1. promote adequate oxygen to the laboring mother and the baby. 2. keep the laboring mother distracted. 3. keep the laboring mother awake. 4. involve the partner in the birth process.	Answer: 1 Rationale: Breathing techniques help keep the mother and her unborn baby adequately oxygenated. Breathing techniques are not intended to distract the laboring mother but to focus her attention. They are not done to keep the laboring mother awake or to involve the partner in the birth process. Implementation Health Promotion and Maintenance Application Learning Objective 13.3
13.8 The nurse is teaching a class to prenatal clients about the benefits of a doula. Which statement by a client demonstrates the need for further teaching? 1. "The doula will deliver the baby." 2. "The doula will assist with the birth." 3. "The doula will provide guidance and encouragement." 4. "The doula will attend to my comfort needs."	Answer: 1 Rationale: The doula is trained to assist with births, but she does not deliver the baby. The doula offers guidance and encouragement and attends to the many comfort needs of the laboring mother and her family. Evaluation Health Promotion and Maintenance Analysis Learning Objective 13.4
13.9 A client having her fourth child is admitted to the labor unit and is accompanied by a doula. The intrapartum nurse expects the doula to assist with 1. fetal monitoring and relaxation techniques. 2. physical and emotional comfort techniques. 3. breathing techniques and labor assessment. 4. massage and vaginal exams.	Answer: 2 Rationale: A doula is a trained lay birth companion, and focuses on helping the mother to relax and increase her comfort. Fetal monitoring, labor assessment, and vaginal exams are performed by nurses and physicians. Planning Health Promotion and Maintenance Analysis Learning Objective 13.4
13.10 During a breastfeeding class, the nurse discusses ways to include the father in the breastfeeding process. The nurse knows that further teaching is necessary when a prospective father states	Answer: 1 Rationale: Feeding the baby a bottle is not an option, so this statement indicates a need for further teaching. Breastfeeding has to be well-established before bottles are introduced to avoid nipple confusion. The father can participate in the breastfeeding process by bringing the baby to the mother for feedings, burping

1. "I can feed the baby a bottle." 2. "I can burp the baby between breasts." 3. "I can rock the baby to sleep after breastfeeding." 4. "When the baby wakes up, I can bring the baby to her mother."	the baby between breasts and/or after feeding, and rocking the baby back to sleep. Evaluation Health Promotion and Maintenance Analysis Learning Objective 13.5
13.11 What content would be appropriate for a nurse to include in an early pregnancy class? 1. the father's role in breastfeeding 2. purchasing of a car seat 3. how to care for an episiotomy 4. methods to cope with stress	Answer: 4 Rationale: Coping with stress is an appropriate topic for an early pregnancy class. The father's role in breastfeeding is a topic for a breastfeeding class. Purchasing a car seat and episiotomy care are topics that are appropriate for later classes (second and third trimesters). Planning Health Promotion and Maintenance Application Learning Objective 13.5
13.12 Following the birth of her infant, a client states that her childbirth classes assisted her in dealing with labor and birth. The nurse understands that current research on childbirth education demonstrates which of the following benefits? 1. Clients develop a strong attachment to the birth attendant. 2. Clients avoid the use of medication for labor. 3. Clients become dependent upon their partners. 4. Clients have a feeling of control over the birthing process.	Answer: 4 Rationale: Current research indicates that parents who participate in childbirth education have a greater sense of control over their labor and birth experience. Childbirth classes do not increase the attachment to the birth attendant, or dependence on the partner. Childbirth education participants may use less medication during labor, but not all will avoid all use of medication. Assessment Health Promotion and Maintenance Analysis Learning Objective 13.3
13.13 A nurse conducts a class on touch relaxation. What is the correct order for the steps of touch relaxation? (Create a five digit number as your answer.) 1. The partner touches the tensed muscles. 2. The woman relaxes the tense muscles in response to her partner's touch. 3. The woman should tense a muscle group. 4. Partner gently strokes the tensed muscle group. 5. The woman releases all the residual tension of the muscle group.	Answer: 31245 Rationale: Touch relaxation increases cooperation and teamwork between the woman and her partner during labor. The steps for this technique using the facial muscles would be: The woman contracts the facial muscles by grimacing, the partner places one hand on either side of the face, the woman releases the tension in the facial muscles as the partner's hands are touching the tense muscles, the partner gently strokes downward over the face and jaw muscles, and the woman releases the residual tension. Evaluation Health Promotion and Maintenance Application Learning Objective 13.6
13.14 A couple discusses their childbirth preparation options with the nurse. They want the father to be actively involved, and for the expectant mother to avoid medications during the birthing process. What is the nurse's best response? 1. "The hospital will follow your wishes." 2. "The Leboyer method will provide what you want."	Answer: 3 Rationale: The Bradley method is referred to as partner- or husband-coached natural childbirth. The Lamaze method involves the breathing techniques that facilitate delivery by relaxing at the proper time. The Leboyer method emphasizes the provision of a gentle and peaceful environment for the birth process. Prenatal education helps couples understand the birth process so that they can express their wishes to hospital staff. Implementation Health Promotion and Maintenance Application Learning Objective 13.7

3. "The Bradley method will meet your needs."
4. "The Lamaze method will be easy to follow."

13.15 A client states that she is not interested in Lamaze classes because she is single and does not want to have natural childbirth. What would be the nurse's best response?
1. "If you practice and learn the Lamaze methods, your pain is minimal."
2. "Lamaze classes teach you relaxation methods and assist you in making decisions."
3. "You are very nervous. I think these classes would be best for you."
4. "Lamaze classes are geared toward couples. You may want to find a different class."

Answer: 2
Rationale: Lamaze teaches relaxation methods by utilizing patterned breathing. Those who are able to use the method require little if any analgesia or anesthesia during delivery. Single women and couples attend Lamaze classes. Therapeutic communication prohibits directing a client, and instead focuses on facilitating a client's decision making.
Implementation
Health Promotion and Maintenance
Analysis
Learning Objective 13.7

CHAPTER 14

14.1 The client is at 36 weeks' gestation. The nurse understands that the pregnancy is progressing normally when she sees which of the following physiologic changes documented on the client's prenatal record? (Select all that apply.)
1. The joints of the pelvis have relaxed, causing hip pain.
2. The cervix is firm and purplish-blue in color.
3. The uterine fundus is at a height of 35 cm above the pubic symphysis.
4. Gastric emptying time is prolonged, and the client complains of gas and bloating.
5. Hair loss is increased, with thinning of the hair.

Answer: 1, 3, 4
Rationale: The pregnancy hormone relaxin creates softening of the ligaments, which in turn can lead to hip or pubic symphysis pain in late pregnancy. The growing fetus causes an enlargement of the uterus; from 20 weeks until delivery, the fundal height measured in cm should be within 2–3 of the number of weeks of gestation. Gas and bloating are seen as the increased progesterone level causes smooth muscle relaxation, which results in delayed gastric emptying and slowed peristalsis. Supine hypotension occurs when the fetus compresses the vena cava against the vertebrae when the mother is supine. Cervical changes during pregnancy include softening and purplish-blue discoloration. Hair loss is slowed during pregnancy, creating a perceived thickening of the hair.
Assessment
Health Promotion and Maintenance
Application
Learning Objective 14.1

14.2 The pregnant client at 16 weeks' gestation has hemoglobin level of 10.5. Her pre-pregnancy hemoglobin level was 13. Which of the following statements should the nurse use to best explain this change to the client?
1. "You are having a problem in pregnancy not making enough red cells."
2. "Because your blood volume has increased, your hemoglobin has dropped."
3. "This change may indicate a serious problem that might harm your baby."
4. "You are not eating nearly enough iron-rich foods like meat."

Answer: 2
Rationale: The blood volume expands rapidly during pregnancy in order to oxygenate the fetus. Physiologic anemia of pregnancy is a normal finding, and occurs during the mid-trimester in women who are not taking supplemental iron. The blood volume expands faster than the erythrocytes can be manufactured, which creates a temporary anemia. No harm will come to the fetus because of this physiologic change.
Implementation
Health Promotion and Maintenance
Application
Learning Objective 14.1

14.3 The nurse is interviewing clients in their third trimester of pregnancy. Which of the following client complaints would be expected? (Select all that apply.)
1. Her chest circumference has increased by 5 cm during the pregnancy.
2. She has a widened subcostal angle.
3. She is using thoracic breathing.
4. She has a respiratory rate of 30.
5. She has a productive cough.

Answer: 1, 2, 3
Rationale: Early in pregnancy, the respiratory rate increases to meet the oxygen demands of the growing fetus. Thoracic breathing is one mechanism that facilitates increased oxygen intake. As the fetus grows, the lower rib cage expands, leading to a widened subcostal angle and an increased chest circumference. The respiratory rate will increase slightly, but 30 breaths per minute is tachypnea. A productive cough is never a normal finding.
Assessment
Health Promotion and Maintenance
Application
Learning Objective 14.2

14.4 It is one week before a pregnant client's due date. The nurse notes on the chart that the client's pulse rate was 74–80 before pregnancy. Today, the client's pulse rate at rest is 90. The nurse should take which of the following actions?
1. Chart the findings.
2. Notify the physician of tachycardia.
3. Repeat the assessment in 60 minutes.
4. Prepare the client for transport to the hospital.

Answer: 1
Rationale: The pulse rate will increase by 10–15 beats per minute during pregnancy due to the increased blood volume during pregnancy. Charting normal findings is appropriate. It is not necessary to repeat the assessment in 60 minutes, nor is it necessary for the client to be hospitalized.
Assessment
Health Promotion and Maintenance
Application
Learning Objective 14.2

14.5 The nurse is planning a presentation about early pregnancy. What should the nurse include as a presumptive change of pregnancy?
1. amenorrhea
2. constipation
3. fetal heart tones
4. a positive pregnancy test

Answer: 1
Rationale: Presumptive signs of pregnancy are those subjective signs that may indicate pregnancy, but are not diagnostic of pregnancy. Amenorrhea can occur due to other causes, such as rapid weight loss, therefore is considered a presumptive change. Constipation is not a change of pregnancy. Fetal heart tones and a positive pregnancy test are both positive or diagnostic changes.
Planning
Health Promotion and Maintenance
Application
Learning Objective 14.3

14.6 The nurse has completed a community presentation about the changes of pregnancy. Which statement by a community member indicates that learning has occurred? "One probable or objective change of pregnancy is
1. enlargement of the uterus."
2. hearing the baby's heart rate."
3. increased urinary frequency."
4. nausea and vomiting."

Answer: 1
Rationale: Objective or probable changes of pregnancy are those that the examiner can detect, but are not diagnostic, because they can be caused by issues other than pregnancy. Enlargement of the uterus is a probable change. Increased urinary frequency and nausea/vomiting are presumptive changes, while hearing the fetal heart rate is positive or diagnostic.
Evaluation
Health Promotion and Maintenance
Application
Learning Objective 14.3

14.7 A client who is experiencing her first pregnancy has just completed the initial prenatal examination with a certified nurse-midwife. Which statement indicates that the client needs additional information?
1. "Because we heard the baby's heart beat, I am undoubtedly pregnant."
2. "Since I haven't felt the baby move yet, we don't know if I'm pregnant."
3. "My last period was two months ago, which means I'm two months along."
4. "The increased size of my uterus means that I am finally pregnant."

Answer: 2
Rationale: Hearing the fetal heart rate is a positive or diagnostic change of pregnancy. Increased uterine size is a probable or objective change, while amenorrhea and fetal movement are presumptive or subjective changes.
Evaluation
Health Promotion and Maintenance
Analysis
Learning Objective 14.3

14.8 The client is at six weeks' gestation, and is spotting. The client had an ectopic pregnancy one year ago. The nurse anticipates that the physician will order

1. a urine pregnancy test.
2. the client to be seen next week for a full examination.
3. a serum pregnancy test.
4. an ultrasound to be done within four weeks.

Answer: 3

Rationale: A client with a history of an ectopic pregnancy is at risk for another ectopic pregnancy, and spotting is a common symptom of ectopic pregnancy. A serum quantitative beta hCG test will be performed and repeated in 48 hours to check for a doubling of the value. Urine pregnancy tests are not quantifiable. An ultrasound may be used to diagnose an ectopic pregnancy, but would not be needed now.

Planning

Health Promotion and Maintenance

Application

Learning Objective 14.4

14.9 A woman telephones the clinic to say that it has been six weeks since her last menstrual period, but that her home pregnancy test was negative today. She asks, "Do you think I could be pregnant?" After determining that the test was performed correctly, what would be the nurse's best reply?

1. "Probably not. These tests rarely give a false-negative result."
2. "You might be. If you haven't started your period in one week, you should repeat the test and call the clinic again."
3. "You probably are. There are a lot of false-negative results with these tests."
4. "You may have an ectopic pregnancy. You should be seen by a doctor in the next few days."

Answer: 2

Rationale: Current home pregnancy tests are quite accurate when used correctly. Some can detect pregnancy as early as the first day of the missed period. If a woman has delayed menses and suspects pregnancy, but the home pregnancy test is negative, she should wait one week and repeat the home test. Ectopic pregnancy diagnosis requires a serum quantitative Beta hCG test.

Implementation

Health Promotion and Maintenance

Analysis

Learning Objective 14.4

14.10 The 20-year-old client at ten weeks' gestation is preparing for her first prenatal visit. She confides, "This pregnancy was unplanned. I'm not sure if I want to be pregnant or not. I haven't even told my boyfriend I'm pregnant. And I haven't decided if I'm going to continue the pregnancy." Which of the following statements should the nurse make next?

1. "It's really unusual for a pregnant woman to feel this way early in the pregnancy."
2. "These thoughts are because your mother died when you were four years old."
3. "You should go to a pregnancy support group to be a goodmother."
4. "It's common to feel ambiguous about pregnancy in the first trimester."

Answer: 4

Rationale: Ambivalence toward the pregnancy is very common in the first trimester. Fathers might not be told immediately about the diagnosis of pregnancy. No psychopathology is present, thus a support group is not indicated. Loss of the client's own mother at a young age would not affect the occurrence of ambivalence in the third trimester.

Implementation

Health Promotion and Maintenance

Application

Learning Objective14.5

14.11 A 25-year-old woman is in the second trimester of her pregnancy. During the interview, you ask her partner what changes they have noticed during the pregnancy. Which of the following answers would indicate a typical response to pregnancy?

Answer: 2

Rationale: In the first trimester, pregnant women tell their partners of the pregnancy, and explore their relationship with their mother and think about their own role as a mother. They also may fear miscarriage, and may feel ambivalence or anxiety about the pregnancy and the changes that a child will bring to their life. The second trimester brings increased introspection and consideration of how she will parent. The needs of the newborn typically are not considered until

---

1. "She is very body-conscious and hates every little change."
2. "She daydreams about what kind of parent she is going to be."
3. "I haven't noticed anything. I just found out she was pregnant."
4. "She has been having dreams at night about misplacing the baby."

the third trimester, but dreams of misplacing the baby or being unable to get to the baby are common during this period.
Assessment
Health Promotion and Maintenance
Analysis
Learning Objective 14.5

14.12 At a second-trimester prenatal visit, a married couple is discussing their new roles as parents with the nurse. The father comments that he really wants to be a good father to their new baby. The nurse should explain that, in developing the fatherhood role, the most important thing is to
1. participate actively in as many aspects of childbearing and childrearing as possible.
2. identify a father he admires and try to develop a fathering role similar to that.
3. decide with his partner on a fathering role that is mutually agreeable to both of them.
4. begin by examining the basic pattern of fathering that his father used with him.

Answer: 3
Rationale: A mutually-developed fathering role will reduce anxiety and miscommunication. Participation in childrearing and especially childbearing is culturally determined, and may not be viewed as desirable. Fathering may be imitated from either one's own father or another admired father, but it is important for the couple to discuss and agree upon the tasks the father will assume to prevent miscommunication and promote family cohesiveness.
Implementation
Health Promotion and Maintenance
Analysis
Learning Objective 14.6

14.13 The nurse is caring for a pregnant client who speaks little English. Which of the following actions should the nurse take to make certain that the client understands the plan of care?
1. Write all of the instructions down and send them home with the client.
2. Obtain a medical interpreter for the client's language.
3. Ask a housekeeper who speaks this language to interpret.
4. Use gestures and facial expressions to get the plan across.

Answer: 2
Rationale: Women of all cultures and all language backgrounds deserve quality prenatal care. When working with a woman who speaks little or no English, a trained medical interpreter should be obtained. Using family members, friends, or other staff to interpret may be problematic because few people understand medical terminology, and it can lead to confidentiality issues. Writing English is not helpful, because verbal fluency usually develops before written fluency when learning a language.
Implementation
Health Promotion and Maintenance
Application
Learning Objective 14.6

14.14 The pregnant client at 14 weeks' gestation is in the clinic for a regular prenatal visit. Her mother also is present. The grandmother-to-be states that she is quite uncertain about how she can be a good grandmother to this baby, because she works full-time, and her own grandmother was retired and always available when she was needed by a grandchild. What would be the nurse's best response to this concern?
1. "Don't worry. You'll be a wonderful grandmother. It will all work out fine."
2. "Grandmothers are supposed to be available. You should retire from your job."

Answer: 4
Rationale: As society has changed to encourage a more active lifestyle in the aging population, the role of grandparents has also. Grandparenting can take many forms. Some grandparents are young and employed full-time, while others are retired and have more free time. Encouraging open communication between grandparents-to-be and the parents-to-be can avoid miscommunication of expectations. Grandparenting classes are one way that these roles can be explored. It is important to avoid clichés and placing guilt on clients to promote effective therapeutic communication.
Implementation
Health Promotion and Maintenance
Analysis
Learning Objective 14.6

3. "As long as there is another grandmother available, you don't have to worry."
4. "What are your thoughts on what your role as grandmother will include?"

14.15 The pregnant client has moved to the United States from another country. She states that her grandmother has provided herbs for her to take during pregnancy. The client asks the nurse if the herbs are safe. How should the nurse respond?
1. "Some herbs are not safe for use during pregnancy."
2. "Herbal supplements during pregnancy do not cause problems."
3. "Your grandmother wouldn't give you anything that was dangerous."
4. "Natural supplements should not be used during pregnancy or labor."

Answer: 1
Rationale: Some herbs are oxytoxic, cause uterine contractions, and thus should be avoided during pregnancy. Some herbs, however, are safe for use during pregnancy and labor. The nurse cannot assume that the client's grandmother is a knowledgeable herbalist.
Implementation
Health Promotion and Maintenance
Application
Learning Objective 14.1

CHAPTER 15

15.1 The nurse is obtaining information from a pregnant client. Which of the following pieces of information would indicate this client is at risk for preterm labor?
1. The client smokes two packs per day and delivered her last child at 34 weeks.
2. The client has group B streptococcus in her urine, and is primiparous.
3. The client had congenital hip dysplasia as a child and is 15 pounds overweight.
4. The client lives in a second-floor apartment without stairs, and walks to work.

Answer: 1
Rationale: Smoking is a risk factor for preterm birth and low birth weight. Nicotine is a vasoconstrictor, and causes the arterioles in the placenta and the uterus to constrict, decreasing blood flow to the uterine musculature as well as the fetus. During and after smoking a cigarette, both the maternal and fetal oxygen saturation drop, and the carbon monoxide found in cigarette smoke also will decrease fetal oxygenation. The presence of group B streptococcus puts the newborn at risk for sepsis after delivery. Neither hip dysplasia nor being 15 pounds overweight predisposes a woman to developing preterm labor. Walking is considered moderate-intensity exercise, and is a healthy practice during pregnancy.
Assessment
Health Promotion and Maintenance
Application
Learning Objective 15.1

15.2 While completing the medical and surgical history during the initial prenatal visit, the 16-year-old primigravida client states, "Why are you asking me all these questions? What difference does it make?" Which of the following statements would best answer the client's questions? "We ask these questions to
1. detect anything that happened in your past that might affect the pregnancy."
2. see if you can have prenatal visits less often than most clients."
3. make sure that our paperwork and records are complete and up to date."
4. look for any health problems in the past that might affect your parenting."

Answer: 1
Rationale: The medical and surgical histories of a new prenatal client must be accurate and complete to detect conditions that may be exacerbated during pregnancy or delivery, to ensure safety of both the mother and the fetus. Prenatal visits follow a set schedule for normal clients without complications. Paperwork is a lower priority than client care. The psychological history of a client, not the medical or surgical histories, may indicate potential problems with parenting.
Implementation
Health Promotion and Maintenance
Analysis
Learning Objective 15.1

15.3 A multigravida gave birth to an 18-week fetus last week. She is in the clinic for follow-up, and notices that her chart states she has had one abortion. The client is upset over the use of this word. How can the nurse best explain this terminology to the client?

1. "Abortion is the medical term for all pregnancies that end before 28 weeks."
2. "Abortion is the word we use when someone has miscarried."
3. "Abortion is how we label pregnancies that end in the second trimester."
4. "Abortion is what we call all babies who are stillborn."

Answer: 1
Rationale: Abortions are fetal losses prior to the onset of the third trimester, and include elective induced (medical or surgical) abortions, ectopic pregnancies, and spontaneous abortions or miscarriages. Third trimester losses are considered fetal death in utero, and the term abortion is not used.
Implementation
Health Promotion and Maintenance
Application
Learning Objective 15.2

15.4 Which of the following clients would be considered a primigravida?

1. a client at 18 weeks' gestation who had a spontaneous loss at 12 weeks
2. a client at 13 weeks' gestation who had an ectopic pregnancy at eight weeks
3. a client at 14 weeks' gestation who has a three-year-old daughter at home
4. a client at 15 weeks' gestation who has never been pregnant before

Answer: 4
Rationale: Primigravida can be broken down into the Latin prefix and root: primi (prime, or first) and gravida (pregnancy). So a primigravida is a pregnant woman who has never been pregnant before. A pregnant woman who has had a pregnancy end before 20 weeks is considered a primipara. A pregnant woman who has been pregnant before is called a multigravida.
Assessment
Health Promotion and Maintenance
Application
Learning Objective 15.2

15.5 The nurse is preparing a class for couples who are planning pregnancy. Which statement should the nurse include? "Prior to your becoming pregnant it is important for you to talk to your provider if (Select all that apply.)

1. the father of the baby has any medical problems."
2. the baby's father has other children from a previous marriage."
3. anyone in the family has had surgery."
4. you are going to move or change jobs."
5. you take medications or herbs on a daily basis."

Answer: 1, 5
Rationale: If the baby's father has an inheritable medical condition, the couple should receive genetic counseling prior to conception. Some medications are teratogenic, and should thus be avoided during pregnancy, while some herbs are known to be oxytoxic, and can lead to miscarriage. Whether or not the father has other children, a history of any kind of surgery in the family, and moving or changing jobs are not essential for the doctor to know prior to conception.
Planning
Health Promotion and Maintenance
Application
Learning Objective 15.3

15.6 The clinic nurse is assisting with an initial prenatal assessment. The following findings are present: spider nevi present on lower legs; dark pink, edematous nasal mucosa; mild enlargement of the thyroid gland; mottled skin and pallor or palms and nail beds; heart rate 88 with murmur present. What is the best action for the nurse to take based on these findings?

1. Document the findings on the prenatal chart.
2. Have the physician see the client today.

Answer: 2
Rationale: Mottling of the skin is indicative of poor oxygenation and a circulation problem. Skin and nail bed pallor can indicate either hypoxia or anemia. These abnormalities must be reported to the physician immediately. Spider nevi are common in pregnancy due to the increased vascular volume and high estrogen levels. Nasal passages can be inflamed during pregnancy from edema, caused by increased estrogen levels. The thyroid gland increases in size during pregnancy due to hyperplasia.
Assessment
Health Promotion and Maintenance
Analysis
Learning Objective 15.4

3. Instruct the client to avoid direct sunlight. 4. Analyze previous thyroid hormone lab results.	
15.7 A 25-year-old primigravida is 20 weeks pregnant. At the clinic, her nurse begins a prenatal assessment and obtains the following vital signs. Which finding would require the nurse to contact the physician? 1. pulse 88/min 2. respirations 30/min 3. temperature 37.4°C (99.3°F) 4. blood pressure 134/82	Answer: 2 Rationale: Tachypnea is not a normal finding, and requires medical care. A slight increase in pulse and temperature are expected findings during pregnancy due to the increased oxygen consumption to support fetal metabolism. The blood pressure is within normal limits. Implementation Health Promotion and Maintenance Application Learning Objective 15.4
15.8 A woman tells the clinic nurse that her last normal menstrual period was September 8. The nurse would calculate her due date to be: _____.	Answer: June 15 Rationale: Using Naegele's rule, you take the first day of the last menstrual period, subtract three months, and add seven days. Subtracting three months from September is June, adding seven days to the 8th is the 15th. Assessment Health Promotion and Maintenance Application Learning Objective 15.5
15.9 The nurse is assisting a physician during a prenatal examination. The physician seeks to estimate the adequacy of the client's pelvis for birth. The nurse understands that the physician will need to perform which measurement vaginally? 1. true conjugate 2. diagonal conjugate 3. transverse outlet diameter 4. obstetrical conjugate	Answer: 2 Rationale: The diagonal conjugate is measured from the lower edge of the symphysis to the sacral promontory. The true conjugate and obstetrical conjugate are measurements of the pelvic inlet, and cannot be directly measured. The transverse outlet diameter is measured externally. Planning Health Promotion and Maintenance Application Learning Objective 15.6
15.10 The nurse is planning an early pregnancy class. Which of the following findings should be explained as a normal psychosocial stage in the first trimester of pregnancy? 1. an unlisted telephone number or no telephone 2. reluctance to tell partner of the pregnancy 3. parental disapproval of the woman's partner 4. ambivalence regarding the pregnancy	Answer: 4 Rationale: Ambivalence about a pregnancy is a common psychosocial adjustment in early pregnancy. An unlisted phone number or no telephone does not indicate psychosocial adjustment, nor does parental disapproval of a client's partner. Reluctance to tell the partner of the pregnancy may be related to ambivalence or may indicate that the client anticipates disapproval. Planning Health Promotion and Maintenance Application Learning Objective 15.7
15.11 When doing a prenatal assessment of parenting, which of the following comments by a woman would the nurse recognize as needing further investigation? 1. "I have so much to learn about taking care of a baby. I've bought a couple of books already." 2. "When will I be able to feel my baby move?"	Answer: 3 Rationale: A newborn requires a great deal of time and care; not anticipating how a baby will change one's life indicates a lack of understanding and knowledge, and presents risk factors for ineffective parenting and postpartum depression. Wanting to learn about fetal movement and baby care are expected, as is announcing the pregnancy to family and friends. Evaluation Health Promotion and Maintenance Analysis Learning Objective 15.7

3. "I work and have an active social life; I don't see how a baby will change it all that much."
4. "We've already told our parents we're expecting, and our friends and the people at work, too."

15.12 Which of the following third-trimester women would you suspect may be having difficulty with psychological adjustments to her pregnancy?
1. a woman who says, "Either a boy or a girl will be fine with me"
2. a woman who puts her feet up and listens to some music for 15 minutes when she is feeling too stressed
3. a woman who was a smoker, but who has quit at least for the duration of her pregnancy
4. a woman who has not investigated the kind of clothing or feeding methods the baby will need

Answer: 4
Rationale: By the third trimester, the client should be making plans for obtaining the equipment needed for the newborn (such as clothing) and should have made a decision on a feeding method. Acceptance of gender, using stress reduction techniques, and quitting smoking are indicative of healthy adaptation to pregnancy.
Assessment
Health Promotion and Maintenance
Analysis
Learning Objective 15.7

15.13 The client at 38 weeks' gestation calls the prenatal clinic nurse to report that her baby has not moved today. Which statement should the nurse give to the client?
1. "Your blood pressure might be increasing. Check it and call me back."
2. "Babies do that sometimes. Don't worry—everything is fine."
3. "Are you having pain with urination or blood in your urine also?"
4. "You should come in so we can check the baby as soon as possible."

Answer: 4
Rationale: Lack of fetal movement can be indicative of fetal hypoxia or fetal death. The fetus needs to be assessed via a nonstress test and possibly ultrasound as well. Increased blood pressure would not directly cause a lack of fetal movement. There is no correlation between UTI and lack of fetal movement. Lack of fetal movement is not a normal finding. This client's fetus requires assessment as soon as possible. Therapeutic communication requires avoiding clichés.
Implementation
Health Promotion and Maintenance
Application
Learning Objective 15.8

15.14 The client has delivered her first child at $37\frac{1}{2}$ weeks. The nurse would explain this to the client as what type of delivery?
1. preterm
2. postterm
3. term
4. near term

Answer: 1
Rationale: Term births are those that occur from 37 completed weeks of pregnancy to 42 weeks. Preterm are those that occur between 20 weeks and 37 completed weeks. Postterm are birth that occur after 42 weeks. Near term is not terminology used to describe birth.
Implementation
Health Promotion and Maintenance
Application
Learning Objective 15.2

15.15 The client is in the physician's office for an initial prenatal examination. The client has indicated that she had a blood transfusion three years ago following a car crash and surgery. The client asks "Why is it important to know if I've ever had a blood transfusion?" The nurse's best answer is, "We ask because
1. most women who have had transfusions are unable to carry a fetus to term."

Answer: 3
Rationale: Transfusion reactions can include antibody production; some antibodies cause fetal hemolysis. A history of a transfusion is not a risk factor for preterm delivery. There is no association between a previous transfusion and an increased risk of postpartum bleeding. Rh_O (D) immune globulin (Rhogam) is given to prevent Rh sensitization, not as treatment after antibodies are formed.
Implementation
Health Promotion and Maintenance
Analysis
Learning Objective 15.1

---

2. that means you might need another transfusion after you deliver."

3. your body might make antibodies that are harmful to your baby."

4. you will need to have Rh$_O$ (D) immune globulin (Rhogam) now to prevent problems."

CHAPTER 16

16.1 The nurse is working with a student nurse. Which step of the nursing process should the nurse encourage the student to use when creating an appropriate educational session for families who are considering pregnancy?
1. assessment
2. planning
3. implementation
4. evaluation

Answer: 2
Rationale: Planning determines which intervention is appropriate, while implementation is enacting the plan. Assessment is data gathering. A nursing diagnosis is formed from the assessed data. During evaluation, the nurse determines if what was intended to occur in fact did take place.
Implementation
Health Promotion and Maintenance
Application
Learning Objective 16.1

16.2 The nurse is caring for a pregnant client. The client's husband has come to the prenatal visit. Which question is best for the nurse to use to assess the adaptation to pregnancy by the father-to-be?
1. "What kind of work do you do?"
2. "What furniture have you gotten for the baby?"
3. "How moody has your wife been lately?"
4. "How are you feeling about becoming a father?"

Answer: 4
Rationale: The adaptation of a husband to pregnancy includes his feelings about impending fatherhood. What kind of work the husband does, what furniture has been obtained, and the husband's perception of his wife's moodiness are not indicators of his adaptation.
Planning
Health Promotion and Maintenance
Application
Learning Objective 16.2

16.3 The pregnant client has asked the nurse what kinds of medications cause birth defects. Which statement would best answer this question?
1. "Birth defects are very rare. Don't worry; your doctor will watch for problems."
2. "To be safe, don't take any medication without talking to your doctor."
3. "Too much vitamin C is one of the most common issues, but is avoidable."
4. "Almost all medications will cause birth defects in the first trimester."

Answer: 2
Rationale: Teratogens are substances that cause birth defects. Alcohol is one example, as are warfarin (Coumadin) and isotretinoin (Accutane). The greatest risk is during the first trimester, but not all medications are teratogenic. Those medications with clear evidence of teratogenicity are classified in Pregnancy Category X, and should be avoided when conception is being attempted and during the first trimester. Vitamin C can cause rebound scurvy, but is not teratogenic. The nurse should avoid a "don't worry" answer to ensure therapeutic communication, but it is appropriate to instruct the client to talk to the doctor about medications.
Implementation
Health Promotion and Maintenance
Application
Learning Objective 16.6

16.4 A Navajo client who is 36 weeks pregnant meets with the tribe's medicine man as well as her physician. The nurse understands this to mean that the client
1. is seeking spiritual direction.
2. does not trust her physician.
3. will not adapt to mothering well.
4. is experiencing complications of pregnancy.

Answer: 1
Rationale: As a result of the introspection that develops, pregnant women often will seek spiritual guidance from their preferred spiritual leader. This does not indicate any type of pathology or complications, nor does it indicate mistrust of the provider, or parenting ability. The nurse has a professional responsibility to promote clients' spiritual well-being. Understanding the belief systems of the client population will facilitate intercultural communication, and will help the nurse provide appropriate information using appropriate teaching methods.

Assessment
Health Promotion and Maintenance
Analysis
Learning Objective 16.3

16.5 A Chinese woman who is 16 weeks pregnant reports to the nurse that ginseng and bamboo leaves help to reduce her anxiety. How should the nurse respond to this client?
1. Advise the client to avoid the use of all herbs.
2. Assess the amount and frequency with which the client is using the remedy.
3. Tell the client that her remedies have no scientific foundation.
4. Assess where the client obtains her remedy, and investigate the source.

Answer: 2
Rationale: Use of herbs is a common alternative health care practice for many women. Pregnant women are often taught "secret family recipes" for avoiding or minimizing the discomforts of pregnancy. It is appropriate to assess the amount and frequency of the client's use of the herbs. Because some herbs have negative effects on pregnancy, using a reliable reference to determine the actions of the herbs can educate both the nurse and the client. Some remedies do have scientific foundation, so it is not appropriate to instruct the client that none do. It is outside the nurse's scope to assess the source of the herbs.
Implementation
Health Promotion and Maintenance
Application
Learning Objective 16.3

16.6 The primiparous client has told the nurse that she is afraid that she will develop hemorrhoids during pregnancy, because her mother did. Which of the following statements would be best for the nurse to make?
1. "It is not unusual for women to develop hemorrhoids during pregnancy."
2. "Most women don't have any problem until after they've delivered."
3. "If your mother had hemorrhoids, you will get them too. Get used to the idea."
4. "If you get hemorrhoids, you probably will need surgery to get rid of them."

Answer: 1
Rationale: Hemorrhoids are anal varicose veins. The increased weight of the gravid uterus, combined with constipation, can result in the varicosities prolapsing. Many pregnant women will develop hemorrhoids either during pregnancy or after delivery from the pushing efforts of the second stage of labor. Topical relief agents such as Preparation H or Tucks pads can provide relief of the itching and burning sensations. Although there is a familial tendency to develop varicosities, including hemorrhoids, a family history does not automatically mean that a client will develop the condition. Most hemorrhoids will resolve spontaneously and will not require surgical intervention.
Implementation
Health Promotion and Maintenance
Application
Learning Objective 16.4

16.7 A 38-year-old client in her second trimester states a desire to begin an exercise program to decrease her fatigue. Which of the following would be the most appropriate nursing response?
1. "Fatigue should resolve in the second trimester, but walking daily might help."
2. "Avoid a strenuous exercise regimen at your age. Drink coffee TID."
3. "Avoid an exercise regimen due to your pregnancy. Try to nap daily."
4. "Fatigue will increase as pregnancy progresses, but jogging daily may help."

Answer: 1
Rationale: Mild to moderate exercise during pregnancy is healthy for moms and babies. The increased stamina that correlates with physical fitness can help decrease fatigue in pregnancy, but the second trimester will bring greater fatigue, as fetal metabolism creates demands on the maternal system. The age of 38 is not too old to begin an exercise routine, but during pregnancy, a client should not begin a new type of extremely strenuous or high-impact activity. Those clients who have regularly engaged in strenuous or high-impact activities prior to pregnancy can continue that practice unless they develop pregnancy complications that contraindicate exercise.
Implementation
Health Promotion and Maintenance
Application
Learning Objective 16.5

16.8 The client in her first trimester of pregnancy is experiencing nausea. To promote self-care, the nurse should help the pregnant client understand that the nausea may be relieved by
1. eating spicy foods.

Answer: 3
Rationale: The nausea of pregnancy can be exacerbated by ketosis, fatigue, and certain foods, such as those containing caffeine or spices. Eating dry carbohydrates prior to rising and avoiding severe hunger by eating small, frequent meals throughout the day can help to prevent or decrease the severity of the nausea. Carbonated beverages may be helpful in decreasing nausea.

2. not eating until two hours after rising. 3. eating small, frequent meals. 4. avoiding carbonated beverages.	Planning Health Promotion and Maintenance Application Learning Objective 16.5
16.9 A pregnant client who swims three to five times per week asks the nurse if she should stop this activity. What is the appropriate nursing response? 1. "You should decrease the number of times you swim per week." 2. "You should continue your exercise program, because it would be beneficial." 3. "You should discontinue your exercise program immediately." 4. "You should increase the number of times you swim per week."	Answer: 2 Rationale: Thirty minutes of moderate-intensity exercise daily is recommended for pregnant women, but even mild exercise is helpful. Women who exercise regularly have better muscle tone, self-image, bowel function, energy levels, sleep, and postpartum recovery than do those who are sedentary. Implementation Health Promotion and Maintenance Application Learning Objective 16.6
16.10 The nurse is teaching a prenatal education class about positions for sexual intercourse during later pregnancy. What position should the nurse teach as an appropriate position for intercourse during the third trimester? 1. lithotomy 2. Fowler's 3. supine 4. side-lying	Answer: 4 Rationale: As the abdomen increases in girth during later pregnancy, changes in position may need to be utilized for sexual activity. Side-lying reduces pressure on the abdomen, and avoids supine hypotension. Lithotomy, Fowler's, and supine positions will increase discomfort. Planning Health Promotion and Maintenance Application Learning Objective 16.7
16.11 The nurse is planning a community presentation about pregnancy after age 35. Which statement should the nurse include? "Pregnancy over the age of 35 is (Select all that apply.) 1. becoming more common due to expanded career options for women." 2. extremely dangerous and should be avoided when possible." 3. due solely to the increased availability and success of infertility treatment." 4. sometimes because of increased housing costs for families." 5. planned in order to allow grandparents to retire before the birth of grandchildren."	Answer: 1, 4 Rationale: Pregnancy after age 35 is increasing in frequency, and accounts for about 14% of pregnancies. Many of these pregnancies are spontaneous, and not only due to infertility treatment. Causes for this trend includes delaying childbirth to obtain education and establish a career, to have time to save money for a house, and an increasing number of partners in second and subsequent marriages desiring biological children together. Although complications of pregnancy increase with age, pregnancy after 35 is not considered extremely dangerous. The employment of grandparents is not a goal of the trend toward later childbearing. Planning Health Promotion and Maintenance Analysis Learning Objective 16.8
16.12 The pregnant client is in her 21st week of pregnancy, and is planning a vacation with her family. She asks the nurse which method of travel would be recommended for her to use. How should the nurse respond? "The safest method of travel is to 1. take an automobile. 2. fly on an airplane. 3. travel by train. 4. not travel this late in pregnancy.	Answer: 3 Rationale: In the latter half of pregnancy, frequent movement is recommended for pregnant women, both to increase comfort and to decrease venous pooling, which can lead to thrombophlebitis. The train allows the most movement for the traveling pregnant woman. Neither automobile nor airplane travel allow for frequent enough movement. It is not necessary to cease travel altogether. Planning Health Promotion and Maintenance Application Learning Objective 16.6

16.13 The nurse is presenting a class to women who are currently pregnant or are planning pregnancy in the near future. Which client's statement indicates that additional teaching is required?

1. "The older a woman is when she conceives, the safer the pregnancy is."
2. "Pregnant teens may have additional nutritional needs."
3. "A woman whose sisters all had hypertension will be watched carefully."
4. "Pregnancy may be more difficult to achieve spontaneously in my 40s."

Answer: 1
Rationale: The health risks associated with pregnancy vary by age. Young teens who are still growing need additional calories and protein. Hypertension and gestational diabetes are more common in women over 35. Spontaneous pregnancy is more difficult in the 40s, and infertility treatment becomes more likely to be required to achieve pregnancy.
Evaluation
Health Promotion and Maintenance
Analysis
Learning Objective 16.9

16.14 The nurse is explaining the importance of fetal activity assessment to the client. What should the nurse do to best reinforce the significance of fetal kick counting to the client?

1. Perform daily phone calls to the client at work or home.
2. Review the client's written record of fetal movement at each visit.
3. Ask the client to remember to count the fetal movements.
4. Explain the rationale for counting fetal movement to the client.

Answer: 2
Rationale: Clients should be instructed to begin counting fetal movement between 24–28 weeks. A fetus that has been active and has a sudden decrease in movements may be conserving energy due to hypoxia. Movements are counted in a specified time period, such as for one hour after each meal, or beginning with arising in the morning. Writing down the count is more accurate than the client simply remembering. When the nurse examines the written record the client has kept, it reinforces the importance of the record, and improves the likelihood of continued record keeping. Daily phone calls would take emphasis away from the importance of the client's counting of fetal movement. Knowing the reasons for the counting will increase understanding of the process, but will not reinforce its significance of the task.
Planning
Health Promotion and Maintenance
Application
Learning Objective 16.6

16.15 A client in her third trimester of pregnancy reports frequent leg cramps. What strategy would be most appropriate for the nurse to suggest?

1. point the toes of the affected leg
2. increase intake of protein-rich foods
3. limit activity for several days
4. flex the foot to stretch the calf

Answer: 4
Rationale: Leg cramps are a common problem in pregnancy, resulting from an imbalance in the calcium-phosphorus ratio; pressure on nerves or decreased circulation in the legs from the enlarged uterus; or fatigue. Dorsiflexing the foot will allow stretching of the calf muscles and will help relieve the cramps. Pointing the toes will exacerbate leg cramps. Protein intake does not affect leg cramps. Limiting activity is not appropriate.
Planning
Health Promotion and Maintenance
Application
Learning Objective 16.5

CHAPTER 17

17.1 The pregnant 16-year-old is seeing the nurse during a prenatal visit. Based on the client's developmental level, which statement would the nurse expect the client to make?

1. "My friends and I all wear totally different styles of clothing."
2. "Having a baby will change my college plans."
3. "I drink alcohol at parties most weekends."
4. "My mom is my best friend."

Answer: 3
Rationale: Middle adolescence (15–17) is a time of experimentation, including drinking alcohol, using other drugs, and smoking. Early adolescents (under 14) conform to group standards by wearing the same types of clothing as friends wear, as do middle adolescents. Late adolescence (18–19) is when the ability to think about the future develops, including understanding the impact that a baby will have on acquiring education. From early adolescence and on, friends have an increasingly important role in the search for independence, which includes friends replacing parents as the primary source of support.
Assessment
Psychosocial Integrity
Analysis
Learning Objective 17.2

17.2 The nurse is teaching a pregnant 14-year-old client at ten weeks' gestation about the expected body changes that will occur during pregnancy. Which statement indicates that additional information is needed?

1. "My breasts are going to get even bigger than they've gotten over the past couple of years."
2. "My belly will gradually get more round, especially from the middle of pregnancy and on."
3. "My hair will feel thicker until I deliver, and then I'll lose more hair than usual for a few weeks."
4. "My skin won't change and I'll look just as good in a bikini next year as I did last summer."

Answer: 4
Rationale: Skin changes of pregnancy are common, and include darkening of the linea nigra, darkened areas on the skin of the face and neck (chloasma), and striae or stretch marks. Breasts will enlarge, as will the belly. Hair decreases shedding during pregnancy, which results in the perception of thicker hair, but after delivery the shedding rate increases until it is back to what was normal prior to conception.
Evaluation
Health Promotion and Maintenance
Analysis
Learning Objective 17.1

17.3 The school nurse is planning a presentation on pregnancy for 13- and 14-year-olds who are currently pregnant. What should the nurse keep in mind when planning the content of this presentation? These teens are

1. working on independence and autonomy.
2. no longer developing a sense of achievement.
3. confident in their own identity.
4. in long-term, intimate relationships.

Answer: 1
Rationale: The developmental tasks of adolescence include: developing an identity, gaining autonomy and independence, developing intimacy in a relationship, developing comfort with one's own sexuality, and developing a sense of achievement. Early adolescence will not have achieved all of these tasks yet, and the relationships are typically short-term.
Planning
Health Promotion and Maintenance
Application
Learning Objective 17.3

17.4 The pregnant 19-year-old begins a job to "save money for the baby." The nurse acknowledges that this statement indicates that the adolescent

1. is striving to gain autonomy and independence.
2. has completed development of a sense of identity.
3. is nearing attainment of a sense of achievement.
4. has developed an intimate relationship.

Answer: 1
Rationale: There are several developmental tasks of adulthood: gaining confidence in one's sexuality, developing intimate relationships, gaining independence and autonomy, and developing a sense of identity and sense of achievement. Having a job is how most pregnant teens in late adolescence develop financial independence and autonomy.
Assessment
Health Promotion and Maintenance
Application
Learning Objective 17.2

17.5 The nurse is working at a clinic for pregnant teens. What developmental-related issues will the nurse expect to encounter in most of the pregnant clients?

1. peer pressure to stop using alcohol once pregnancy is diagnosed
2. contraception failure resulted in this pregnancy
3. the father of the baby being emotionally supportive to the client
4. feeling that she can't live up to her parents' expectations

Answer: 4
Rationale: Pregnant teens face risk factors based on the developmental tasks of adolescence. These include adopting a negative identity if she feels she cannot live up to parental expectations, peer pressure to engage in substance use, sexual activity without contraception due to lack of a future orientation, and sexual activity as experimentation without emotional intimacy.
Planning
Health Promotion and Maintenance
Application
Learning Objective 17.1

17.6 The nurse counseling a group of middle-school girls about pregnancy avoidance should include which of the following statements?
1. "Although sexuality is common in the media, the peer pressure to have sex is not an important factor."
2. "It has become far less acceptable to give birth during your teenage years than it used to be."
3. "Although condom use is growing, there is still an increasing rate of STDs among teens."
4. "You have learned enough from your friends and families to understand how pregnancy occurs."

Answer: 3
Rationale: Condom use is increasing, but the rate of STD infections, including HIV, is also rising. Images of sexuality are common in American society: in music lyrics and videos, in advertising, in television shows and movies. Peer pressure to have sex is also common, and is a strong influence on when a teen becomes sexually active. Society has become more accepting of teen pregnancy, and there are fewer stigmas attached to being a young mother. Formal education about the physiology of the body and conception will decrease the myths and misunderstandings that abound among teens and undereducated adults.
Planning
Health Promotion and Maintenance
Application
Learning Objective 17.4

17.7 Which of the following statements would a pregnant teenager likely make at the first prenatal visit? (Select all that apply.)
1. "I didn't know I could get pregnant the first time I had sex."
2. "Several of my friends go to clinics to get contraception."
3. "It's no big deal; two of my best friends have babies, too."
4. "We have plenty of money at home to buy diapers and stuff."
5. "I'll have to drop out of school because I don't have day care for my baby."

Answer: 1, 3
Rationale: There are several contributing factors for the United States having a higher adolescent pregnancy rate than any other developed nation in the world. These factors include lack of knowledge about conception; difficulty accessing contraception; decreased social stigma of being a young and single mother; younger age at onset of sexual activity; poverty; and early childhood sexual abuse. Lack of support from the partner and parents is common, especially when the pregnancy is first diagnosed and disclosed, but in some cultural groups early pregnancy is a norm. Poverty is commonly experienced by adolescents during their pregnancy and after birth, as is lowered educational achievement. Some school districts are attempting to impact this aspect of teen pregnancy by providing day care at schools for teen parents.
Assessment
Health Promotion and Maintenance
Analysis
Learning Objective 17.5

17.8 The nurse is preparing an in-service presentation for a group of middle school nurses. Which statements, if made by a school nurse, would indicate the nurse's understanding of the role of culture in adolescent pregnancy? (Select all that apply.)
1. "Eighty-five percent of teen mothers are middle class, and give birth to gain adult status."
2. "Teens who have a lot of time without adult supervision are more sexually active."
3. "Young teens that have a child are more likely to have another while still a teen."
4. "Most pregnant teens do not have relatives who had their first child as teens."
5. "Rape is the leading cause of teen pregnancy in the United States."

Answer: 2, 4
Rationale: Poor teens tend to have a lower self-image, see fewer choices for the future, and have less access to contraception. When teens in poverty become pregnant, they are more likely to maintain the pregnancy and view the birth as a way to be seen as an adult. Middle class teens are more likely to have future education and career goals, use contraception, and seek therapeutic abortion if they become pregnant. The pregnancy rate for African-American teens between the ages of 15 and 17 has dropped by 15%, but Hispanic- and African-American teens have a disproportionately large number of adolescent births. Teens who participate in after-school activities are less likely to be sexually active, and therefore have fewer pregnancies; conversely, teens that spend more time without adult supervision are more likely to be sexually active and to become pregnant. When the first birth occurs in the early teen years, the next birth also is likely to occur prior to adulthood. Having a mother or a sister who had her first child during adolescence is a risk for a teen to become pregnant. Unprotected consensual sex is the leading cause of teen pregnancy.
Evaluation
Health Promotion and Maintenance
Analysis
Learning Objective 17.5

17.9 A 20-week-gestation adolescent client states that it is important not to have a baby that weighs too much. She states this has been her rationale for limiting calories. Her weight

Answer: 4
Rationale: Teens might not understand the physiology behind the profound body changes of pregnancy. Pregnant adolescents are just adapting to a new body image created by the changes of puberty, when the pregnancy produces rapid and substantial body changes. The desire to maintain a socially-desirable figure

has decreased from 110 pounds to 106 pounds. What would be the best nursing response?
1. "You are causing harm to your baby."
2. "It's OK to want a small baby when you're a teen."
3. "You shouldn't be worrying about your figure."
4. "Your baby needs adequate nutrition to develop."

can lead to nutritional deficits. The first role of the nurse is to explain why food is important to the growing fetus, specifying what each food group will help the fetus develop. Next, the nurse must assist the pregnant adolescent to plan foods that she likes to eat from each food group. Anticipatory guidance in the body changes of pregnancy will assist the adolescent's adjustment to them. Although many teens are anxious, this teen is expressing a direct nutritional deficit.
Implementation
Health Promotion and Maintenance
Application
Learning Objective 17.6

17.10 Which of the following statements, if made by the pregnant adolescent, indicates that she understands her increased risk of physiologic complications during pregnancy?
1. "It's no big deal that I started prenatal care in my seventh month."
2. "My anemia and eating mostly fast food are not important."
3. "I need to take good care of myself so my baby doesn't come early."
4. "Smoking and using crack cocaine won't harm my baby."

Answer: 3
Rationale: Early and regular prenatal care is the best intervention to prevent complications or to detect them early, to minimize the harm to both the teen and her fetus. Pregnant adolescents are at high risk for complications such as pregnancy-induced hypertension, anemia, preterm birth, low-birth-weight infants, and fetal harm from cigarette smoking, alcohol consumption, or the use of street drugs.
Assessment
Health Promotion and Maintenance
Application
Learning Objective 17.6

17.11 The nurse seeks to involve the adolescent father in the prenatal care of his girlfriend. The rationale for this nursing strategy includes
1. increasing the self-care behaviors of the pregnant teen.
2. avoiding conflict between the adolescent father and pregnant teen.
3. improving the long-term outcome of the relationship.
4. avoiding legal action by the adolescent father's family.

Answer: 1
Rationale: The nurse first must explore what the relationship is between the pregnant teen and the father. Relationships between adolescents tend to be short-lived, and pregnancy is an added stressor for the couple. If the client desires the participation of her partner, the nurse should provide education and support appropriate to the age, knowledge, and developmental level of the adolescent father. Involving the partner of a pregnant adolescent helps the mom-to-be feel more confident in her decision making and improves her self-confidence and self-esteem, which in turn will improve positive self-care behaviors. Involving the client's partner in prenatal care will not decrease the likelihood that this relationship will be short term.
Assessment
Psychosocial Integrity
Application
Learning Objective 17.7

17.12 Which of the following statements from the mother of a pregnant 13-year-old would be an expected response?
1. "We had such high hopes for you."
2. "But she was always an easygoing child."
3. "I told you that boy was up to no good."
4. "This is just one of those things that happen."

Answer: 1
Rationale: When an adolescent pregnancy is first revealed to the teen's mother, the result is often anger, shame, or disappointment. The degree of negative response will be determined by the age of the teen, the family expectations for the teen, and presence or absence of other teen pregnancies in the family or support network. In early adolescents, the teen's mother frequently accompanies her daughter to prenatal examinations. The role of the nurse is to facilitate communication between mother and daughter, and provide education for both.
Assessment
Psychosocial Integrity
Analysis
Learning Objective 17.8

17.13 The nurse is working in a teen pregnancy clinic. In order to give the pregnant adolescent a role in her prenatal care, the nurse should allow the teen to
1. choose the type of prenatal vitamin she takes.

Answer: 2
Rationale: Having the client weigh herself and record her weight provides her with information that indicates she is growing a healthy fetus. Prenatal vitamins are prescribed by the Certified Nurse-Midwife or the physician. Many formulations exist, and some may not be indicated for this client due to her nutritional practices and lab results. In addition, if the client is a member of a Health Maintenance Organization, only certain medications (including prenatal

2. measure and record her weight at each visit. 3. choose the schedule of her prenatal visits. 4. decide if she wants her labor to be induced.	vitamins) are accepted for coverage. Prenatal visit schedules are set to detect developing complications of pregnancy. Induction of labor is a medical decision, and should not be taken lightly. Planning Health Promotion and Maintenance Analysis Learning Objective 17.9
17.14 A 16-year-old is making her first prenatal visit to the clinic in her fourth month of pregnancy. The nurse's first responsibility would be to 1. contact the social worker. 2. develop a trusting relationship. 3. schedule the client for prenatal classes. 4. teach the client about proper nutrition.	Answer: 2 Rationale: The most important goal for the nurse caring for a pregnant adolescent is to be open-minded and nonjudgmental in order to foster trust between the adolescent and the nurse. Through a trusting relationship, the nurse can provide counseling and education to the mother-to-be, both about her body and the fetus. A social worker might be able to provide assistance with financial program eligibility, support groups, or obtaining baby items such as furniture and car seats. Prenatal classes specifically designed for teen moms and attended by only teen moms facilitate both learning and support for the teens. Although nutrition is an important physiologic need, without a trusting relationship, little teaching will occur, because the teen will often "tune out" adults that she does not trust. Planning Psychosocial Integrity Application Learning Objective 17.9
17.15 The nurse is planning a community adolescent pregnancy prevention program. Which of the following strategies should the program include in order to be effective? 1. role models from similar cultural and racial backgrounds 2. planning executed by the planner and organizer only 3. short-term, informal programs available twice per year 4. focus on the expectations of the adolescents' parents	Answer: 1 Rationale: The National Campaign to Prevent Teen Pregnancy's task forces found that the programs most effective at preventing teen pregnancy provide models from similar cultural and racial backgrounds as the participants. They also include adolescents in the planning of activities, are both long-term and intensive, and focus on adolescent males and not just females. Planning Health Promotion and Maintenance Analysis Learning Objective 17.10

CHAPTER 18

18.1 The nurse is presenting a preconceptual counseling class. The nurse instructs the participants that niacin intake should increase during pregnancy to promote metabolic coenzyme activity. The nurse would know that teaching has been effective if a client suggests which of the following foods as a source of niacin? 1. fish 2. apples 3. broccoli 4. milk	Answer: 1 Rationale: Dietary sources of niacin include meats, fish, and enriched grains. Apples, broccoli, and milk will provide sources of other vitamins; however, they do not contain significant niacin. Evaluation Physiologic Integrity Application Learning Objective 18.1
18.2 The nurse evaluates the diet of a pregnant client, and finds that it is low in zinc. The nurse knows that zinc intake should increase during pregnancy to promote protein metabolism. Which of the following foods should the nurse suggest in order to increase intake of zinc?	Answer: 1 Rationale: Zinc is found in greatest concentration in meats and meat byproducts. Enriched grains also tend to be high in zinc. Bananas, yogurt, and cabbage are high in other nutrients but do not have significant levels of zinc. Implementation Physiologic Integrity Application Learning Objective 18.1

1. shellfish
2. bananas
3. yogurt
4. cabbage

18.3 The breastfeeding mother is concerned that her milk production has decreased. The nurse knows that further client teaching is needed based on which statement?
1. "I am drinking a minimum of eight to ten glasses of liquid a day."
2. "I have started cutting back on my protein intake."
3. "At least three times a day, I am drinking a glass of milk."
4. "I try to take a nap in the morning and afternoon when the baby is sleeping."

Answer: 2
Rationale: The breastfeeding mother must consume a minimum of eight to ten glasses of liquid per day, and increase her protein and calcium intake. It has also been found that adequate rest is necessary for the body to maintain its production of milk. The decreased intake of protein will decrease milk production.
Evaluation
Physiologic Integrity
Analysis
Learning Objective 18.2

18.4 The nurse is preparing for a postpartum home visit. The client has been home for a week, is breastfeeding, and experienced a third-degree perineal tear after vaginal delivery. The nurse should assess the client for
1. dietary intake of fiber and fluids.
2. dietary intake of folic acid and prenatal vitamins.
3. return of the hemoglobin and hematocrit levels to baseline.
4. return of protein and albumin to pre-delivery levels.

Answer: 1
Rationale: This mother needs to avoid the risk of constipation. She might be hesitant to have a bowel movement due to anticipated pain from the perineal tear, and constipation will decrease the healing of the laceration. Dietary intake of prenatal vitamins is important while breastfeeding, but folic acid is important prior to conception and in the first weeks of pregnancy to prevent neural tube defects. It will take several months for the laboratory levels to return to normal.
Planning
Physiologic Integrity
Analysis
Learning Objective 18.2

18.5 The pregnant client was assessed at her initial prenatal visit, and her diet was found to be low in nutrients. Prenatal supplements were prescribed by the Certified Nurse-Midwife. At her second prenatal visit the client states that she does not want "to take all these supplements." What recommendation should the nurse make for the client? (Select all that apply.)
1. "Folic acid has been found to be essential for minimizing the risk of neural tube defects."
2. "You do not have to take these supplements if you think you are healthy enough."
3. "These medications do the same thing I will call your Certified Nurse-Midwife to cancel one of your medications."
4. "You can trust your Certified Nurse-Midwife. Don't worry about taking the supplements."
5. "You need the supplements because your dietary intake is not adequate for fetal development."

Answer: 1, 5
Rationale: Research has shown such a strong correlation between decreased folic acid/folate intake and the risk of neural tube defects that all women who are considering becoming pregnant are encouraged to begin taking a 400 mcg supplement beginning two months before attempting conception and continue through the first trimester. Iron is essential because most pregnant women do not have adequate intake of iron before pregnancy. The client must take both supplements. Therapeutic communication requires addressing the client's concern, and not giving a cliché for an answer. One role of the nurse is educator, and this client needs additional information on why she needs the supplements.
Implementation
Physiologic Integrity
Analysis
Learning Objective 18.3

18.6 A pregnant client who is of normal pre-pregnancy weight is now 30 weeks pregnant. She asks the nurse what is an appropriate weight gain. The nurse's best response is
1. "25–28 pounds."
2. "20–22 pounds."
3. "17–18 pounds."
4. "less than 15 pounds."

Answer: 2
Rationale: The method for calculating weight gain is based on the expectation that a pregnant woman will gain three to five pounds for the first trimester and then one pound each week thereafter. Therefore, a 30-week pregnancy should end with a weight gain of 17 + 3–17 + 5, which is 20–22 pounds.
Implementation
Physiologic Integrity
Application
Learning Objective 18.4

18.7 A pregnant client who follows a strict vegan diet asks the nurse to assist her with her diet. The nurse should assess intake of which nutrient?
1. iron
2. vitamin C
3. vegetables
4. fruits

Answer: 1
Rationale: Vegans do not eat meat or any animal products, and consequently tend to have low iron levels. It is difficult for vegan clients to have adequate intake of iron and proteins prior to pregnancy. This problem increases with the pregnancy and the infant's needs for iron stores. Vegans only eat fruits and vegetables; therefore, they usually have adequate vitamin C intake.
Planning
Physiologic Integrity
Application
Learning Objective 18.10

18.8 A client has achieved a 20-pound weight loss over the past year. She now is at the antepartum clinic. Her pregnancy test is positive. She is concerned about gaining the weight back, and asks the nurse if she can remain on her diet. The nurse's best response would be
1. "As long as you supplement your diet with the prenatal vitamins, the amount of weight you gain in pregnancy is not significant."
2. "I understand that gaining weight after such an accomplishment must not look attractive, but weight gain during pregnancy is important for proper fetal growth."
3. "Dieting during pregnancy is considered child neglect."
4. "Excessive weight in pregnancy is due to water retention, so weight loss following birth will not be an issue."

Answer: 2
Rationale: Supplementation with vitamins is important, but maintaining weight gain within the respected parameters is more important. Good nutrition is essential for the health and well-being of the mother and the fetus. Adequate weight gain is an indicator of adequate nutrition. Child neglect can apply only after the child has been born. Weight gain during pregnancy typically is not water-related except with disease processes. Excess weight gain can be difficult to lose.
Implementation
Physiologic Integrity
Application
Learning Objective 18.6

18.9 The pregnant client cannot tolerate milk or meat. What should the nurse recommend to the client to assist in meeting protein needs?
1. wheat bread and pasta
2. ice cream and peanut butter
3. eggs and tofu
4. beans and potatoes

Answer: 3
Rationale: The best selection of food choices that are non-dairy and complete proteins are eggs and tofu. Wheat bread and pasta are not sources of complete protein. Ice cream is a milk byproduct, and would not be tolerated by this client. Beans and potatoes would not provide the client with adequate protein.
Implementation
Physiologic Integrity
Application
Learning Objective 18.6

18.10 When preparing nutritional instruction, which of the following pregnant clients would the nurse consider highest priority?
1. 40-year-old gravida 2
2. 22-year-old primigravida
3. 35-year-old gravida 4
4. 15-year-old nulligravida

Answer: 4
Rationale: Adolescent clients typically are still in their own growth cycle. Suddenly, they have to supply nutrition for themselves and the fetus. This places them at highest risk for malnutrition. The 22-year-old, the 40-year-old, and the 35-year-old have completed their growth cycles, and their bodies can focus on diverting the nutritional needs to the fetus.
Planning
Physiologic Integrity

be included in a teaching plan for this client? 1. Exercise either just before meals or wait until two hours after a meal. 2. Carry hard candy (or other simple sugar) when exercising. 3. If your blood sugar is 120 mg/dL, eat 20 g of carbohydrate. 4. If your blood sugar is more than 120 mg/dL, drink a glass of whole milk.	Implementation Health Promotion and Maintenance Analysis Learning Objective 19.2
19.5 The client with β-thalassemia intermedia has a hemoglobin level of 9.0. The nurse is preparing an education session for the client. Which statement should the nurse include? 1. "You need to increase your intake of meat and other iron-rich foods." 2. "Your low hemoglobin could put you into preterm labor." 3. "Increasing your vitamin C intake will help your hemoglobin level." 4. "You should not take iron or folic acid supplements."	Answer: 4 Rationale: β-thalassemia intermedia is due to an abnormal red blood cell structure, which leads to microcytic anemia with normal ferritin and iron levels. Iron supplements should be avoided to prevent iron overload. Because the iron levels are normal, increasing dietary iron intake will not affect the hemoglobin. Vitamin C increases iron absorption, but a client with thalassemia does not need additional iron. Planning Physiologic Integrity Application Learning Objective 19.3
19.6 The client at 20 weeks' gestation has had an ultrasound that reveals that her fetus has a neural tube defect. The client's hemoglobin level is 8.5. The nurse should include which statement when discussing these findings with the client? 1. "Your low iron intake has caused anemia, which leads to the neural tube defect." 2. "You should increase your vitamin C intake to improve your anemia." 3. "You are too picky about food. Your poor diet caused your baby's defect." 4. "You haven't had enough folic acid in your diet. You should take a supplement."	Answer: 4 Rationale: Folic acid deficiency can cause both neural tube defects and megaloblastic anemia, in which the red cells are immature and abnormally large. Low hemoglobin does not cause neural tube defects. Vitamin C will increase iron absorption, but this client is deficient in folic acid. Therapeutic communication must avoid judgmental statements. Implementation Health Promotion and Maintenance Analysis Learning Objective 19.3
19.7 During the history, the client admits to being HIV-positive and knows that she is about 16 weeks pregnant. Which statements made by the client indicate an understanding of the plan of care both during the pregnancy and postpartally? (Select all that apply.) 1. "During labor and delivery, I can expect the zidovudine (AZT) to be given in my IV." 2. "After delivery, the dose of zidovudine (AZT) will be doubled to prevent further infection." 3. "My baby will be started on zidovudine (AZT) within 12 hours of delivery." 4. "My baby's zidovudine (AZT) will be given in a cream form."	Answer: 1, 3 Rationale: All HIV-positive clients are prescribed a three-part therapy after the first trimester. The initial treatment is zidovudine (AZT) orally every day. In order to keep the level consistent, it is recommended that dosages be taken consistently. During the labor and delivery process, the doses will be given intravenously. Finally, within 8–12 hours after delivery, the infant is administered oral zidovudine (AZT) and kept on the medication a minimum of six weeks. The mother will continue with her oral dosage of zidovudine (AZT) after delivery just as prior to delivery. Evaluation Health Promotion and Maintenance Analysis Learning Objective 19.4

5. "My baby will not need zidovudine (AZT) if I take it during my pregnancy."

19.8 A woman is 32 weeks pregnant. She is HIV-positive but asymptomatic. What would be important in managing her pregnancy and delivery?
1. an amniocentesis at 30 and 36 weeks
2. weekly nonstress testing beginning at 32 weeks' gestation
3. application of a fetal scalp electrode as soon as her membranes rupture in labor
4. administration of intravenous antibiotics during labor and delivery

Answer: 2
Rationale: Clients who are HIV-positive are considered high-risk pregnancies. Therefore, beginning at about 32 weeks, these clients have weekly nonstress tests to assess for placental function and an ultrasound every two to three weeks to assess for intrauterine growth retardation (IUGR). All invasive procedures are avoided that would expose the uninfected infant to the HIV virus. Antibiotics would be ineffective for either the mother or the infant who is HIV-positive.
Planning
Health Promotion and Maintenance
Analysis
Learning Objective 19.4

19.9 A pregnant woman is married to an intravenous drug user. She had a negative HIV screening test just after missing her first menstrual period. What would indicate that the client needs to be retested for HIV?
1. hemoglobin of 11 g/dL and a rapid weight gain
2. elevated blood pressure and ankle edema
3. shortness of breath and frequent urination
4. unusual fatigue and recurring Candida vaginitis

Answer: 4
Rationale: The client who is HIV-positive would have a suppressed immune system and would experience symptoms of fatigue and opportunistic infections such as Candida vaginitis. The client would be anemic and anorexic, with a decrease in blood pressure and no ankle edema. Shortness of breath and frequent urination do not indicate a need to retest for HIV.
Assessment
Health Promotion and Maintenance
Application
Learning Objective 19.4

19.10 A 21-year-old is 12 weeks pregnant with her first baby. She has cardiac disease, class III, as a result of having had childhood rheumatic fever. During a prenatal visit, the nurse reviews the signs of cardiac decompensation with her. The nurse will know that the client understands these signs and symptoms if she states, "I would notify my doctor if I have
1. a pulse rate increase of ten beats per minute."
2. breast tenderness."
3. mild ankle edema."
4. a frequent cough."

Answer: 4
Rationale: With the increased workload of the heart with pregnancy and the increase in blood volume, this client is at risk for developing congestive heart failure. This would result in a frequent cough. The majority of pregnant clients will develop breast tenderness, and the heart rate will increase. The client with rheumatic heart disease will have a much higher pulse rate. Also, the client with rheumatic heart disease who develops congestive heart failure would have severe ankle edema.
Evaluation
Health Promotion and Maintenance
Analysis
Learning Objective 19.5

19.11 A 21-year-old woman is 12 weeks pregnant with her first baby. She has cardiac disease, class III, as a result of having had childhood rheumatic fever. Which planned activity would indicate to the nurse that the client needs further teaching?
1. "I will be sure to take a rest period every afternoon."
2. "I would like to take childbirth education classes in my last trimester."
3. "I will have to cancel our trip to Disney World."

Answer: 4
Rationale: The client with class III heart disease will experience an increased heart rate and become symptomatic with the slightest amount of exertion. Therefore, she should not establish a new exercise program. Because of the class III of the heart disease, this client should be encouraged to get adequate rest. Childbirth classes would be helpful for the client, as long as she is aware not to overexert herself. Travel during the pregnancy would be based upon the tolerance of the client. However, a trip to Disney World would involve a large amount of activity and would stress the client.
Evaluation
Health Promotion and Maintenance
Analysis
Learning Objective 19.5

---

4. "I am going to start my water aerobics classes next week."

19.12 The client was found to have hepatitis B surface antigen (HBsAG) early in her pregnancy. The nurse is explaining to the client what will happen during labor and birth because the client is contagious for hepatitis B. Which statement by the client indicates that additional teaching is needed?
1. "An internal fetal monitor will be applied as soon as possible during labor."
2. "My baby will get a bath as soon as its temperature is stable."
3. "Two shots will be given to my baby to prevent transmission of hepatitis B."
4. "Breastfeeding is a good feeding method for my baby."

Answer: 1
Rationale: The presence of hepatitis B surface antigen (HBsAG) indicates that the client is contagious for and capable of transmitting hepatitis B. Perinatal transmission is most likely to occur at the time of birth, thus measures are taken to prevent exposing the fetus to the mother's blood and body fluids and to clean the baby's skin thoroughly of fluids as soon as possible after birth. An internal fetal monitor will be avoided. Breastfeeding is not contraindicated in a client with HBsAG. A newborn of a mother with HBsAG will receive an injection of hepatitis B immune globulin and a hepatitis B vaccine injection.
Evaluation
Health Promotion and Maintenance
Analysis
Learning Objective 19.6

19.13 A 26-year-old multipara is 26 weeks pregnant. Her previous births include two large-for-gestational-age babies and one unexplained stillbirth. Which tests would the nurse anticipate as being most definitive in diagnosing gestational diabetes?
1. a 50 g, one-hour glucose screening test
2. a single fasting glucose level
3. a 100 g, one-hour glucose tolerance test
4. a 100 g, three-hour glucose tolerance test

Answer: 4
Rationale: A client with a history of LGA infants or gestational diabetes will be given the 100 g of glucose and three-hour glucose tolerance test. All women get the initial 50 g of glucose and a one-hour screening. A single fasting glucose level is not an adequate indicator of the glucose level in relation to food, nor is the 100 g, one-hour tolerance test.
Planning
Health Promotion and Maintenance
Application
Learning Objective 19.2

19.14 A client is 12 weeks pregnant with her first baby. She has class III cardiac disease. She states that she had been taking sodium warfarin (Coumadin), but her physician changed her to heparin (Hepalean). She asks the nurse why this was done. The nurse's response should be
1. "Heparin may be given by mouth, while warfarin must be injected."
2. "Heparin is safer because it does not cross the placenta."
3. "They are the same drug, but heparin is less expensive."
4. "Warfarin interferes with iron absorption in the intestines."

Answer: 2
Rationale: Heparin (Hepalean) is safest for the client to take, because it does not cross the placental barrier, and therefore will not increase the fetal clotting time. Warfarin (Coumadin) is teratogenic. Heparin (Hepalean) is injected and warfarin (Coumadin) is taken orally. Heparin (Hepalean) does not cost less. Warfarin (Coumadin) does not interfere with iron absorption in the intestines.
Implementation
Health Promotion and Maintenance
Application
Learning Objective 19.5

19.15 The nurse is doing preconceptual counseling with a 28-year-old woman with no prior pregnancies. Which of the following statements made by the client indicates to the nurse that the client has understood the teaching?
1. "I can continue to drink alcohol until I am diagnosed as pregnant."

Answer: 2
Rationale: Women should discontinue drinking alcohol when they start to attempt pregnancy. It is not known how much alcohol will cause fetal damage; therefore, alcohol during pregnancy is contraindicated. Alcohol passes readily into breast milk; therefore, it should be avoided, or the milk should be pumped and dumped after alcohol consumption.
Evaluation
Health Promotion and Maintenance

---

2. "I need to stop drinking alcohol completely when I start trying to get pregnant."
3. "A beer once a week will not damage the fetus."
4. "I can drink alcohol while breastfeeding since it doesn't pass into breast milk."

Application
Learning Objective 19.1

CHAPTER 20

20.1 A woman is 16 weeks pregnant. She has had cramping, backache, and mild bleeding for the past three days. Her physician determines that her cervix is dilated to 2 centimeters, with 10% effacement, but membranes are still intact. She is crying, and says to the nurse, "Is my baby going to be okay?" In addition to acknowledging the client's fear, the nurse should also say

1. "Your baby will be fine. Don't worry. We'll start an IV, and get this stopped in no time at all."
2. "Your cervix is beginning to dilate. That is a serious sign. We will continue to monitor you and the baby."
3. "You are going to miscarry. But most miscarriages are the result of abnormalities in the fetus."
4. "I really can't say. However, when your physician comes, you can ask her to talk to you about it."

Answer: 2
Rationale: A cerclage can be performed in the first trimester and early into the second trimester. Many interventions can be attempted to prevent further dilation and effacement. This is a serious situation. The client should not be offered false hope of everything being fine. The nurse should avoid justification of the miscarriage. The nurse should not defer the conversation to someone else, such as the physician.
Implementation
Health Promotion and Maintenance
Analysis
Learning Objective 20.2

20.2 A client who is 11 weeks pregnant presents to the emergency room with complaints of dizziness, lower abdominal pain, and right shoulder pain. Laboratory tests reveal a beta-hCG at a lower than expected level for this gestational age. An adnexal mass is palpable. Ultrasound confirms no intrauterine gestation. The client is crying, and asks what is happening. The nurse knows that the most likely diagnosis is an ectopic pregnancy. Which statement should the nurse include?

1. "The dizziness you feel is because the pregnancy is compressing your vena cava."
2. "The pain is due to the baby putting pressure on nerves internally."
3. "The baby is in the fallopian tube; the tube has ruptured and is causing bleeding."
4. "This is a minor problem. The doctor will be right back to explain it to you."

Answer: 3
Rationale: Dizziness and abdominal pain with shoulder pain are symptoms of internal bleeding. A lower than expected beta-hCG indicates either an ectopic pregnancy or a pregnancy that is miscarrying; in this case, it is from the pregnancy being ectopic. The ultrasound confirmation of a lack of intrauterine pregnancy is another indication the pregnancy is ectopic. Dizziness from vena cava compression occurs in the third trimester when women are supine. The fetus is too small to be putting pressure on nerves. Therapeutic communication requires giving the client an answer and not referring the client to speak with someone else.
Planning
Health Promotion and Maintenance
Analysis
Learning Objective 20.1

20.3 A woman has had her hydatidiform mole (molar pregnancy) evacuated, and is prepared for discharge. The nurse should make certain that the client understands that it is essential that she

1. not become pregnant for at least one year.
2. receive Rh$_o$ (D) Immune Globulin RhoGAM with her next pregnancy and birth.
3. have her blood pressure checked weekly for the next 30 days.
4. seek genetic counseling with her partner before the next pregnancy.

Answer: 1
Rationale: Hydatidiform mole (molar pregnancy) is the result of an empty ovum being fertilized or two sperm fertilizing one egg. For one year after the pregnancy, hCG levels are monitored to assess for carcinoma growth. Clients are advised not to get pregnant due to potential confusion regarding tumor growth or pregnancy. There is no indication for the administration of Rh$_o$ (D) Immune Globulin (RhoGAM). There is no indication of blood pressure problems or preeclampsia. This is not a genetic defect, so genetic counseling is not indicated.
Planning
Health Promotion and Maintenance
Application
Learning Objective 20.1

20.4 A pregnant woman at 16 weeks' gestation is diagnosed with hyperemesis gravidarum. She has been admitted to the floor from the emergency department. Which issue should receive priority for the nurse planning care?

1. fluid volume deficit
2. constipation
3. decreased pulse rate
4. knowledge deficit

Answer: 1
Rationale: The newly-admitted client with hyperemesis gravidarum has been experiencing excessive vomiting and is in a fluid volume deficit state. Because no preexisting cardiac condition is present, the body has compensated for this fluid loss. Constipation is more likely to be a problem in later pregnancy; however, if constipation were present, it would be a lower priority than the fluid volume deficit. The pulse rate would be increased due to hypovolemia. Knowledge deficit is a psychosocial need, and therefore will not be a top priority when providing care to this client.
Assessment
Health Promotion and Maintenance
Application
Learning Objective 20.3

20.5 A woman is experiencing preterm labor. The client asks why she is on betamethasone (Celestone). The best response by the nurse would be, "This medication

1. will halt the labor process, until the baby is more mature."
2. will relax the smooth muscles in the infant's lungs so the baby can breathe."
3. is effective in stimulating lung development in the preterm infant."
4. is an antibiotic that will treat your urinary tract infection, which caused preterm labor."

Answer: 3
Rationale: Betamethasone (Celestone) has been found to induce pulmonary maturation, and thereby decrease the risk of respiratory problems in the preterm infant. It has no effect on the labor process or on the smooth muscles in the lungs. This medication is not an antibiotic, and therefore will not help resolve a urinary tract infection.
Implementation
Health Promotion and Maintenance
Application
Learning Objective 20.4

20.6 A woman is 30 weeks pregnant. She has come to the hospital because her membranes have ruptured spontaneously. The labor and delivery nurse explains what will be done for the client and her fetus. Which statement should the nurse include?

1. "We will give you medication to help the baby's lungs mature."
2. "Infection is not an issue, but we'll monitor you for infection."
3. "An IV will be started to increase your intravascular fluid volume."
4. "Since you are coping fine, we'll transfer you to the high-risk floor."

Answer: 1
Rationale: Because of the rupture of membranes and the preterm status, an attempt will be made to mature the fetal lungs and maintain the pregnancy for as long as possible. Therefore, the greatest risk is for infection. This client is not at risk for fluid volume deficit. There is not enough information to determine how she is coping.
Planning
Health Promotion and Maintenance
Analysis
Learning Objective 20.4

20.7 A woman is being treated for preterm labor with magnesium sulfate. The nurse is concerned that the client is experiencing early drug toxicity. What assessment finding by the nurse indicates early magnesium sulfate toxicity?

1. patellar reflexes are weak or +1
2. complaints by the client of feeling flushed and warm
3. respiratory rate of 16
4. fetal heart rate of 120

Answer: 1
Rationale: Early signs of magnesium sulfate toxicity are related to a decrease in deep tendon reflexes. The peripheral vasodilation will cause flushing and a feeling of warmth; this is a side effect, not a toxic effect. Late signs of toxicity are a respiratory rate less than 12, urine output less than 30 cc/hr, and confusion. Magnesium typically has no effect on fetal heart rate.
Assessment
Health Promotion and Maintenance
Application
Learning Objective 20.5

20.8 A client has preeclampsia. She is 36 weeks pregnant, and comes to the high-risk screening center for a contraction stress test. The nurse should explain to the client that the contraction stress test is being done to determine

1. what effect her hypertension has had on the fetus.
2. if the fetus will be able to tolerate labor.
3. if fetal movement increases with contractions.
4. what effect contractions will have on her blood pressure.

Answer: 2
Rationale: Contraction stress tests are performed to assess the ability of the fetus to tolerate labor. The effect of contractions on blood pressure would be noted, but this is not the purpose. With contractions, the nurse is assessing for a heart rate response, not movement. The fetal heart rate response to movement is assessed in a nonstress test.
Implementation
Health Promotion and Maintenance
Application
Learning Objective 20.5

20.9 During her first prenatal visit to the clinic at seven weeks' gestation, a 24-year-old primiparous client comments, "My blood type is A negative, and my husband's blood type is B positive. Will that cause problems with my pregnancy?" The nurse's best response would be

1. "There is no danger to your baby, but there could be a few minor complications for you. Let's talk about what we can do to prevent those."
2. "We will do a blood test to see if your body is responding to the baby's blood type. If so, we will give the baby some medication to prevent harm."
3. "Because your partner is positive and you are negative, there is some risk to the baby, but because this is your first pregnancy the risks are very small."
4. "If you were O negative, you might have ABO incompatibility because of your partner's blood type; but since you are type A, there should be no problem."

Answer: 3
Rationale: This client is at risk for Rh incompatibility because she is Rh negative and the father of the baby is Rh positive. Because this is her first pregnancy, it is extremely unlikely that she has been exposed to Rh positive blood, which would stimulate the development of antibodies. These antibodies cross the placenta, and cause fetal hemolysis which can lead to severe anemia that could cause fetal loss. It is recommended that a Coombs' blood test be drawn to assess for antibody formation at the first prenatal visit and again at 28 weeks. Rh_o (D) Immune Globulin (RhoGAM) will be given to the mother (not the fetus) at 28 weeks, and again after delivery if the baby is Rh positive, to prevent antibody formation. ABO incompatibility is not present.
Implementation
Health Promotion and Maintenance
Analysis
Learning Objective 20.6

20.10 The nurse identifies the following assessment findings on a client with preeclampsia: blood pressure 158/100; urinary output 50 mL/hour; lungs clear to auscultation; urine protein 1+ on dipstick; and edema of the hands, ankles, and feet. On the next hourly assessment, which of the following new assessment findings would be an indication of worsening of the preeclampsia?

1. blood pressure 158/104
2. urinary output 20 mL/hour
3. reflexes 2+
4. platelet count 150,000

Answer: 2
Rationale: The decrease in urine output is an indication of decrease in GFR, which indicates a loss of renal perfusion. The blood pressure has not had a significant rise, the reflexes are normal at 2+, and the platelet count is normal, though it is at the lower end. The assessment finding most abnormal and life-threatening is the urine output change.
Assessment
Health Promotion and Maintenance
Application
Learning Objective 20.5

20.11 The client presents to the clinic for an initial prenatal examination. She asks the nurse if there might be a problem for her baby because she has type B Rh positive blood and her husband has type O Rh negative blood, or because her sister's baby had ABO incompatibility. What is the nurse's best answer? (Select all that apply.)

1. "Your baby would be at risk for Rh problems if your husband was Rh negative."
2. "Rh problems only occur when the mother is Rh negative and the father is not."
3. "ABO incompatibility occurs only after the baby is born."
4. "We don't know for sure, but we can test for ABO incompatibility."
5. "Your husband being type B puts you at risk for ABO incompatibility."

Answer: 3,4
Rationale: Rh incompatibility is a possibility when the mother is Rh negative and the father is Rh positive. ABO incompatibility occurs when the mother is type O and the baby is type A or B or AB at the time the placenta delivers. There is no prenatal testing for ABO incompatibility because it is a postnatal problem. The husband's blood type is not an issue for ABO incompatibility, which causes hemolysis and jaundice in babies and does not affect mothers.
Planning
Health Promotion and Maintenance
Analysis
Learning Objective 20.7

20.12 The client at 36 weeks' gestation requires an appendectomy. The nurse has performed the preoperative teaching. Which statement made by the client indicates a need for additional information?

1. "I will be tilted to my left side to prevent the baby from compressing a major blood vessel and causing my blood pressure to drop."
2. "It may be more difficult for the surgeon to find my appendix because the uterus is enlarged from the baby."
3. "Coughing and deep breathing after surgery will help prevent me from developing pneumonia."
4. "I can take off these anti-embolism stockings as soon as I am awake from the anesthesia."

Answer: 4
Rationale: Due to the increased estrogen level of pregnancy and immobility, the risk for developing thrombophlebitis is higher than in a non-pregnant state. Anti-embolism stockings will be used until the client is ambulatory. Vena cava syndrome can occur if the client in the third trimester is positioned supine, therefore a left lateral tilt is used. The enlarged uterus can make it difficult to reach other abdominal organs in the third trimester. Clients will be encouraged to cough and deep breathe to prevent atelectasis and pneumonia.
Evaluation
Health Promotion and Maintenance
Analysis
Learning Objective 20.8

20.13 The client at 32 weeks' gestation slipped on the ice and fell, and landed on her abdomen and outstretched arms. She has a broken left wrist that is splinted. She is in the obstetrical triage unit to assess fetal wellbeing. Which statement should the nurse include when explaining procedures to the client?

1. "It's very rare for the pregnancy to be affected when you land on your abdomen."
2. "Since your wrist is broken, there is a danger that the uterus has ruptured."
3. "Advanced pregnancy affects balance, which can lead to more falls on slippery surfaces like ice."
4. "We'll just take your vital signs, then you'll return to the orthopedist."

Answer: 3
Rationale: Advanced pregnancy affects balance and coordination, which results in more falls, especially in slippery conditions. Landing on the abdomen can cause the placenta to abrupt. A ruptured uterus would lead to severe internal bleeding, which would manifest as abdominal pain, and hypovolemic shock. There is no correlation between fractures and uterine rupture. The fetus must be evaluated by electronic fetal monitoring, and occasionally with an ultrasound examination as well. Just taking vital signs does not assess the fetus.
Implementation
Health Promotion and Maintenance
Analysis
Learning Objective 20.9

20.14 The client at 34 weeks' gestation has been stabbed in the low abdomen by her boyfriend. She is brought to the emergency room for treatment. Which statement indicates that the client understands the treatment being administered? (Select all that apply.)

1. "The baby needs to be monitored to check the heart rate."
2. "My bowel has probably been lacerated by the knife."
3. "I may need an ultrasound to look at the baby."
4. "The catheter in my bladder will prevent urinary complications."
5. "The IV in my arm will replace the amniotic fluid if it is leaking."

Answer: 1, 3
Rationale: Penetrating trauma to the abdomen during advanced pregnancy often results in ruptured membranes, with external leaking of fluid. The baby will be evaluated with electronic fetal monitoring and ultrasound examination to determine the hemodynamic stability of the fetus and look for injuries of the fetus. The pregnancy usually sustains the majority of the damage, sparing the bowel from injury. Fetal mortality after penetrating trauma to the abdomen ranges from 59% to 80%. The Foley catheter is placed to assess for hematuria. The IV will replace intravascular volume, not amniotic fluid.
Evaluation
Health Promotion and Maintenance
Analysis
Learning Objective 20.9

20.15 A woman is 10 weeks pregnant. Her initial prenatal laboratory screening test for rubella showed an antibody titer of less than 1:6. The woman calls the clinic and tells the nurse that she has been exposed to rubella. The nurse's best response is

1. "Since you are in your first trimester of pregnancy, there is not likely to be a problem."
2. "Would you like to see a counselor to talk about your options for the remainder of your pregnancy?"
3. "You should come to the clinic in the next day or two for further evaluation."
4. "You need to have a rubella vaccination immediately. Can you get a ride to the clinic today?"

Answer: 3
Rationale: The best advice for the client would be to come to the clinic in the next day or two to talk with the nurse and physician about her options. Exposure to rubella in the first trimester has the greatest risk for causing congenital anomalies. Clients are not vaccinated during the pregnancy. It is not therapeutic to send the client to a counselor.
Implementation
Physiologic Integrity
Application
Learning Objective 20.10

21.1 The client with an abnormal quadruple screen is scheduled for an ultrasound. Which of the following statements indicate that the client understands the need for this additional antepartal fetal surveillance?

1. "After the ultrasound, my partner and I will decide how to decorate the nursery."
2. "During the ultrasound we will see which of us the baby looks most like."
3. "The ultrasound will show if there are abnormalities with the baby's spine."
4. "The blood test wasn't run correctly and now we need to have the sonogram."

Answer: 3

Rationale: Ultrasound is used to detect neural tube defects. However, parents often try to identify the baby's sex, and which parent the fetus most resembles during an ultrasound.

An abnormal serum quadruple screen is not a result of a lab error, and can indicate either an open neural tube defect, or trisomy 18 or 21.

Evaluation

Health Promotion and Maintenance

Analysis

Learning Objective 21.1

21.2 The nurse is assisting with a transabdominal ultrasound procedure to determine fetal age. The nurse should

1. ask the woman to sign an operative consent form prior to the procedure.
2. have the woman empty her bladder before the test begins.
3. assist the woman into a supine position on the examining table.
4. instruct the woman to not eat two hours before the scheduled test time.

Answer: 3

Rationale: Clients are placed in a supine position for transabdominal ultrasounds. Transabdominal ultrasounds are not invasive procedures, and do not require a consent form. The recommendation is that the client has a full bladder to help elevate the uterus out of the pelvic cavity for better visualization. Dietary intake is not relevant to an ultrasound of pregnancy.

Planning

Health Promotion and Maintenance

Application

Learning Objective 21.2

21.3 The nurse is returning phone calls from clients. Which client does the nurse anticipate would not require a serum Beta hCG?

1. a client with a risk of ectopic pregnancy
2. a client with spotting during pregnancy
3. a client with previous pelvic inflammatory disease
4. a client with a previous history of twins

Answer: 4

Rationale: A history of twins does not increase the risk of ectopic pregnancy. Beta human chorionic gonadatropin (hCG) will double every two days in a normally implanted pregnancy. An ectopic pregnancy will not double in two days. Clients at risk for developing an ectopic are those with a history of a previous ectopic, and history of pelvic inflammatory disease. Spotting during pregnancy can indicate ectopic pregnancy, although about one-third of women with normal pregnancies will also experience spotting.

Planning

Health Promotion and Maintenance

Analysis

Learning Objective 21.3

21.4 A woman is at 32 weeks' gestation. Her fundal height measurement at this clinic appointment is 26 centimeters. After reviewing the ultrasound results, the healthcare provider asks the nurse to schedule the client for a series of sonograms to be done every two weeks. The nurse should make sure that the client understands that the main purpose for this is to

1. assess for congenital anomalies.
2. evaluate fetal growth.
3. determine fetal presentation.
4. rule out a suspected hydatidiform mole.

Answer: 2

Rationale: A pregnant client at 32 weeks' gestation should measure 32 cm of fundal height. When a discrepancy between fundal height and measurement exists, the purpose of serial ultrasounds is to monitor fetal growth. Assessment of anomalies or of fetal presentation, or ruling out a hydatidiform mole, would require only one ultrasound.

Implementation

Health Promotion and Maintenance

Application

Learning Objective 21.4

21.5 At 32 weeks' gestation, a woman is scheduled for a second nonstress test (in addition to the one she had at 28 weeks' gestation). Which response by the client would indicate an adequate understanding of this procedure?
1. "I can't get up and walk around during the test."
2. "I'll have an IV started before the test."
3. "I must avoid drinks containing caffeine for 24 hours before the test."
4. "I need to have a full bladder for this test."

Answer: 1
Rationale: The purpose of the nonstress test is to determine fetal heart rate response to fetal movement. The client will have to lie still on her side during the procedure. There is no IV needed to administer medications. Caffeine might cause the infant to be more active. Clients usually are asked to have their bladders full only for first and second trimester ultrasounds.
Evaluation
Health Promotion and Maintenance
Analysis
Learning Objective 21.5

21.6 Each of the following pregnant women is scheduled for a 14-week antepartal visit. In planning care, the nurse should give priority teaching about the serum quadruple screen including alpha-fetoprotein amniotic (AFP) to which client?
1. 28-year-old with history of rheumatic heart disease
2. 18-year-old with exposure to HIV
3. 20-year-old with a history of preterm labor
4. 35-year-old with a child with spina bifida

Answer: 4
Rationale: Alpha-fetoprotein (AFP) is one component of the quadruple screen. AFP levels are elevated in multigestational pregnancies, in pregnancies with neural tube defects (such as spina bifida), and Down syndrome. The 35-year-old is considered to be of advanced maternal age, and is at risk for having a child with Down syndrome. Considering this client's past history of a child with spina bifida, she would be highly encouraged to have the AFP screening. The client with rheumatic heart disease would need to be monitored for pregnancy and the stressors it places on the client. The client with HIV exposure needs HIV testing and protection education. The client with a history of preterm labor needs education on prevention and signs and symptoms of preterm labor.
Planning
Health Promotion and Maintenance
Application
Learning Objective 21.5

21.7 A 27-year-old married woman is 16 weeks pregnant, and has an abnormally low maternal serum alpha-fetoprotein test. Which of the following statements indicates that the couple understands the implications of this test result?
1. "We have decided to have an abortion if this baby has Down syndrome."
2. "If we hadn't had this test, we wouldn't have to worry about this baby."
3. "I'll eat plenty of dark green leafy vegetables until I have the ultrasound."
4. "The ultrasound should be normal because I'm under the age of 35."

Answer: 1
Rationale: A low maternal serum alpha-fetoprotein test can indicate trisomy 18 or trisomy 21 (Down syndrome). Many couples will abort a fetus that has a genetic abnormality that significantly affects quality of life or has multiple medical problems. The condition begins in very early fetal life. Dark green leafy vegetables contain folic acid. Low folic acid levels in the first trimester can lead to neural tube defects, which would cause a high maternal serum alpha-fetoprotein screen. Down syndrome is more likely to occur in women over the age of 35 at delivery, but is not limited to this age group.
Evaluation
Health Promotion and Maintenance
Analysis
Learning Objective 21.6

21.8 The client and her partner are carriers of sickle cell disease. They are considering prenatal diagnosis with either amniocentesis or chorionic villus sampling (CVS). Which statements indicate that further teaching is needed on these two diagnostic procedures? (Select all that apply.)
1. "Chorionic villus sampling carries a lower risk of miscarriage."
2. "Amniocentesis can be done earlier in my pregnancy than CVS."
3. "Neither test will conclusively diagnose sickle cell disease in our baby."

Answer: 4, 5
Rationale: CVS is performed at 8–12 weeks' gestation and amniocentesis is performed at 11–14 weeks. Both are equally diagnostic, but because CVS is performed earlier in pregnancy and the results are usually back in about 24 hours, the greatest advantage to CVS is earlier diagnostic information. CVS carries twice the risk of spontaneous abortion compared to amniocentesis. Both tests will diagnose genetic disorders.
Evaluation
Health Promotion and Maintenance
Analysis
Learning Objective 21.7

4. "The diagnosis comes sooner if we have CVS, not amniocentesis."
5. "Amniocentesis is more accurate in diagnosis than the CVS."

21.9 For which client is the physician most likely to order a cervico-vaginal fetal fibronectin test?
1. 34-weeks' gestation with gestational diabetes
2. 32-weeks' gestation with regular uterine contractions
3. 37-weeks' multi-fetal gestation
4. 20-weeks' gestation with ruptured amniotic membranes

Answer: 2
Rationale: Fetal fibronectin is tested by swabbing the cervico-vaginal secretions. The presence of this substance is a strong predictor of preterm delivery, and thus is performed on women at risk for preterm delivery. Regular uterine contractions can be preterm labor. The client experiencing preterm contractions should be tested for the presence of fetal fibronectin. Gestational diabetes does not predispose a client toward preterm labor. Multi-fetal pregnancies often experience preterm delivery, but 37 weeks is at term. A pregnancy at 20 weeks has not reached the point of viability, and is treated as an impending spontaneous abortion, not preterm labor.
Assessment
Health Promotion and Maintenance
Application
Learning Objective 21.8

21.10 The client at 14 weeks' gestation has undergone a transvaginal ultrasound to assess cervical length. The ultrasound revealed cervical funneling. How should the nurse explain these findings to the client? "Your cervix
1. has become cone-shaped and more open at the end near the baby."
2. is shortened, and you will deliver your baby prematurely."
3. is short, and has become wider at the end that extends into the vagina."
4. was beginning to open but now is starting to close up again."

Answer: 1
Rationale: Transvaginal ultrasound involves inserting a small transducer into the vagina to perform the ultrasound exam. Cervical funneling is a widening of the portion of the cervix that attaches to the uterus. The outer os of the cervix can be closed, while the upper portion is dilating. This can be an indicator of an incompetent cervix or preterm labor. Cervical change in pregnancy is progressive, and the cervix does not spontaneously constrict or close again until after delivery.
Planning
Health Promotion and Maintenance
Application
Learning Objective 21.8

21.11 A 28-year-old woman has been an insulin-dependent diabetic for ten years. At 36 weeks' gestation she has an amniocentesis. A lecithin/sphingomyelin (L/S) ratio test is performed on the sample of her amniotic fluid. Since she is a diabetic, the 2:1 ratio obtained indicates that the fetus
1. may or may not have immature lungs.
2. has an intrauterine infection.
3. has a neural tube defect.
4. is at risk for hyperglycemia.

Answer: 1
Rationale: The fetal lungs mature more slowly in diabetics, especially those on insulin. An intrauterine infection would create cloudy amniotic fluid, with the presence of white blood cells. Neural tube defects are screened with the maternal serum alpha-fetoprotein test, and diagnosed with ultrasound. After birth, infants of diabetic mothers are at risk for hypoglycemia, not hyperglycemia.
Evaluation
Health Promotion and Maintenance
Analysis
Learning Objective 21.9

21.12 The client is being seen for her first prenatal appointment at 14 weeks' gestation. She is sure of her last menstrual period (LMP). The fundal height is measured at 20 centimeters. Which test would the nurse anticipate that the certified nurse-midwife will order for this client?
1. amniocentesis for fetal genetic anomaly
2. ultrasound to determine the number of fetuses
3. beta hCG to detect the location of the pregnancy

Answer: 2
Rationale: A significantly larger fundal height than expected during pregnancy can be an indicator of a multi-fetal pregnancy. Ultrasound in the second trimester will detect the number of fetuses present. Genetic anomalies would not create an overly large fundal height, nor does Down syndrome. Two or more Beta hCG tests are ordered in the first trimester to rule out ectopic pregnancy.
Planning
Health Promotion and Maintenance
Application
Learning Objective 21.4

---

4. maternal serum alpha fetoprotein for Down syndrome

21.13 A woman at 28 weeks' gestation is asked to keep a fetal activity diary and to bring the results with her to her next clinic visit. One week later, she calls the clinic and anxiously tells the nurse that she has not felt the baby move for over 30 minutes. What would be the most appropriate initial comment by the nurse?
1. "You need to come to the clinic right away for further evaluation."
2. "Have you been smoking?"
3. "When did you eat last?"
4. "Your baby may be asleep."

Answer: 4
Rationale: A lack of fetal activity for 30 minutes typically is insignificant and only means the infant is sleeping. After meals, typically an infant is active and moving. Smoking also typically will decrease fetal movements temporarily. The mother would need to come to the clinic only if there had been no fetal activity for several hours. If the mother truly is concerned, in 30 minutes, she could eat a complex carbohydrate snack. This may stimulate the fetus, and the mother should have fetal activity. But at present, this is an indicator that the fetus is sleeping.
Assessment
Health Promotion and Maintenance
Application
Learning Objective 21.5

21.14 A pregnant woman is having a nipple-stimulated contraction stress test (CST). Which result indicates hyperstimulation?
1. The fetal heart rate decelerates when three contractions occur within a ten-minute period.
2. The fetal heart rate accelerates when contractions last up to 60 seconds.
3. There are more than five fetal movements in a ten-minute period.
4. There are more than three uterine contractions in a ten-minute period.

Answer: 3
Rationale: Uterine hyperstimulation is characterized by contractions closer than or equal to every two minutes, or lasting longer than 90 seconds. Three contractions in ten minutes is the desired outcome of a contraction stress test to determine fetal well-being, and thus is not hyperstimulation. Decelerations are considered a positive contraction stress test. The acceleration of the heart rate and the fetal movement are considered a negative contraction stress test.
Evaluation
Health Promotion and Maintenance
Analysis
Learning Objective 21.5

21.15 The client at 24 weeks' gestation is experiencing painless vaginal bleeding after intercourse. The physician has ordered a transvaginal ultrasound examination. Which of the following statements made by the client indicates an understanding of why this exam has been requested? "This ultrasound (Select all that apply.)
1. will show what gender the baby is."
2. might cause a miscarriage of my baby."
3. carries a risk of creating a uterine infection."
4. can determine the location of my placenta."
5. may detect if the placenta is detaching prematurely."

Answer: 4, 5
Rationale: Painless bleeding in the second and third trimesters can be symptoms of placenta previa, or the placenta covering the cervix. Transvaginal ultrasound will determine the placental location. Ultrasound is noninvasive, and does not increase the risk for either fetal loss or uterine infection. Although gender can sometimes be detected with second trimester ultrasound, that is never the primary reason for the procedure.
Evaluation
Health Promotion and Maintenance
Analysis
Learning Objective 21.4

CHAPTER 22

22.1 A clinic nurse is preparing diagrams of pelvic shapes. Which pelvic shapes should the nurse describe as considered favorable for childbirth? (Select all that apply.)
1. android
2. anthropoid
3. gynecoid
4. platypelloid

Answer: 2, 3
Rationale: The gynecoid pelvis is the most common female pelvis, and like the anthropoid pelvis, all of the diameters are adequate for childbirth. The android and playtpelloid pelvis types are not favorable for childbirth.
Planning
Health Promotion and Maintenance
Application
Learning Objective 22.1

22.2 The client is asking about the fontanelles of her fetus. What should the nurse include when teaching about the similarities between the anterior and posterior fontanelles of a newborn? "Anterior and posterior fontanelles

1. are approximately the same size."
2. close within 12 months of birth."
3. are used in labor to identify station."
4. allow for molding of the head."

Answer: 4
Rationale: The anterior fontanelle measures approximately 2 3 cm, and closes around the eighteenth month. The posterior fontanelle is much smaller, and closes between 8 to 12 weeks after birth. In labor, the presenting part is used to identify station, not the fontanelles.
Planning
Health Promotion and Maintenance
Application
Learning Objective 22.1

22.3 The nurse is caring for a laboring client. To identify the duration of a contraction, the nurse should

1. start timing from the beginning of one contraction to the completion of the same contraction.
2. time from the beginning of one contraction to the beginning of the next contraction.
3. palpate the uterus through the lower abdomen at the peak of a contraction for the intensity.
4. time from the beginning of one contraction to the peak of the same contraction.

Answer: 1
Rationale: Contraction duration is measured from the beginning of a contraction to the completion of the same contraction. Frequency is the time from the start of one contraction until the start of the next contraction. The nurse will obtain information on contraction intensity by palpating contractions through the maternal abdomen. The time from the beginning of the contraction to the peak of the same contraction is not significant.
Assessment
Health Promotion and Maintenance
Analysis
Learning Objective 22.2

22.4 The primiparous client in early labor asks the nurse what the contractions are like as labor progresses. The nurse responds, "In normal labor, as the uterine contractions become stronger, they usually also become

1. less frequent."
2. less painful."
3. longer in duration."
4. shorter in duration."

Answer: 3
Rationale: The uterine contractions of labor will achieve cervical change only as the contractions become longer, stronger, and thus more painful over time.
Implementation
Health Promotion and Maintenance
Application
Learning Objective 22.2

22.5 The primiparous client at 39 weeks' gestation calls the clinic and reports increased bladder pressure but easier breathing and irregular, mild contractions. She also states that she just cleaned the entire house. Which statement should the nurse make?

1. "You shouldn't work so much at this point in pregnancy."
2. "What you are describing is not commonly experienced in the last weeks."
3. "Your body may be telling you it is going into labor soon."
4. "If the bladder pressure continues, come in to the clinic tomorrow."

Answer: 3
Rationale: One of the premonitory signs of labor includes lightening: The baby drops lower into the pelvis, which creates increased pelvic and bladder pressure but less pressure on the diaphragm, which makes breathing easier. Lightening is a common and expected finding, and does not indicate pathology, therefore there is no need to come to the clinic if the symptoms continue. There is no indication that the client should decrease her work schedule.
Implementation
Health Promotion and Maintenance
Analysis
Learning Objective 22.3

22.6 The nurse is teaching a prenatal class about false labor. The nurse should teach clients that false labor most likely will include which of the following? (Select all that apply.)

Answer: 1, 4
Rationale: True labor results in progressive dilation, an increase in vaginal secretions, increased intensity and frequency of contractions, and pain beginning low in the abdomen and radiating upward or into the back. True labor contractions intensify while walking.

1. contractions that do not intensify while walking 2. an increase in the intensity and frequency of contractions 3. progressive cervical effacement and dilatation 4. pain in the abdomen that does not radiate 5. increased thin vaginal secretions	Assessment Health Promotion and Maintenance Application Learning Objective 22.4
22.7 Four minutes after the birth of a client's baby, there is a sudden gush of blood from the client's vagina and about eight inches of umbilical cord slides out of her vagina. What action should the nurse take first? 1. Place the bed in Trendelenberg position. 2. Watch for the emergence of the placenta. 3. Prepare for the delivery of an undiagnosed twin. 4. Roll her onto her left side.	Answer: 2 Rationale: As the placenta separates from the uterine wall, the umbilical cord that extends out of the vagina will lengthen, and a gush of blood occurs. Delivery of the placenta is the third stage of labor. Trendelenberg position is used for hypotensive clients. The first placenta usually does not deliver before the birth of the second twin. Pregnant women are placed on the left side to facilitate uterine blood flow. Planning Health Promotion and Maintenance Analysis Learning Objective 22.5
22.8 The nurse has determined through digital exam that the client's cervix is 8 cm dilated. The client has a slight urge to push. The nurse should encourage the mother to not bear down until after the cervix is completely dilated to prevent (Select all that apply.) 1. maternal exhaustion. 2. cervical edema. 3. tearing and bruising of the cervix. 4. enhanced perineal thinning. 5. lack of pain control.	Answer: 1, 2, 3 Rationale: If the client pushes before the cervix is completely dilated, cervical edema, tearing and bruising of the cervix, and maternal exhaustion can occur. Perineal thinning will not occur until the presenting part is on the perineum in the second stage of labor. Some clients experience decreased pain in the second stage and some have increased pain, but premature pushing can be very uncomfortable. Implementation Health Promotion and Maintenance Application Learning Objective 22.5
22.9 While caring for a labor client, the nurse determines during a vaginal exam that the baby's head has internally rotated. This information is given to the family. The labor support person asks the nurse, "What other position changes will the baby undertake during labor and birth?" How should the nurse describe the rest of the cardinal movements for a baby in a vertex presentation? 1. flexion, extension, restitution, external rotation, and expulsion 2. expulsion, external rotation, and restitution 3. restitution, flexion, external rotation, and expulsion 4. extension, restitution, external rotation, and expulsion	Answer: 4 Rationale: The fetus changes position in the following order: descent, engagement, flexion, internal rotation, extension, restitution, external rotation, expulsion. Planning Health Promotion and Maintenance Application Learning Objective 22.8
22.10 During the fourth stage of labor, your client's assessment includes a BP of 110/60, pulse 90, and the fundus is firm midline and halfway between the	Answer: 4 Rationale: The client's assessment data is normal for the fourth stage of labor, so monitoring is the only action necessary. During the fourth stage of labor, the mother experiences a slight drop in blood pressure and a slightly increased

symphysis pubis and the umbilicus. The priority action of the nurse should be to
1. turn the client onto her left side.
2. place the bed in Trendelenburg position.
3. massage the fundus.
4. continue to monitor.

pulse. Trendelenburg or a left lateral position is not necessary with a BP of 110/60 and a pulse of 90. The uterus should be midline and firm; massage is not necessary.
Implementation
Health Promotion and Maintenance
Application
Learning Objective 22.6

22.11 The labor and birth nurse is preparing a prenatal class about facilitating the progress of labor. Which of the following frequent responses to pain should the nurse indicate is most likely to impede progress in labor?
1. increased pulse
2. elevated blood pressure
3. muscle tension
4. increased respirations

Answer: 3
Rationale: Muscle tension can impede labor progress by increased oxygen and calorie consumption, and by creating a mechanical obstruction that the uterine contractions must overcome to achieve labor progress. Increased pulse, respiration, and blood pressure all are manifestations of pain but do not impede labor.
Planning
Planning
Application
Learning Objective 22.7

22.12 A client is admitted to the labor unit with contractions 1.5 to 2 minutes apart and lasting 60 to 90 seconds. The client is apprehensive and irritable. This nurse understands this information to indicate that the client is most likely in what phase of labor?
1. active
2. transition
3. latent
4. second

Answer: 2
Rationale: During the transition phase of labor, contractions have a frequency of about every 1.5 to 2 minutes with a duration of 60 to 90 seconds. The woman may become apprehensive and irritable during this stage. The active phase is characterized by contractions every 2 to 3 minutes; there is a sense of fear of loss of control during this phase, but it's not as pronounced as in the transition stage. The latent phase is characterized by mild contractions that progress from a frequency of 10 to 20 minutes to 5 to 7 minutes. In the latent stage, the woman is excited that labor has begun. The second stage is the pushing stage, and the woman may feel relieved that the birth is near and she can push. The second stage is not a phase of labor.
Assessment
Health Promotion and Maintenance
Analysis
Learning Objective 22.7

22.13 The nurse has just palpated a laboring woman's contractions. The uterus cannot be indented during a contraction. The nurse compares the consistency of the uterus during a contraction with that of the forehead. The intensity of these contractions would best be identified as
1. weak.
2. mild.
3. moderate.
4. strong.

Answer: 4
Rationale: Strong contractions are not indentable, and feel similar to the forehead. Weak contractions are not identified. Mild contractions are easily indented during the peak of the contraction, and are similar to the consistency of the nose. Moderate are similar to the consistency of the chin.
Assessment
Health Promotion and Maintenance
Analysis
Learning Objective 22.6

22.14 A nurse is aware that labor and birth will most likely proceed normally when the fetal position is
1. occiput posterior.
2. mentum anterior.
3. occiput anterior.
4. mentum posterior.

Answer: 3
Rationale: The most common fetal position is occiput anterior. When this position occurs, labor and birth are likely to proceed normally. Positions other than occiput anterior are more frequently associated with problems during labor and are called malpositions.
Planning
Health Promotion and Maintenance
Application
Learning Objective 22.8

22.15 A nurse needs to evaluate the progress of a woman's labor. The nurse obtains the following data: cervical dilatation 6 cm; contractions mild in intensity, and occur every five minutes,

Answer: 1
Rationale: Cervical dilatation of 6 cm indicates the active phase of labor. The active phase of labor is usually characterized by moderately strong contractions that occur every three to four minutes, and last 45 to 60 seconds.

---

with a duration of 30 to 40 seconds. Which cue in this data does not fit the pattern suggested by the rest of the cues?
1. cervical dilatation 6 cm
2. mild contraction intensity
3. contraction frequency every two minutes
4. contraction duration 30 to 40 seconds

Assessment
Health Promotion and Maintenance
Analysis
Learning Objective 22.2

CHAPTER 23

23.1 The primigravida has been pushing for three hours, and the fetus is making slow descent. The partner asks the nurse if pushing for this long is normal. How should the nurse respond?
1. "Your baby is taking a little longer than average, but is making progress."
2. "First babies take a long time to be born; the next baby will be easier."
3. "The birth would go faster if you had taken prenatal classes and practiced."
4. "Every baby is different; there really are no norms for labor and birth."

Answer: 1
Rationale: The appropriate nursing response is to say that although the baby is taking a little longer than average, the baby is making progress. Giving factual and reassuring advice using therapeutic communication techniques is best. Although subsequent childbirth is usually shorter and faster, telling the partner this does not answer the partner's question. Prenatal classes teach relaxation, which may affect the overall length of labor, but not the second stage. Labor norms do exist for primigravidas and multigravidas.
Implementation
Health Promotion and Maintenance
Application
Learning Objective 23.2

23.2 The nurse is admitting a client to the birthing unit. What question should the nurse ask to gain a better understanding of the psychosocial status of the client?
1. "How did you decide to have your baby at this hospital?"
2. "Who will be your labor support person?"
3. "Have you chosen names for your baby yet?"
4. "What feeding method will you use?"

Answer: 2
Rationale: Labor support is important for laboring client. In some cultures, the father of the baby will be the support person; while in other cultures men are not involved with birth, and older women who have given birth themselves provide labor support. Why the client is delivering at this facility is not an indication of psychosocial status. Feeding method and naming the infant are influenced by culture, but neither indicates psychosocial status during labor.
Planning
Health Promotion and Maintenance
Application
Learning Objective 23.1

23.3 During the initial intrapartal assessment of a client in early labor, the nurse performs a vaginal examination. The client's partner asks the nurse why this pelvic exam needs to be done. The nurse should explain that the purpose of the vaginal exam is to obtain information about the (Select all that apply.)
1. uterine contraction pattern.
2. fetal position.
3. presence of the mucous plug.
4. cervical dilation and effacement.
5. presenting part.

Answer: 4, 5
Rationale: The vaginal examination of a laboring client obtains information about the fetal presenting part, the station of the presenting part, and the dilation and effacement of the cervix. A vaginal exam would not provide information about the uterine contraction pattern nor the mucous plug. Fetal position is assessed with Leopold's maneuvers.
Implementation
Health Promotion and Maintenance
Application
Learning Objective 23.1

23.4 A primigravida client has just arrived in the birthing unit. What steps would be most important for the nurse to perform to gain an understanding of the physical status of the client and her fetus? (Select all that apply.)
1. Check for ruptured membranes, and apply a fetal scalp electrode.
2. Auscultate the fetal heart rate between and during contractions.

Answer: 2, 3
Rationale: Fetal heart rate auscultation gives information about the physical status of the fetus. Contraction palpation provides information about the frequency, duration, and intensity of the contractions. A fetal scalp electrode can only be applied if membranes have ruptured and the cervix is at least 3 cm dilated, and is indicated for high risk pregnancies. Vital signs do not provide information on the well-being of the fetus, nor do Leopold's maneuvers or a vaginal exam.
Planning
Health Promotion and Maintenance

3. Palpate contractions and resting uterine tone.
4. Assess the blood pressure, temperature, respiratory rate, and pulse rate.
5. Perform a vaginal exam for cervical dilation, and perform Leopold's maneuvers.

Application
Learning Objective 23.1

23.5 A 32-year-old gravida 2 comes to the birthing area in labor. The contractions are every three minutes, and last 60 seconds. Her membranes are intact, and the cervix is 5 cm dilated and 75% effaced, with the vertex at a 1 station. During the admission interview, the client tells the nurse that she has type I diabetes, and that she gave birth to a term stillborn infant two years ago. The nurse decides that in this situation, the best method for assessing fetal well-being is
1. intermittent fetal heart rate auscultation with a fetoscope.
2. internal uterine pressure catheter.
3. continuous electronic fetal monitoring.
4. biophysical profile.

Answer: 3
Rationale: Diabetes and a term stillbirth are both conditions that make this client high-risk. This client needs continuous electronic fetal monitoring. Intermittent auscultation with a fetoscope will not provide enough information. An intrauterine pressure catheter gives information about contractions, not the fetus. A biophysical profile is not performed during labor.
Assessment
Health Promotion and Maintenance
Application
Learning Objective 23.3

23.6 The nurse is explaining to a student nurse how to determine fetal presentation and position by performing Leopold's maneuvers. The nurse should explain that the second maneuver in this procedure is used to determine
1. whether the fetal head or buttocks occupies the uterine fundus.
2. the location of the fetal back.
3. whether the head or buttocks lies in the pelvic inlet.
4. the descent of the presenting part into the pelvis.

Answer 2
Rationale: The second Leopold's maneuver determines the location of the fetal back. The first maneuver determines what part of the fetus is in the fundus. The third maneuver determines which fetal part is in the pelvic inlet, and the fourth maneuver determines the flexion of the fetal neck and descent into the pelvis.
Assessment
Health Promotion and Maintenance
Application
Learning Objective 23.4

23.7 Which of the following, if seen on an electronic fetal monitoring strip, would the nurse explain to a laboring client as a change in the baseline fetal heart rate?
1. acceleration
2. late deceleration
3. sinusoidal pattern
4. tachycardia

Answer: 4
Rationale: Bradycardia and tachycardia are changes in the fetal heart rate baseline. Late decelerations, accelerations, and a sinusoidal pattern are all periodic changes of the fetal heart rate.
Implementation
Health Promotion and Maintenance
Application
Learning Objective 23.5

23.8 The labor and delivery nurse is assigned to four clients in early labor. Which of the following electronic fetal monitoring findings would require immediate intervention?
1. early decelerations with each contraction
2. variable decelerations that recover to the baseline
3. late decelerations with minimal variability
4. accelerations

Answer: 3
Rationale: Late decelerations are considered a nonreassuring fetal heart rate (FHR) pattern, and therefore require immediate intervention. Early decelerations are usually benign. Variable decelerations indicate cord compression, but those that recover to the baseline indicate that the fetus is tolerating the decelerations. Accelerations of the fetal heart rate indicate good oxygen reserve.
Assessment
Health Promotion and Maintenance
Application
Learning Objective 23.7

23.9 The nurse notices that a fetal heart rate begins to decline from its baseline of 130 beats per minute (bpm) to 110 bpm after the acme of each contraction. The wave is smooth and uniform, with a shape that reflects the contraction. The first action of the nurse should be to
1. give the laboring client oxygen via a mask.
2. prepare the room and client for imminent delivery.
3. reposition the client into semi-Fowler's position.
4. start a large-bore IV of lactated Ringer's solution.

Answer: 1
Rationale: This fetal heart rate pattern is a late deceleration. The first priority of the nurse is to give the client oxygen. Delivery is not imminent. Left lateral position would be the preferred position. An IV of lactated Ringer's solution is not indicated.
Implementation
Health Promotion and Maintenance
Analysis
Learning Objective 23.10

23.10 The primigravida in labor asks the nurse to explain the electronic fetal heart rate monitor strip. The fetal heart rate baseline is 150 with accelerations to 165, variable decelerations to 140, and moderate long-term variability. Which statement indicates that the client understands the nurse's teaching? "The most important part of fetal heart monitoring is the
1. absence of variable decelerations."
2. presence of variability."
3. fetal heart rate baseline."
4. depth of decelerations."

Answer: 2
Rationale: Variability is an indicator of the interplay between the sympathetic nervous system and the parasympathetic nervous system. Variable decelerations indicate cord compression. Neither the fetal heart rate baseline nor the depth of decelerations indicates central nervous system function.
Evaluation
Health Promotion and Maintenance
Analysis
Learning Objective 23.8

23.11 A woman is in labor. The fetus is in vertex position. When the client's membranes rupture, the nurse sees that the amniotic fluid is meconium-stained. The nurse should immediately
1. change the client's position in bed.
2. notify the physician that birth is imminent.
3. administer oxygen at two liters per minute.
4. begin continuous fetal heart rate monitoring.

Answer: 4
Rationale: Meconium-stained amniotic fluid is an abnormal fetal finding, and is an indication for continuous fetal monitoring. Changing the client's position is not indicated, nor is oxygen administration. Meconium-stained amniotic fluid does not indicate that birth is imminent.
Assessment
Health Promotion and Maintenance
Application
Learning Objective 23.8

23.12 The nurse has detected repetitive variable decelerations in the fetal heart rate. What should the nurse do first?
1. Give the laboring client oxygen via nasal cannula.
2. Prepare the room and client for imminent delivery.
3. Reposition the client onto her left side.
4. Start a large-bore IV of lactated Ringer's solution.

Answer: 3
Rationale: Variable decelerations are indicative of cord compression. Repositioning the client to her left side will get the baby off of the cord and reduce the compression of the cord. Oxygen and an IV are not indicated. Variable decelerations do not indicate imminent delivery.
Implementation
Health Promotion and Maintenance
Analysis
Learning Objective 23.9

23.13 A woman is in active labor. Her cervical dilation is 6 cm. The nurse notes that the fetal heart rate (FHR) slows from its baseline of 144 beats per minute (bpm) to 126 bpm with the

Answer: 2
Rationale: The fetal heart rate pattern described is an early deceleration, which is indicative of fetal head compression. Fetal hypoxia causes decreased variability, while deterioration of the placenta and maternal hypoxia create late decelerations.

acme of the contraction. The FHR then returns to its baseline by the end of the contraction. The nurse understands that this indicates

1. fetal hypoxia.
2. fetal head compression.
3. deterioration of the placental unit.
4. maternal hypoxia.

Assessment
Health Promotion and Maintenance
Application
Learning Objective 23.7

23.14 The laboring client's fetal heart rate baseline upon admission was 145, with accelerations and moderate long-term variability present. Three hours later, the baseline is 160, variability is absent, and late decelerations are present. What should the nurse do first?

1. Get the client to the bathroom to void.
2. Take the client's temperature.
3. Place the client in a supine position.
4. Encourage the client to increase oral intake of clear liquids.

Answer: 2
Rationale: Late decelerations, tachycardia, and lack of variability are all aspects of a nonreassuring fetal heart rate pattern. Taking the client's temperature will determine if maternal fever is the cause of the tachycardia. Supine positioning is contraindicated with late decelerations due to vena cava compression, which will worsen fetal hypoxia. Increased oral intake is contraindicated because a cesarean birth may be indicated.
Planning
Health Promotion and Maintenance
Analysis
Learning Objective 23.10

23.15 The primigravida client is in the second stage of labor. The fetal heart rate baseline is 170, with minimal variability present. The nurse performs fetal scalp stimulation. The client's partner asks why the nurse did that. What is the best response by the nurse? "I stimulated the top of the baby's head to

1. wake him up a little."
2. try to get his heart rate to accelerate."
3. calm the baby down before birth."
4. find out if he is in distress."

Answer: 2
Rationale: Fetal scalp stimulation is done when there is a question regarding fetal status. When an acceleration occurs, fetal well-being is present. When no acceleration occurs, further measures should be undertaken, because lack of acceleration does not diagnose acidemia. Waking up or calming a baby is not the goal or outcome of fetal scalp simulation.
Implementation
Health Promotion and Maintenance
Application
Learning Objective 23.11

CHAPTER 24

24.1 The laboring primiparous client is at 7 cm, with the vertex at a +1 station. Her birth plan indicates that she and her partner took Lamaze prenatal classes, and they have planned on having a natural, unmedicated birth. Her contractions are every three minutes, and last 60 seconds. She has used relaxation and breathing techniques very successfully in her labor until the last 15 minutes. Now during contractions she is writhing on the bed, and screaming. Her labor partner is rubbing the client's back and speaking to her quietly. Which nursing diagnosis should the nurse incorporate into the plan of care for this client?

1. health seeking behaviors related to increased pain level
2. acute pain related to contractions and the birth process
3. compromised family coping related to birth process

Answer: 2
Rationale: The client is exhibiting signs of acute pain, which is both common and expected in the transitional phase of labor. The client is not asking questions; therefore health seeking behaviors does not fit. No evidence is present regarding the family's coping, only the client's coping with the pain. The client used breathing and relaxation techniques earlier in labor, thus has demonstrated a knowledge of them.
Diagnosis
Health Promotion and Maintenance
Analysis
Learning Objective 24.1

4. deficient knowledge related to lack of information about relaxation

24.2 A multiparous client is admitted to the labor and delivery unit with contractions that are regular, two minutes apart, and that last 60 seconds. She reports that her labor began about six hours ago, and she had bloody show earlier that morning. A vaginal exam reveals a vertex presenting, her cervix is 100 percent effaced and 8 cm dilated. The client asks what part of labor she is in. The nurse should inform the client that she is in the
1. early phase.
2. active phase.
3. transition phase.
4. fourth stage.

Answer: 1
Rationale: The transition phase begins with 8 cm of dilatation, and is characterized by contractions that are closer and more intense. Early and active are not correct because dilatation is less than 8 cm, and contractions are less frequent and are of shorter duration. The fourth stage is not correct, because the fourth stage occurs after delivery of the placenta.
Assessment
Health Promotion and Maintenance
Analysis
Learning Objective 24.2

24.3 By inquiring about the expectations and plans that a laboring woman and her partner have for the labor and birth, the nurse is primarily
1. recognizing the client as an active participant in her own care.
2. attempting to correct any misinformation the client may have received.
3. acting as an advocate for the client.
4. establishing rapport with the client.

Answer: 1
Rationale: Couples often invest a great deal of time and energy in learning about pregnancy and birth and then making plans for their birth experience. The correct answer choice is that the nurse is recognizing the client as an active participant in her own care. Understanding the expectations and plans that a couple has made for their birth is necessary to provide optimal nursing care that facilitates the best possible birth experience. Any misinformation the family has can be corrected, but that is not the primary focus. The nurse may use the information about plans and expectations to act as an advocate for the client as the labor progresses. Rapport and a therapeutic relationship are important for all nurse-client interactions, but are not best addressed by asking about plans and expectations for the birth.
Assessment
Health Promotion and Maintenance
Application
Learning Objective 24.4

24.4 The labor and birth nurse is admitting a client. The nurse's assessment questions include asking the client who she would like to have present for the labor and birth, and what the client would prefer to wear. The client's partner asks the nurse why these questions were asked. The best responses of the nurse would be (Select all that apply.)
1. "These questions are asked of all women. It's no big deal."
2. "I'd prefer that your partner asks me all the questions, not you."
3. "A client's preferences for her birth are important for me to understand."
4. "Many women have beliefs in childbearing that impact these choices."
5. "I'm gathering information that the nurses will use after the birth."

Answer: 3, 4
Rationale: The nurse assesses the family's expectations into the plan of care to be culturally appropriate and to best facilitate the birth. Although this information is asked of all clients, it is purposefully gathered. It is not therapeutic communication to tell the partner to not ask questions. The information gathered will be used during the labor and birth, not after delivery.
Implementation
Health Promotion and Maintenance
Analysis
Learning Objective 24.4

24.5 The laboring client presses the call light and reports that her water just broke. The nurse's first action should be to
1. check fetal heart tones.
2. encourage the mother to go for a walk.
3. change the bed linen.
4. call the physician.

Answer: 1
Rationale: Fetal heart tones should be checked after rupture of the membranes to assess for cord compression. If the presenting part is not engaged, the laboring client should not be allowed to walk because there is a risk of cord prolapse once the membranes have ruptured. The bed linen can be changed after assessing the heart rate. The physician does not need to be called after rupture of the membranes unless there is a change in fetal or client status.
Assessment
Health Promotion and Maintenance
Application
Learning Objective 24.6

24.6 Breathing techniques used in labor provide which of the following? (Select all that apply.)
1. a form of anesthesia
2. a source of relaxation
3. an increased ability to cope with contractions
4. a source of distraction
5. a type of sedation

Answer: 2, 3, 4
Rationale: When used correctly, breathing techniques can increase the woman's pain threshold, permit relaxation, provide a source of distraction, enhance the ability to cope with contractions, provide a sense of control, and allow the uterus to function more effectively. Breathing techniques do not provide a form of anesthesia or sedation.
Planning
Health Promotion and Maintenance
Application
Learning Objective 24.6

24.7 Before applying a cord clamp, the nurse assesses the umbilical cord. The mother asks why the nurse is looking at the umbilical cord. The nurse should reply, "I'm checking the blood vessels in the cord to see if it has
1. one artery, one vein."
2. two arteries, one vein."
3. two veins, one artery."
4. two veins, two arteries."

Answer: 2
Rationale: Two arteries and one vein are present in a normal umbilical cord. None of the other answer choices are characteristics of a normal umbilical cord.
Assessment
Health Promotion and Maintenance
Application
Learning Objective 24.7

24.8 At one minute after birth, the infant has a heart rate of 100 bpm and is crying vigorously. His limbs are flexed, his trunk is pink, and his feet and hands are cyanotic. The infant cries easily when the soles of his feet are stimulated. How would the nurse document this infant's Apgar score?
1. 7
2. 8
3. 9
4. 10

Answer: 3
Rationale: Two points each are scored in the categories of heart rate, respiratory effort, muscle tone, and reflex irritability. One point is scored in the category of skin color. The total Apgar would be 9.
Assessment
Health Promotion and Maintenance
Analysis
Learning Objective 24.7

24.9 Oxytocin (Pitocin) 20 units was given intramuscularly to the client at the time of the delivery of the placenta. The nurse should explain that this was done primarily to
1. contract the uterus and minimize bleeding.
2. decrease breast milk production.
3. decrease maternal blood pressure.
4. increase maternal blood pressure.

Answer: 1
Rationale: Oxytocin (Pitocin) is given to contract the uterus and minimize bleeding. Oxytocin does not have an effect on maternal blood pressure or breast milk production.
Implementation
Physiologic Integrity
Application
Learning Objective 24.8

24.10 Upon delivery of the newborn, the nursing intervention that best promotes parental attachment is

Answer: 2
Rationale: Placing the baby on the maternal abdomen promotes attachment and bonding, and gives the mother a chance to interact with her baby immediately.

---

1. placing the newborn under the radiant warmer.	The other answer choices all involve separating the baby from the mother, which does not promote interaction.
2. placing the newborn on the maternal abdomen.	Implementation
3. allowing the mother a chance to rest immediately after delivery.	Health Promotion and Maintenance
4. taking the newborn to the nursery for the initial assessment.	Application Learning Objective 24.9

24.11 The nurse understands that there are different admission considerations for an adult woman in labor versus an adolescent in labor. Given this knowledge, what is the nurse's assessment priority for an adolescent in labor? 1. cultural background 2. plans for keeping the infant 3. support persons 4. developmental level	Answer: 4 Rationale: It is important to identify the adolescent's level of development so that a plan of care is consistent with the adolescent's abilities. Knowing the adolescent's level of development will help to plan nursing care for the adolescent who is keeping her infant. Cultural background and support person(s) are important to planning anyone's care, but not more important than identifying developmental level in an adolescent in labor. Planning Health Promotion and Maintenance Application Learning Objective 24.10

24.12 A client's labor has progressed so rapidly that a precipitous birth is occurring. The nurse should 1. go to the nurse's station and immediately call the physician. 2. run to the delivery room for an emergency birth pack. 3. stay with the client and ask for auxiliary personnel for assistance. 4. try to delay the delivery of the infant's head until the physician arrives.	Answer: 3 Rationale: If birth is imminent, the nurse must not leave the client alone. The nurse can direct auxiliary personnel to contact the physician and retrieve the emergency birth pack. The nurse should not hold the infant's head back from delivering, but should apply gentle pressure against the head to prevent it from popping out rapidly. Planning Health Promotion and Maintenance Analysis Learning Objective 24.11

24.13 The client who wishes to have an unmedicated birth is in the transition stage. She is very uncomfortable and turns frequently in the bed. Her partner has stepped out momentarily. In which of the following ways can the nurse be most helpful? 1. Talk to her the entire time. 2. Turn on the television to distract her. 3. Stand next to the bed with hands on the railing next to her. 4. Sit silently in the room away from the bed.	Answer: 3 Rationale: Standing next to the bed is supportive without being irritating. Clients in the transition phase of labor are usually very uncomfortable, and may find sounds and physical contact annoying. Both talking and turning on the television may irritate the client. Sitting silently away from the client can lead to her feeling abandoned. Implementation Health Promotion and Maintenance Application Learning Objective 24.6

24.14 The client presents to labor and delivery stating that her water broke two hours ago. Barring any abnormalities, what information should the nurse give the client about how often the nurse expects to take the client's temperature? 1. every hour 2. every two hours 3. every four hours 4. every shift	Answer: 1 Rationale: Once the membranes are ruptured, the maternal temperature is taken every hour. If elevated, it may be taken every thirty minutes. Every two hours, every four hours, and every shift are too long. Assessment Health Promotion and Maintenance Application Learning Objective 24.6

24.15 The primiparous client is being admitted to the birthing unit. As the nurse begins the assessment, the client's partner asks why the baby's heart rate is going to be monitored. After the explanation, the client's partner makes a statement. Which statement indicates a need for further teaching?

1. "The baby's heart rate will vary between 110 and 160."
2. "The heart rate is monitored to see if the baby is tolerating labor."
3. "By listening to the heart, we can tell the gender of the baby."
4. "After listening to the heart rate you will contact the midwife."

Answer: 3
Rationale: Fetal heart rate is not predictive of gender. A normal fetal heart rate is 110–160. The outcome of assessing the fetal heart rate is to determine the fetal tolerance to the physiologic stresses of labor. Once the admission is complete, the nurse will contact the client's provider with the assessment findings.
Evaluation
Health Promotion and Maintenance
Analysis
Learning Objective 24.2

CHAPTER 25

25.1 A client has just been admitted to the labor and delivery unit. She is having mild contractions every 15 minutes that last 30 seconds. The client wants to have a medication-free birth. When discussing alternatives to medication use, the nurse should be sure the client understands that

1. in order to respect her wishes, the nurse will make certain that no medication will be given.
2. the use of pain relief will allow the client to have a more enjoyable birth experience.
3. the use of medications can allow the client and her partner to rest and be less fatigued for the birth.
4. maternal pain and stress can have a more adverse effect on the fetus than a small amount of analgesia.

Answer: 4
Rationale: The decision not to medicate should be an informed one, and it is possible that the client does not know about the effects pain and stress can have on the fetus. Once the effects are explained, it is still the client's choice whether to receive medication. It is important to respect the client's wishes when possible. While pain relief can lead to a more enjoyable experience and allow the mother to be less fatigued, that may be the view of the nurse and not the mother.
Implementation
Physiologic Integrity
Application
Learning Objective 25.1

25.2 The laboring client rates her pain with contractions at 10 out of 10. The nurse administers an analgesic medication intravenously to the client. The nurse would evaluate the medication as effective if the

1. client dozes between contractions.
2. contractions decrease in intensity.
3. contractions decrease in frequency.
4. the client rates the pain during contractions at a 9.

Answer: 1
Rationale: Increasing pain interferes with the mother's ability to cope. Analgesics decrease discomfort and increase relaxation, which can facilitate dozing between contractions. The medication would not be considered effective if the client rates her pain nearly the same as before the medication was administered. While the intensity and frequency of the contractions may be affected, the intent is to help the mother be able to cope with the contractions
Evaluation
Physiologic Integrity
Analysis
Learning Objective 25.2

25.3 After receiving nalbuphine hydrochloride (Nubain), a client's labor progresses rapidly and the baby is born less than one hour later. Which medication should the nurse have prepared to give to the newborn in case the baby exhibits signs of respiratory depression?

1. fentanyl (Sublimaze)
2. butorphanol tartrate (Stadol)

Answer: 3
Rationale: Naloxone (Narcan) is the only choice that is an opiate antagonist, which would reverse the effects of the nalbuphine hydrochloride (Nubain). Fentanyl (Sublimaze), butorphanol tartrate (Stadol), and pentobarbital (Nembutal) are all opioid analgesics.
Planning
Physiologic Integrity
Application
Learning Objective 25.2

3. naloxone (Narcan)
4. pentobarbital (Nembutal)

25.4 A primigravida who is dilated to 5 cm has just received an epidural for pain. She complains of feeling lightheaded and dizzy within ten minutes after the procedure. Her blood pressure before the procedure was 120/80 and is now 80/52. A bolus of IV fluids has been given. Which medication should the nurse be prepared to administer to increase her blood pressure? 1. epinephrine injection, USP 1:10,000 (0.1 mg/mL) 2. terbutaline (Bricanyl) 3. ephedrine (Ephedra) 4. diphenhydramine (Benoject)	Answer: 1 Rationale: Epinephrine injection is the medication of choice to increase maternal blood pressure. Terbutaline, ephedrine, and diphenhydramine are not used for this purpose. Implementation Physiologic Integrity Application Learning Objective 25.3
25.5 A client received an epidural anesthesia during the first stage of her labor. The epidural is discontinued immediately after delivery. The nurse should be prepared to assess the client for which of the following during the fourth stage of labor? 1. nausea 2. bladder distention 3. uterine atony 4. hypertension	Answer: 2 Rationale: Bladder distention may be a result of decreased bladder sensation in the fourth stage. The epidural is discontinued after delivery, decreasing the likelihood of nausea. Uterine atony is not the result of an epidural. Hypotension, not hypertension, is an early side effect of epidurals. Assessment Physiologic Integrity Application Learning Objective 25.3
25.6 The nurse is working with a client in active labor. The client has requested an epidural for analgesia. Which of the following nursing actions should the nurse be prepared to implement to prevent or detect common side effects of epidural anesthesia? 1. Preload the client with a rapid infusion of IV fluids. 2. Use intermittent fetal heart rate monitoring so the client can use the birthing ball. 3. Place an intrauterine pressure catheter. 4. Warm the room temperature slightly.	Answer: 1 Rationale: Hypotension can be prevented by preloading with rapid IV infusion followed by continuous IV infusion. Variability of fetal heart rate may decrease and late decelerations may occur if maternal hypotension occurs. Continuing fetal heart rate monitoring is essential. Although a decrease in the intensity and/or frequency of uterine contractions can occur, an intrauterine pressure catheter is not indicated at this time. There is no need to change the room temperature. Planning Physiologic Integrity Analysis Learning Objective 25.3
25.7 The client in active labor is requesting pain relief. The physician orders an epidural anesthetic for the client. Which of the following actions should the nurse be prepared to make immediately after administration of the epidural? The nurse should assess 1. the blood pressure. 2. for headache. 3. for urinary retention. 4. the maternal pulse rate.	Answer: 1 Rationale: The most common complication of an epidural is maternal hypotension. Headaches are a complication that occurs after the delivery. Urinary retention is common after the epidural, but is not as important as blood pressure. Maternal pulse rate is not affected by an epidural. Assessment Physiologic Integrity Application Learning Objective 25.4

25.8 A laboring client has received an order for epidural anesthesia. In order to prevent the most common complication associated with this procedure, the nurse would expect to do which of the following?

1. Observe fetal heart rate variability.
2. Rapidly infuse 500–1000 mL of intravenous fluids.
3. Place the client in the semi-Fowler's position.
4. Teach the client appropriate breathing techniques.

Answer: 2

Rationale: Administering a fluid bolus prior to an epidural generally prevents maternal hypotension, which is the most common complication associated with the procedure. Fetal heart rate variability must be assessed prior to administration of a narcotic, not an epidural. The client will be positioned either sitting on the edge of the bed, or lying on her side. Breathing techniques are used to help avoid the need for analgesia.

Planning

Health Promotion and Maintenance

Application

Learning Objective 25.4

25.9 The laboring client requests pain medication. Her contractions last 20–30 seconds and occur every 8–20 minutes. The nurse should explain that analgesics given at this time would likely cause

1. fetal respiratory depression.
2. decreased analgesic effectiveness at the end of labor.
3. maternal hypotension.
4. prolonged labor.

Answer: 4

Rationale: Pain medication given before labor becomes established is likely to prolong the labor process. Pain medication given before established labor does not cause fetal respiratory depression unless the mother delivers within an hour of receiving the medication. This is not likely if labor is not established. Medication given early in the labor process does not become less effective at the end of labor. Analgesics may lower the blood pressure, but this effect does not cause the contraction pattern to be altered.

Implementation

Health Promotion and Maintenance

Application

Learning Objective 25.2

25.10 The nurse is providing preoperative teaching for a client who has a cesarean birth under general anesthesia scheduled for the next day. Which statement indicates that the client requires additional information? "General anesthesia

1. can be accomplished with inhaled gases."
2. usually involves giving medication into my IV."
3. will provide good pain relief after the birth."
4. takes effect faster than an epidural."

Answer: 3

Rationale: General anesthesia provides no pain relief after birth as regional anesthesia does, but takes effect very quickly. General anesthesia can be accomplished via inhalation, intravenous injection, or a combination of the two.

Evaluation

Physiologic Integrity

Analysis

Learning Objective 25.5

25.11 A cesarean section is ordered for the laboring client the nurse has worked with all shift. The client will receive general anesthesia. The nurse knows education has been successful if the client lists which of the following as potential complications of general anesthesia? (Select all that apply.)

1. fetal depression that is directly proportional to the depth and duration of the anesthesia
2. poor fetal metabolism of anesthesia which inhibits use with preterm infants
3. uterine relaxation that causes increased blood loss
4. increased gastric motility that causes increased appetite
5. itching of the face and neck

Answer: 1, 2, 3

Rationale: A primary danger of general anesthesia is fetal depression because the medication reaches the fetus in about two minutes. The depression is directly proportional to the depth and duration of anesthesia. The drugs cause depression of vasomotor, respiratory, and other centers of the brain. There is poor fetal metabolism of the anesthesia agent, especially if the fetus is premature, which contraindicates its use in premature delivery. Uterine relaxation prevents uterine contraction after delivery, which causes an increased maternal blood loss. Decreased gastric motility causes food to remain undigested. Itching of the face and neck is not associated with general anesthesia.

Evaluation

Physiologic Integrity

Analysis

Learning Objective 25.6

25.12 The client with a normal pregnancy had an emergency cesarean birth under general anesthesia two hours ago. The client now has a respiratory rate of 30, has pale blue nail beds, a pulse rate of 110, a temperature of 102.6°F, and is complaining of chest pain. The nurse understands that the client is most likely experiencing
1. pulmonary embolus.
2. pneumococcal pneumonia.
3. pneumonitis.
4. gastroesophageal reflux disease.

Answer: 3
Rationale: Pneumonitis that results from aspiration of gastric secretions during general anesthesia is also referred to as Mendelson syndrome. Women with emergency cesareans are at greatest risk for this complication. Pulmonary embolus does not cause fever. General anesthesia does not cause pneumococcal pneumonia. Gastroesophageal reflux disease does not cause a fever or cyanosis.
Assessment
Physiologic Integrity
Application
Learning Objective 25.6

25.13 The nurse is inducing the labor of a client with severe preeclampsia. As labor progresses, fetal intolerance of labor develops. The induction medication is turned off, and the client is prepared for cesarean birth. Which statement should the nurse include in her preoperative teaching? "Because of your preeclampsia
1. you are at higher risk for hypotension after an epidural anesthesia."
2. you may develop hypertension after a spinal anesthesia."
3. your baby might have decreased blood pressure after birth."
4. your husband will not be allowed into the operating room."

Answer: 1
Rationale: The vasoconstriction of severe preeclampsia results in a lowered blood volume; the vasodilation of regional anesthesia then is more likely to result in hypotension. Hypertension is not associated with spinal anesthesia. Preeclampsia does not affect the baby's blood pressure, nor prevent the husband from being present at the birth.
Implementation
Health Promotion and Maintenance
Analysis
Learning Objective 25.7

25.14 The nurse is working with a laboring client who has requested an epidural for analgesia. Prior to administration of the lumbar epidural anesthesia, the nurse should anticipate placing the client in which of the following positions? (Select all that apply.)
1. on her right side in the center of the bed, curled in a fetal position
2. lying prone with a pillow under her chest
3. on her left side with the bottom leg straight and the top leg slightly flexed
4. sitting on the edge of the bed with her back slightly curved and her feet on a stool
5. supine on the side of the bed

Answer: 1, 4
Rationale: Sitting on the edge of the bed with the back slightly curved and the feet on a stool allows the epidural spaces to be accessed easier, as does lying on the side and curling into a fetal position. None of the other positions facilitate access to the epidural spaces.
Planning
Physiologic Integrity
Application
Learning Objective 25.3

25.15 The nurse is caring for a laboring client with thrombocytopenia. During labor, it is determined that the client requires a cesarean delivery. The nurse is preparing the client for surgery, and is performing preoperative teaching. The nurse should instruct the client that which method of anesthesia is recommended?

Answer: 1
Rationale: General anesthesia will be recommended. A client with thrombocytopenia is at risk for increased bleeding, and therefore all regional anesthetics (including spinal and epidural anesthesia) are contraindicated for her.
Implementation
Physiologic Integrity
Application
Learning Objective 25.7

1. general anesthesia
2. epidural anesthesia
3. spinal anesthesia
4. regional anesthesia

CHAPTER 26

26.1 A woman has been having contractions since 4:00 A.M. At 8:00 A.M, her cervix is dilated to 5 cm. Contractions are frequent, and mild to moderate in intensity. Cephalopelvic disproportion (CPD) has been ruled out. After giving the mother some sedation so she can rest, the nurse should anticipate preparing for
1. oxytocin (Pitocin) induction of labor.
2. amnioinfusion.
3. increased intravenous infusion.
4. cesarean section.

Answer: 1
Rationale: Hypertonic labor patterns result in frequent ineffectual contractions that exhaust the mother. Sedation is used to let the mother rest and stop the ineffective contractions. If sedation does not stop the ineffective contractions, oxytocin (Pitocin) may be used to establish more effective contractions. Increasing the IV infusion and amnioinfusion are not methods that would change the ineffective labor pattern. Since CPD has been ruled out, a cesarean section is not anticipated.
Planning
Health Promotion and Maintenance
Application
Learning Objective 26.2

26.2 A laboring multipara is having intense uterine contractions with incomplete uterine relaxation between contractions. Vaginal examinations reveal rapid cervical dilation and fetal descent. The nurse should
1. notify the physician of these findings.
2. place the woman in knee-chest position.
3. turn off the lights to make it easier for the woman to relax.
4. assemble supplies to prepare for a cesarean birth.

Answer: 1
Rationale: This client's contraction pattern and rapid cervical change are indicative of a precipitous birth. The best action by the nurse is to notify the physician and prepare for delivery. Knee-chest position is used for back labor or prolapsed cord. Turning off the lights may prevent the nurse from assessing a crowning perineum. It is inappropriate for the nurse to leave a client that will deliver soon.
Implementation
Health Promotion and Maintenance
Analysis
Learning Objective 26.3

26.3 The client at 42 weeks pregnancy is admitted for induction of her labor. Which statement indicates that she understands the indications for the induction?
1. "If I go too overdue, my baby's amniotic fluid volume can decrease."
2. "Since I am so tired of being pregnant, I am being induced."
3. "My health can be affected if I don't deliver soon."
4. "My baby took longer to grow, and now it's ready to be born."

Answer: 1
Rationale: Risks to the postterm fetus include oligohydramnios, which leads to meconium aspiration or even intrauterine fetal demise. The mother's health is not affected by postterm pregnancy, although the psychological aspect of waiting can be difficult to endure. A postterm fetus has had accurate dating, and does not take longer to grow.
Evaluation
Health Promotion and Maintenance
Analysis
Learning Objective 26.4

26.4 A client has just given birth. During labor, the fetus was in a brow presentation, but after a prolonged labor, the fetus converted to occiput presentation, and was delivered vaginally with vacuum extractor assistance. The nurse should explain to the parents that
1. the infant will need to be observed for meconium aspiration.
2. molding of the head will subside in a few days.

Answer: 2
Rationale: Prolonged labor, malpresentation, and use of vacuum or forceps can lead to molding of the head. There is no mention of meconium-stained fluid that would cause the nurse to assess for meconium aspiration. There is no reason to delay breastfeeding or to place the infant on antibiotics.
Implementation
Health Promotion and Maintenance
Analysis
Learning Objective 26.5

3. the infant will have prophylactic antibiotics. 4. breastfeeding will need to be delayed for a day or two.	
26.5 The client vaginally delivers an infant that weighs 4750 g. Moderate shoulder dystocia occurred during the birth. During the initial assessment of this infant, the nurse should look for 1. Bell's palsy. 2. bradycardia. 3. Erb's palsy. 4. petechiae.	Answer: 3 Rationale: Macrosomic newborns should be inspected for cephalohematoma, Erb's palsy, and fractured clavicles. Bell's palsy and bradycardia are not associated with macrosomia. Petechiae may occur with shoulder dystocia, but are not as significant as Erb's palsy. Assessment Health Promotion and Maintenance Application Learning Objective 26.6
26.6 The client is carrying monochorionic-monoamniotic twins. The nurse teaches the client what this is, and the implications of this finding. The nurse knows that further information is required if the client makes which statement? 1. "My babies came from two eggs." 2. "About two-thirds of twins have this amniotic sac formation." 3. "My use of a fertility drug led to this issue." 4. "My babies have about a 50% chance of surviving to term."	Answer: 4 Rationale: Monochorionic-monoamniotic twins are both in one amniotic sac, and are also monozygotic, or identical, coming from one ovum. About 2% of twins are of this type. Fertility drugs lead to an increase in dizygotic twinning, not monochorionic-monoamniotic. Because the umbilical cords can tangle or knot, there is a 50% mortality rate. Evaluation Health Promotion and Maintenance Analysis Learning Objective 26.7
26.7 The nurse is planning an in-service educational program to talk about disseminating intravascular coagulation (DIC). The nurse should include which of the following as risk factors for developing DIC? (Select all that apply.) 1. diabetes mellitus 2. abruptio placentae 3. prolonged retention of a fetus after demise 4. multiparity 5. preterm labor	Answer: 2, 3 Rationale: Abruptio placentae leave intrauterine arteries open and bleeding. This results in release of thromboplastin into the maternal blood supply, and triggers the development of DIC. In prolonged retention of the fetus after demise, thromboplastin is released from the degenerating fetal tissues into the maternal blood stream, which activates the extrinsic clotting system. This triggers the formation of multiple tiny clots which deplete the fibrinogen and factors V and VII and result in DIC. Diabetes, multiparity, and preterm labor do not cause the same release of thromboplastin that triggers DIC. Planning Health Promotion and Maintenance Application Learning Objective 26.8
26.8 The client at 30 weeks' gestation is admitted with painless late vaginal bleeding. The nurse understands that expectant management includes 1. limiting vaginal exams to only one per 24-hour period. 2. evaluating the fetal heart rate with an internal monitor. 3. monitoring blood loss, pain, and uterine contractibility. 4. assessing blood pressure every two hours.	Answer: 3 Rationale: Placenta previa is painless bleeding. If the pregnancy is less than 37 weeks' gestation, expectant management is employed to allow the fetus to mature. Vaginal exams are contraindicated. Blood loss, pain, and uterine contractibility need to be assessed. Fetal heart rate monitoring will be done with an external fetal monitor. Blood pressure measurements every two hours are unnecessary. Planning Health Promotion and Maintenance Application Learning Objective 26.8
26.9 The nurse examines the client's placenta, and finds that the umbilical cord is inserted at the placental margin. The client comments that the placenta and cord look different than with her	Answer: 4 Rationale: Battledore placenta has the cord inserted at or near the edge of the placenta. Placenta accrete is a placenta that grows into the uterine wall. Circumvallate placenta has a fold of the amnion and chorion on the placental

first two births. The nurse should explain that this variation in placenta and cord is called a
1. placenta accrete.
2. circumvallate placenta.
3. succenturiate placenta.
4. battledore placenta.

surface. Succenturiate placenta has at least one extra lobe attached to the edge of the placenta.
Implementation
Health Promotion and Maintenance
Application
Learning Objective 26.9

26.10 The nurse is admitting a client who was diagnosed with hydramnios. The client asks why she has developed this condition. The nurse should explain that hydramnios is sometimes associated with (Select all that apply.)
1. chest pain, dyspnea, tachycardia, and hypotension.
2. postmaturity syndrome.
3. renal malformation or dysfunction.
4. maternal diabetes.
5. large for gestational age infants.

Answer: 1, 2, 4
Rationale: Chest pain, dyspnea, tachycardia, and hypotension are symptoms of amniotic embolism, which occurs more commonly with hydramnios. Hydramnios occurs in 10–20% of pregnant diabetics. Renal malformation or dysfunction and postmaturity can cause oligohydramnios. Large for gestational age infants and placenta previa are not associated with hydramnios.
Implementation
Health Promotion and Maintenance
Analysis
Learning Objective 26.10

26.11 A pregnant client was in an auto accident. She presents to the labor suite from the emergency room after she presented there with a deep gash to her forearm from the auto accident. She had no seatbelt on and was traveling at a high rate of speed. She seems very agitated, is walking continuously, and is talking very rapidly. The nurse should suspect that the client has what type of psychological disorder?
1. schizophrenia
2. bipolar, manic phase
3. social anxiety disorder
4. obsessive-compulsive disorder

Answer: 2
Rationale: Agitation, constant movement, and rapid talking are symptoms of the manic phase of bipolar disorder. Schizophrenia is characterized by withdrawal and altered perception of reality, often with hallucinations or delusions. Social anxiety disorder is fear of social activities like being in a group. Obsessive-compulsive disorder is characterized by the repetitive performing of a ritual activity.
Assessment
Psychosocial Integrity
Application
Learning Objective 26.1

26.12 The 26-year-old primiparous client is having her initial prenatal appointment. The client reports to the nurse that she suffered a pelvic fracture in a car accident three years ago. The client asks the nurse if her pelvic fracture might affect her ability to have a vaginal delivery. What response by the nurse is best?
1. "It depends on how your pelvis healed."
2. "You will need to have a cesarean birth."
3. "Please talk to your doctor about that."
4. "You will be able to delivery vaginally."

Answer: 1
Rationale: Displaced pelvic fractures can heal in such a way that leads to a contracture or diminished diameter of the pelvis. Non-displaced fractures can heal and maintain adequate diameters for birth. Not all clients will be able to deliver vaginally, but not all will need cesarean birth. It is not therapeutic to tell a client to talk to someone else.
Implementation
Health Promotion and Maintenance
Analysis
Learning Objective 26.11

26.13 The client delivered thirty minutes ago. Her blood pressure and pulse are stable. Scant vaginal bleeding is taking place. The nurse should prepare for which procedure?
1. abdominal hysterectomy
2. manual removal of the placenta
3. repair of perineal lacerations
4. foley catheterization

Answer: 2
Rationale: Retained placenta is the lack of placental delivery within 30 minutes of birth. Manual removal of the placenta is then performed. Abdominal hysterectomy is not required. Repair of perineal lacerations would not ensue until after the placenta is delivered. There is no indication of urinary retention that requires a Foley catheter.
Planning
Health Promotion and Maintenance
Analysis
Learning Objective 26.12

26.14 The client has delivered a 4200 g fetus. The physician performed a midline episiotomy, which extended into a third-degree laceration. The client asks the nurse where she tore. Which response is best? "The episiotomy extended and tore
1. through your rectal mucosa."
2. up near your urethra."
3. into the muscle layer."
4. through your rectal sphincter."

Answer: 4
Rationale: A third-degree laceration includes the rectal sphincter. A fourth-degree laceration is through the rectal mucosa. A periurethral laceration is near the urethra. A first-degree laceration involves only the skin. A second-degree laceration involves skin and muscle.
Implementation
Health Promotion and Maintenance
Application
Learning Objective 26.12

26.15 The client at 37 weeks' gestation comes to the labor triage unit crying and distraught. She says, "I haven't felt my baby move today, and I just know that it died." The nurse should prepare the client for what procedure?
1. internal fetal monitoring
2. ultrasound examination
3. amniocentesis
4. induction of labor

Answer: 2
Rationale: Fetal demise is diagnosed with ultrasound examination when no fetal heart tones are present. Internal fetal monitoring requires a dilated cervix and ruptured membranes. Amniocentesis will provide information about fetal viability. Induction of labor may be undertaken after fetal death is diagnosed and the family has been informed.
Planning
Health Promotion and Maintenance
Analysis
Learning Objective 26.13

CHAPTER 27

27.1 The client is seeing the Certified Nurse-Midwife for prenatal care. Her first pregnancy was delivered by cesarean birth. The client is hoping for a vaginal birth after cesarean (VBAC) for this pregnancy. Which statement indicates that this client requires additional information regarding VBAC?
1. "I can try a vaginal birth because my uterine incision is a low segment transverse incision."
2. "The up-and-down scar on my skin doesn't mean that the scar on my uterus is in the same direction."
3. "There is about a 90% chance of successfully giving birth vaginally after having a cesarean."
4. "Because the hospital I go to has surgery staff on call 24 hours a day, I can try a VBAC there."

Answer: 3
Rationale: The VBAC success rate is about 60–80% unless the primary cesarean birth was done due to dystocia, in which the rate of success drops to 50–70%. Only low segment transverse uterine incisions are recommended for attempting a VBAC. Abdominal skin incision and uterine incision are not always the same. VBAC should only be attempted at facilities that have 24-hour coverage of operating room staff and anesthesia.
Evaluation
Health Promotion and Maintenance
Analysis
Learning Objective 27.10

27.2 The client had a classical uterine incision for her cesarean birth. The nurse knows that the client understands implications for future pregnancies that are secondary to her classical uterine incision when the client states
1. "the next time I have a baby, I can try to deliver vaginally."
2. "the risk of rupturing my uterus is too high for me to have any more babies."
3. "every time I have a baby, I will have to have a cesarean delivery."
4. "i can only have one more baby."

Answer: 3
Rationale: A classical uterine incision is made in the upper uterine segment, and holds an increased risk of rupture in subsequent pregnancy, labor, and birth. Attempting a vaginal birth is contraindicated, and future births will be planned cesareans. Future pregnancies are neither prohibited nor are future pregnancies limited to one.
Evaluation
Health Promotion and Maintenance
Analysis
Learning Objective 27.9

27.3 After being in labor for several hours with no progress, the client is diagnosed with cephalopelvic disproportion (CPD), and must have a cesarean section. The client is being prepared for a cesarean delivery in the operating room. The doctor is present. The nurse knows that the last assessment the nurse should make just prior to the client being draped for surgery is

1. maternal temperature.
2. maternal urine output.
3. vaginal exam.
4. fetal heart tones.

Answer: 4
Rationale: Fetal heart tones are assessed just prior to the start of surgery because the supine position can lead to fetal hypoxia. Maternal temperature is monitored by anesthesia personnel. Maternal urine output is not significant at this point. Vaginal exam is unnecessary when cephalopelvic disproportion (CPD) is present.
Assessment
Health Promotion and Maintenance
Analysis
Learning Objective 27.9

27.4 The client has been pushing for two hours, and is exhausted. The fetal head is visible between contractions. The physician informs the client that a vacuum extractor could be used to facilitate the delivery. Which statement indicates that the client needs additional information about vacuum extraction assistance?

1. "A small cup will be put onto the baby's head and a gentle suction will be applied."
2. "I can stop pushing and just rest if the vacuum extractor is used."
3. "The baby's head might have a bruise from the vacuum cup."
4. "Vacuum will be applied for a total of ten minutes or less."

Answer: 2
Rationale: Vacuum extraction is an assistive delivery, and the client must continue with pushing efforts to accomplish the birth. The vacuum extractor is a small cup-shaped device that is applied to the scalp for up to ten minutes total, and may leave a bruise on the scalp where the device was placed.
Evaluation
Health Promotion and Maintenance
Analysis
Learning Objective 27.8

27.5 The physician responsible for the care of the client has determined the need for the use of forceps. The client asks why this is needed. The nurse should explain that the client's indication for the use of forceps is

1. because her support person is exhausted.
2. due to premature placental separation.
3. to shorten the first stage of labor.
4. to prevent fetal distress.

Answer: 2
Rationale: Forceps are applied during the second stage of labor. Indications for use of forceps include premature placental separation, nonreassuring fetal heart rate, and to shorten the second (not the first) stage of labor in cases of maternal exhaustion or regional anesthesia. Exhaustion of the support person is not an indication for use of forceps.
Implementation
Health Promotion and Maintenance
Application
Learning Objective 27.7

27.6 The client requires vacuum extraction assistance. To provide easier access to the fetal head, the physician cuts a mediolateral episiotomy. After delivery, the client asks what kind of episiotomy was performed. What is the best response for the nurse to make? "The episiotomy

1. goes straight back toward your rectum."
2. is from your vagina toward the urethra."
3. is cut diagonally away from your vagina."
4. extends from your vagina into your rectum."

Answer: 3
Rationale: Mediolateral episiotomy is angled from the vaginal opening toward the buttock. Midline episiotomy is straight back from the vagina toward the rectum, but extension into the rectum is a fourth-degree laceration. Episiotomies are not cut anteriorly toward the urethra unless the client has had a female circumcision.
Implementation
Health Promotion and Maintenance
Application
Learning Objective 27.6

27.7 The client is recovering from delivery that included a midline episiotomy. Her perineum is swollen and sore. The client is asking for her ice pack to be refreshed. The best response from the nurse is

1. "I'll get you one right away."
2. "You only need to use one ice pack."
3. "You need to leave it off for at least 20 minutes and then reapply."
4. "I'll bring you an extra so that you can change it when you are ready."

Answer: 3
Rationale: Optimal effects from the use of an ice pack occur when it is applied for 20–30 minutes and then removed for at least 20 minutes before being reapplied. Providing an additional ice pack before 20 minutes have passed would increase the perineal edema. More than one ice pack must be used in order to apply ice for 20 minutes on followed by 20 minutes off. An ice pack that is provided now for use in 20 minutes would be melted before being used.
Implementation
Health Promotion and Maintenance
Application
Learning Objective 27.6

27.8 The client is having fetal heart rate decelerations. An amnioinfusion has been ordered for the client in an attempt to alleviate the decelerations. The nurse understands that the type of decelerations that will be alleviated by amnioinfusion is

1. early decelerations.
2. moderate decelerations.
3. late decelerations.
4. variable decelerations.

Answer: 4
Rationale: Amnioinfusion can be used when cord compression is presenting as variable decelerations. Early decelerations require no intervention, and late decelerations are consistent with head compression. Amnioinfusion does not relieve head compression. Moderate is not a descriptor used to identify decelerations.
Assessment
Health Promotion and Maintenance
Application
Learning Objective 27.5

27.9 The nurse performs a Bishop's prelabor score for a client prior to induction of labor. The client asks for an explanation of the Bishop's score. The nurse should describe the Bishop's score as a system for cervical readiness that includes (Select all that apply.)

1. fetal station.
2. cervical dilation.
3. fetal presenting part.
4. fetal movement.
5. fetal heart rate baseline.

Answer: 1, 2
Rationale: Fetal station, and cervical dilation, effacement, consistency, and position are the components of the Bishop's score. Fetal presenting part, fetal movement, and fetal heart baseline are not part of the scoring system for the Bishop's score.
Implementation
Health Promotion and Maintenance
Application
Learning Objective 27.4

27.10 The client presents for cervical ripening in anticipation of labor induction tomorrow. What should the nurse include in her plan of care for this client?

1. Apply an internal fetal monitor.
2. Allow the client to void prior to insertion of dinoprostone (Cervidil) gel.
3. Withhold oral intake and start intravenous fluids.
4. Place the client in a semi-Fowler's position.

Answer: 2
Rationale: The client should void before insertion of the dinoprostone (Cervidil). It is recommended that the client stay in bed for one hour after insertion, and should void prior to the insertion for comfort. An internal fetal monitor cannot be applied until adequate cervical dilatation has occurred and the membranes are ruptured. Until labor begins, there is no rationale for withholding oral intake. The client will be positioned supine with a wedge under the right hip to maintain maximal gel contact with the cervix.
Implementation
Health Promotion and Maintenance
Application
Learning Objective 27.4

27.11 A laboring client's obstetrician has suggested amniotomy as a method for creating stronger contractions and facilitating birth. The client asks, "What are the advantages to doing this?" What should the nurse cite in response? (Select all that apply.)

1. "Contractions elicited are similar to those of spontaneous labor."
2. "Decreases the chance of prolapsed cord."

Answer: 1
Rationale: Contractions after amniotomy are similar to spontaneous labor. Blood pressure is not increased, as can happen with oxytocin. A disadvantage is the increased chance of prolapsed cord, especially if the fetal presenting part is not well-applied against the cervix. There is no correlation between amniotomy and episiotomy.
Implementation
Health Promotion and Maintenance
Analysis
Learning Objective 27.3

3. "Blood pressure is not affected."
4. "The client won't need an episiotomy."

27.12 Your client tells you that she has come to the hospital so that her baby's position can be changed. Which information should the nurse include when teaching the client about the upcoming procedure? (Select all that apply.) 1. If the fetus is breech or transverse, an external version may be attempted. 2. A version is usually done between the 20th and 30th weeks of gestation. 3. The success rate for versions is 95%. 4. Terbutaline sulfate (Bricanyl) may be given prior to beginning the version.	Answer: 1 Rationale: If breech or shoulder (transverse lie) is detected prior to the onset of labor and after 36 weeks' gestation, an external version is done. Experience of the clinical professional affects the success rates, but overall rates are about 68%. Multiparous clients have a higher success rate, especially when terbutaline sulfate (Bricanyl) 0.25 mg is given subcutaneously 20 to 30 minutes prior to beginning the version. Implementation Health Promotion and Maintenance Application Learning Objective 27.2
27.13 The laboring client participated in childbirth preparation classes that strongly discouraged the use of medications and intervention during labor. The client has been pushing for two hours, and is exhausted. The provider requests that a vacuum extractor be used to facilitate the birth. The client first states that she wants the birth to be normal, then allows the vacuum extraction. Following this, what should the nurse assess the client for after the birth? 1. elation, euphoria, and talkativeness 2. a sense of failure and self-disappointment 3. questions about whether or not to circumcise 4. uncertainty surrounding the baby's name	Answer: 2 Rationale: Clients who participate in childbirth classes that stress the normalcy of birth often feel as though they have failed the class if an intervention is used during their labor or birth. Elation euphoria, and talkativeness are expected after birth. Decisions on circumcision and naming are often encountered after birth, and are not correlated with the use of intervention. Assessment Health Promotion and Maintenance Analysis Learning Objective 27.1
27.14 The client is undergoing an emergency cesarean birth for fetal bradycardia. The partner of the client has not been allowed to be present in the operating room. What can the nurse do to alleviate the partner's emotional distress? (Select all that apply.) 1. Allow the partner to wheel the baby's crib to the newborn nursery. 2. Take digital pictures of the newborn and show them to the partner. 3. Have the partner wait in the client's postpartum room. 4. Encourage the partner to be in the nursery for the initial assessment. 5. Teach the partner how to take the client's blood pressure.	Answer: 1, 2, 4 Rationale: When the partner cannot be present at the birth, they often feel left out, disappointed, and/or fearful. Encouraging any interaction between the partner and the infant will decrease these negative feelings. Effective measures include bringing the baby to the nursery and being present for the initial assessment, and taking digital pictures for the partner to view until the baby is stable. The nurse must take the blood pressure as part of assessing the client. Implementation Health Promotion and Maintenance Application Learning Objective 27.1
27.15 The nurse is explaining induction of labor to a client. The client asks what the indications for labor induction are. Which of the following should the nurse include when answering the client?	Answer: 4 Rationale: A client with hypertension is appropriate for labor induction. Suspected placenta previa, breech presentation, and prolapsed umbilical cord are contraindications to labor induction.

1. suspected placenta previa	Implementation
2. breech presentation	Health Promotion and Maintenance
3. prolapsed umbilical cord	Application
4. hypertension	Learning Objective 27.4

CHAPTER 28

28.1 The nurse has assessed four newborns' respiratory rates immediately following birth. Which of the following respiratory rates would require further assessment by the nurse? 1. 60 breaths per minute 2. 70 breaths per minute 3. 64 breaths per minute 4. 28 breaths per minute	Answer: 4 Rationale: The normal range for respirations of a newborn within two hours after birth is 60 to 70 breaths per minute. If respirations drop below 30 breaths per minute when the infant is at rest, the nurse should notify the physician. Assessment Health Promotion and Maintenance Application Learning Objective 28.1
28.2 The pediatric clinic nurse is evaluating lab results with a two-month-old infant's mother. The infant's hemoglobin has decreased since birth. Which statement indicates that the mother needs additional teaching? 1. "My baby isn't getting enough iron in my breast milk." 2. "Babies undergo physiologic anemia of infancy." 3. "This results from dilution by the increased plasma volume." 4. "Delaying the cord clamping did not cause this to happen."	Answer: 1 Rationale: Breast milk is low in iron, but the bioavailability of the iron is high. At two months of age, infants increase their plasma volume, which results in a dilutional physiologic anemia. Early or delayed cord clamping will not affect hemoglobin levels at this age. Evaluation Health Promotion and Maintenance Analysis Learning Objective 28.2
28.3 The nurse is planning care for a newborn. Which of the following nursing interventions would best protect the newborn from the most common form of heat loss? 1. placing the newborn away from air currents 2. pre-warming the examination table 3. drying the newborn thoroughly 4. removing wet linens from the isolette	Answer: 3 Rationale: The most common form of heat loss is evaporation. Evaporation occurs when water is converted to a vapor. Drying the newborn thoroughly immediately after birth or after a bath will prevent heat loss by evaporation. Placing the newborn away from air currents reduces heat loss by convection. Pre-warming the examination table reduces heat loss by conduction. Removing wet linens from the isolette that are not in direct contact with the newborn reduces heat loss by radiation. Planning Health Promotion and Maintenance Application Learning Objective 28.3
28.4 A telephone triage nurse gets a call from a postpartum client who is concerned about jaundice. The client's newborn is 37 hours old. What data should the nurse gather first? 1. stool characteristics 2. fluid intake 3. skin color 4. bilirubin level	Answer: 3 Rationale: Yellow coloration of the skin and sclera are signs of physiologic jaundice that appear after the first 24 hours postnatally. Inspection of the skin would be the first step in assessing for jaundice. Skin color begins to appear yellow once the serum levels of bilirubin are about 4 to 6 mg/dL. The stool characteristic of green coloration indicates excretion of bilirubin. Inadequate fluid intake can predispose an infant toward becoming jaundiced, and is best determined by the number of wet diapers per day. Assessment Health Promotion and Maintenance Application Learning Objective 28.4
28.5 The mother of a three-day-old infant calls the clinic and reports that her baby's skin is turning slightly yellow. The nurse should explain to the mother that	Answer: 1 Rationale: Physiologic jaundice peaks about the third day of life, as a result of the infant breaking down and excreting red blood cells (RBCs). The liver of an infant is not fully mature at this point, and conjugates the bilirubin so it then is excreted

1. physiologic jaundice is normal and peaks at this age.
2. the newborn's liver is not working as well as it should.
3. the baby is yellow because the bowels are not excreting bilirubin.
4. the yellow color indicates that brain damage may be occurring.

through the bowels. A severely jaundiced infant can have a very high bilirubin level that can lead to brain damage. An infant with severe jaundice would have a high level of yellow skin color, but this infant is only slightly yellow.
Implementation
Health Promotion and Maintenance
Analysis
Learning Objective 28.5

28.6 The home care nurse is examining a three-day-old infant. The child's skin on the sternum is yellow when blanched with a finger. The parents ask the nurse why jaundice occurs. The best response from the nurse is
1. "The liver of an infant is not fully mature, and doesn't conjugate the bilirubin for excretion."
2. "The infant received too many red blood cells after delivery because the cord was not clamped immediately."
3. "The yellow color of your baby's skin indicates that you are breastfeeding too often."
4. "This is an abnormal finding related to your baby's bowels not excreting bilirubin as they should."

Answer: 1
Rationale: Physiologic jaundice is a common occurrence, and peaks on day three or four. It happens in part because of the RBC destruction that infants experience combined with liver immaturity, which leads to less efficient conjugation of bilirubin for excretion. Bilirubin binds to the proteins in breastmilk and formula for excretion through the bowels. Frequent feeding, therefore, will decrease jaundice.
Implementation
Health Promotion and Maintenance
Application
Learning Objective 28.6

28.7 The parents of a newborn are receiving discharge teaching. The nurse explains that the infant should have several wet diapers per day. Which statement by the parents indicates that further education is necessary?
1. "Our baby was born with kidneys that are too small."
2. "A baby's kidneys don't concentrate urine well for several months."
3. "Feeding our baby frequently will help the kidneys function."
4. "Kidney function in an infant is very different from an adult."

Answer: 1
Rationale: Size of the kidneys is rarely an issue. Counting wet diapers indicates urine output in relation to fluid intake. Frequent feeding helps maintain the fluid volume. The ability to concentrate urine develops by three to four months of age. The inability to concentrate urine due to limited tubular reabsorption and lower glomerular filtration rate are the main differences in kidney function between a newborn and normal adult kidney function.
Evaluation
Health Promotion and Maintenance
Analysis
Learning Objective 28.7

28.8 The parents of a newborn who is being treated for bacterial septicemia ask the nurse why their baby didn't seem very ill. The best response of the nurse is
1. "A newborn's immune system isn't mature, so symptoms are vague."
2. "You would have seen more symptoms if you had been looking closely."
3. "A fever will be present in sick newborns, including your baby."
4. "A mother's immunity usually protects the infant from illness."

Answer: 1
Rationale: Newborns have vague and nonspecific symptoms of illness because of their immature immune system and limited inflammatory response. Hypothermia is more common in ill infants than hyperthermia. Maternal immune globulin crosses the placenta and gives the newborn a limited acquired immunity to many illnesses, but will not prevent all illness from developing.
Implementation
Health Promotion and Maintenance
Application
Learning Objective 28.8

28.9 The student nurse notices that the newborns sleep peacefully in the nursery, although the environment is noisy and well-lit. The nursing instructor explains that this newborn behavior is

Answer: 1
Rationale: Habituation is the newborn's ability to process and respond to visual and auditory stimulation. The capacity to ignore repetitive disturbing stimuli is a newborn defense mechanism readily apparent in the noisy, well-lit nursery.

---

1. habituation. 2. orientation. 3. self-quieting. 4. due to sleep-alert states.	Orientation is the newborn's ability to be alert to, follow, and fixate on complex visual stimuli that are appealing and attractive. Self-quieting ability is the newborn's ability to quiet and comfort herself by sucking on her fist. Habituation can occur during both the deep sleep state and the active rapid eye movement (REM) sleep state. Assessment Health Promotion and Maintenance Application Learning Objective 28.9
28.10 The client's partner is holding the day-old infant and talking quietly to him. The client asks if it is possible for the newborn to focus on his father's eyes. The nurse's best response is, "Yes. Your infant is exhibiting 1. habituation." 2. orientation." 3. self-quieting." 4. behavior that is due to sleep-alert states."	Answer: 2 Rationale: Orientation is the newborn's ability to be alert to, follow, and fixate on complex visual stimuli that are appealing and attractive, such as a mother's eyes. Habituation is the newborn's ability to process and respond to visual and auditory stimulation. Self-quieting ability is the newborn's ability to quiet and comfort himself by sucking on his fist. This is an example of the wide awake alert state, not a sleep-alert state. Assessment Health Promotion and Maintenance Application Learning Objective 28.9
28.11 A postpartum client calls the nursery to report that her three-day-old newborn has passed a bright green stool. The nurse's best response is 1. "Take your newborn to the pediatrician." 2. "There may be a possible food allergy." 3. "Your newborn has diarrhea." 4. "This is a normal occurrence."	Answer: 4 Rationale: By the third day of life, the newborn's stools appear a thin, brown color to green in color. It is not necessary for the client to take her newborn to the pediatrician. The green color of stool is not due to food allergies or characterized as diarrhea, but is a transitional stool that consists of part meconium and part fecal material. Implementation Health Promotion and Maintenance Analysis Learning Objective 28.6
28.12 The nurse is planning the care of a one-day-old infant. Which of the following nursing interventions would protect the newborn from heat loss by convection? 1. placing the newborn away from air currents 2. pre-warming the examination table 3. drying the newborn thoroughly 4. removing wet linens from the isolette	Answer: 1 Rationale: Placing the newborn away from air currents reduces heat loss by convection. Drying the newborn thoroughly immediately after birth or after a bath will prevent heat loss by evaporation. Pre-warming the examination table reduces heat loss by conduction. Removing wet linens from the isolette that are not in direct contact with the newborn reduces heat loss by radiation. Planning Health Promotion and Maintenance Analysis Learning Objective 28.3
28.13 The student nurse notices that a newborn weighs less today compared with the newborn's birth weight three days ago. The nursing instructor explains that newborns lose weight following birth due to 1. a shift of intracellular water to extracellular spaces. 2. loss of meconium stool. 3. a shift of extracellular water to intracellular spaces. 4. the sleep-wake cycle.	Answer: 1 Rationale: A shift of intracellular water to extracellular space accounts for the 5% to 10% of weight loss during the first few days of life. Loss of meconium stool and the sleep-wake cycle do not affect this amount of weight loss. Assessment Health Promotion and Maintenance Analysis Learning Objective 28.1
28.14 The new mother is holding her two-hour-old son. The delivery occurred on the due date. Apgar scores were 9 at both one and five minutes. The mother asks the nurse why her son was so wide	Answer: 2 Rationale: The first alert phase lasts about 30 minutes after birth, followed by decreased activity and then sleep that will last about two to four hours. Six hours of sleep at this point is not an expected finding. Although this infant's behavior is

awake right after birth, and now is sleeping so soundly. Which statement is best for the nurse to make?

1. "Don't worry at all; babies go through a lot of these little phases."
2. "Your son is in the second alert phase. He'll wake up soon."
3. "Your son is exhausted from being born, and will sleep six more hours."
4. "Your breastfeeding efforts have caused excessive fatigue in your son."

expected, nurses must avoid using clichés in therapeutic communication. Breastfeeding will not cause fatigue in a normal term newborn.
Implementation
Health Promotion and Maintenance
Application
Learning Objective 28.9

28.15 The nurse is teaching a group of new parents about newborn behavior. Which statement made by a parent would indicate a need for additional information?

1. "Sleep and alert states cycle throughout the day."
2. "We can best bond with our child during an alert state."
3. "About half of the baby's sleep time is in active sleep."
4. "Babies will sleep during the night right from birth."

Answer: 4
Rationale: Sleep and alert states are noticeable behaviors in infants, beginning immediately after birth with the first period of alert activity. The diurnal sleep-wake patterns, in which the baby sleeps at night and is more awake during the daytime, develop over time. Bonding between infant and parents takes place with interaction during alert states. From 45–50% of a newborn's time sleeping will take place in the active sleep state, and 35–45% will take place in the deep sleep state.
Evaluation
Health Promotion and Maintenance
Analysis
Learning Objective 28.9

CHAPTER 29

29.1 The student nurse has performed a gestational age assessment of an infant, and finds the infant to be at 32 weeks. Which set of characteristics are most likely to be found?

1. lanugo mainly gone, little vernix across the body
2. prominent clitoris, enlarging minora, anus patent
3. full areola, 5 to 10 mm bud, pinkish-brown in color
4. skin is opaque, has cracking at wrists and ankles, no vessels visible

Answer: 2
Rationale: Labia minora enlarge as the infant achieves greater gestational age, and the clitoris will be covered at term. Lanugo and vernix disappear as the infant approaches term. Areolas develop greater size with advancing gestational age. Skin of a preterm infant is translucent, and vessels are visible through the skin.
Assessment
Health Promotion and Maintenance
Application
Learning Objective 29.1

29.2 The nurse is completing the gestational age assessment on a newborn while in the mother's postpartum room. During the assessment, the mother asks the nurse what aspects of the baby are being checked during this assessment. Which response by the nurse is best?

1. "I'm checking to make sure the baby has all of its parts."
2. "This looks both at physical aspects and the nervous system."
3. "This checks the baby's brain and nerve function."
4. "Don't worry. We perform this check on all of the babies."

Answer: 2
Rationale: The gestational age assessment incorporates external physical characteristics and neurologic or neuromuscular development evaluations. The assessment immediately after birth would assess for grossly intact physiology (such as presence of the anus, location of the urethra, number of cord vessels, gender of genitalia, etc.). Nurses must always use therapeutic communication, and giving a "don't worry" answer dismisses the client's question or concern.
Assessment
Health Promotion and Maintenance
Application
Learning Objective 29.1

29.3 Before the nurse begins to dry the newborn off after birth, which of the following assessment finings should the nurse document to ensure an accurate

Answer: 1
Rationale: Drying the baby after birth will disturb the vernix and potentially alter the score when using the Ballard gestational assessment tool. The nurse first should document the amount and coverage of the vernix before drying the

gestational rating on the Ballard gestational assessment tool?
1. amount and area of vernix coverage
2. creases on the sole
3. size of the areola
4. body surface temperature

newborn. Creases on the sole and size of the areola are not affected by drying the newborn. Body surface temperature is not part of the Ballard gestational assessment tool.
Assessment
Health Promotion and Maintenance
Application
Learning Objective 29.2

29.4 During an assessment of a 12-hour-old newborn, the nurse notices pale pink spots on the nape of the neck. The nurse documents this finding as
1. nevus vasculosus.
2. nevus flammeus.
3. telangiectatic nevi.
4. a Mongolian spot.

Answer: 3
Rationale: Telangiectatic nevi (stork bites) are pale pink or red spots that appear on the eyelids, nose, lower occipital bone, or the nape of the neck. Nevus vasculosus (strawberry mark) is a capillary hemangioma. Nevus flammeus (port-wine stain), a capillary angioma, is located directly below the epidermis. Mongolian spots are macular areas of bluish-black pigmentation on the dorsal area of the buttocks.
Assessment
Health Promotion and Maintenance
Application
Learning Objective 29.2

29.5 The student nurse attempts to take the vital sign of the newborn, but the newborn is crying. What nursing action would be appropriate?
1. Place a gloved finger in the newborn's mouth.
2. Take the vital signs.
3. Wait until the newborn stops crying.
4. Place a hot water bottle in the isolette.

Answer: 1
Rationale: To soothe a newborn during assessment or other procedures, place a gloved finger into the newborn's mouth. Crying will increase heart rate and respiratory rate, so vitals should not be taken when the newborn is crying. However, assessment of vitals needs to be done at regularly-timed intervals, so waiting until the newborn stops crying may be too long of a delay. A hot water bottle should not be placed next to the newborn because of a potential risk for burns.
Assessment
Health Promotion and Maintenance
Application
Learning Objective 29.5

29.6 The student nurse assesses the pinna of the newborn's ears, and finds them to be parallel with the outer canthus of the eye. The nursing instructor should explain this finding to be
1. a normal position.
2. a possible chromosomal abnormality.
3. facial paralysis.
4. prematurity.

Answer: 1
Rationale: The top of the ear (pinna) should be parallel to the outer and inner canthus of the eye in the normal newborn. Low-set ears may indicate a chromosomal abnormality. Facial paralysis would not affect ear placement. Gestational age does not affect ear placement.
Assessment
Health Promotion and Maintenance
Application
Learning Objective 29.3

29.7 A new parent reports to the nurse that the baby looks cross-eyed several times a day. The nurse teaches the parents that this finding should resolve in
1. two months.
2. two weeks.
3. one year.
4. four months.

Answer: 4
Rationale: The newborn might demonstrate transient strabismus that is caused by poor neuromuscular control of the eye muscles. This will gradually regress in three to four months.
Assessment
Health Promotion and Maintenance
Application
Learning Objective 29.3

29.8 A new mother is concerned about a mass on her newborn's head. The nurse assesses this, and finds it to be a cephalhematoma. Which of the following characteristics would indicate a cephalhematoma? (Select all that apply.)
1. The mass appeared on the second day after birth.
2. The mass appears larger when the newborn cries.

Answer: 1, 4
Rationale: A cephalhematoma is a collection of blood resulting from ruptured blood vessels between the surface of a cranial bone and the periosteal membrane, and is often visible as a purplish mass. It can appear between the first and second day after birth and does not increase in size when the newborn cries. Cephalhematomas can be unilateral or bilateral but do not cross the suture lines. Molding causes the head to appear asymmetrical; this is due to the overriding of cranial bones during labor and birth.
Assessment
Health Promotion and Maintenance

3. The head appears asymmetrical. 4. The mass is purplish in color. 5. The mass overrides the suture line.	Analysis Learning Objective 29.3
29.9 The nurse is making an initial assessment of the newborn. The findings include a chest circumference of 32.5 cm, and a head circumference of 33.5 cm. Based on these findings, which action should the nurse take first? 1. Notify the physician. 2. Elevate the newborn's head. 3. Document the findings in the chart. 4. Assess for hypothermia immediately.	Answer: 3 Rationale: None of the findings indicate hypothermia, and none are out of the ordinary; thus, documentation is the appropriate first step. A physician would only be notified if abnormal findings are present. There is no indication that the newborn's head should be elevated. No data on temperature is given. The average circumference of the head at birth is 32 to 37 cm. Average chest circumference ranges from 30 to 35 cm at birth. The circumference of the head is approximately 2 cm greater than the circumference of the chest at birth. Planning Health Promotion and Maintenance Analysis Learning Objective 29.3
29.10 A nursing instructor is demonstrating an assessment on a newborn for the nursing students, and is using the Ballard gestational assessment tool. The nurse explains that which of the following tests should be performed after the first hour of birth? 1. arm recoil 2. square window sign 3. scarf sign 4. popliteal angle	Answer: 1 Rationale: Recoil time is slower in fatigued newborns. Therefore, arm recoil is best elicited after the first hour of birth so that the newborn can recover from the stress of birth. Square window sign, scarf sign, and popliteal angle are assessments performed by the examiner, whereas arm recoil is a response by the newborn. Assessment Health Promotion and Maintenance Application Learning Objective 29.4
29.11 The nurse attempts to elicit the Moro reflex on a newborn and assesses movement of the right arm only. Based on this finding, the nurse immediately assesses the 1. Ortolani maneuver. 2. Babinski reflex. 3. clavicle. 4. Gallant reflex.	Answer: 3 Rationale: When the Moro reflex is elicited, the newborn will straighten both arms and hands outward while the knees are flexed, then slowly return the arms to the chest, as in an embrace. If this response is not elicited, the nurse will assess the clavicle. If the clavicle is fractured, the response will be demonstrated on the unaffected side only. Ortolani maneuver is an assessment technique that rules out the possibility of congenital hip dysplasia. Babinski reflex tests for upper neuron abnormalities. Trunk incurvation (Gallant reflex) is seen when the newborn is prone and the pelvis is turned to the stimulated side when the spine is stroked. Assessment Health Promotion and Maintenance Analysis Learning Objective 29.4
29.12 The nurse determines the gestational age of an infant to be 40 weeks. Which characteristics are most likely to be found? (Select all that apply.) 1. lanugo abundant over shoulders and back 2. plantar creases over entire sole 3. pinna of ear springs back slowly when folded 4. vernix well-distributed over entire body 5. testes are pendulous and the scrotum has deep rugae.	Answer: 2, 5 Rationale: Plantar creases develop as gestational age advances, until the term infant's entire sole of the foot is covered with these creases. Term male infants have pendulous testes and a scrotum covered with deep rugae. Vernix and lanugo both disappear as the infant reaches term. Pinna springing slowly indicates prematurity; a term infant's pinna would spring back immediately. Assessment Health Promotion and Maintenance Application Learning Objective 29.4
29.13 The nurse wishes to demonstrate to a new family their infant's individuality. Which assessment tool would be most appropriate for the nurse to use?	Answer: 1 Rationale: The Brazelton Neonatal Behavioral Assessment Scale assesses the newborn's state changes, temperament, and individual behavior patterns. The Ballard Maturity Scale and the Dubowitz Gestational Age Scale are tools that assess external physical characteristics and neurological or neuromuscular

1. Brazelton Neonatal Behavioral Assessment Scale
2. Ballard Maturity Scale
3. Dubowitz Gestational Age Scale
4. Ortolani maneuver

development. The Ortolani maneuver is an assessment technique that rules out the possibility of congenital hip dysplasia.
Planning
Health Promotion and Maintenance
Application
Learning Objective 29.5

29.14 The nurse is teaching an infant care class to new parents. Which statement indicates that additional teaching is needed?
1. "The white spots on my baby's nose are called milia, and are harmless."
2. "The cheesy white substance in the creases is vernix, and will be absorbed."
3. "The red spots with a white center on my baby are abnormal acne."
4. "Jaundice might develop in my baby when it is a few days old.

Answer: 3
Rationale: Red spots with a white or yellow center are erythema toxicum, and will disappear within a few hours or days. Milia are exposed sebaceous glands, and appear as white spots, often across the nose. Vernix caseosa is white and cheesy and can remain in the groin and axillary creases after bathing. Physiologic jaundice peaks on about day three.
Evaluation
Health Promotion and Maintenance
Analysis
Learning Objective 29.2

29.15 The parents of a newborn comment to the nurse that their infant seems to enjoy being held, and that holding the baby helps him calm down after crying. They ask the nurse why this happens. After explaining newborn behavior, the nurse assesses the parents' learning. Which statement indicates that teaching was effective?
1. "Some babies are easier to deal with than others."
2. "We are lucky to have a baby with a calm disposition."
3. "Our baby spends more time in the active alert phase."
4. "Cuddliness is a social behavior that some babies have."

Answer: 4
Rationale: The Brazelton Neonatal Behavioral Assessment Scale looks at: habituation, orientation to animate or inanimate visual or auditory stimuli, motor activity, self-quieting, cuddliness or social behaviors, and variations of each of these categories. Easier or more difficult to deal with and describing an infant as having a calm disposition are judgments, not part of an assessment. The active alert phase of the sleep-awake cycle is characterized by motor activity.
Evaluation
Health Promotion and Maintenance
Analysis
Learning Objective 29.5

CHAPTER 30

30.1 The nurse is caring for a client who was given meperidine (Demerol) during labor. In planning care for the client's newborn, the nurse should closely assess the newborn for
1. body temperature.
2. stool pattern.
3. bilirubin level.
4. urine output.

Answer: 1
Rationale: Certain drugs such as meperidine (Demerol) may prevent the metabolism of brown fat. Therefore, when meperidine (Demerol) is given to a laboring woman, the newborn may be at risk for hypothermia. Meperidine (Demerol) does not affect the stool pattern, bilirubin level, or urine output.
Assessment
Health Promotion and Maintenance
Application
Learning Objective 30.1

30.2 The nurse is caring for four newborns who have recently been admitted to the newborn nursery. Which labor event puts the newborn at risk for an alteration of health? The infant's mother had
1. ruptured membranes for 36 hours.
2. an IV of lactated Ringer's solution.
3. a labor that lasted 12 hours.
4. a cesarean birth with her last child.

Answer: 1
Rationale: Prolonged rupture of membranes (greater than 12 hours) increases the risk for maternal endometritis and newborn sepsis. An IV of lactated Ringer's solution will not affect the newborn's blood sugar. A 12-hour labor is normal. Having had a cesarean with her last child gives the mother risk factors during labor, and does not affect this newborn.
Assessment
Health Promotion and Maintenance
Analysis
Learning Objective 30.1

30.3 A two-day-old newborn is asleep, and the nurse assesses the apical pulse to be 88 breaths per minute (bpm). What would be the most appropriate nursing action based on this assessment finding?
1. Call the physician.
2. Administer oxygen.
3. Document the finding.
4. Place the newborn under the radiant warmer.

Answer: 3
Rationale: An apical pulse rate of 88 bpm is within the normal range of a sleeping full-term newborn. Documentation is an appropriate action with a normal finding. The physician is only called with abnormal findings. There is no indication the baby is hypoxic or cold.
Implementation
Health Promotion and Maintenance
Application
Learning Objective 30.2

30.4 The nurse has assessed a newborn's respiratory rate one hour after birth. Which of the following respiratory rates would require further action by the nurse?
1. 60 breaths per minute
2. 35 breaths per minute
3. 55 breaths per minute
4. 25 breaths per minute

Answer: 4
Rationale: The normal range for respirations of a newborn within two hours of birth is 60–70 breaths per minute. If respirations drop below 30 breaths per minute when the infant is at rest, the nurse should notify the physician.
Assessment
Health Promotion and Maintenance
Application
Learning Objective 30.2

30.5 The nurse is supervising a student nurse who is caring for a newborn 30 minutes after birth. During an assessment of respiratory function, the following data is collected. Which of the following assessment findings should the student nurse report as abnormal? (Select all that apply.)
1. periodic breathing with pauses of two to three seconds
2. Chest and abdomen movements are synchronous.
3. grunting on expiration
4. nasal flaring
5. retractions

Answer: 3, 4, 5
Rationale: Grunting, nasal flaring, and retractions are signs of respiratory distress. The normal respiratory rate for a newborn is 40–60 breaths per minute, with an irregular rate, and pauses of several seconds occurring. The chest and abdomen may be synchronous or asynchronous.
Assessment
Health Promotion and Maintenance
Application
Learning Objective 30.3

30.6 The nurse has just assisted the father in bathing the newborn two hours after birth. The nurse explains to the father that the newborn must remain in the radiant warmer after the bath. Which of the following assessment data indicate that this is required?
1. a heart rate of 120
2. temperature 96.8°F
3. respiratory rate 50
4. temperature 99.6°F

Answer: 2
Rationale: After the first bath, the temperature is rechecked. If the temperature falls below 97.5, the nurse returns the newborn to the radiant warmer. The re-warming process is gradual, to prevent hypothermia. Heart rate and respiratory rate are within normal limits for a newborn who is two hours old.
Assessment
Health Promotion and Maintenance
Analysis
Learning Objective 30.3

30.7 The nurse is supervising care of a student nurse. Which of the following nursing actions indicates that the student nurse needs additional education to protect the newborn from heat loss?
1. placing the newborn near the warm air duct
2. pre-warming the examination table
3. drying the newborn thoroughly
4. removing wet linens from the isolette

Answer: 1
Rationale: Placing the newborn near air currents will increase heat loss from convection. The form of heat loss to which the infant is most susceptible is evaporation. Evaporation occurs when water is converted to a vapor. Drying the newborn thoroughly immediately after birth or after a bath will prevent heat loss by evaporation. Pre-warming the examination table reduces heat loss by conduction. Removing wet linens from the isolette that are not in direct contact with the newborn reduces heat loss by radiation.
Evaluation
Health Promotion and Maintenance
Analysis
Learning Objective 30.4

30.8 The new mother is asking the nurse about the baby's cord. Which client statement indicates that teaching has been effective?
1. "The cord will fall off in one to two weeks."
2. "I should keep the cord covered by the diaper."
3. "The clamp will be left on until my son is circumcised."
4. "The cord might smell bad after we get home."

Answer: 1
Rationale: The umbilical cord stump will spontaneously fall off in one to two weeks. The diaper should be kept folded below the cord. The clamp is taken off in about 24 hours, and does not relate to timing of the circumcision. A malodorous cord should be reported to the baby's provider.
Evaluation
Health Promotion and Maintenance
Analysis
Learning Objective 30.4

30.9 At birth, an infant weighed 8 pounds 4 ounces. Three days later the newborn is being discharged. The parents note that the baby now weighs 7 pounds 15 ounces. What explanation should the nurse give for the change in this newborn's weight? "His weight loss is
1. excessive."
2. within normal limits."
3. less than expected."
4. unusual."

Answer: 2
Rationale: This newborn's weight loss is within normal limits. During the first five to ten days of life, caloric intake often is insufficient for weight gain. Therefore, there may be a weight loss of 5 % to 10 % in term newborns.
Implementation
Health Promotion and Maintenance
Analysis
Learning Objective 30.5

30.10 A postpartum client calls the clinic to report that her three-day-old baby girl has a spot of blood on her diaper. The best explanation for the nurse to give is that this finding is due to
1. withdrawal of maternal hormones.
2. a urinary infection.
3. an immature immune system.
4. physiologic jaundice.

Answer: 1
Rationale: As maternal hormones clear the newborn, it is not unusual to find blood on the diapers of a female newborn. This is referred to as pseudomenstruation. A urinary infection or an immature immune system does not cause pseudomenstruation. Physiologic jaundice causes yellow coloring of the skin, not blood in the diaper.
Implementation
Health Promotion and Maintenance
Application
Learning Objective 30.5

30.11 A postpartum mother questions whether the room temperature should be warmer in the baby's room at home. The nurse responds that, yes, the environmental temperature should be warmer for the newborn. This response by the nurse is based on which of the following newborn characteristics? (Select all that apply.)
1. Newborns have little subcutaneous fat.
2. Newborns have a thick epidermis layer.
3. Variable posture of the term newborn
4. Newborns have an increase in subcutaneous fat.
5. Newborns are unable to shiver to produce heat.

Answer: 1, 5
Rationale: The normal newborn will require a higher environmental temperature in order to maintain a thermoneutral environment. Little subcutaneous fat, blood vessels that are close to the skin, a thin epidermis layer, and the inability to shiver all are characteristics that affect the newborn's ability to maintain its temperature. Newborns assume a flexed posture to reduce heat loss by decreasing the surface area that is exposed to the environment.
Implementation
Health Promotion and Maintenance
Application
Learning Objective 30.6

30.12 A postpartum client reports to her nurse that her three-day-old newborn has passed a bright green stool. The nurse's best explanation for this is
1. "Please talk to your pediatrician about this."
2. "There may be a possible food allergy."

Answer: 4
Rationale: By the third day of life, the newborn's stools appear thin brown to green in color. The green color of stool is not due to food allergies or characterized as diarrhea, but is a transitional stool that consists of part meconium and part fecal material. It is not therapeutic to ask the client to talk to someone else about a question.
Implementation
Health Promotion and Maintenance

3. "Your newborn has diarrhea." 4. "This is a normal finding in newborns."	Analysis Learning Objective 30.6
30.13 The newly-delivered primiparous client notices that the newborn seems to focus on her eyes. After discussing this finding with the client, the nurse knows that teaching has been effective if the new mother describes this newborn behavior as 1. habituation. 2. orientation. 3. self-quieting. 4. the sleep-alert state.	Answer: 2 Rationale: Orientation is the newborn's ability to be alert to, follow, and fixate on complex visual stimuli that are appealing and attractive, such as a mother's eyes. Habituation is the newborn's ability to process and respond to visual and auditory stimulation. Self-quieting is the newborn's ability to quiet and comfort himself by sucking on his fist. Sleep and alert states identify the two behavioral states of the newborn. Evaluation Health Promotion and Maintenance Application Learning Objective 30.7
30.14 The nurse is instructing the parents of a newborn about car seat safety. Which statement indicates that the parents need additional information? 1. "The baby should be in the back seat." 2. "Newborns must be in rear-facing car seats." 3. "We need to read the owner's manual before using the car seat." 4. "How the straps go around the baby isn't that important."	Answer: 4 Rationale: Car seats for infants are mandatory in most states. Straps must be snug around the baby in order to be effective in protecting the baby during a crash. The safest place for a newborn is in a rear-facing car seat in the middle of the back seat. Each car seat is different; the owner's manual contains instructions for proper use. Evaluation Health Promotion and Maintenance Application Learning Objective 30.8
30.15 The nurse is discharging a 15-year-old first-time mother. Which statement should the nurse include in the discharge teaching? 1. "Call your pediatrician if the baby's temperature is below 98° F." 2. "Your baby's stools will change to a golden color when your milk comes in." 3. "You can wipe away any eye drainage that may form." 4. "Your infant should wet a diaper at least six times per day."	Answer: 4 Rationale: A minimum of six wet diapers per day indicates adequate fluid intake. Eye drainage is abnormal, and should be reported to the baby's provider. A temp less than 98°F is abnormally low. Stool color turns a golden brown when lactation is established. Implementation Health Promotion and Maintenance Analysis Learning Objective 30.8

CHAPTER 31

31.1 The nurse is teaching a prenatal class about feeding methods. A father-to-be asks the nurse which method, breast or formula, leads to the fastest infant growth and weight gain. Which response by the nurse is best? "In the first three to four months 1. breastfed babies gain weight faster." 2. there is no difference in weight gain." 3. bottle-fed babies grow faster." 4. growth isn't as important as your comfort with the method."	Answer: 1 Rationale: Once feeding is established, breastfed babies tend to gain weight faster than bottle-fed babies, and have a leaner body at the end of the first year. Although comfort with the feeding method is important, the question is specifically about growth and weight gain; it is not therapeutic to change the topic and not answer the question. Implementation Health Promotion and Maintenance Application Learning Objective 31.1
31.2 The community nurse is working with poor women who are formula-feeding their infants. Which statement indicates that the nurse's education session was effective?	Answer: 2 Rationale: Powdered and concentrated formula must be mixed according to manufacturer's guidelines. Formula that is too dilute can cause malnutrition and diarrhea. Formula that is too concentrated can lead to excess sodium intake, which creates increased thirst and overfeeding. Once formula is mixed, it must be used within two hours or refrigerated. Each bottle should contain only enough

1. "I should only use soy-based formula for the first year."
2. "I follow the instructions for mixing the powdered formula exactly."
3. "I can reuse one bottle for several feedings."
4. "The mixed formula can be left on the counter for a day."

formula for one feeding, and any formula left after the feeding should be discarded to prevent bacterial growth. Soy-based formulas are more expensive than whey-based formulas, and are only needed by infants with a milk allergy. No information is provided about milk allergy symptoms. Powdered formula is the cheapest, followed by concentrated formula; ready-to-feed formula is the most expensive.
Evaluation
Health Promotion and Maintenance
Analysis
Learning Objective 31.1

31.3 The client at 20 weeks' gestation has not decided on a feeding method for her infant. She asks the nurse for advice. The nurse presents information about the advantages and disadvantages of formula feeding and breastfeeding. Which statements by the client indicate that the teaching was successful?
1. "Formula feeding gives the baby protection from infections."
2. "Breast milk cannot be stored; it has to be thrown away after pumping."
3. "Breastfeeding is more expensive than formula feeding."
4. "My baby has a lower risk of food allergies if I breastfeed."

Answer: 4
Rationale: Breastmilk provides newborns with immunoglobulins, and reduces the risk of food allergies in children. Formula does not provide the baby with protection from infections, like breastmilk does. Breastmilk can be refrigerated or frozen after pumping. Formula must be purchased and therefore is an expense.
Evaluation
Health Promotion and Maintenance
Analysis
Learning Objective 31.2

31.4 The community nurse is working with a new mother who has a four-week-old infant. The mother states that she is unhappy with breastfeeding because her breasts leak between feedings. Which of the following should the nurse explain may contribute to the letdown reflex in breastfeeding mothers?
1. pain with breastfeeding
2. number of hours passed since last feeding
3. the newborn's cry
4. maternal fluid intake

Answer: 3
Rationale: A newborn's cry can stimulate the letdown reflex in breastfeeding mothers. Pain with breastfeeding is associated with improper positioning. Maternal fluid intake and too many hours between feeding can affect milk supply; these factors will not affect letdown.
Implementation
Health Promotion and Maintenance
Application
Learning Objective 31.2

31.5 A nurse is caring for the one-hour-old infant of a diabetic mother. Which of the following should be included in the nurse's plan of care for this newborn?
1. Take the newborn's temperature hourly.
2. Use formula for all feedings, avoiding 5% dextrose.
3. Evaluate blood glucose levels at 12 hours after birth.
4. Assess for hyperthyroidism.

Answer: 2
Rationale: Newborns of diabetic mothers can require frequent feedings to maintain normal levels of blood glucose. Formula feedings contain protein and will maintain blood sugar better than glucose water alone. The onset of hypoglycemia occurs at one to three hours after birth, and can continue for several days. Blood glucose levels should be checked hourly during the first four hours and then at four-hour intervals until stable normal levels are attained. Hyperthyroidism is not associated with newborns of diabetic mothers.
Planning
Health Promotion and Maintenance
Analysis
Learning Objective 31.3

31.6 A community nurse is visiting a new mother and her newborn in their home. The mother is concerned that her baby is not gaining enough weight. To encourage proper weight gain, the mother should be instructed to

Answer: 2
Rationale: From birth to two months of age, the newborn should take between 6–8 feedings consisting of approximately two to four ounces of formula per 24 hours. When formula is over-diluted, the infant will not receive adequate nutrients to ensure proper weight gain. Formula-fed newborns should be fed

---

1. dilute formula with water.
2. offer 12–32 ounces of formula every 24 hours.
3. offer formula every six to eight hours.
4. provide skim milk exclusively.

every three to four hours but should not go longer than four hours between feedings. Skim milk should not be offered to newborns before one year of age.
Implementation
Health Promotion and Maintenance
Analysis
Learning Objective 31.3

31.7 A nurse is assisting a new mother to breastfeed. Put the following steps for breastfeeding in a logical sequence. Your answer should be a five digit number.
1. Tickle newborn's lips with the nipple.
2. Bring newborn to breast.
3. Newborn opens mouth wide.
4. Have newborn face mother tummy to tummy.
5. Position newborn so the newborn's nose is at level of the nipple.

Answer: 54132
Rationale: To facilitate successful breastfeeding, the nurse may encourage the mother to follow these steps: position newborn so the newborn's nose is at level of the nipple; have newborn face mother tummy to tummy; tickle newborn's lips with the nipple; wait until newborn opens mouth wide; and then bring newborn to breast.
Implementation
Health Promotion and Maintenance
Analysis
Learning Objective 31.3

31.8 The nurse is working with a new mother who has fed her newborn twice in the past 12 hours. The nurse instructs the mother how to encourage a sleepy baby to breastfeed. Which of the following methods should the nurse include in teaching the mother how to get her sleepy baby to feed? (Select all that apply.)
1. Provide skin-to-skin contact.
2. Swaddle the newborn in a blanket.
3. Allow the newborn to feel and smell mother's breast.
4. Give the baby a bottle feeding between breast feedings.
5. Turn the volume of the TV up.

Answer: 1, 3
Rationale: Activities that encourage a sleepy newborn to breastfeed include: unwrapping the newborn; providing skin-to-skin contact between mother and newborn; and allowing the mother to rest with the newborn near her breast so the newborn can feel and smell mother's breast. Breastfed infants should not be offered bottles until lactation is well-established. Talking quietly to the infant may help awaken him, but an infant will habituate to loud noises and continue to sleep.
Evaluation
Health Promotion and Maintenance
Analysis
Learning Objective 31.4

31.9 The nurse is working in a high-risk maternity unit. Which of the following mothers should the nurse counsel against breastfeeding?
1. a mother with a poorly-balanced diet
2. a mother who is overweight
3. a mother who is HIV-positive
4. a mother who has twins

Answer: 3
Rationale: Women with HIV or AIDS are counseled against breastfeeding. A newborn whose mother has a poor diet may need to receive supplements. Mothers who are overweight or have twins are encouraged to breastfeed.
Implementation
Health Promotion and Maintenance
Application
Learning Objective 31.4

31.10 A nurse is evaluating the diet plan of a breastfeeding mother, and determines that her intake of fruits and vegetables is inadequate. The nurse explains that the nutritional composition of the breastmilk can be adversely affected by this aspect of the mother's nutrition. Which of the following strategies should be recommended to the mother?
1. Stop breastfeeding.
2. Provide vitamin supplements to the newborn.
3. Offer whole milk.
4. Supplement with skim milk.

Answer: 2
Rationale: The mother may continue to breastfeed, but the caregiver may choose to prescribe additional vitamins for the newborn. Whole milk and skim milk are not recommended during the first year of life.
Implementation
Health Promotion and Maintenance
Analysis
Learning Objective 31.5

31.11 The triage nurse receives a call from a mother of an obese infant who appears pale, sweaty, and has become increasingly irritable. What data should the nurse gather next?
1. newborn's daily iron intake
2. number of wet diapers a day
3. skin color
4. bilirubin level

Answer: 1
Rationale: An obese newborn that appears pale in color, diaphoretic, and irritable should be suspected of iron deficiency. The number of wet diapers a day would provide information about hydration. Skin color and bilirubin level would provide information about jaundice.
Assessment
Health Promotion and Maintenance
Analysis
Learning Objective 31.5

31.12 A premature newborn is unable to suck at the breast. The nurse arranges for the mother to use an electric pump at least
1. two times in a 24-hour period.
2. four times in a 24-hour period.
3. six times in a 24-hour period.
4. eight times in a 24-hour period.

Answer: 4
Rationale: An electric pump should be used at least eight times a day. This will help a new mother establish and increase her milk supply until the newborn can breastfeed. Not using the pump frequently will lead to an inadequate supply of milk.
Planning
Health Promotion and Maintenance
Application
Learning Objective 31.4

31.13 The nurse is preparing a class on breastfeeding to clients in their first trimesters. The clients are from a variety of cultural backgrounds, and all speak English well. Which statement should the nurse include in this presentation?
1. "Although some cultures believe colostrum is not good for the baby, it provides protection from infections and helps the digestive system to function."
2. "Some women are uncomfortable with exposing their breasts to nurse their infant, but it really isn't a big deal. You will get used to it."
3. "No religion prescribes a feeding method, so you all can choose whatever method makes the most sense to you."
4. "Many cultures consider skinny babies to be healthier than chubby babies; breastfeeding is best for those people."

Answer: 1
Rationale: Although it is true that some cultures believe colostrum to be unhealthy, colostrum contains immune-boosting properties and helps establish normal digestive tract function. It is not therapeutic to downplay a woman's concern by stating, "It's no big deal"; this type of statement should be avoided. The Muslim religion is encouraged by the Qur'an to breastfeed for two years. Many cultures consider chubby babies to be healthier than skinny babies; breastfed babies gain weight faster and therefore breastfeeding will help babies to appear healthier from a cultural perspective.
Planning
Health Promotion and Maintenance
Analysis
Learning Objective 31.6

31.14 The nurse is caring for a new breastfeeding mother who is from Pakistan. The nurse plans her care so that the newborn is offered the breast on the
1. day of birth.
2. first day after birth.
3. third day after birth.
4. two weeks after birth

Answer: 3
Rationale: It is important for the nurse to understand the impact of culture on specific feeding practices. Women from Pakistan do not offer colostrum to their newborns. They begin breastfeeding only after the milk flow has been established, which is typically on the third day after birth.
Planning
Health Promotion and Maintenance
Analysis
Learning Objective 31.6

31.15 The nurse is assisting a mother to bottle-feed her newborn, who has been crying. The nurse suggests that prior to feeding, the mother should
1. offer a pacifier.
2. burp the newborn.
3. unwrap the newborn.
4. stroke the newborn's spine and feet.

Answer: 2
Rationale: If a newborn has been crying prior to feeding, air might have been swallowed; therefore, the newborn should be burped before feeding. Time should be taken to calm the newborn prior to feeding. The newborn's cries are indicative of an issue; a pacifier would not solve the problem. Unwrapping the newborn and stroking the spine and feet stimulate the newborn.
Implementation
Health Promotion and Maintenance
Analysis
Learning Objective 31.3

32.1 A nurse assesses the gestational age of a newborn. She explains to the parents that the newborn is premature. Which of the following findings indicates symptoms of prematurity?
1. Clitoris and labia minora are prominent.
2. There is a strong sucking reflex.
3. Umbilical cord has three vessels.
4. Ears spring back when folded.

Answer: 1
Rationale: Assessment findings that indicate prematurity include a prominent clitoris and labia minora. A strong sucking reflex is found in normal term newborns, as is a pinna that springs back. Two arteries and one vein is the normal finding for an umbilical cord.
Evaluation
Health Promotion and Maintenance
Application
Learning Objective 32.1

32.2 The nurse is caring for a two-hour-old newborn whose mother is diabetic. The nurse assesses that the newborn is experiencing tremors. What nursing action has the highest priority?
1. Obtain a blood calcium level.
2. Take the newborn's temperature.
3. Obtain a bilirubin level.
4. Place a pulse oximeter on the newborn.

Answer: 1
Rationale: Tremors are the classic sign for hypocalcemia. Diabetic mothers tend to have decreased serum magnesium levels at term. This could cause secondary hypoparathyroidism in the infant. Body temperature, bilirubin level, and oxygen saturation do not present with tremors in the newborn.
Assessment
Health Promotion and Maintenance
Analysis
Learning Objective 32.3

32.3 The nurse is working with a new graduate. Which of the following actions by the graduate nurse indicates an understanding of how to support development of a preterm newborn in a NICU? (Select all that apply.)
1. Schedule care throughout the day.
2. Silence alarms quickly.
3. Place a blanket over the top portion of the incubator.
4. Avoid use of a pacifier.
5. Dim the lights.

Answer: 2, 3, 5
Rationale: Silencing alarms quickly, placing a blanket over the top portion of the incubator, and dimming the lights are supportive interventions that can support development of a preterm newborn. Care should be clustered to minimize the number of times the newborn is disturbed. Pacifiers should be offered, because they provide opportunities for development of sucking. Kangaroo care, where the infant is cradled skin-to-skin against the parent's chest, facilitates growth and development.
Evaluation
Health Promotion and Maintenance
Analysis
Learning Objective 32.2

32.4 A 38-week newborn is found to be small for gestational age (SGA). Which of the following nursing interventions should be included in the care of this newborn?
1. Monitor for feeding difficulties.
2. Assess for facial paralysis.
3. Monitor for signs of hyperglycemia.
4. Maintain a warm environment.

Answer: 4
Rationale: Hypothermia is a common complication of the small-for-gestational age (SGA) newborn; therefore, the newborn's environment must remain warm to decrease heat loss. LGA newborns are more likely to have feeding difficulties, and are prone to birth trauma resulting in facial paralysis. SGA newborns are more prone to hypoglycemia.
Implementations
Health Promotion and Maintenance
Analysis
Learning Objective 32.2

32.5 A nurse is caring for a newborn born ten minutes ago to a diabetic mother. Which of the following should be included in the nurse's plan of care for this newborn?
1. Teach the parents exceptionally good skin care.
2. Obtain blood glucose levels hourly.
3. Evaluate bilirubin levels frequently.
4. Assess for hypothermia.

Answer: 2
Rationale: Blood glucose levels should be checked hourly during the first four hours and then at four-hour intervals until stable normal levels are attained. Hypothermia is more common in SGA newborns due to diminished subcutaneous fat. Infants of diabetic mothers tend to have macrosomia. There is no need to provide exceptionally good skin care. Hyperbilirubinemia is not more common among infants of diabetic mothers.
Planning
Health Promotion and Maintenance
Application
Learning Objective 32.3

32.6 Interventions provided by the nurse caring for a postterm newborn can include 1. provision of warmth. 2. frequent monitoring of blood pressure. 3. observation of respiratory status. 4. restriction of breastfeeding.	Answer: 3 Rationale: Provision of warmth, frequent monitoring of blood glucose, and observation of respiratory status are important interventions for post-term newborns. These interventions can help prevent common complications such as hypoglycemia, cold stress, and hypoxia. Weight measurements twice daily are not required, nor are pain medications. Breastfeeding is encouraged. Implementation Health Promotion and Maintenance Analysis Learning Objective 32.4
32.7 A mother of a premature newborn questions why a gavage-feeding catheter is placed in the mouth of the newborn, and not in the nose. What is the nurse's best response? 1. "Most newborns are nose breathers." 2. "The tube will elicit the sucking reflex." 3. "A smaller catheter is preferred for feedings." 4. "Most newborns are mouth breathers."	Answer: 1 Rationale: Most newborns are nose breathers; therefore, an orogastric catheter is preferable. A small catheter is used for a nasogastric tube to minimize airway obstruction. Gavage feedings are used when newborns have a poorly-coordinated suck and swallow reflex, or are ill. Implementation Health Promotion and Maintenance Application Learning Objective 32.5
32.8 In caring for the premature newborn, the nurse must assess hydration status continually. Assessment parameters should include (Select all that apply.) 1. volume of urine output. 2. weight. 3. blood pH. 4. head circumference. 5. bowel sounds.	Answer: 1, 2 Rationale: In order to assess hydration status, volume of urine output, weight, and stools must be evaluated. Blood pH, head circumference, and bowel sounds are not indicators of hydration. Assessment Health Promotion and Maintenance Application Learning Objective 32.5
32.9 The nurse is planning appropriate care for the preterm newborn. Which nursing diagnosis has the highest priority? 1. risk for impaired elimination 2. risk for ineffective airway clearance 3. impaired oxygenation 4. enhanced family coping	Answer: 3 Rationale: Oxygenation is an issue with preterm infants secondary to lung immaturity, and has the highest priority. Impaired elimination may develop if necrotizing fascitis develops. Ineffective airway clearance can also be an issue for preterm infants due to weak respiratory muscles. Family coping is a psychosocial need, and is therefore a lower priority than physiologic needs. Diagnosis Health Promotion and Maintenance Application Learning Objective 32.6
32.10 The nurse manager is working with a newborn with fetal alcohol syndrome (FAS). What should the nurse manager consider when planning this infant's care? 1. Allow extra time for feedings. 2. Assign different personnel to the newborn each day. 3. Place the newborn in a well-lit room. 4. Monitor for hyperthermia.	Answer: 1 Rationale: Newborns with fetal alcohol syndrome have feeding problems. Therefore, extra time and patience are needed for feeding. Provide consistency of staff when working with the newborn, and keep environmental stimuli to a minimum. Newborns with fetal alcohol sy`mia. Planning Health Promotion and Maintenance Analysis Learning Objective 32.7
32.11 The nurse is creating a plan for teaching the parents of an infant with phenylketonuria (PKU) how to care for the infant at home. The nurse should include information about:	Answer: 1 Rationale: Teaching should include information about special diets that limit intake of phenylalanine. Special formulas low in phenylalanine include Lofenalac, Minafen, and Albumaid XP. Cataracts are associated with infants who have galactosemia. The infant with phenylketonuria (PKU) exhibits signs of central

1. special formulas for the infant. 2. cataract problems. 3. respiratory problems. 4. administration of thyroid medication.	nervous system damage if treatment is not started by one month of age, not respiratory problems. Thyroid medication is given to infants with congenital hypothyroidism. Planning Health Promotion and Maintenance Application Learning Objective 32.7
32.12 The nurse is caring for a newborn who was born to a narcotic addicted mother. At the age of 24 hours, which expected assessment findings should the nurse consider when planning care for this newborn? 1. lethargy 2. decreased muscle tone 3. exaggerated reflexes 4. decreased oral secretions	Answer: 3 Rationale: Newborns born to narcotic addicted mothers will begin to exhibit symptoms of withdrawal after 24 hours. Withdrawal symptoms include hyperirritability, exaggerated reflexes, and excessive oral secretions. Decreased muscle tone and lethargy would be seen in infants experiencing drug or alcohol toxicity. Planning Health Promotion and Maintenance Application Learning Objective 32.8
32.13 During discharge planning of a drug-dependent newborn, the nurse explains to the mother that daily care for the infant should include 1. placing the newborn in a prone position. 2. limiting feedings to three a day to decrease diarrhea. 3. continuous operation of a home apnea monitoring system. 4. weaning the newborn off the pacifier.	Answer: 3 Rationale: Drug-dependent newborns are at a higher risk for sudden infant death syndrome (SIDS). Therefore, the newborn should sleep in a supine position, and a home apnea monitoring system should be implemented. Small, frequent feedings are recommended. A pacifier may be offered to provide non-nutritive sucking. Implementation Health Promotion and Maintenance Application Learning Objective 32.8
32.14 A newborn was born to an HIV-positive mother two days ago. The infant will be placed in foster care. The nurse is planning discharge teaching for the foster parents about how to care for the newborn at home. Which of the following instructions should the nurse include? 1. Provide three feedings per day. 2. Place soiled diapers in a sealed plastic bag. 3. Rectal temperatures are preferred. 4. Put the infant in sunlight through a window.	Answer: 2 Rationale: The nurse should instruct the parents about proper handwashing techniques, proper disposal of soiled diapers, and to wear gloves when diapering. Small, frequent feedings are recommended about every two to three hours. Taking rectal temperatures should be avoided, because it may stimulate diarrhea. Placing an infant in the sun through a window is recommended for jaundice, not HIV exposure. Planning Health Promotion and Maintenance Application Learning Objective 32.9
32.15 An infant was born prematurely at 25 weeks' gestation. Due to lung immaturity, the baby has been exposed to prolonged oxygen therapy. The nurse should explain to the parents that their infant is at a higher risk for what condition due to the oxygen therapy? 1. visual impairment 2. hypocalcemia 3. cerebral palsy 4. sensitive gag reflex	Answer: 1 Rationale: Premature infants are at greater risk for developing complications related to prolonged oxygen therapy, such as retinopathy, which can lead to visual impairment. Hypocalcemia is more common in premature infants, as is an absent or decreased gag reflex. Cerebral palsy may be due to decreased oxygen. Assessment Health Promotion and Maintenance Application Learning Objective 32.5

33.1 During newborn resuscitation, effectiveness of bag and mask ventilations can be determined by
1. the rise and fall of the chest.
2. amount of air in bag.
3. placement of hands over newborn's chest.
4. the newborn's heart rate.

Answer: 1
Rationale: With proper resuscitation, effectiveness is observed by visualizing the rise and fall of the chest. Depending upon the type of bag used, total inflation may not occur. This is not an effective sign. Nothing should obscure the view of the newborn's chest while resuscitation is being performed. The newborn's heart rate will only be monitored for effectiveness after breathing has been established.
Evaluation
Health Promotion and Maintenance
Application
Learning Objective 33.1

33.2 A nurse explains to new parents that their newborn has developed respiratory distress syndrome (RDS). The nurse bases this assessment on which of the following data? (Select all that apply.)
1. grunting respirations
2. nasal flaring
3. respiratory rate of 40 during sleep
4. chest retractions
5. temperature 101.0°F

Answer: 1, 2, 4
Rationale: Grunting with respirations, nasal flaring, and chest retractions are characteristics of respiratory distress syndrome (RDS). A respiratory rate of 40 during sleep is normal, as is a heart rate of 110. A fever does not indicate RDS.
Assessment
Health Promotion and Maintenance
Application
Learning Objective 33.2

33.3 A woman in labor is found to have meconium-stained amniotic fluid upon rupture of her membranes. At delivery, the nurse anticipates that the priority nursing intervention is to
1. deliver the neonate on its side with head up, to facilitate drainage of secretions.
2. suction the oropharynx when the head has delivered.
3. prepare for the immediate use of positive pressure to expand the lungs.
4. monitor the woman's temperature.

Answer: 2
Rationale: After the birth of the head, while the shoulders and chest are still in the birth canal, the newborn's oropharynx is suctioned by the birth attendant. If the oropharynx is not adequately suctioned with the head on the perineum, respiratory or resuscitative efforts will push meconium into the airway and into the lungs. Stimulation of the newborn should be avoided to minimize respiratory movements that will pull meconium deeper into the airways. Use of high-pressure ventilation may be required later if the infant develops meconium aspiration syndrome. The newborn is at risk, not the mother, so monitoring maternal temperature is not the priority.
Planning
Health Promotion and Maintenance
Analysis
Learning Objective 33.2

33.4 Which of the following assessment findings by the nurse would require obtaining a blood glucose level on the newborn?
1. jitteriness of the newborn
2. newborn sucking on fingers
3. lusty cry
4. rectal temperature of 98.8°F

Answer: 1
Rationale: Jitteriness of the newborn is associated with hypoglycemia, and would require close monitoring of blood glucose levels. A rectal temperature of 98.8°F is normal. Newborn sucking on fingers, holding the body in a flexed posture, a lusty cry, and the presence of vernix in body creases are normal newborn findings; therefore, there is no need to obtain blood glucose levels with these findings.
Assessment
Health Promotion and Maintenance
Application
Learning Objective 33.3

33.5 The visiting nurse evaluates a three-day-old breastfed newborn at home, and notes that the baby appears jaundiced. When explaining jaundice to the parents, the nurse should tell them
1. "Jaundice is nothing to worry about."
2. "Some newborns require phototherapy."
3. "Jaundice is a medical emergency."
4. "Jaundice is always a sign of liver disease."

Answer: 2
Rationale: Physiologic jaundice is a normal process that may occur after 24 hours of life in about half of healthy newborns. Physiologic jaundice may require phototherapy. It is not a sign of liver disease nor is it a medical emergency.
Implementation
Health Promotion and Maintenance
Application
Learning Objective 33.4

33.6 The nurse is preparing an educational in-service presentation about jaundice in the newborn. What content should the nurse include in this presentation? (Select all that apply.)
1. Physiologic jaundice occurs after 24 hours of age.
2. Pathologic jaundice occurs after 24 hours of age.
3. Phototherapy is required when bilirubin levels exceed 14.
4. The need for phototherapy depends on the bilirubin level and age of the infant.
5. Kernicterus causes irreversible neurological damage.

Answer: 1, 4, 5
Rationale: Jaundice that occurs after 24 hours is physiologic, while jaundice that appears within 24 hours is pathologic. Phototherapy need is determined by the bilirubin level and age of the infant. Kernicterus is the build-up of bilirubin in the gray matter cells of the brain, and causes irreversible neurological damage. Exchange transfusions may be undertaken when the bilirubin level exceeds 20.
Planning
Health Promotion and Maintenance
Analysis
Learning Objective 33.4

33.7 The nurse assesses a 12-hour-old newborn's serum bilirubin level, and finds it to be 14 mg/dL. What nursing intervention would be included in the plan of care for this newborn?
1. Continue to observe.
2. Begin phototherapy.
3. Begin blood exchange transfusion.
4. Stop breastfeeding.

Answer: 2
Rationale: Jaundice within 24 hours of birth is due either to Rh incompatibility or ABO incompatibility, and requires phototherapy. Continued observation is only appropriate with normal findings. Newborns with a bilirubin of 20 mg/dL or above might need an exchange transfusion. Newborns under phototherapy should continue to breastfeed.
Planning
Health Promotion and Maintenance
Analysis
Learning Objective 33.5

33.8 The nurse is evaluating the effectiveness of phototherapy on a newborn. Which of the following evaluations indicates a therapeutic response to phototherapy?
1. The newborn maintains a normal temperature.
2. bilirubin level of 14 mg/dL
3. decreased reflexes
4. skin blanches less yellow

Answer: 4
Rationale: Expected outcomes of phototherapy include bilirubin levels less than 6 mg/dL, normal reflexes, and skin that does not appear yellow. A normal temperature reading is not related to phototherapy.
Evaluation
Health Promotion and Maintenance
Analysis
Learning Objective 33.6

33.9 The nurse assesses that a newborn's skin has a ruddy appearance and the peripheral pulses are decreased. The nurse suspects polycythemia. Which of the following findings might support the presence of polycythemia?
1. venous hematocrit of 70%
2. venous hemoglobin level less than 12 g/dL
3. blood glucose level of 64 mg/dL
4. history of prolonged rupture of membranes

Answer: 1
Rationale: A venous hematocrit level of 70% indicates polycythemia. A venous hemoglobin level less than 12 g/dL indicates anemia. Blood glucose of 64 is within the normal range. A history of ruptured membranes is not a risk factor for developing polycythemia.
Assessment
Health Promotion and Maintenance
Application
Learning Objective 33.7

33.10 Antibiotics have been ordered for a newborn with an infection. Which of the following interventions should the nurse prepare to implement? (Select all that apply.)
1. Obtain sterile urine specimen for culture.
2. Restrict parental visits.
3. Evaluate bilirubin levels.

Answer: 1, 3, 4
Rationale: The assessments the nurse will undertake for an infant with sepsis include: sterile urinary catheterization for culture, evaluate bilirubin levels, and administer oxygen as ordered. The nurse will encourage parents to visit. Hypoglycemia, not hyperglycemia is not seen in sepsis.
Implementation
Health Promotion and Maintenance
Analysis
Learning Objective 33.8

4. Administer oxygen as ordered.
5. Observe for signs of hyperglycemia.

33.11 The newborn of a mother who is suffering a primary infection of genital herpes simplex has vaginally delivered a full-term infant. During the initial newborn assessment, the nurse notices that the infant has small clusters of vesicular lesions over most of the body. The mother of the infant asks what the presence of the lesions indicates. Which statement by the nurse is best? "The lesions

1. may be a sign that your baby has disseminated herpes."
2. might lead to the baby becoming jaundiced."
3. are not related to the herpes infection that you have."
4. indicate that your baby will have neurologic abnormalities."

Answer: 1
Rationale: The presence of small clusters of vesicular lesions over most of the body in a newborn whose mother delivered with active herpes lesions indicates that the baby also has a herpes infection, which can become a disseminated infection. Jaundice may develop from the hepatic involvement of disseminated herpes, but is no evidence is given that the infant is presently jaundiced. Neurologic abnormalities occur in some (but not all) infants with disseminated herpes infection.
Implementation
Health Promotion and Maintenance
Analysis
Learning Objective 33.9

33.12 The nurse is planning care for four infants who were born this shift. Which infant will require the most detailed assessment? An infant whose mother

1. has a history of obsessive-compulsive disorder (OCD).
2. has chlamydia.
3. has six other children.
4. has a urinary tract infection (UTI).

Answer: 2
Rationale: Infants born to mothers with chlamydia infections are at risk for neonatal pneumonia and conjunctivitis, thus require close observation of the respiratory status and eyes. Obsessive-compulsive disorder (OCD) is not a risk for the infant, nor is the presence of multiple siblings. An infant whose mother has an active untreated urinary tract infection (UTI) may have been exposed to pathogens, but it is not known if the mother is on antibiotics or not. Assuming that the mother is not on antibiotics is reading into the question.
Planning
Health Promotion and Maintenance
Analysis
Learning Objective 33.9

33.13 The parents of a preterm newborn desire to visit their baby in the neonatal intensive care unit (NICU). Which of the following statements by the nurse will support the parents as they visit their newborn?

1. "Stroking the newborn will help with stimulation."
2. "Visits must be scheduled between feedings."
3. "The baby's grandparents should not visit."
4. "Talking could startle the baby."

Answer: 1
Rationale: Statements that encourage the parents to touch and stroke the newborn will help parents become more familiar and bond with their preterm newborn. Comments that personalize the baby will tell the parents their baby is unique and special. The nurse always should encourage parents to visit and get to know their newborn, even in the neonatal intensive care unit (NICU). Talking quietly to the infant can be reassuring to both the infant and the parents. Visits do not need to be between feedings. Discouraging involvement of the grandparents does not support the parents.
Implementation
Health Promotion and Maintenance
Application
Learning Objective 33.10

33.14 The parents of an infant born at 27 weeks are at the bedside of the baby. The neonatal intensive care unit (NICU) nurse is performing an assessment of the newborn's respiratory status. The mother says, "Stop it! You're hurting our baby! You pressed so hard on the stethoscope that you left marks on his skin!" The nurse understands

1. the mother does not know how to use a stethoscope.

Answer: 2
Rationale: Parents with sick babies who require neonatal intensive care unit (NICU) admission experience anger, and often direct the anger at the nurses and physicians rather than at the infant. Although the mother may not know that using a stethoscope frequently leaves ring-shaped marks on the skin, that is not the best answer. Denial would manifest as not believing the nurses or doctors.
Assessment
Health Promotion and Maintenance
Analysis
Learning Objective 33.11

2. is experiencing anger and is directing the anger at the nurse.
3. is in denial of her infant's unstable condition.
4. is probably overly tired and therefore irritable.

33.15 The nurse is caring for a newborn with jaundice. The parents question why the newborn is not under the phototherapy lights. The nurse explains that the fiber optic blanket is beneficial because (Select all that apply.)
1. the lights can be turned off intermittently.
2. the eyes do not need to be covered.
3. the lights will need to be removed for feedings.
4. newborns do not get overheated.
5. weight loss is not a complication of this system.

Answer: 2, 4, 5
Rationale: Benefits of the fiber optic blanket are that newborns do not get overheated, the eyes do not have to be covered, and the lights can stay on during feedings. In addition to these benefits, weight loss is not a complication of the fiber optic blanket system. It is not appropriate to use phototherapy intermittently.
Implementation
Health Promotion and Maintenance
Application
Learning Objective 33.6

CHAPTER 34

34.1 The nurse is caring for a client who delivered yesterday. The nurse understands that the best method to assess the healing of the uterus at the placental site is by assessing
1. hemoglobin and hematocrit lab values.
2. blood pressure and pulse rate.
3. presence or absence of orthostatic hypotension.
4. type, amount, and consistency of lochia.

Answer: 4
Rationale: The type, amount, and consistency of lochia determines the stage of healing of the placenta site, which occurs by a process of exfoliation. Hemoglobin and hematocrit values will only detect excessive blood loss after it has occurred. Blood pressure varies slightly in the normal postpartal woman. Like hemoglobin and hematocrit, blood pressure only changes after significant amounts of blood have been lost, which is more likely related to involution than the placental site. Orthostatic hypotension is an indicator of hypovolemia, not of placental site healing.
Implementation
Health Promotion and Maintenance
Application
Learning Objective 34.1

34.2 The nurse weighs a postpartum client. The client expresses dismay that she has only lost ten pounds. What is the best response by the nurse?
1. "Ten to 12 pounds is the usual initial weight loss after delivery."
2. "Most people lose more weight than you have."
3. "Most people lose less than ten pounds."
4. "You seem to be obsessed with your weight."

Answer: 1
Rationale: Ten to 12 pounds is the usual initial weight loss. This weight is lost with the birth of the infant and the expulsion of the placenta and the amniotic fluid. It is not therapeutic to tell a client they are obsessed with their weight, even if the nurse suspects a body image disturbance. It is also not therapeutic to say that most people lose more weight.
Implementation
Health Promotion and Maintenance
Analysis
Learning Objective 34.1

34.3 The nurse assesses the postpartum client, and finds that she has inflamed hemorrhoids on the day of birth. Which of the following nursing interventions would be appropriate?
1. Encourage warm baths.
2. Position the client in the supine position.
3. Avoid stool softeners.
4. Decrease fluid intake.

Answer: 1
Rationale: Encouraging warm baths is the correct approach because moist heat decreases inflammation and provides for comfort. Positioning the client in a supine position would just increase the pressure on the hemorrhoids. Avoiding stool softeners would put the client at risk for constipation and increase the likelihood of increased inflammation. Decreasing fluid intake also would put the client at risk for constipation.
Implementation
Health Promotion and Maintenance
Application
Learning Objective 34.1

34.4 On the first postpartum day, the nurse teaches the client about breastfeeding. Two hours later, the mother seems to remember very little of the teaching. The nurse understands that this memory lapse is due to
1. the taking-hold phase.
2. postpartum hemorrhage.
3. the taking-in phase.
4. epidural analgesia.

Answer: 3
Rationale: The taking-in phase, which occurs during the first day or two following birth, is characterized by a passive and dependent affect. The mother also might be in need of rest, and often will not remember teaching. The taking-hold phase occurs by the second or third day, when the mother is ready to resume control of life and is open to teaching. Postpartum hemorrhage is a serious complication, and will need medical intervention. Epidural analgesia does not affect memory.
Assessment
Psychosocial Integrity
Application
Learning Objective 34.2

34.5 The nurse is preparing a prenatal class session about maternal role attainment. Which statement should the nurse include?
1. The formal stage occurs after delivery when the mother looks to her own mother and other role models.
2. The informal stage is reached when the mother develops her own personal style of mothering that works for her.
3. The anticipatory stage begins when the child is about two years of age, when the mother is looking inward.
4. The personal stage is characterized by trying to act as the mother believes others expect her to act.

Answer: 2
Rationale: The informal stage is reached when the mother develops her own personal style of mothering that works for her. The anticipatory stage occurs during pregnancy, and is characterized by looking to role models, especially one's own mother. The personal stage is when the mother is comfortable with herself in the role of "mother."
The formal stage begins when the child is born, and is characterized by trying to act as the mother believes others expect her to act.
Planning
Psychosocial Integrity
Application
Learning Objective 34.2

34.6 The community nurse is working with a client from Asia who has delivered her first child. Her mother has come to live with the family for several months. The nurse understands that the main role of the grandmother while visiting is to
1. do the cooking and cleaning so the new mother can feed the baby and rest.
2. teach her son-in-law the right way to be a father since this is his first child.
3. make sure that her daughter does not become abusive toward the infant.
4. pass on the cultural values and beliefs to the newborn grandchild.

Answer: 1
Rationale: It is common in Asian and African families who have childbearing families in the United States and extended family abroad to have the mother of the wife come and live with the new family in the United States for several months. The main role of the grandmother is to facilitate adaptation to the mothering role by freeing the mother from the demands of cooking, cleaning, laundry, and the like. Often, cultural beliefs include specific foods that should be eaten or avoided during the first month postpartum. The new father may be taught some skills either directly or indirectly through observation, but this is not the most important role of the grandmother. The new grandmother does not presume that her daughter will be abusive toward the infant. An infant is too young to be taught values and beliefs.
Assessment
Health Promotion and Maintenance
Analysis
Learning Objective 34.3

34.7 The nurse is caring for a postpartum client who delivered two hours ago. The nurse determines the client's fundus to be boggy. The first step that the nurse should take to
1. document the findings.
2. catheterize the client.
3. massage the fundus gently.
4. call the physician immediately.

Answer: 3
Rationale: The appropriate intervention is to massage the fundus gently to prevent postpartum hemorrhage. Documentation of findings would come after the reassessment and evaluation. Catheterizing the client may be indicated if assessment reveals a full bladder and inability to void, but not as an initial intervention. Calling the physician immediately is not necessary until more data are obtained.
Implementation
Health Promotion and Maintenance
Application
Learning Objective 34.4

34.8 Which of the following behaviors noted in the postpartum client would require the nurse to assess further?
1. Responds hesitantly to infant cries.
2. Expresses satisfaction about the sex of the baby.
3. Numerous friends visit the client and give advice.
4. Talks to and cuddles with the infant frequently.

Answer: 1
Rationale: Responding hesitantly to infant cries might need further assessment to determine what the mother is feeling. She might not know what to do, and needs assistance to guide her. Expressing satisfaction about the sex of the baby is usually a positive sign. Numerous friends who visit the client and give advice can provide a strong support system for her, and assessment can be done on her reactions to the advice. Talking to and cuddling with the infant frequently is a behavior that facilitates attachment.
Assessment
Psychosocial Integrity
Application
Learning Objective 34.6

34.9 The nurse is caring for a postpartal client who is experiencing afterpains following the birth of her third child. Which of the following comfort measures should the nurse implement to decrease the client's pain? (Select all that apply.)
1. Offer warm blankets for her abdomen.
2. Call the physician to report this finding.
3. Inform her that this is not normal, and she will need an oxytocic agent.
4. Massage the fundus of the uterus gently and observe lochia for clots.
5. Administer a nonsteroidal anti-inflammatory drug (NSAID).

Answer: 1, 4, 5
Rationale: The nurse should offer comfort measures that address the discomfort of afterpains; warm blankets and NSAIDs will decrease pain. Massaging out any clots present will decrease the afterpains, which will often increase if the bladder is full, therefore the client should be reminded to void every one to two hours. It is not necessary to call the physician. This is a normal finding, and the client does not need an oxytocic agent.
Implementation
Health Promotion and Maintenance
Analysis
Learning Objective 34.4

34.10 The community nurse is working with a client whose only child is eight months old. Which statement does the nurse expect the mother to make?
1. "I have a lot more time to myself than I thought I would have."
2. "My confidence level in my parenting is higher than I anticipated."
3. "I am constantly tired. I feel like I could sleep for a week."
4. "My baby likes everyone, and never fusses when she's held by a stranger."

Answer: 3
Rationale: Fatigue is a common issue with new mothers due to the demands of nighttime care. Most women have difficulty finding time for themselves. Feelings of incompetence at parenting are also common. At eight months, infants develop stranger anxiety, and will cry when held by people other than the parents.
Assessment
Health Promotion and Maintenance
Analysis
Learning Objective 34.5

34.11 The nurse assesses the postpartum client who has not had a bowel movement by the third postpartum day. Which of the following nursing interventions would be appropriate?
1. Encourage patience; it will happen soon.
2. Instruct the client to eat a low-fiber diet.
3. Encourage the client to decrease her fluid intake.
4. Obtain an order for a stool softener.

Answer: 4
Rationale: Obtaining an order for a stool softener is the correct intervention if no bowel movement has occurred by the third day. The client may fear having a bowel movement due to perineal soreness, and stool softeners would increase bulk and moisture in the fecal material, allowing for more comfortable evacuation. Encouraging patience; it will happen soon does not address the client's needs, and could increase the chance for constipation. Eating a low-fiber diet would not increase bulk or moisture in the stool. Decreasing fluid intake would decrease moisture in the fecal material, and worsen constipation.
Implementation
Health Promotion and Maintenance
Application
Learning Objective 34.5

34.12 Every time the nurse enters the room of a postpartum client who gave birth three hours ago, the client asks

Answer: 2
Rationale: Review documentation of the birth experience and discuss it with her so that the client can integrate the experience. Three hours after birth, the mother needs to talk about her perceptions of her labor and delivery. Answering

something else about her birth experience. The nurse should

1. answer questions quickly and try to divert her attention to other subjects.
2. review documentation of the birth experience and discuss it with her.
3. contact the physician to warn him that the client might want to file a lawsuit due to her preoccupation with her birth experience.
4. submit a referral to social services because you are concerned about obsessive behavior.

questions quickly and trying to divert her attention to other subjects trivializes her questions and does not allow her to sort out the reality from her fantasized experience. Contacting the physician to warn him that the client might want to file a lawsuit is an incorrect action. Preoccupation with the birth experience is normal behavior. Submitting a referral to social services because you are concerned about obsessive behavior is an incorrect action, because this behavior is normal.
Implementation
Health Promotion and Maintenance
Analysis
Learning Objective 34.5

34.13 The community nurse is meeting a new mother for the first time. The client delivered her first child five days ago after a 12-hour labor. Neither the mother nor the infant had any complications during the birth or postpartum period. Which statement from the client would indicate to the nurse that the client is experiencing postpartum blues?

1. "I am so happy and blessed to have my new baby."
2. "One minute I'm laughing and the next I'm crying."
3. "My husband is helping out by changing the baby at night."
4. "Breastfeeding is going quite well now that the engorgement is gone."

Answer: 2
Rationale: Postpartum blues is a transient period of mild depressive symptoms that is self-limiting within about two weeks. Manifestations include mood swings, anger, weepiness, lack of appetite, feeling let down, and difficulty sleeping. Feeling happy is not a symptom of postpartum blues, nor is successful lactation. The husband's assistance does not relate to postpartum blues.
Assessment
Health Promotion and Maintenance
Analysis
Learning Objective 34.4

34.14 The nurse is preparing a class for mothers and their partners who have just recently delivered. One topic of the class is infant attachment. Which statement indicates that the class participants understand this concept? (Select all that apply.)

1. "We should avoid holding the baby too much."
2. "Looking directly into the baby's eyes might frighten him."
3. "Talking to the baby is good because he'll recognize our voices."
4. "Holding the baby so we have direct face to face contact is good."
5. "We should expect the baby to smile when we talk to him."

Answer: 3, 4
Rationale: Attachment behaviors include holding the baby in the en face position, making eye contact, holding the infant with the whole arm (not just the hands), and talking to the baby (especially in a high-pitched voice). Smiling as a response will not develop until the child is about three months old.
Evaluation
Health Promotion and Maintenance
Application
Learning Objective 34.6

34.15 The nurse is providing discharge teaching to a woman who has delivered her first child two days ago. The nurse understands that additional information is needed if the client makes which statement? (Select all that apply.)

1. "I should expect a lighter flow next week."
2. "The flow will increase if I am too active."

Answer: 3
Rationale: Lochia should gradually diminish in amount and change to a lighter brownish or pinkish color. This will lead to a noticeably lighter flow a week after delivery compared to the lochia on the second postpartum day. By the second postpartum day, the lochia should no longer be bright red. Too much activity will often lead to an increase in the amount and a more red lochia. By the end of the three to six weeks that lochia is shed, the amount is very small and requires only a pantiliner for protection. The amount of lochia on the third postpartum day will require a sanitary pad.
Evaluation

---

3. "My bleeding will remain red for about a month." 4. "I will be able to use a pantiliner by tomorrow."	Health Promotion and Maintenance Analysis Learning Objective 34.1

CHAPTER 35

35.1 The postpartum nurse is planning discharge teaching of the postpartal client. Which of the following adult learning principles should the nurse include to most actively involve the client during teaching? 1. demonstration of skills 2. classroom lectures and one-on-one teaching 3. use of television and videos 4. sensory involvement and active participation	Answer: 4 Rationale: Sensory involvement and active participation are two of the keys in adult learning, because they actively involve the clients in the learning. Demonstration of skills is done by the nurse, and classroom lectures, one-on-one teaching, and use of television and videos—while helpful when used as part of the teaching plan—do not actively involve the client in learning. Planning Health Promotion and Maintenance Application Learning Objective 35.1
35.2 Which of the following statements by the nursing student would require further teaching concerning rubella vaccine? 1. "Clients should be assessed for allergies to eggs." 2. "Breastfeeding mothers should not receive the vaccine." 3. "Clients should avoid pregnancy for three months following vaccination." 4. "Some clients develop a slight rash after vaccination."	Answer: 2 Rationale: The nursing student needs to review the purpose of rubella vaccine, which is to increase the immunity in the mother. It does not affect either breastfeeding or the infant. Exposure to rubella in a nonimmune mother who is in her first trimester can result in multiple congenital defects and fetal death. Assessing clients for allergies to eggs, instructing clients to avoid pregnancy for three months following vaccination, and instructing clients that they may develop a slight rash after vaccination are teaching points when administering rubella vaccine. Evaluation Health Promotion and Maintenance Analysis Learning Objective 35.1
35.3 On the second day postpartum, the client experiences engorgement. To relieve her discomfort, the nurse should encourage the client to 1. remove her bra. 2. apply heat to the breasts. 3. apply ice packs to the breasts. 4. limit breastfeeding to twice per day	Answer: 3 Rationale: Applying ice packs to the breasts relieves discomfort through the numbing effect of ice. Removing her bra and applying heat will only increase breast milk. Limiting breastfeeding to twice per day would eventually decrease the flow of breast milk and would not serve to decrease the mother's discomfort. Implementation Health Promotion and Maintenance Application Learning Objective 35.2
35.4 The client who delivered two hours ago tells the nurse that she is exhausted but feels guilty because her friends told her how euphoric they were after giving birth. How should the nurse respond to the client? 1. "Everyone is different and both responses are normal." 2. "Most mothers do feel euphoria; I don't know why you don't." 3. "It's good for me to know that because it might indicate a problem." 4. "Let me bring your baby to the nursery so that you can rest."	Answer: 1 Rationale: Both euphoria and exhaustion are normal feelings after birth. The nurse should not imply that a mother's emotional response is not expected. Fatigue after birth is not indicative of a problem. The client may want to be with her newborn, and the nurse should not encourage unnecessary separation of mother and child. Implementation Health Promotion and Maintenance Analysis Learning Objective 35.3
35.5 The nurse is preparing to discharge a postpartum client. Which	Answer: 2 Rationale: Fatigue in the first weeks at home after delivery is common, and napping is an appropriate response to the fatigue. Long walks will increase the

statement should the nurse include in the discharge teaching?

1. "You may want to take a long walk each day to get your energy back."
2. "Many new mothers need to nap once or twice a day during the first weeks."
3. "If you become too fatigued, you should switch from breastfeeding to formula."
4. "Exhaustion indicates that your nutritional intake is not adequate."

exhaustion. Although breastfeeding does require energy expenditure, breastfeeding should be encouraged for the health of the infant. Early postpartal exhaustion is not an indicator of poor nutritional intake.
Implementation
Health Promotion and Maintenance
Analysis
Learning Objective 35.3

35.6 The breastfeeding client asks the nurse about appropriate contraception methods while lactating. What is the best answer for the nurse to give?

1. "Most breastfeeding mothers do not resume sexual activity."
2. "Intrauterine devices (IUDs) are easy to use and easy to insert prior to sexual intercourse."
3. "Breastfeeding hampers ovulation, but to be safe, use condoms."
4. "Breastfeeding prevents ovulation, so no contraception is needed."

Answer: 3
Rationale: Breastfeeding increases the hormone prolactin, which decreases the release of the hormonal feedback system that induces ovulation. However, breastfeeding does not completely prevent ovulation, and a barrier method such as condoms should be used. Stating that intrauterine devices (IUDs) are easy to use and easy to insert prior to sexual intercourse is incorrect, because IUDs can only be placed by a healthcare provider in a clinic situation. It is untrue that breastfeeding mothers do not resume sexual activity. The possible effect of breastfeeding on intercourse is that some women experience vaginal dryness, and some leak milk during orgasm.
Implementation
Health Promotion and Maintenance
Application
Learning Objective 35.4

35.7 The new grandmother comments that, when her children were born, they stayed in the nursery. The grandmother asks the nurse why her daughter's baby stays mostly in the room instead of the nursery. How should the nurse respond?

1. "Babies like to be with their mothers more than being in the nursery."
2. "Contact between parents and babies increases attachment."
3. "Budget cuts have decreased the number of nurses in the nursery."
4. "Why do you ask? Do you have concerns about your daughter's parenting?"

Answer: 2
Rationale: Contact between parents and their newborns facilitates attachment. Although most newborns cry less when held than when in their cribs, this is not the most important reason for encouraging mothers to spend time with their babies. Budget cuts are not a reason for babies being in the nursery less than in the past. It is not therapeutic to use the word "why." The grandmother has not indicated that she has any concerns about her daughter's parenting.
Implementation
Health Promotion and Maintenance
Application
Learning Objective 35.4

35.8 The multiparous client delivered her first child vaginally two years ago, and delivered this infant by cesarean yesterday due to breech presentation. Which statement would the nurse expect the client to make?

1. "I can't believe how much more tired I was with the first baby."
2. "The pain I'm having is significantly more than with my last birth."
3. "It is disappointing that I can't breastfeed because of the cesarean."
4. "Getting in and out of bed feels more comfortable than last time."

Answer: 2
Rationale: Cesarean birth recovery is longer and involves more pain and fatigue than a vaginal birth due to the physiologic requirements of healing. Breastfeeding is not contraindicated with cesarean birth. Getting in and out of bed is more painful after cesarean birth than after vaginal birth.
Assessment
Health Promotion and Maintenance
Application
Learning Objective 35.5

35.9 The nurse is caring for two clients: one who had a cesarean birth four hours ago, and one who delivered vaginally

Answer: 1, 3, 5
Rationale: Administering analgesics as needed; encouraging leg exercises every two hours; encouraging the client to cough and deep-breathe every two

---

four hours ago. Which of the following interventions would be appropriate for the nurse to implement for the mother who experienced a cesarean birth? (Select all that apply.)

1. Administer analgesics as needed.
2. Encourage her to ambulate to the bathroom to void.
3. Encourage leg exercises every two hours.
4. Encourage client to cough and deep-breathe every eight hours.
5. Encourage the use of breathing, relaxation, and distraction.

hours; and encouraging the use of breathing, relaxation, and distraction all address the client's nursing care needs, which are similar to those of other surgical clients. Encouraging her to ambulate to the bathroom to void might be an intervention done on the first or second day postpartum, but not in the first four hours.
Implementation
Health Promotion and Maintenance
Analysis
Learning Objective 35.5

35.10 The nurse is supervising a student nurse who is working with a 14-year-old client who delivered her first child yesterday. Which statement indicates that the nursing student needs additional information before caring for this client? "Because of her age, this client will

1. need less teaching because she will have gotten the information in school."
2. require less frequent fundal checks to assess for postpartum hemorrhage."
3. most likely need extra teaching about the terminology for her anatomy."
4. need to have her mother provide daycare and help raise the baby."

Answer: 3
Rationale: The physiologic needs of an adolescent after delivery are the same as an adult. Additional teaching is often required due to the developmental level of the client, especially about terminology, anatomy, and physiology. Although the adolescent will require daycare to continue with her education, the assistance does not have to come from the client's mother.
Evaluation
Health Promotion and Maintenance
Analysis
Learning Objective 35.6

35.11 The nurse is planning care for three newly-delivered adolescents and their babies. What should the nurse keep in mind when planning their care?

1. The baby's father should be encouraged to participate in teaching.
2. A class for all the adolescents would decrease teaching effectiveness.
3. The schools that the adolescents attend will provide teaching on bathing.
4. Adolescents understand the danger signals in newborns.

Answer: 1
Rationale: Adolescent fathers should be encouraged to participate in all educational offerings. Classes are effective for teaching groups of adolescents. The nurse should never assume that basic newborn care education will be provided to a client elsewhere. Adolescents may need more teaching than adults about the danger signals in newborns and when it is necessary to call the doctor.
Planning
Health Promotion and Maintenance
Application
Learning Objective 35.6

35.12 The nurse is caring for a client who plans to relinquish her baby for adoption. The nurse should implement which of the following approaches to care? (Select all that apply.)

1. Encourage the client to see and hold her infant.
2. Encourage the client to express her emotions.
3. Respect any special requests for the birth.

Answer: 2, 3, 4
Rationale: Encouraging the client to express emotions, respecting any special request for the birth, acknowledging the grieving process, and allowing for access to the infant at the client's requests all are aspects of providing care for the client who decides to relinquish her infant. Encouraging the client to see and hold her infant does not respect the client's right to refuse interaction, and might make her feel guilty for not wanting to see the infant. Discouraging contact between the mother's family and the infant does not respect the client's wishes.
Implementation
Health Promotion and Maintenance
Analysis
Learning Objective 35.7

---

4. Acknowledge the grieving process in the client.
5. Discourage the client from holding the infant.

35.13 The nurse assesses the postpartum client, and finds her to have moderate lochia rubra with clots. Which of the following nursing actions should the nurse undertake first?
1. Assess the fundus and bladder status.
2. Catheterize the client.
3. Administer methylergonovine maleate (Methergine) IM per order.
4. Contact the physician immediately.

Answer: 1
Rationale: Assess the fundus and bladder status first. Moderate lochia, even with clots, might be due to the client's supine position for several hours, or to other factors. Catheterizing the client may be an intervention if the bladder is full and the client is unable to void, but is not the initial intervention. It is not necessary to administer methylergonovine maleate (Methergine) IM per order or contact the physician immediately, because the situation does not warrant these interventions.
Implementation
Health Promotion and Maintenance
Analysis
Learning Objective 35.2

35.14 Which client is appropriate for an early discharge at 24 hours after delivery?
1. multipara, has had two successful breast feedings
2. primipara, bottle-feeding, has not voided since delivery
3. multipara, twins delivered at 35 weeks, bottle-feeding
4. primipara, cesarean birth performed for fetal distress

Answer: 1
Rationale: A client must be physiologically stable, and the infant must be physiologically stable to be appropriate for early discharge. Feeding successfully is one of the physiologic needs of the infant, just as voiding is a physiologic need of the mother. Preterm infants and infants who experienced distress in labor are not appropriate for early discharge.
Assessment
Health Promotion and Maintenance
Application
Learning Objective 35.8

35.15 The client that delivered twelve hours ago desires early discharge. The client is breastfeeding successfully. Which patient education point should the nurse include that is not given to clients who go home at 48 hours?
1. "Your baby requires newborn screening blood work. The doctor's office will collect the blood sample."
2. "Your baby will eat more than you expect, and feedings should be spaced out to prevent the baby getting gas."
3. "If your bleeding becomes heavier and brighter red, put your feet up and rest for a while."
4. "Your going home early means that an appointment with the lactation consultant is not possible."

Answer: 1
Rationale: Newborn metabolic screening blood work cannot be obtained until the baby has digested protein, which will not happen until the mother's milk supply is established. Feedings should be on demand; spacing out feedings will lead to an inadequate intake. Frequent feedings do not cause gas. An increase in lochia that saturates a pad in an hour or more indicates postpartum hemorrhage, which is a medical emergency that requires immediate treatment. Returning to see the lactation consultant is not prohibited by early discharge.
Implementation
Health Promotion and Maintenance
Analysis
Learning Objective 35.8

CHAPTER 36

36.1 A client and her newborn are discharged when her infant is 12 hours of age. The community nurse is making a home visit to collect a blood sample for the normal screening tests for newborns. These tests are usually completed before a newborn and mother are discharged from the hospital on the second day after delivery. What information should the nurse give the family?

Answer: 3
Rationale: The normal screening tests for newborns are done to detect disorders that cause mental retardation, physical handicaps, or death if left undiscovered. The testing will not prevent any disorders, and will not detect hypertension or diabetes.
Implementation
Health Promotion and Maintenance
Application
Learning Objective 36.6

---

1. The tests will prevent infants from developing phenylketonuria.
2. The tests will detect disorders such as hypertension and diabetes.
3. The tests will detect disorders that cause mental retardation, physical handicaps, or death if left undiscovered.
4. The tests will prevent sickle cell anemia, galactosemia, and hemocysteinuria.

36.2 The nurse should explain to new parents that their infant's position should be changed periodically during the early months of life to prevent
1. muscle contractures.
2. respiratory distress.
3. permanently flattened areas of the skull.
4. esophageal reflux.

Answer: 3
Rationale: Permanently flattened areas of the skull can occur if the infant is consistently in one position, because the skull bones are soft in the early months of life. Muscle contractures would not occur with periodic changing of the infant's position. Respiratory distress and esophageal reflux would indicate complications, and may not be affected by periodic position changes.
Implementation
Health Promotion and Maintenance
Application
Learning Objective 36.6

36.3 The nurse is meeting with a client for the first time during a home visit. The client delivered her first child three days ago. She had a normal pregnancy, and a vaginal delivery. The infant is breastfeeding. Which client statement indicates that the client needs more information about the home visit? "You are (Select all that apply.)
1. going to check my baby's weight."
2. going to watch me nurse the baby and give me tips."
3. going to teach my mother about the baby."
4. checking for safety issues when my son starts crawling."
5. going to take a blood sample from me and from my son."

Answer: 1, 2
Rationale: The components of a postpartum home visit typically include weighing the infant, asking about elimination, assessing a feeding if possible, checking for immediate safety issues (such as infant sleeping positions), assessment of the infant's color, and assessing the mother's uterine involution. The mother's weight is not usually assessed. Safety when the infant crawls should be assessed later. Not all home visits require blood draws; with no pregnancy or birth complications, there is no need to draw blood from the mother. Teaching of family members may occur, but the main purpose of the visit is to assess the infant's physiologic stability.
Evaluation
Health Promotion and Maintenance
Analysis
Learning Objective 36.2

36.4 The nurse is phoning a client to arrange a home visit of a three-day-old infant and the family. The client asks the nurse what the visit will entail, and what the nurse will be doing. What is the best answer from the nurse?
1. "I'll be coming to make sure your older children are safely adapting to the new baby."
2. "Some babies get jaundiced, so I'll assess your baby's color, feeding, and elimination."
3. "Weighing your baby is my main priority for the home care visit."
4. "I will be checking to see how you and your baby are doing overall."

Answer: 4
Rationale: The primary reason for the home visit is to verify the physiologic stability of the newborn and the mother. Neither weight nor jaundice are the only factors to be assessed. Although adaptation of the family is a part of the home visit, adaptation of the older siblings is a psychosocial issue and therefore not the most important.
Implementation
Health Promotion and Maintenance
Analysis
Learning Objective 36.3

36.5 The nurse is presenting an educational in-service presentation for new community nurses. The topic of the presentation is safety. Which of the following objects should the nurse tell the nurses is most important for safety when making home visits?
1. personal handgun
2. cellular phone
3. can of mace
4. map of the area

Answer: 2
Rationale: Cellular phones provide a means of contact; therefore, the nurse should carry a cellular phone. A map of the area should be checked before leaving for a visit, and the route traced, but this is not the most important object for a home visit. Personal handguns and mace are not permissible or legal for nurses to carry on home visits.
Planning
Health Promotion and Maintenance
Application
Learning Objective 36.4

36.6 The nurse is planning a home care visit to a mother who just recently delivered, and her baby. Their neighborhood is known to have a significant crime rate. Which of the following should the nurse do when planning this visit to facilitate personal safety?
1. Plan the visit at nighttime.
2. Wait to find the location until you arrive in the neighborhood.
3. Put personal possessions in the trunk when leaving the office.
4. Wear flashy jewelry to garner respect.

Answer: 3
Rationale: Maintaining safety during home visits should include making visits during daylight hours whenever possible, knowing the exact address and locating the home on a map prior to leaving the office, driving around the neighborhood before the visit to identify potential cues to violence, wearing a name tag and carrying identification, placing personal possessions in the trunk before arriving at the home, and avoid wearing expensive or flashy jewelry.
Planning
Health Promotion and Maintenance
Analysis
Learning Objective 36.4

36.7 Which step should the nurse include when preparing for a postpartal home visit to establish a caring relationship?
1. Ask family members how they want to be addressed.
2. Do a portion of what you say that you will do for the family, to avoid overwhelming them.
3. Speak directly to the father when asking questions.
4. Present information to the family instead of asking questions.

Answer: 1
Rationale: Establishing a caring relationship starts with introducing oneself and asking how the client/family would like to be addressed. It is important to ask questions instead of talking at the family, and allow the mother to be the spokesperson. Trust will only be built if the nurse follows through and does whatever is promised.
Implementation
Health Promotion and Maintenance
Application
Learning Objective 36.5

36.8 To prevent sudden infant death syndrome (SIDS), the nurse encourages the parents of a term infant to place the infant in what position when the infant is sleeping?
1. on the parents' waterbed
2. swaddled in the infant swing
3. on his back
4. on his stomach

Answer: 3
Rationale: The infant should be placed on his back when sleeping. Research has shown that sleeping on the back decreases the risk of sudden infant death syndrome (SIDS). Placing the infant on the parents' waterbed, on his stomach, or swaddled in the infant swing can increase the risks of SIDS.
Implementation
Health Promotion and Maintenance
Analysis
Learning Objective 36.6

36.9 The new mother hesitantly asks the nurse at the six-week postpartum visit about resumption of sexual activity. To promote comfort during sex, the nurse suggests
1. the female superior position.
2. using Vaseline for lubrication.
3. the male superior position.
4. douching before and after intercourse.

Answer: 1
Rationale: The female superior position puts the least amount of pressure against the healing perineum, and creates more control of movement for the woman. Using Vaseline for lubrication is not recommended. A water soluble lubricant, such as KY Jelly, are recommended. The male superior position creates more pressure on the perineum. Douching is never recommended.
Implementation
Health Promotion and Maintenance
Application
Learning Objective 36.7

36.10 On the third day postpartum, the client experiences engorgement. To relieve her discomfort, the nurse should encourage the client to (Select all that apply.)
1. remove her bra.
2. apply heat to the breasts.
3. apply tea leaves to the breasts.
4. take a nonsteroidal anti-inflammatory drug (NSAID).

Answer: 4
Rationale: Nonsteroidal anti-inflammatory drugs (NSAIDs) are very helpful in reducing the discomfort of engorgement. Removing her bra will not decrease engorgement. Applying ice packs to the breasts relieves discomfort through the numbing effect of ice; heat may increase milk production. Many women find that applying cabbage leaves to their breasts helps decrease engorgement; tea leaves are not used for engorgement.
Implementation
Health Promotion and Maintenance
Analysis
Learning Objective 36.8

36.11 The breastfeeding postpartum client reports sore nipples to the nurse who is making a home visit. The highest priority information that the nurse needs to collect is
1. infant positioning.
2. use of the breast shield.
3. use of breast pads.
4. type of soap used.

Answer: 1
Rationale: Infant positioning is a critical factor in nipple soreness. Changing positions alters the focus of greatest stress and promotes more complete breast emptying. Use of the breast shield and the use of breast pads are not critical factors in alleviating nipple soreness. Although the breastfeeding client should be instructed to avoid using soap on her nipples, the type of soap used is not as important to sore nipples as infant positioning.
Assessment
Health Promotion and Maintenance
Application
Learning Objective 36.8

36.12 The nurse is making an initial visit to a postpartum family's home. The mother states that she is having difficulty with breastfeeding. Which resource should the nurse tell the family about?
1. the lactation consultant at the hospital
2. free immunizations through the county public health department clinics
3. sources of free formula at a local food pantry
4. a support group for mothers who are experiencing postpartum depression

Answer: 1
Rationale: When the client specifies a problem with breastfeeding, the best resource that the nurse should inform the family about is the lactation consultant. Free immunizations do not help with breastfeeding. Providing a mother with formula undermines her breastfeeding efforts, and sends a message that she will not be successful with breastfeeding. There is no evidence that the client is experiencing postpartum depression.
Implementation
Health Promotion and Maintenance
Application
Learning Objective 36.9

36.13 The nurse is presenting a community educational presentation about the controversy regarding length of the hospital stay for postpartum clients. Which statement indicates that a participant needs additional information?
1. "Congress passed a bill in 1996 that requires insurance to pay for a 48-hour stay after an uncomplicated birth."
2. "Shortened lengths of stays were implemented by insurance companies to decrease healthcare costs."
3. "Early discharge became more popular in the 1980s as an alternative to having a home birth."
4. "With current length-of-stay laws, newborns have no problems at home and get recommended follow-up care."

Answer: 4
Rationale: Congress passed a bill in 1996 that requires insurance to pay for a 48-hour stay after an uncomplicated birth and a 96-hour stay after cesarean birth. Early discharge became more popular in the 1980s as an alternative to having a home birth. This shorter length-of-stay trend became an insurance company policy to decrease healthcare costs. However, even with the current length-of-stay laws, many newborns still do not receive the recommended follow-up care when they go home early.
Evaluation
Health Promotion and Maintenance
Application
Learning Objective 36.1

36.14 The nurse is at the home of a postpartum client for an initial assessment. The client gave birth by cesarean section one week earlier. Which statement should the nurse include? (Select all that apply.)
1. "Because you had a cesarean, I'd like to assess your incision."
2. "You aren't having any problems nursing, right?"
3. "How rested do you feel since you came home?"
4. "Since you are bottle feeding, I won't assess your breasts."
5. "You should remain at home for the first three weeks after delivery."

Answer: 1, 3
Rationale: The home care nurse should assess the cesarean incision and rest/sleep and fatigue. Therapeutic communication prohibits asking leading questions. Breasts should be assessed for engorgement even for bottle-feeding moms. New mothers should be instructed to match their activities to their energy level.
Implementation
Health Promotion and Maintenance
Assessment
Learning Objective 36.7

36.15 It is July, and a new father asks the nurse who is making a postpartum home visit about taking the baby to a family outing this weekend. The nurse should encourage the father to
1. cover the infant with dark blankets to block the sun.
2. protect the infant with light clothing.
3. uncover the infant's head to prevent hyperthermia.
4. avoid taking the infant outdoors for six months.

Answer: 2
Rationale: Protecting the infant with light clothing is enough to prevent overheating and damaging effects from the sun. Covering the infant with dark blankets to block the sun would cause overheating, and is not necessary. Uncovering the infant's head to prevent hyperthermia could actually cause hypothermia, because infants lose much of their body heat through the head. Avoiding taking the infant outdoors for six months is not necessary or practical.
Implementation
Health Promotion and Maintenance
Analysis
Learning Objective 36.6

CHAPTER 37

37.1 The nurse is planning an in-service presentation about perinatal loss. Which statements should the nurse include in this presentation? "Perinatal loss (Select all that apply.)
1. refers to third trimester fetal death in utero."
2. occurs more frequently in assisted reproduction."
3. rates have declined in the United States over the past few years."
4. is most frequent in the last four weeks of pregnancy."
5. rarely causes an emotional problem for the family."

Answer: 2, 3
Rationale: Perinatal loss rates have decreased in industrialized nations. The term perinatal loss refers to all fetal loss from conception until the infant is 28 days old. Perinatal loss occurs more frequently in pregnancies that were accomplished by assisted reproductive technology than in spontaneously-occurring pregnancies. Over 80% of perinatal loss occurs prior to the fetus reaching term. Perinatal losses are grieved by most couples and families like any other death, and like other grief, can become overwhelming.
Planning
Psychosocial Integrity
Application
Learning Objective 37.1

37.2 The nurse has returned from working as a maternal-child nurse volunteer for a nongovernmental organization. Upon completion of a community presentation about her experiences, the nurse knows that learning has occurred when a participant states
1. "Malaria is a chronic disease and rarely causes fetal loss."
2. "Escherichia coli bacteria can cause diarrhea but not stillbirth."

Answer: 3
Rationale: Infections play a significant role in fetal death in underdeveloped nations. A first case of malaria during pregnancy frequently leads to fetal loss. Escherichia coli and Group B streptococci can cause ascending infections prior to or after rupture of membranes. Viral infections are also frequent causes of fetal death.
Evaluation
Psychosocial Integrity
Analysis
Learning Objective 37.1

3. "Group B streptococci can cause infection and death of the fetus."
4. "Viral infections don't cause fetal death in underdeveloped nations."

37.3 The client at 37 weeks' gestation calls the clinic nurse to report that neither she nor her partner have felt fetal movement for the past 48 hours. The nurse anticipates that the physician would order which test to assess fetal viability? 1. ultrasound 2. serum progesterone levels 3. computed tomography (CT) scan 4. contraction stress test	Answer: 1 Rationale: Ultrasound is used to detect the presence or absence of fetal heart motion when fetal demise is suspected. Serum estriol levels drop during fetal demise, but progesterone levels are not measured. A computed tomography (CT) scan is not indicated. Contraction stress tests are used to determine if a fetus will tolerate the stresses of labor. Assessment Psychosocial Integrity Application Learning Objective 37.1
37.4 The nurse is working with a family who experienced a stillbirth of their son two months ago. Which statement by the mother would be expected? 1. "I seem to keep crying for no reason." 2. "The death of my son hasn't changed my life." 3. "I have not visited my son's gravesite." 4. "I feel happy all of the time."	Answer: 1 Rationale: Weeping is a frequent response to grief. Visiting the gravesite is a common coping mechanism to adjust to a fetal loss. A fetal loss is devastating to parents, and results in significant life changes. Happiness is not an expected part of mourning. Assessment Psychosocial Integrity Application Learning Objective 37.2
37.5 The nurse is working with a laboring family who has a known intrauterine fetal demise. To facilitate the family's acceptance of the fetal loss, after delivery the nurse should encourage the parents to 1. look at the infant from across the room. 2. hold the infant in their arms. 3. have the nurse bring the infant to the morgue immediately. 4. call family members and inform them of the birth.	Answer: 2 Rationale: Attachment theory states that human beings are biologically predisposed to bond with emotionally significant persons in their lives. The grief response, as per attachment theory, is a state of separation anxiety that is brought on by the disruption in the attachment bond. Holding the infant makes the experience real to the parents, and facilitates appropriate grief and mourning. Looking at the infant from a distance would not be helpful; nor would avoiding contact with the fetus. Calling family members would not be helpful. Planning Psychosocial Integrity Analysis Learning Objective 37.2
37.6 The postpartum unit nurse is caring for a family who delivered a term stillborn infant yesterday. The mother is heard screaming at the nutrition services worker, "This food is horrible! You people are incompetent and can't cook a simple edible meal!" The nurse understands this as 1. an indication the mother is in the anger phase of grief. 2. an abnormal response to the loss of the child. 3. reactive stress management techniques are being used. 4. denial of the death of the child she delivered yesterday.	Answer: 1 Rationale: Anger is a common and normal response to the grief of perinatal loss, and is often directed at members of the healthcare team. Reactive stress management techniques do not exist. Denial of the loss would manifest as believing that she still has a live fetus in utero. Assessment Psychosocial Integrity Application Learning Objective 37.2

37.7 The 15-year-old client delivered a 22-week stillborn fetus. The nurse is presenting the client with information about a fetal loss support group for clients of all ages that can be joined without a fee. The nurse should encourage the client to attend based on an understanding that

1. grieving a fetal loss will manifest with very similar behaviors regardless of the age of the clients.
2. teens tend to withhold emotions and need older adults with the same type of loss to help process the experience.
3. most teens have had a great deal of contact with death and loss and will have an established method of coping.
4. communication styles vary within families, and teens whose families are extremely busy may have little support at home.

Answer: 4
Rationale: Chaotic families may not have open communication patterns, and the teen may have little support. Grieving behaviors will be very different in teens and in those in their 30s. Teens will rely more on their peers than other adults for emotional support. Most teens have had little experience with death, and the fetal loss is often the first time a teen is personally impacted by loss and grief.
Planning
Psychosocial Integrity
Application
Learning Objective 37.3

37.8 The community nurse has identified that the mother who gave birth to a stillborn baby last week is an intuitive griever. Which behavior would the nurse have encountered that would lead to this assessment? The mother

1. has verbalized that her problem-solving skills have been helpful during this process.
2. repeatedly talks about her thoughts, feelings, and emotions about losing her child last week.
3. talks little about her experience, and appears detached and unaffected by the loss of her child.
4. has asked her close friends, co-workers, and relatives to please not call her and to not visit.

Answer: 2
Rationale: Intuitive grievers tend to feel their way through the loss with emphasis on emotional and psychosocial support, and will seek support from non-judgmental friends. Instrumental grievers tend to use problem-solving skills in the grief process, and often appear detached and unaffected by the experience.
Assessment
Psychosocial Integrity
Analysis
Learning Objective 37.3

37.9 The nurse is caring for a client who experienced the birth of a stillborn son earlier in the day. The client comes from a culture that is heavily paternalistic, and emphasizes the importance of male children over female. What behavior would the nurse expect in this client?

1. The client is crying inconsolably.
2. The client expresses feelings of failure as a woman.
3. The client requests for family members to be present.
4. The client shows little emotion.

Answer: 2
Rationale: When a woman belongs to a culture that emphasizes the importance of males, she often sees that her main role as an adult is to produce children. A fetal death will often result in feelings of failure as a woman in these cultures. Inconsolable crying is not a sign of a paternalistic culture, nor is the presence of multiple family members. Showing little emotion indicates a stoic culture, which may or may not be paternalistic.
Planning
Psychosocial Integrity
Application
Learning Objective 37.3

37.10 The nurse is present when a mother and her partner are told that their 35-week fetus has died. Which

Answer: 1
Rationale: The top priority for the nurse is to encourage open communication between the mother, her partner, and the healthcare team members, which will

nursing intervention should the nurse do first?

1. Encourage open communication with the family and the healthcare team.
2. Ask the family to withhold their questions until later the next day.
3. Request that another nurse come and care for this family.
4. Contact a local funeral home to help the family with funeral plans.

contribute to a realistic understanding of the medical condition and its associated treatments. Requesting that the couple not ask questions does not facilitate communication, nor does requesting that another nurse care for the family. Funeral plans can be made later.
Planning
Psychosocial Integrity
Application
Learning Objective 37.4

37.11 The labor and delivery nurse is caring for a client whose labor is being induced due to fetal death in utero at 35 weeks' gestation. In planning intrapartum care for this client, which nursing diagnosis is most likely to be used?

1. powerlessness
2. ineffective elimination
3. effective family coping
4. energy field disturbance

Answer: 1
Rationale: Powerlessness is commonly experienced by families who face fetal loss. Ineffective elimination and energy field disturbance are not related to fetal loss. Ineffective family coping is more likely to occur than effective family coping.
Diagnosis
Psychosocial Integrity
Analysis
Learning Objective 37.4

37.12 The nurse is supervising care by a new graduate nurse who is working with a couple who have experienced a stillbirth. Which statement made by the new graduate nurse indicates that further instruction is necessary?

1. "I should stay out of their room as much as possible."
2. "The parents may express their grief differently."
3. "My role is to help the family communicate and cope."
4. "Hopelessness may be expressed by this family."

Answer: 1
Rationale: Families experiencing perinatal loss need support, and the nurse must be in the room as much as the parents need her to be in order to provide that support. Partners often express grief very differently. Families need to communicate to cope effectively. Hopelessness is commonly experienced by families experiencing perinatal loss.
Evaluation
Psychosocial Integrity
Analysis
Learning Objective 37.4

37.13 The mother of a client who has experienced a term stillbirth arrives at the hospital and goes to the nurses' desk. The mother asks what she should say to her daughter in this difficult time. Which answer should the nurse provide? (Select all that apply.)

1. "Use clichés; your daughter will find the repetition comforting."
2. "Remind her that she is young and can have more children."
3. "Keep talking about other things to keep her mind off the loss."
4. "Express your sadness, and sit silently with her if she doesn't respond."
5. "Encourage her to talk about the baby whenever she wants to."

Answer: 4, 5
Rationale: Silence is commonly needed, and simply saying, "I'm sorry for your loss" may help to facilitate communication. Talking is a way for a client experiencing grief to begin to come to terms with what has happened, and is important for resolution of grief.
Clichés are inappropriate with someone experiencing grief. Reminding her that she is young enough to have other children downplays the importance of this baby. Nonstop talking does not allow the client to express her emotions and feelings, which is a necessary step in the grief process.
Implementation
Psychosocial Integrity
Analysis
Learning Objective 37.5

37.14 The community nurse is planning care for a family that experienced the loss of twins at 20

Answer: 2
Rationale: Maintaining belief that the family can get through this experience is an attribute of caring theory. Care for a family experiencing perinatal loss must be

---

weeks. Which of these steps should be a part of the nurse's care of this family?

1. Base care on the reactions of previous clients who experienced stillbirth.
2. Express the belief that the family will be able to get through this experience.
3. Encourage the couple to keep their feelings to themselves.
4. Honor the birth by reminding the couple that their baby is happy in heaven.

individualized; no two couples will respond in the same way. Communication should be encouraged. Clichés are to be avoided.
Planning
Psychosocial Integrity
Analysis
Learning Objective 37.5

37.15 The nurse is anticipating the arrival of a couple in the labor unit. The couple's 37-week fetus has been determined to have died in utero from unknown causes. What should the nurse include in her plan of care for this family?

1. Allow the family to adjust to the labor unit in the waiting area.
2. Place the family in a labor room at the end of the hall and an empty room next door.
3. Encourage the father to go home and rest for a few hours.
4. Contact the mother's emergency contact person and explain the situation.

Answer: 2
Rationale: A family who is experiencing fetal loss should be allowed to remain together as much as they desire, and should be placed in a labor room as far away from other laboring families as possible. The family should not be put into a waiting area where others who are anticipating a birth may be. According to HIPPA, the nurse cannot give medical information to any person without the express permission of the client.
Planning
Psychosocial Integrity
Analysis
Learning Objective 37.5

CHAPTER 38

38.1 The nurse suspects that a client has developed a perineal hematoma. What assessment findings would the nurse have detected to lead to this conclusion?

1. facial petechiae
2. large, soft hemorrhoids
3. tense tissues with severe pain
4. elevated temperature

Answer: 3
Rationale: Tenseness of tissues that overlay the hematoma are characteristic signs of perineal hematomas. An elevated temperature can be due to a variety of reasons, such as dehydration or mastitis. Facial petechiae do not indicate perineal hematoma. Large, soft hemorrhoids are not indicative of perineal hematoma.
Assessment
Health Promotion and Maintenance
Application
Learning Objective 38.1

38.2 The postpartum client is being tested for a diagnosis of renal failure. Which assessment would the nurse most likely perform to provide data for the physician to confirm this diagnosis? (Select all that apply.)

1. urine pH
2. calculation of output
3. urine-specific gravity
4. calculation of intake
5. clean catch urinalysis

Answer: 2, 3
Rationale: Urine-specific gravity and output will be assessed to determine if a client has renal failure. Urine pH, calculation of intake, and clean-catch urinalysis do not assist in the diagnosis of renal failure.
Assessment
Health Promotion and Maintenance
Application
Learning Objective 38.1

38.3 A nurse suspects that a postpartum client has mastitis. Which of the following assessments provides the data to support this assessment? (Select all that apply.)

Answer: 1, 2, 3, 5
Rationale: Mastitis is characterized by late onset nipple pain, followed by shooting pain during and between feedings. The sudden onset of fever to 102°F is common. The skin of the affected breast may become pink, with flaking and

1. shooting pain in her nipple during breastfeeding
2. late onset of nipple pain
3. pink and flaking skin of the affected breast
4. nipple soreness when the infant latches on
5. sudden onset of fever

itching. It is common for breastfeeding mothers to experience latch on pain; this finding does not indicate mastitis.
Assessment
Health Promotion and Maintenance
Application
Learning Objective 38.1

38.4 The client delivered vaginally two hours ago after receiving an epidural analgesia. She has a slight tingling sensation in both lower extremities but normal movement. She sustained a second-degree perineal laceration. Her perineum is edematous and ecchymotic. What should the nurse include in the plan of care for this client?
1. Assist client to the bathroom in two hours to void.
2. Place a Foley catheter now.
3. Apply warm packs to perineum three times a day.
4. Allow client to rest for the next eight hours.

Answer: 1
Rationale: This client is at risk for urinary retention and bladder over-distention from both the perineal edema and the effects of the epidural. Assisting the client to the bathroom is the most likely intervention that will prevent urinary retention. If the client is unable to void soon, a straight in-and-out catheter may be used. A Foley catheter is not indicated at this time. Cold packs will help decrease the perineal edema; warm packs would increase the edema. Waiting eight hours to reassess the bladder is too long.
Planning
Health Promotion and Maintenance
Analysis
Learning Objective 38.2

38.5 The nurse is teaching the client about the risk of infection after delivery. Which action should the nurse teach the client to perform to prevent the development of postpartum endometritis?
1. Void every two hours.
2. Change peri-pads frequently.
3. Avoid over-hydration.
4. Report symptoms of uterine cramping.

Answer: 2
Rationale: Changing peri-pads frequently prevents contamination of the perineum and risk of infection. Wiping from front to back and good hygiene practices also are important. Reporting symptoms of uterine cramping and voiding frequently would not be preventive actions for infection. Avoiding over-hydration would actually increase the risk for infection by not providing adequate fluids to flush the kidneys and bladder.
Implementation
Health Promotion and Maintenance
Application
Learning Objective 38.2

38.6 The postpartum client is concerned about mastitis because she experienced it with her last baby. The nurse discusses preventive measures with the client. Which client statement indicates that teaching was effective? "To prevent mastitis, I should:
1. Wear a tight-fitting bra."
2. Limit feedings to four times per day."
3. Breastfeed frequently."
4. Force myself to drink fluids."

Answer: 3
Rationale: Frequent breastfeeding is important because complete emptying of the breasts prevents engorgement and stasis. Wearing a tight-fitting bra would mechanically suppress lactation, as would limiting feedings to four times per day. Forcing fluids is not necessary.
Implementation
Health Promotion and Maintenance
Application
Learning Objective 38.5

38.7 The client has experienced a postpartum hemorrhage at six hours postpartum. After controlling the hemorrhage, the client's partner asks what would cause a hemorrhage. How should the nurse respond?
1. "Sometimes the uterus relaxes and excessive bleeding occurs."
2. "The blood collected in the vagina, and poured out when your partner stood up."

Answer: 1
Rationale: Uterine atony, in which the uterus relaxes, is the most common cause of early postpartum hemorrhage (within the first 24 hours after delivery.) Although blood may pool in the vagina and thus pour out when the client stands, this does not cause a hemorrhage. Although breastfeeding stimulates the release of oxytocin which causes the uterus to contract, bottle feeding does not cause hemorrhage. Had the placenta embedded abnormally (as in placenta accreta) the hemorrhage would have occurred immediately after the placenta delivered.
Implementation
Health Promotion and Maintenance
Application
Learning Objective 38.3

---

3. "Bottle feeding prevents the uterus from getting enough stimulation to contract."
4. "The placenta had embedded into the uterine tissue abnormally."

38.8 The nurse is caring for a postpartum client who had an estimated blood loss of 500 mL following a vaginal birth. The client does not have an IV in place. The nurse understands that the most reliable clinical measure of the client's actual blood loss is estimated by:
1. The clinical estimation of blood loss at the time of birth.
2. A decrease in the hematocrit of ten points between admission and after the birth.
3. The amount of saturation of the linens during and after the birth.
4. Decreased blood pressure and increasing pulse after birth.

Answer: 2
Rationale: A decrease in the hematocrit of ten points between the time of admission and after the birth is seen by many clinicians as more reliable in estimating the actual blood loss. The clinical estimation of blood loss at the time of birth often is obscured by blood mixing with amniotic fluid and oozing onto the sterile drapes or getting sponged away. The amount of saturation of the linens during and after the birth is incorrect for this reason. A decrease in blood pressure and an increasing pulse rate after birth do not appear until as much as 1800-2100 mL have been lost, and shortly before the woman becomes hemodynamically unstable.
Assessment
Health Promotion and Maintenance
Analysis
Learning Objective 38.3

38.9 The nurse is assessing a client who is three days post-op from a cesarean birth. She has tenderness, localized heat, and redness of the left leg. She is afebrile. As a result of these symptoms, she most likely will be
1. encouraged to ambulate freely.
2. given aspirin 650 mg by mouth.
3. given methylergonovine maleate (Methergine) IM.
4. placed on bedrest.

Answer: 4
Rationale: These symptoms indicate the presence of superficial thrombophlebitis, so the client should be placed on bedrest. The treatment for superficial thrombophlebitis involves bedrest, elevating the affected limb, analgesics, and use of elastic support hose. The client should not be encouraged to ambulate freely because that would increase the inflammation. Aspirin has anticoagulant properties but usually is not necessary unless complications occur. Methylergonovine maleate (Methergine) is administered only for postpartum hemorrhage.
Assessment
Health Promotion and Maintenance
Application
Learning Objective 38.4

38.10 The client who is one month postpartum states that she does not understand why she does not enjoy being with her baby. Based on this statement, the nurse should be concerned about
1. postpartum psychosis.
2. postpartum infection.
3. postpartum depression.
4. postpartum blues.

Answer: 3
Rationale: Postpartum depression is characterized by feelings of failure and self-accusation, and lack of enjoyment of the baby and lack of enjoyment in general. Postpartum psychosis is more severe, and includes hallucinations and irrationality that is not represented in this situation. Postpartum infection has nothing to do with this situation. The postpartum blues is characterized by mild depression interspersed with happier feelings, and is self-limiting to two weeks.
Assessment
Health Promotion and Maintenance
Application
Learning Objective 38.4

38.11 The client delivered her second child one day ago. The client's temperature is 101.4°F, her pulse is 100, and her blood pressure is 110/70. Her lochia is moderate, serosanguinous, and malodorous. She is started on IV antibiotics. The nurse provides education for the client and her partner. Which statement indicates that teaching has been effective?
1. "This condition is called parametritis."

Answer: 3
Rationale: A postpartum infection of the uterus is endometritis, and when it develops within 36 hours after delivery is most commonly caused by Beta-strep. Parametritis or pelvic cellulitis, is an ascending complication of endometritis, and involves infection of more extensive tissue. Gonorrhea is not a common cause of endometritis, and especially early onset endometritis. Walking would prevent deep vein thrombophlebitis, not endometritis.
Evaluation
Health Promotion and Maintenance
Analysis
Learning Objective 38.4

---

2. "Gonorrhea is the most common organism that causes this type of infection."
3. "My Beta-strep culture being positive may have contributed to this problem."
4. "If I had walked more yesterday, this probably wouldn't have happened."

38.12 The client delivered by cesarean birth three days ago, and is being discharged. Which statement should the nurse include in the discharge teaching? 1. "If your incision becomes increasingly painful, call the doctor." 2. "It is normal for the incision to ooze greenish discharge in a few days." 3. "Increasing redness around the incision is a part of the healing process." 4. "A fever is to be expected because you had a surgical delivery."	Answer: 1 Rationale: The client should call the doctor if the incision becomes increasingly painful. Cesarean wound infections are characterized by fever, increased pain, increasing redness in the peri-wound area, and purulent drainage. A fever is never an expected finding. Implementation Health Promotion and Maintenance Application Learning Objective 38.5
38.13 The client delivered her second child yesterday, and is preparing to be discharged. She expresses concern to the nurse because she developed an upper urinary tract infection (UTI) after the birth of her first child. Which statement indicates that the client needs additional teaching about this issue? 1. "If I start to have burning with urination, I need to call the doctor." 2. "Drinking eight glasses of water each day will help prevent another UTI." 3. "I will remember to wipe from front to back after I move my bowels." 4. "Voiding two or three times per day will help prevent a recurrence."	Answer: 4 Rationale: Voiding only two or three times per day is not sufficient to prevent recurrence of a urinary tract infection (UTI). Upper urinary tract infections (pyelonephritis) are most often caused by ascending bacteria from a lower UTI. Burning with urination is a common symptom of a UTI. Drinking eight or more glasses of water per day, voiding every two to three hours, and wiping from front to back after bowel movements will all help to prevent the development of a UTI. Evaluation Health Promotion and Maintenance Analysis Learning Objective 38.5
38.14 The postpartum client who is being discharged from the hospital experienced severe postpartum depression after her last birth. What should the nurse include in the plan of care for this client? 1. one visit from a home care nurse, to take place in two days 2. two visits from a public health nurse over the next month 3. an appointment with a mental health counselor within ten days 4. follow-up with the obstetrician in six weeks	Answer: 3 Rationale: Postpartum depression has a high recurrence rate. Setting the client up with a mental health appointment within ten days is the best option for detecting the onset of postpartum depression symptoms. A home visit in two days will be helpful to assess feeding, but is too early to detect signs of postpartum depression. Two home visits in a month are too sporadic to accurately pick up postpartum depression. Following up with the obstetrician in six weeks is too long of a time. Planning Health Promotion and Maintenance Application Learning Objective 38.6
38.15 A postpartal client experienced a deep vein thrombosis (DVT) after delivery. The community health nurse is making an initial home visit. The nurse has taught the client about activities to engage in and to avoid. Which statement	Answer: 1 Rationale: The client should take frequent walks to promote venous return; staying in bed most of the day would lead to venous pooling. Taking a daily aspirin increases anticoagulant activity, and should be avoided if the client is being treated with other anticoagulants. Avoiding long car trips is not necessary.

indicates that teaching was effective? "I should

1. take frequent walks."
2. take a daily aspirin dose of 650 mg."
3. avoid long car trips."
4. stay in bed most of the day."

The client should be told to take frequent breaks during car trips, but not to avoid them entirely.
Evaluation
Health Promotion and Maintenance
Analysis
Learning Objective 38.6

PRENTICE HALL NURSING MEDIALINK DVD-ROM

CHAPTER 1

DVD-ROM
Audio Glossary
NCLEX Review

Companion Website
Additional NCLEX ReviewCase Study: *Cord Blood Banking*
Case Study: *Cord Blood Banking*
Care Plan Activity: *Request for Second Trimester Abortion*
Applications: *Scope of Practice; Standards of Care*
Critical Thinking

CHAPTER 2

DVD-ROM
Audio Glossary
NCLEX Review

Companion Website
Additional NCLEX Review
Case Study: *Family Assessment*
Care Plan Activity: *Effects of Hispanic Culture on Infant Feeding Practices*
Applications: *Ethnocentrism and Health Care—Providing Culturally Sensitive Care; Examine Your Cultural Influences*
Critical Thinking

CHAPTER 3

DVD-ROM
Audio Glossary
NCLEX Review
Video: *Massage for Pregnancy*

Companion Website
Additional NCLEX Review
Case Study: *Complementary Therapies*
Care Plan Activity: *Use of CAM in High-Risk Adolescent Pregnancy*
Applications: *Complementary Therapies; Internet Information on Complementary Therapies*
Critical Thinking

CHAPTER 4

DVD-ROM
Audio Glossary
NCLEX Review

Companion Website
Additional NCLEX Review
Case Study: *Premenstrual Girl*
Care Plan Activity: *Bone Injuries in a Postmenopausal Woman*
Applications: *Teaching Adolescents How to Keep a Period Calendar; Menopause*
Critical Thinking

CHAPTER 5

DVD-ROM
Audio Glossary
NCLEX Review
Oral Contraceptive Animation
Videos: *Vasectomy; Through the Eyes of a Nurse—Welcoming the New Arrival at the Postpartal Visit*

Companion Website
Additional NCLEX Review
Case Study: *Family Planning*
Care Plan Activity: *Fertility Awareness*
Applications: *Abstinence Support Resources; Contraceptive Services for Minors*
Critical Thinking

CHAPTER 6

DVD-ROM
Audio Glossary
NCLEX Review

Companion Website
Additional NCLEX Review
Case Study: *Pediculosis Pubis*
Care Plan Activity: *Gynecologic Infection*
Applications: *Sexually Transmitted Infections; Preventing Urinary Tract Infections*
Critical Thinking

CHAPTER 7

DVD-ROM
Audio Glossary
NCLEX Review
Video: *Breast Self-Examination*

Companion Website
Additional NCLEX Review
Case Study: *Toxic Shock Syndrome*
Care Plan Activity: *Irregular Bleeding in Perimenopausal Woman*
Applications: *Preparing an Adolescent for Her First Pelvic Examination; Cystocele*
Critical Thinking

CHAPTER 8

DVD-ROM
Audio Glossary
NCLEX Review

Companion Website
Additional NCLEX Review
Case Study: *Social Issues Affecting Women*
Care Plan Activity: *Pregnancy in a Disabled Client*
Applications: *How to Find Good Day Care; Elder Abuse*
Critical Thinking

ANSWERS TO CRITICAL THINKING IN ACTION ACTIVITY QUESTIONS

CHAPTER 1

CRITICAL THINKING IN ACTION: CULTURALLY COMPETENT CARE

You are working as a prenatal nurse in a local clinic. Before entering a client's room, you review the chart for pertinent information such as cultural background, significant family members, weeks of gestation, test results, birth plan, and education for health promotion. You greet each client and family members by name and ask how they are coping with the pregnancy. Depending on the trimester of the pregnancy, you review the discomforts or concerns of the mother/family and what they may expect. You examine the mother, including fundal height, fetal heart rate and fetal position if appropriate, maternal blood pressure, weight gain, and urine analysis. With each client, you discuss the community resources available such as prenatal classes, lactation consultants, and prenatal exercise/yoga classes. Based upon the information you obtain, you might refer the mother to social services or the WIC program as appropriate. At the end of the clinic session, you review the clients with the collaborating physician.

1. How would you define the terms *family* and *family-centered care?*	Answer: Family is those persons defined by the mother. For example, the family of a single mother may include her mother, her sister, another relative, a close friend, a lesbian partner, or the father of the child. Many cultures also recognize the importance of extended families, and several family members may provide care and support.
	Family-centered care is characterized by an emphasis on the family and the family's choices about their birth experience. Fathers and partners are active participants; siblings are encouraged to visit and meet the newest family member, and they may even attend the birth. Care is designed to meet the emotional, social, and developmental needs of children and families seeking health care.
2. Describe how the nursing process provides the framework for the delivery of direct nursing care.	Answer: The nurse assesses the mother and identifies the nursing diagnoses that describe the responses of the individual and family to the pregnancy or illness. The nurse then implements and evaluates nursing care. The care is designed to meet specific physical and psychosocial needs.
3. How would you describe the concept of community-based care?	Answer: A "seamless" system of family-centered, comprehensive, coordinated health care, health education, and social services. The system requires coordination as clients move from primary care services to acute care facilities and then back into the community.
4. How would you describe culturally competent care?	Answer: Culture develops from socially learned beliefs, lifestyles, values, and integrated patterns of behavior that are characteristic of the family, cultural group, and community. Conflicts can occur within a family when traditional rituals and practices of the family do not conform with current healthcare practices. Nurses need to be sensitive to the potential implications for the client's health care. When cultural values are not part of the nursing care plan, the client may be forced to decide whether the family's beliefs should take priority over the healthcare professional's guidance.

CHAPTER 2

CRITICAL THINKING IN ACTION: CULTURAL BELIEFS AND HEALTH PRACTICES

While working in an inner-city clinic for adolescents, you meet a new client, a 14-year-old Latina girl named Juanita. She is accompanied by her parents. None of them speak English. Through a translator, Juanita tells you that she recently moved here with her parents. They have brought her here today because she has a sore throat. The curandero they took her to see prescribed the herbal remedy *Echinacea*, but her throat is still sore. The rapid test you perform for strep throat is positive, and the nurse practitioner prescribes an antibiotic.

1. According to the national standards for culturally and linguistically appropriate services in health care set by the government, what are examples of important standards of care you as the nurse can provide in the care of this adolescent?	Answer: You should provide respectful care in their preferred language (getting an interpreter if needed), attend ongoing cultural sensitivity training, provide language brochures in their preferred language, and evaluate if the client is satisfied with the services you provided.

2. How can you, as the nurse, take steps to achieve cultural competence?	Answer: The first step is to evaluate your own feelings about people from other cultures. You can also examine your own personal background to determine what values and beliefs you have. This will help identify what values and beliefs you have that are similar to and different from other cultures.
3. How would you, as the nurse, be able to address some of the disparities that can exist when this client comes to the clinic?	Answer: You can prevent any barriers to the access of health care in your clinic. The barriers this family may encounter are lack of health insurance, hours available, transportation problems, and providing a trusting relationship.
4. What are some examples of common food preferences in the Latino-American culture?	Answer: The use of corn, cheese, beans, and rice is common in this population.

CHAPTER 3

CRITICAL THINKING IN ACTION: COMPLEMENTARY AND ALTERNATIVE THERAPIES

Rommy Startorius, a 24-year-old woman who has never been pregnant, is being seen for her annual gynecologic examination. As part of the health history you ask her whether she is using any forms of treatment for her health that are new since she was seen last year. Initially she reports that she has been getting massage therapy for low back pain and then, as the conversation progresses, she reports that she has been having acupuncture as well. She asks you how "regular" doctors feel about acupuncture and other forms of alternative therapy.

1. How would you describe the role of CAM in health care today?	Answer: In current medical practice, the integration of CAM with traditional western medicine is more and more becoming the norm. In 1992, the National Institute of Health (NIH) established the Office of Alternative Medicine. More and more healthcare practitioners are recognizing the benefits of combination therapies.
2. What information could you provide about the use of acupuncture?	Answer: Acupuncture uses fine metal needles to stimulate specific points based on the client's medical assessment and diagnosis. Six to twelve needles are placed in specific sites to get a desired response. Acupuncture is more common in the East and can be used to stimulate labor contractions or aid in pain relief during vaginal births. Clients should be encouraged to seek accredited practitioners and check local, state, and national organizations for verification of credentialing.
3. She asks you how she can learn about CAM therapies that have some research support for their effectiveness. How would you reply?	Answer: The National Center of Complementary and Alternative Medicine (NCCAM) is a division of the NIH that provides research funding for complementary and alternative therapies. Clients may access the NCCAM website on the Internet at *http://nccam.nih.gov.*

CHAPTER 4

CRITICAL THINKING IN ACTION: PREMENSTRUAL SYNDROME

Linda Knoll, 35 years old, presents to you at the GYN clinic for her annual physical and pelvic exam. You obtain the following menstrual history: LMP 8 days ago. Periods occur every 29 days and last 5 days. She tells you that she uses superabsorbent tampons during the first 2 days of her period and then changes to regular absorbency tampons for the duration, and that she currently has an IUD in place for contraception. She tells you that her husband has been complaining for the last few months that she seems irritable, tense, and moody near "that time of the month." Linda admits that she doesn't feel well before her period and describes having low pelvic discomfort, breast tenderness, "bloating," and some constipation. She seems to cry easily 2 to 3 days before her period. She has noticed this pattern over the last 4 or 5 months. You recognize these symptoms as related to premenstrual syndrome (PMS). Linda asks you if these changes are due to female hormones.

1. How would you answer Linda's question concerning female hormones?	Answer: Although there is no known cause for PMS, one study suggests there is a complex interrelationship among ovarian hormones and stress-related hormones. Many women believe PMS to be psychologic, but the result of the study provided information that actual physiologic changes occur.
2. After reviewing Linda's diet with her, what would you recommend to help?	Answer: Counsel Linda to restrict her intake of foods containing methylxanthines, such as chocolate, cola, and coffee; restrict her intake of alcohol, nicotine, red meat, and foods containing salt and sugar; increase her intake of complex carbohydrates and protein; and increase the frequency of meals.

3. Linda has an IUD in place. What other type of contraceptive might help reduce the symptoms of PMS?	Answer: Low-dose oral contraceptives.
4. What other activities can you suggest to help Linda reduce PMS symptoms?	Answer: A program of aerobic exercises such as fast walking, jogging, or aerobic dancing is generally beneficial.
5. What should you tell Linda about using tampons during heavy menstrual flow?	Answer: Tampons should be used during the day; change to pads at night when flow is lighter to decrease the risk of toxic shock syndrome.

CHAPTER 5

CRITICAL THINKING IN ACTION: REDUCING ANXIETY DURING A FIRST PELVIC EXAM

You are working at a local clinic when Joy Lang, age 20, presents for her first pelvic exam. You obtain the following GYN history: LMP 6-12, menarche age 12, menstrual cycle 28–30 days lasting 4–5 days, heavy one day, then lighter. She tells you that she needs to use superabsorbent tampons on the first day of her period and then she switches to a regular absorbency tampon for the remaining days. She confirms that she changes the tampon every 6 to 8 hours, never leaving it in overnight. She denies premenstrual syndrome, dysmenorrhea, or medical problems and says that she is not taking any medication on a regular schedule. She tells you that she recently got married, but would like to wait before getting pregnant. She'd like to discuss birth control methods. Joy tells you that doctors make her nervous and she admits to being anxious about her first pelvic exam.

1. What steps would you take to reduce Joy's anxiety relating to the pelvic exam?	Answer: Perform the head-to-toe exam leaving the pelvic exam for last to establish trust. Involve Joy as an active participant in the examination. Explain the sensations she may feel. Use the opportunity to teach about the body and its function. Invite Joy to visualize her external and internal genitalia by using a mirror.
2. What position is best to relax Joy's abdominal muscles for the pelvic exam?	Answer: Assist Joy in the semi-sitting position with her hands either at her sides or over her chest. The stirrups should be at a comfortable length for her height.
3. What precaution should be taken when obtaining a Pap smear?	Answer: No lubricant is used with the speculum as it can interfere with the laboratory results.
4. Explain the purpose of the Pap smear.	Answer: The purpose of the test is to screen for the presence of cellular abnormalities by obtaining a sample containing cells from the cervix and the endocervical canal.
5. What factors do you include in a discussion of the type of birth control that Anita could practice?	Answer: The discussion should explore available choices, advantages, disadvantages, effectiveness, side effects, contraindications, and long-term effects. Outside factors influence the choice of contraception such as cultural practices, religious beliefs, attitudes and personal preferences, cost effectiveness, misinformation, practicality of method, and self-esteem.

CHAPTER 6

CRITICAL THINKING IN ACTION: GONORRHEA IN WOMEN

Cherelle Latkowski, age 24, was just diagnosed with gonorrhea by the nurse practitioner at the clinic where you work. Although she had been asymptomatic, she had come in for evaluation after her boyfriend was diagnosed with gonorrhea and started on antibiotics. Cherelle is treated with ceftriaxone administered intramuscularly plus doxycycline by mouth.

1. Cherelle asks you why she received two medications. How would you reply?	Answer: Since chlamydia and gonorrhea commonly co-exist, the Center for Disease Control (CDC) recommends treating both infections when one of these infections has been diagnosed.
2. Cherelle asks you whether she is now immune to gonorrhea. Is she?	Answer: No, since gonorrhea is a bacterium, gonorrhea can reoccur, and commonly does if reinfection with the bacterium occurs.
3. Cherelle asks whether she can now have sex with her boyfriend. Can she do so?	Answer: No. Cherelle and her boyfriend should refrain from intercourse until both are treated and recultured. Once both have negative cultures, they may resume intercourse, but should be advised to consistently use condoms. If the cultures remain positive after 7–14 days, retreatment and another set of repeat cultures may be needed.

CHAPTER 7

CRITICAL THINKING IN ACTION: FIBROCYSTIC BREAST CHANGES

Mercedes de Martini is a 32-year-old gravida 2 para 2 who has a well documented history of fibrocystic breast changes. Mercedes' breast symptoms typically increase premenstrually, when her breasts become markedly nodular and dense. She is being seen today because she has a palpable "lump" in her left breast that she describes as painful and easily moveable. Mercedes reports that her menses is due in 5 days. Based on history and physical examination, the physician suspects that Mercedes has developed a cyst and decides to complete a fine-needle aspiration.

1. Identify findings on examination that might help distinguish a cyst from breast cancer.	Answer: Cysts are typically painful, tender, and sometimes occur with nipple discharge. Fibrocystic breast changes commonly increases and then decrease in size in relation to the menstrual cycle. Small cysts can present as a localized tender area instead of a discrete encapsulated area. Cysts tend to be mobile and do not cause skin retraction. Malignant masses tend to cause pulling in the surrounding tissue (skin retraction) and are usually fixed in one site and nonmobile. Breast cancer masses tend to be nontender, can result in nipple inversion, can change the size or shape of the breast, can be accompanied by erosion or skin ulceration, and can co-exist with an auxiliary lump.
2. Why is a fine-needle aspiration done?	Answer: A fine needle aspiration can be performed as a diagnostic test to determine if a mass is malignant. If a mass is determined to be malignant, a plan of care based on the findings can be determined. A needle aspiration can also be performed on benign cysts to provide relief from painful or tender cysts.
3. What steps can Mercedes take to help decrease the discomfort associated with her fibrocystic breast changes?	Answer: Fibrocystic breast changes typically occur as a result of hormonal changes during the menstrual cycle. Women can decrease sodium intake the week prior to menses and may benefit from Vitamin B6 and E supplements. Evening primrose oil supplements can also decrease breast tenderness. Women can also try decreasing caffeine intake. Oral contraceptives may also decrease fibrocystic breast changes. Rarely, danazol or bromocriptine can be prescribed in severe cases. Ibuprofen is often helpful in decreasing breast tenderness.

CHAPTER 8

CRITICAL THINKING IN ACTION: DOMESTIC VIOLENCE IN THE ELDERLY

Grace Abbey, an 83-year-old woman presents for irregular bleeding to the gynecologist. Mrs. Abbey, a widow, has been living with her son, a 54-year-old unemployed retail manager, for the last 2 years when her husband died. Her son accompanies her to the visit and is reluctant to leave his mother's side. You ask the son to wait in the waiting room and begin your assessment of Mrs. Abbey. When you roll up her sleeve to take her blood pressure, you note bruises on her wrist and forearm. When you question her about the etiology of the bruises, she looks down at the floor and avoids making eye contact. She then states she cannot remember how the bruises occurred. After obtaining her vital signs, you escort her into the exam room and note additional bruises on her back as you assist her with her gown. When you question her about those bruises, she breaks down sobbing, saying "Don't say anything. Don't tell my son you saw them."

1. Discuss how you would assess Mrs. Abbey for other forms of elder abuse?	Answer: Provide privacy and a nonjudgmental approach to ask Mrs. Abbey sensitive questions. Begin by asking more general, nonthreatening questions before asking her more specific questions regarding issues of elder abuse. Assess all types of elder abuse including psychological, physical, and financial abuse along with neglect and abandonment.
2. Mrs. Abbey describes physical violence that started occurring after her son lost his job and his wife left him. She admits "I have been more trouble with my health problems lately." What factors can increase the risk of elder abuse?	Answer: Risk factors include being cared for by a family member, older (over the age of 80) women, shared living arrangements, family history of violence, lack of financial resources, dependence, isolation, poor health, and cognitive impairment. Black women are more likely to be abandoned than white women. Asian and Hispanic elderly populations are the least likely to be victims of elder abuse. Risk factors for abusers include substance abuse and stress.
3. Mrs. Abbey begins crying and says "I know this has never happened to anyone else. I don't understand why this is happening." What is your reply?	Answer: Elder abuse is a common occurrence. It is estimated that there are 550,000 cases annually in the United States. Reassure Mrs. Abbey that she is not alone and it is not her fault. Provide resources and referrals.

CHAPTER 9

CRITICAL THINKING IN ACTION: COUNSELING THE SURVIVOR OF DOMESTIC VIOLENCE

Marishka Devonowski, a 28-year-old G2P2 has a 6-year-old son and a 3-year-old daughter at home. Mrs. Devonowski has been seen at the Emergency Department several times for a variety of problems including a broken arm, sprained ankle, and multiple contusions from reportedly "walking into a door" when she got up during the night but did not turn on a light. She describes herself as clumsy and accident-prone. At each visit her husband, a computer analysist, who appears thoughtful and protective of his wife, accompanies her.

Today she is being seen for a severe laceration of her cheek and a mild concussion. You observe that she also has a black eye and bruising of her upper arm and chest. At each previous visit the nurse had managed to spend time alone with Mrs. Devonowski and had asked specifically about domestic violence. However, Marishka denied it vehemently each time. Today, when you are alone with her you ask about abuse. This time she admits that her husband caused her injuries. She states, "His job is so stressful and sometimes he just loses his temper. But he seems to get more angry no matter what I do. I hate it but I can't leave him. I don't know how I would manage alone."

1. In talking with Marishka, what information would you focus on initially?	Answer: Initially, a complete assessment should be performed to identify the types of abuse she has encountered besides physical abuse. Many women exhibit a variety of physical and psychological signs and symptoms of as a result of abuse. Information should be obtained by asking open ended, nonjudgmental questions. A warm supportive approach can make the woman feel more comfortable in answering questions.
2. What specific information should you share about preparing an exit or safety plan?	Answer: The woman should be counseled to establish an exit or safety plan. The woman should prepare certain items for herself and children (if she has any). This should include a change of clothing, toilet articles, and an extra set of house and car keys. The woman should be advised to have money, important documents (driver's license, social security card, checkbook, savings account information, financial records, children's medical and school records). The woman should also have an established escape route and emergency telephone numbers, including the local police, domestic violence shelters, and a local hotline number.

CHAPTER 10

CRITICAL THINKING IN ACTION: TALKING WITH A TEENAGE GIRL ABOUT MENSTRUATION

You are working in the OB/GYN clinic when Sally Smith, a 17-year-old teenager, comes in complaining of irregular menses. She believes her periods are really "messed up" and interfering with her active schedule. She wants them to be more regular and asks you for birth control. She tells you that she is a member of the swimming team and is a senior in high school. She says she is planning to start community college next year to obtain an associate degree in computer technology. You assess Sally's history as follows: menarche began at age 12; periods occur every 28 to 32 days. She usually experiences cramping in the first 2 days and the flow lasts 4 to 5 days. She uses an average of 4 to 5 tampons a day during her period. She has never been hospitalized, has no prior medical problems, and is up to date on her immunizations except for meningitis.

1. Based on your knowledge of menstruation, how would you describe Sally's menstrual cycle?	Answer: Sally has described a normal menstrual cycle. While there is some variability in frequency, it is not outside the normal range for a teenager.
2. What is your primary goal in discussing Sally's menstrual cycle with her?	Answer: It is important to reassure Sally that her menstrual cycle is normal. Your role is to provide accurate information and assist in clarifying misconceptions so that Sally will develop a positive self-image.
3. What information would you give Sally relating to her menstrual cycle?	Answer: The menstrual cycle length is determined from the first day of one menses to the first day of the next. Normal length is 25 to 35 days. The amount of flow is approximately 30 mL per period. Flow is heavier at first and lightens toward the end of the period. The length of menses may last 2 to 8 days.
4. What important request does Sally have?	Answer: Of utmost importance is the request for birth control. Sally may be considering becoming sexually active and needs contraception. Teenagers often have difficulty asking for what they really want. This is an ideal situation to bring up issues of sexuality.
5. Sally expresses problems dealing with the cramping she experiences with the first 2 days of her menses. What would you suggest to Sally to cope with the discomfort?	Answer: Relief may be obtained with oral contraception, prostaglandin inhibitors such as ibuprofen, aspirin, naproxen, and measures such as regular exercise, rest, heat, and good nutrition with emphasis on vitamins B and E.

CHAPTER 11

CRITICAL THINKING IN ACTION: VULNERABILITY OF THE UNBORN CHILD TO MATERNAL ILLNESS

You are working at the local clinic when Frances, a 28-year-old G2 P1001 at 11 weeks' gestation comes in to the office. Frances tells you that early in the first trimester, her husband experienced a flulike syndrome and that he was later diagnosed with cytomegalovirus (CMV) pneumonia. She tells you that his physician found an enlarged supraclavicular lymph node and an ulcer on one tonsil. Laboratory testing revealed elevated liver enzymes. Further testing led to the discovery of positive cytomegalovirus (CMV) IgM levels. She has come today with symptoms including night sweats, persistent sore throat, joint pain, headache, vomiting, and fatigue. You obtain vital signs of temperature 99°F, pulse 90, respirations 14, BP 110/70. Her physical exam is normal; no lymphadenopathy are present. Her weight gain is 2 lb even with nausea and some vomiting. She is worried that her husband's illness could be related to her current symptoms.

1. How would you respond to Frances's concern?	Answer: Frances's symptoms may be attributable to normal pregnancy or possibly to a flu virus. The physician will probably order serologic tests for CMV IgM and IgG. The test will determine if Frances has been exposed to CMV, has an acute or recent infection, or is immune.
2. Frances asks you if her baby is formed. How would you discuss the three stages of development?	Answer: The preembryonic stage consists of the first 14 days after the ovum is fertilized, the embryonic stage covers the period from day 15 until the end of the eighth week, and the fetal stage extends from the end of the eighth week until birth.
3. Frances asks when her baby is most vulnerable for abnormal growth or structure. How would you answer?	Answer: During the embryonic stage when tissues differentiate into essential organs and the main external features develop, the embryo is most vulnerable.
4. Frances asks what stage her baby is in. What would you tell her?	Answer: At 11 weeks your baby is considered a fetus and all the organs are present.

CHAPTER 12

CRITICAL THINKING IN ACTION: BASAL BODY TEMPERATURE (BBT) METHOD OF FERTILITY AWARENESS

Marie Neives, age 19, presents while you are working at a Planned Parenthood Clinic. She is there for a GYN exam and tells you that she is sexually active with her boyfriend but doesn't want to become pregnant. Since she lives at home with her parents, she does not want to use "the pill" because her mother might find out. Marie asks you for information concerning fertility awareness. You obtain a menstrual history as follows: menarche age 12, cycle every 28 days, dysmenorrhea the first 2 days with moderate flow. She has had one sexual partner. She states her boy friend doesn't like to use condoms and that she has been lucky so far in not getting pregnant. You assist the nurse practitioner with a physical and pelvic exam. The results show that Marie is essentially healthy. The nurse practitioner asks you to review with Marie the basal body temperature (BBT) method of fertility awareness.

1. Explore with Marie "natural family planning." How would you explain this to her?	Answer: Natural family planning is based on an understanding of the changes that occur throughout a woman's ovulatory cycle. This method requires periods of abstinence and recording of certain events throughout the cycle; cooperation of the partners is important.
2. Briefly explain why the basal body temperature (BBT) method can predict ovulation.	Answer: Basal temperature for the woman in the preovulatory phase is usually below 36°C. As ovulation approaches, production of estrogen peaks and may cause a slight drop, then a rise in the basal temperature. After ovulation, progesterone production rises. It causes a 0.3°C to 0.6°C sustained rise in basal temperature. Just before or coincident with the onset of menses, the temperature falls below 36°C.
3. Describe to Marie the procedure for obtaining BBT.	Answer: Using a BBT thermometer, the woman chooses one site (oral, vaginal, or rectal) which she uses consistently. She takes her temperature for 5 minutes every day before arising and before starting any activity, including smoking. The result is recorded on a BBT chart, and the temperature dots are connected to form a graph. She shakes the thermometer down and cleans it in preparation for use the next day.
4. To avoid conception, when do you tell Marie to abstain from unprotected intercourse?	Answer: If her periods are regular, she should abstain or use protection (condoms) 3 days before and 3 days after the anticipated day of ovulation.

CHAPTER 13

CRITICAL THINKING IN ACTION: BIRTH PLANS WITH EXPECTANT PARENTS

Terry Dole, a 38-year-old G1, P0000, at 6 weeks' gestation, presents to you at the OB clinic for her first prenatal visit with the certified nurse-midwife (CNM). One of the first decisions facing Terry is the selection of a healthcare provider. The midwife explains the various options available to Terry at the clinic related to the differences in educational preparation, skill level, practice characteristics, and general philosophy of CNMs and obstetricians. Terry tells you that she has been married for 6 years and works as a massage therapist. You obtain the following data: BP 110/70, temperature 97°F, pulse 76, respirations 12, weight 140 lb, height 5′7″. The physical and pelvic exams are essentially normal. The CNM asks you to teach Terry about birth plans.

1. Discuss the advantages of a birth plan.	Answer: A birth plan helps couples set priorities. It identifies areas that they want to incorporate into their own birth experience. By writing down preferences, prospective parents identify aspects of the childbearing experience that are most important to them.
2. Discuss the disadvantages of a birth plan.	Answer: At times expectations cannot be met because of the unavailability of some choices in the community, limitations set by insurance providers, or unexpected problems during pregnancy or birth.
3. Explain the role of a doula.	Answer: Doula roles and responsibilities include providing specific labor support skills; offering guidance and encouragement; assisting mothers to cover gaps in their care; building a team relationship; and encouraging communication between patient, nursing staff, and medical caregivers.
4. What gender differences are there in moving toward parenthood?	Answer: Women, especially working women, experience appreciably more change than do men in the transition to parenthood. Women tend to feel responsible for their children's success and happiness. They also internalize the distress experienced by those to whom they are closest, particularly family members.

CHAPTER 14

CRITICAL THINKING IN ACTION: PRENATAL EDUCATION: NAUSEA, URINARY FREQUENCY, AND EXERCISE SAFETY

Twenty-two-year-old Jean Simmons is an aerobic instructor, G0, P0000 in her first trimester of pregnancy. She presents to you at the local clinic complaining of frequent nausea, urinary frequency, and fatigue. You obtain her vital signs as 108/60, 97°F P68, R12, weight 125 lb, height 64 inches. Her urine tests negative for ketones, albumin, leukocytes, and sugar. You note that Jean has lost 3 lbs. since her last visit. You assist the certified nurse-midwife with a physical exam, the findings of which are essentially normal. Jean says that while she knows it could become an issue, she would like to continue working as an aerobic instructor for as long as she possibly can during the pregnancy. You identify Jean's complaints as normal discomforts of pregnancy, and proceed with prenatal education.

1. What advice would you suggest to cope with the nausea of pregnancy?	Answer: Eat crackers or dry toast before arising; avoid causative foods and odors; eat small, frequent meals and dry foods with fluids between meals; avoid greasy or highly seasoned foods.
2. What advice might you suggest to cope with urinary frequency?	Answer: Do not cut back on fluid; void when urge is experienced; increase fluid intake during the day.
3. What teaching would be important relating to exercise in pregnancy?	Answer: Decrease intensity of exercise as pregnancy progresses and stop when fatigued. Avoid high-risk activities or activities that require good balance and coordination. Avoid prolonged overheating. Keep heart rate at or below 140 beats per minute. Wear supportive shoes and supportive bra.
4. What symptoms related to exercise should Jean report to her physician?	Answer: Extreme fatigue, dizziness or faintness, sudden sharp pain, difficulty in breathing, nausea and vomiting, pain, vaginal bleeding, and excessive muscle soreness.

CHAPTER 15

CRITICAL THINKING IN ACTION: HEALTH PREGNANCY SIGNS

Wendy Stodard, age 40, G3, P0020 comes to the obstetrician's office where you are working for a prenatal visit. Wendy had experienced two spontaneous abortions followed by a D & C at 14 and 15 weeks' gestation during the previous year. She has a history of *Chlamydia* infection 3 years ago which was treated with azithromycin. She is at 10 weeks' gestation. Wendy tells you that she is afraid of losing this pregnancy as she did previously. She says she has been experiencing some mild nausea, breast tenderness, and fatigue which did not occur with her other pregnancies. You assist the obstetrician with an ultrasound. The gestational sac is clearly seen, fetal heartbeat is observed, and crown-to-rump measurements are consistent with gestational age of 10 weeks. The pelvic exam demonstrates a closed cervix, and positive Goodell's, Hegar's, and Chadwick's signs. You discuss with Wendy the signs of a healthy pregnancy.

1. What signs are reassuring with this pregnancy?	Answer: The ultrasound showed a gestational sac with a fetus consistent with gestational age, and the fetus has a heartbeat. Breast tenderness, nausea, and fatigue confirm a pregnancy hormone level consistent with a normal pregnancy.
2. What symptoms should be reported to the obstetrician immediately?	Answer: Vaginal bleeding or cramping, painful urination, severe vomiting or diarrhea, fever higher than 101°F, low abdominal pain located on either side or in the middle of the abdomen, lightheadedness, and dizziness, particularly if accompanied by shoulder pain.
3. What is the frequency of antepartal visits?	Answer: Every 4 weeks for the first 28 weeks' gestation; every 2 weeks until 36 weeks' gestation; after week 36, every week until childbirth.

CHAPTER 16

CRITICAL THINKING IN ACTION: THIRD TRIMESTER PREGNANCY DISCOMFORTS

Thirty-seven-year-old Cathy Sommers, G1, P0000, presents to you, with her husband, at the OB physician's office at 32 weeks' gestation. Cathy tells you that she and her husband are practicing lawyers with their own firm. The couple delayed starting a family because it has been important to them to advance their careers and establish their firm. Cathy had an amniocentesis at 18 weeks' gestation because of her advanced maternal age, and the results ruled out chromosomal abnormalities. The couple knows that the baby is a boy and are anticipating a vaginal birth. Cathy tells you that she is experiencing more fatigue, leg cramps, and shortness of breath when climbing stairs. The physical exam including a negative Homans' sign is within normal limits with the exception of slight ankle edema. Her weight is 150 lb, temperature 98.6°F, pulse 88, respirations 16, BP 126/70. You discuss pregnancy discomforts in the third trimester with Cathy and her husband.

1. What measures can you suggest to cope with fatigue?	Answer: Encourage adequate sleep and rest periods. Explore ways to arrange work to allow frequent rest periods. Encourage good posture, wearing of low-heeled shoes, and pelvic rock exercises to ease backaches. Suggest ways to reduce insomnia with the use of pillows and raising the head of the bed.
2. Discuss measures to decrease leg cramps.	Answer: Avoid stretching her legs, pointing her toes, walking excessively, and lying on her back. Demonstrate how to massage legs and buttocks to her husband.
3. Discuss the physiologic changes underlying dyspnea.	Answer: The uterus presses up against the abdominal organs and diaphragm, preventing full expansion of the lungs. Relief will occur in the ninth month when the baby drops into the pelvis.
4. Review Braxton Hicks contractions.	Answer: Around the sixth month, the uterus begins painless irregular contractions. No cervical dilatation occurs. The contractions may increase the tone of the uterine muscle in preparation for labor.

CHAPTER 17

CRITICAL THINKING IN ACTION: PSYCHOLOGIC AND CULTURAL FACTORS IN TEENAGE PREGNANCY

Sixteen-year-old Linda Perez and her mother present to you at the OB clinic for Linda's first prenatal visit. You determine that Linda is 20 weeks pregnant. Her weight is 135 lb, height 5'4", T 98°F, P 80, R 14, BP 100/64. You assess that Linda's mother has type 2 diabetes, and that her siblings are healthy. Linda admits to having one sexual partner and says she has never been hospitalized. Her immunizations are up to date and she's never used tobacco or recreational drugs. To date, the father of the baby is not involved. Mrs. Perez is clearly upset over the fact that Linda's pregnancy is so far advanced without her knowledge. Linda is very quiet and speaks only when questioned directly. You do your best to try to establish a trusting relationship with Linda and her mother by providing an atmosphere where issues can be discussed.

1. What psychologic factors contribute to teenage pregnancy?	Answer: "Magical thinking," feelings of invincibility, and limited abstract thought processes contribute to the incidence of unplanned pregnancy.
2. Explore reasons why teenagers delay prenatal care.	Answer: Teenagers deny signs and symptoms of pregnancy, feel embarrassed to admit their inability to use birth control, or misuse birth control.
3. Linda's mother asks you what factors facilitate adolescent pregnancies.	Answer: Adolescent pregnancies can be related to cultural norms, peer interaction, immature cognitive abilities, psychologic needs, increasing societal acceptance, and unprotected coitus.
4. You assess that Linda has some anxiety concerning the birth process. She states she is not interested in prenatal classes because she is single and does not want to have natural childbirth. Your best response would be:	Answer: Prenatal classes can teach you relaxation methods and benefits and risks of pain relief methods. This will help you to make the best decision for you. You can bring whoever is going to be with you in labor—a friend, the father of the baby, or your mother.

CHAPTER 18

CRITICAL THINKING IN ACTION: NUTRITIONAL NEEDS OF MOTHER AND FETUS DURING PREGNANCY

Sandra Hill is a 17-year-old at 19 weeks' gestation with her first pregnancy. She presents to you accompanied by her mother. Her mother tells you that Sandra is an active teenager who plays sports and has been taking dance lessons for 5 years. She maintains a "B+" in school. Sandra voices concern about potential weight gain during pregnancy. She tells you that this was not a planned pregnancy and she has ambivalent feelings about it. You become concerned as she tells you that she has reduced her caloric intake over the last few months to try to keep her weight down and camouflage her pregnancy. You do a nutritional assessment and find that she is deficient in calcium, iron, and protein. Sandra seems to have irregular eating patterns and she admits to often skipping breakfast. She asks why she has to gain so much weight when you explain the nutritional needs of her baby during the pregnancy.

1. Discuss weight distribution in pregnancy.	Answer: The average distribution is as follows: 11 lb fetus, placenta, and amniotic fluid; 2 lb uterus; 4 lb increased blood volume; 3 lb breast tissue; and 5–10 lbs maternal stores.
2. Discuss foods that will increase calcium, protein, and iron in her diet.	Answer: A diet that includes 4 cups of milk or servings of fortified orange juice, legumes, nuts, dried fruit, and dark green leafy vegetables will increase calcium. Red meat or dairy products will increase protein. She should take prenatal vitamins to ensure adequate iron and folate intake.
3. Explain why folate supplementation is important.	Answer: Prenatal folate supplementation significantly reduces the risk of neonatal neural tube defects.
4. What criteria will measure adequate caloric intact during pregnancy?	Answer: A satisfactory weight gain.

CHAPTER 19

CRITICAL THINKING IN ACTION: HIV TRANSMISSION TO THE FETUS DURING LABOR: PREVENTION

Jane Adams, a 23-year-old, G3 P2, at 37 weeks' gestation, presents to you in the birthing unit complaining of "vaginal pressure" but no contractions. You assess her and find that her history includes being HIV positive for 2 years, second-trimester cocaine and marijuana use, missed appointments, anemia (Hct 28%), and a positive syphilis serology. Jane tells you that she has other children and that they are being cared for by her mother, who has legal custody of them. You admit Jane and place her on the fetal monitor for evaluation of fetal well-being and contraction patterns. The monitor shows you that the fetal heart rate baseline is 120 to 130 with no decelerations; contractions are mild and irregular lasting 20 to 30 seconds. You obtain vital signs of BP 130/88, temperature 97.0°F P 88 R 14. A vaginal exam determines that Jane is 7 cm dilated at +1 station with intact membranes. She asks you if being HIV positive will affect her labor.

1. Discuss the prophylactic regimen for the prevention of HIV transmission to the fetus during labor.	Answer: To prevent transmission of the HIV virus to the neonate, a loading dose of Zidovudine is given; followed by a continuous infusion of the medication until delivery.
2. Discuss the transmission of HIV to the fetus during pregnancy and birth.	Answer: Transmission of HIV to the fetus can occur antenatally through the placenta, or intrapartum through contact with infected maternal blood or secretions.
3. Identify the emotional impact of HIV infection or other STIs on the woman.	Answer: Their story is often one of fear, anxiety, frustration, anger, shame, and guilt.
4. On postpartum day 2, you inform Jane that her infant is HIV antibody positive. How would you clarify the results?	Answer: Because of placental passage of antibodies, infants born to HIV seropositive mothers will test positive for HIV antibodies whether or not the neonate is actually infected. Positive viral blood cultures are necessary to confirm the diagnosis of HIV infection in the newborn.

CHAPTER 20

CRITICAL THINKING IN ACTION: BED REST AND THE LEFT-SIDE LYING POSITION

Carol Smith, a 40-year-old, single, G2, P0010 presents to you while you are working in the birthing unit, at 32 weeks' gestation. Her chief complaint is severe headache, nausea, and trouble seeing. She describes "blackened areas" in her visual fields bilaterally. Her pre-natal record reveals long-term substance abuse, depression, and hypertension currently treated with nifedipine 60 mg by mouth once in the morning. You note that she has had two prenatal visits with this pregnancy. You determine her blood pressure to be 170/110; deep tendon reflexes are 3+, clonus negative. She has general edema and 3+ proteinuria. You place Carol on the external fetal mon-itor to observe for fetal well-being and any contractions. You position her on her left side with her head elevated and use pillows for comfort. You observe that the fetal heart rate is 143–148 with decreased long-term variability. No fetal heart rate decelerations or ac-celerations are noted. The uterus is soft, and no contractions are palpated or noted on the fetal monitor. Carol asks you why she should stay on her left side.

1. How would you explain the importance of the left-side lying position when on bed rest?	**Answer:** This position decreases pressure on the vena cava, increasing venous return, circu-latory volume, and placenta and renal perfusion. Improved renal flow helps to decrease an-giotension II levels, promotes diuresis, and lowers blood pressure.
2. You administer nifedipine 10 mg sublingual and a loading dose of magnesium sulfate 4 gm IV piggyback to the main IV line of Ringer's lactate. What findings would indicate that Carol has therapeutic levels of magnesium?	**Answer:** You observe for diminished reflexes, decreased respiratory rate, slurring of speech, awkwardness of movement, and decreased appetite.
3. What signs of magnesium toxicity should you monitor Carol for?	**Answer:** Absent deep tendon reflexes, difficulty swallowing, drooling, respirations below 10 and decreased urine output less than 30 cc hour. Calcium gluconate should be at the bedside to reverse magnesium toxicity.
4. Carol asks if magnesium sulfate will affect her infant. How would you answer her?	**Answer:** The newborn may exhibit poor muscle tone, suppressed respiratory effort at birth, and poor sucking. These effects subside as the newborn excretes the drug over 3 to 4 days.
5. Which signs of premature labor would you ask Carol to notify you of if she experiences?	**Answer:** Uterine contractions that occur every 10 minutes or less with or without pain; mild menstrual-like cramps low in the abdomen; constant or intermittent feeling of pelvic pres-sure that feels like the baby is pressing down; rupture of membranes; or constant or inter-mittent low back pain.

CHAPTER 21

CRITICAL THINKING IN ACTION: BIOPHYSICAL PROFILE (BPP) FOR FETAL WELL-BEING

Patricia Adams is a 20-year-old, married, G2, P0010 at 36 weeks' gestation with gestational diabetes. She presents to you during her prenatal visit with a complaint of decreased fetal movement for the "last day or so." Her OB history includes a 13 lb weight gain, hematocrit of 29%, diastolic BP ranging 80–96 mm Hg, and 1+ proteinuria. A 19-week ultrasound demonstrated no fetal anatomic defects. A hemoglobin A1c at 23 weeks was 5.8%. Patricia has had weekly NST since 28 weeks' gestation. You place Patricia on the fetal monitor for a NST. You obtain vital signs of T 97°F, P 88, R 14, BP 130/88. After 30 minutes you observe that the fetal heart rate baseline is 160–165, long-term variability is decreased, and repetitive variable decelerations are occurring. No contractions are noted. The fetus is very active. You notify the physician of the fetal heart rate baseline and unsatisfactory NST. The physician orders a biophysical profile (BPP) for fetal well-being. You describe and explain the biophysical profile test to Patricia.

1. How would you describe and explain the biophysical profile test?	**Answer:** The BPP provides additional information about fetal health. Real-time ultrasound allows visualization of the fetus in its environment and fetal activities. The BPP measures acute and chronic markers of fetal well-being. The five biophysical characteristics are fetal breathing movements, gross body movements, fetal tone reactive, fetal heart rate, and amniotic fluid volume. These five characteristics are evaluated and scored as present (2) or absent (0). Patricia's baby's highest score could only be 8 because of the unsatisfactory NST.

2. To heighten Patricia's awareness of fetal movement, how would you instruct her to do a daily fetal movement record (FMR)?	Answer: For consistency, the FMC should be done the same time each day. Most fetal movement tends to be in the evening. Start by recording the day and time; then lie in the left lateral position, preferably after a meal or when the baby is most active. Place your hand over the abdomen to feel the baby's movement. Mark every movement the baby makes. Remain in this position until you have counted 10 movements. Record the end time. Bring the card with you to your next visit.
3. Explain when Patricia should contact her care provider.	Answer: If 10 movements are not obtained within 3 hours; if overall the fetus's movements are slowing, and it takes much longer each day to note 10 movements; if there are no movements in the morning; or if there are fewer than 3 movements in 8 hours.
4. Discuss the significance of fetal movement.	Answer: Maternal perception of fetal movement correlates with fetal well-being. From 24 weeks until term, frequency of fetal movement is consistent if the fetus is not compromised. Decreased fetal movement is associated with more complications during the intrapartum period or in the newborn after birth.
5. Explore factors that decrease fetal movements.	Answer: Fetal and placental factors that influence fetal movement include congenital abnormalities, decreased placenta perfusion due to maternal disease, and fetal demise. Maternal use of barbiturates, alcohol, methadone, narcotics, or cigarettes will decrease fetal movements. Decreased movement may also be due to fetal sleep cycles or to inactivity during a particular time of day.

CHAPTER 22

CRITICAL THINKING IN ACTION: CERVICAL RIPENING USING PROSTAGLANDIN GEL

Ann Nelson, a 28-year-old, G2, P0010 at 41 weeks' gestation, is admitted to the birthing unit where you are working. She is here for cervical ripening and induction of labor due to postdate pregnancy and decreased amniotic fluid volume. A review of her prenatal chart reveals a pertinent history of infertility (Clomid-induced pregnancy) and asthma (treated with inhalers on a PRN basis). The Doppler picks up a fetal heart rate of 120 bpm. You place Ann on the electronic fetal monitor and obtain the following data: BP 126/76, T 98°F, P 82, R 16; vaginal exam reveals a 20% effaced cervix, 1 cm dilatation in the posterior position, and vertex at –2 station. The fetal monitor shows a fetal heart rate baseline of 120 to 128 with occasional variable decelerations, accelerations to 140 with fetal activity. No contractions are noted on the monitor or palpated. Ann asks you what to expect with "cervical ripening" using prostaglandin gel.

1. Discuss the action of prostaglandin gel.	Answer: The prostaglandin gel is expected to soften and efface the cervix, change the cervix from posterior to midposition, and provide cervical dilatation. If uterine activity is initiated, it is expected to improve the fetal station as well.
2. Ann asks you why cervical ripening and induction of labor are recommended for her and her baby. How would you best respond to her?	Answer: Postdate pregnancy is associated with perinatal morbidity and mortality such as neonatal jaundice, neonatal low blood sugar, temperature instability, respiratory distress, meconium aspiration syndrome, birth trauma secondary to macrosomia, and neonatal asphyxia.
3. Ann asks how she will know if she is getting contractions. How would you answer her?	Answer: Uterine contractions are felt in the lower abdominal wall and in the area over the lower lumbar and upper sacrum region. It may start in the front and radiate to the back, or start in the back and radiate to the front. In the latent stage, it may feel like cramping.
4. Discuss the difference between mild, moderate, and strong contractions.	Answer: During the peak of the contraction, the uterine fundus is palpated to estimate the intensity of the contraction. During mild contraction, the uterine wall can be indented easily; during a strong contraction, the uterine wall cannot be indented. A contraction of moderate intensity falls between mild and strong.
5. Describe the latent phase of labor.	Answer: The latent phase of labor starts with the beginning of regular uterine contractions which are usually mild, lasting 30 seconds with a frequency of 10 to 20 minutes. The contractions progress to moderate ones, lasting 30 to 40 seconds with a frequency of 5 to 7 minutes. The cervix begins to efface and dilate.

CHAPTER 23

CRITICAL THINKING IN ACTION: BENEFITS OF AMBULATION DURING LABOR

Cindy Bell, a 20-year-old Gravida 2 para 1, 40 weeks gestation, presents to you in the birthing unit with contractions every 5 to 7 minutes. She is accompanied by her husband. Spontaneous rupture of membranes occurred 2 hours prior to admission. Cindy tells you that the fluid was colorless and clear. You orient Cindy and her family to the birthing room, and perform a physical assessment, documenting the following data: Vital signs are normal. A vaginal exam reveals that the cervix is 75% effaced, 4 cm dilated with a vertex at −1 station in the LOP position. You place Cindy on an external fetal monitor. The fetal heart rate baseline is 140–147 with accelerations to 156, no decelerations are noted. Contractions are 5–6 minutes apart, of moderate intensity and lasting 40 to 50 seconds. Cindy states she would like to stay out of bed as long as possible because lying down seems to make the contractions more painful, especially in her back.

1. Discuss the benefits of ambulation in labor.	Answer: Ambulation may assist in labor progression by stimulating contractions and allowing gravity to help with the descent of the fetus. Ambulating may be more comfortable for the woman and may give her a sense of independence and control.
2. Cindy would like her daughter to be present for the baby's birth. What would you discuss with her about the impact of having a young sibling present during labor and birth?	Answer: It is important that a young child have her own support person whose sole responsibility is tending to the child's needs. This person must be prepared to interpret what is happening for the child and to intervene when necessary. Being present at the birth seems to increase siblings' acceptance of the new baby.
3. What fetal heart rate assessment will best ensure fetal well-being during the period Cindy is ambulating?	Answer: Perform intermittent auscultation every 15 minutes with an ultrasound or a fetoscope. Listen to the fetal heart during a contraction and 30 seconds after the contraction to identify nonreassuring heart pattern.
4. When a nonreassuring fetal heart pattern is detected, what remedial nursing intervention is carried out?	Answer: Change position, preferably on the left side, give IV fluids, administer oxygen by tight-fitting mask, discontinue oxytocics, and notify the physician.
5. What are indications for continuous fetal monitoring in labor?	Answer: Indications include previous history of a stillbirth at 38 or more weeks' gestation, presence of a complication of pregnancy, induction of labor, preterm birth, decreased fetal movement, nonreassuring fetal status, meconium-stained amniotic fluid, and trial of labor following a previous cesarean birth.

CHAPTER 24

CRITICAL THINKING IN ACTION: LABOR STRESS AND ANXIETY REDUCTION

Anita Grey, a 22-year-old primigravida at 40 weeks' gestation, is admitted to you in the birthing center in labor. Anita was sent from her physician's office after being evaluated at her prenatal visit. While in the office, she was assessed to be 4 cm dilated, 100% effaced, vertex at 0 station with bulging membranes. She tells you that her husband is on his way to the birthing center and she is anxious for him to arrive. A review of her prenatal record shows no complications affecting this pregnancy. Anita's vital signs are within normal limits. You assess the fetal heart rate and contraction pattern with the fetal monitor and observe a fetal heart rate of 140 to 150 bpm with accelerations to 160s. Contractions are every 3 to 4 minutes × 30 seconds of moderate intensity by palpation. Anita seems to be tolerating the contractions well, but still seems anxious about her husband's arrival.

1. What steps can you take to reduce the stress and anxiety of the laboring woman and her family?	Answer: You introduce yourself and escort the woman and her family to the birthing room and provide an orientation which includes location of restrooms, public phones, and nurse call or emergency call system. You explain the monitor equipment and other unfamiliar technology. You provide an environment which is quiet and feels safe.
2. When you notify the physician/midwife, what pertinent information should the report contain?	Answer: Pertinent information includes parity, cervical dilatation and effacement, station, presenting part, status of membranes, contraction pattern, fetal heart rate, abnormal vital signs, any significant prenatal history, and her preference for pain relief.

3. What support measures can you give in the active phase of labor?	Answer: Support and encourage breathing patterns, provide a quiet environment, provide reassurance, keep couple informed of progress. Promote comfort with back rubs, sacral pressure, and cool cloths. Assist with position changes, support with pillows, and effleurage. Provide ice chips for dry mouth. Encourage to void every 1–2 hours. Offer shower/whirlpool/warm bath if available.
4. What measures can be used to decrease discomfort/pain as labor progresses?	Answer: Ensure general comfort, provide information to decrease anxiety, use specific supportive relaxation techniques, encourage controlled breathing, and administer pharmacologic agents as ordered by physician/CNM.
5. What observations reflect the physiologic manifestations of pain?	Answer: Assess for increased pulse and respiratory rates, dilated pupils, increased blood pressure, and muscle tension.

CHAPTER 25

CRITICAL THINKING IN ACTION: REGIONAL ANALGESIA DURING LABOR AND BIRTH

Sandra, a 26-year-old G1 P0000, is in active labor when she presents to you at the birthing center. She has been in labor for 5 hours and is clearly tired and seems to be having difficulty coping with the pain. Her contractions are occurring every 2 to 4 minutes lasting 50 to 60 seconds, and are moderate to strong in intensity. You assess the fetal heart rate of 120 to 130 with early decelerations; moderate long-term variability is present. Sandra's vital signs are stable and her laboratory results are within normal limits. She is requesting an epidural analgesia for pain control. A vaginal exam demonstrates the cervix is 100% effaced, 6 cm dilated with the vertex at 0 station in the LOT position. You notify the physician of Sandra's wish for pain relief and labor progress. You review the client's record for written consent for regional analgesia and assist the anesthesiologist with the procedure.

1. Discuss the advantages of regional analgesia.	Answer: Regional analgesia relieves discomfort during labor and birth. The woman is fully awake and can participate in the birth process.
2. Describe the nursing responsibility during the administration of regional analgesia.	Answer: Provide hydration with 500–100 mL of intravenous solution and encourage the woman to void prior to starting the procedure; assist her with positioning during and after the procedure; monitor and assess maternal vital signs and respiratory status; monitor analgesic effect and determine fetal well-being. Provide reassurance and thorough explanations to help decrease anxiety and fear.
3. Discuss the side effects of regional analgesia.	Answer: The anesthetic agents may interfere with blood pressure stability, leg movements, and the ability to void. Some women experience pruritus, nausea, and vomiting.
4. What are the absolute contraindications for an epidural block?	Answer: Contraindications are client refusal, infection at the site of needle puncture, coagulopathies, specific drug allergies to the agents being used, and hypovolemic shock.
5. How do you assist Sandra with the second stage of labor when she cannot feel her contractions?	Answer: Help her to get into a pushing position and place her hand on her abdomen to feel when a contraction begins. Instruct her to bear down with the contraction. Give her extra assistance by holding her legs up and apart. Inform her when the contraction is over and encourage her to lay back and rest until the next contraction begins.

CHAPTER 26

CRITICAL THINKING IN ACTION: OXYTOCIN LABOR INDUCTION OR AUGMENTATION

June Dice, a 25-year-old G3, P1011, is admitted to you in labor and delivery at 38 weeks with a moderate amount of dark red vaginal bleeding. June's prenatal history is significant for late prenatal care (20 weeks' gestation by ultrasound) and cocaine abuse. An ultrasound is done upon admission which demonstrates a marginal placenta abruption. You place June on the fetal monitor and observe a fetal heart rate baseline of 146 to 155 with accelerations to 166 with fetal movement. There are occasional mild variable decelerations with a quick return to baseline. Contraction pattern is interpreted as an irritable uterus. An intravenous infusion with Ringer's lactate is started with a #18 intracath. June's vital signs are within normal limits. Her hematocrit is 29%. You assist the physician with a vaginal exam to rupture membranes and insert a fetal scalp electrode and intrauterine pressure catheter. A small amount of light yellow-green amniotic fluid is observed. The exam shows June is 4 cm dilated, 50% effaced, vertex at −1 station. You follow protocol and start an oxytocin induction/augmentation. June is asking why oxytocin is needed.

1. Explain the goal of labor induction/augmentation in response to June's question.	Answer: The goal of oxytocin augmentation/induction is to establish an adequate contraction pattern that would promote cervical dilatation. A contraction pattern of three contractions in 10 minutes lasting 40 to 60 seconds with an intensity of 25 to 75 mm Hg intrauterine pressure is adequate for labor progression.

2. Explain potential risk factors associated with oxytocin induction of labor.	Answer: Observe for uterine hyperstimulation (contractions occurring more frequently than every 2 minutes or lasting longer than 90 seconds), uterine hyperactivity (tachysystole, skewed contractions, polysystole, coupled contractions, tetanic contractions), uterine hypertonus (elevated resting tone, 20 mm Hg), uterine rupture, and nonreassuring fetal heart rate patterns.
3. You observe a nonreassuring fetal heart rate of 144 to 150 with decreased variability, and persistent late decelerations with each contraction. What interventions would you immediately take?	Answer: Assist the woman to turn to a left lateral position, increase the rate of the IV infusion, discontinue oxytocin, and administer oxygen by tight face mask. Perform a vaginal examination for fetal scalp stimulation to obtain further information about the condition of the fetus. Notify the physician of your observations.
4. What supportive actions are taken to decrease the risk of hypofibrinogenemia?	Answer: You would obtain blood work for type and crossmatch for blood transfusions, evaluating the blood clotting mechanism (pt, ptt, and fibrin index), platelet and hemoglobin counts, and provide intravenous fluids.
5. What complications might be present in the newborn at birth?	Answer: Anemia and hypoxia.

CHAPTER 27

CRITICAL THINKING IN ACTION: CEPHALIC VERSION PROCEDURE (EXTERNAL)

Betsy Jones, a 28-year-old G1 P0 at 39 weeks' gestation, and her husband present to you in the labor suite for an external cephalic version procedure by her obstetrician. You introduce yourself and review her record for any significant risk factors or contraindications to the version procedure. Her prenatal chart is significant in that the fetus has been in a persistent frank breech position. You encourage Betsy and her husband to express their understanding and expectations of the procedure. You discuss certain criteria to be met prior to the procedure and obtain vital signs as follows: T 98.8°F, P 88, R 14, BP 110/80, urine screening negative for sugar, albumin, and ketones. You place Betsy on the external electronic fetal monitor which demonstrates a fetal heart rate baseline of 140 to 152 with moderate long-term variability. There are no contractions observed by the monitor or Betsy. After explaining how to record fetal movement on the monitor, you proceed with an NST.

1. Explain the contraindications to the version procedure.	Answer: The woman has no pregnancy problems such as uterine anomalies, uncontrolled preeclampsia, or third-trimester bleeding. There are no complications of pregnancy such as ruptured membranes, oligohydramnios, hydramnios, or placenta previa present. There is no previous cesarean birth or other significant uterine surgery. The pregnancy is a singleton gestation with no fetal abnormalities such as intrauterine growth restriction, nuchal cord, or nonreassuring fetal heart rate.
2. Discuss the criteria that should be met prior to performing external version.	Answer: The pregnancy is 36 weeks' gestation or more. The fetal breech is not engaged. An ultrasound is done to locate the placenta and confirm fetal presentation. A nonstress test is reactive.
3. How would you explain to Betsy and her husband what to expect during the version procedure?	Answer: Explain that before the version begins, you will help her into a comfortable semisitting position on the labor bed. You will start an intravenous line to give her medications if necessary. She will receive an injection of terbutaline to relax the uterus. If she has severe pain or there is a significant slowing or deceleration of the fetal heart rate, the procedure will be discontinued. There is the possibility of failure of the version and slight risk of cesarean birth if the fetal heart rate becomes nonreassuring.
4. What support would you give Betsy during the procedure?	Answer: You continue to monitor maternal blood pressure, pulse, and comfort level frequently. Fetal well-being is ascertained before, intermittently during, and for 30 minutes following the procedure, using electronic fetal monitoring, ultrasound, or both. Because the procedure can be uncomfortable, encourage the mother to take slow deep breaths and relax her abdominal muscles. Use distractions and speak in a calm reassuring voice to help decrease fear and anxiety.
5. Explain postversion discharge teaching.	Answer: Explain to the mother how to monitor for contractions. Describe mild, moderate, and strong contractions. Teach the mother to observe and record fetal kick counts. Advise the mother to notify her physician if her water breaks or if she experiences any vaginal bleeding or signs of labor.

CHAPTER 28

CRITICAL THINKING IN ACTION: NEWBORN ASSESSMENT

Sandra Dee, a 21-year-old, G1, P0000, at 36 weeks' gestation, has been in labor for the last 12 hours and is fully dilated with caput visible on the perineum. The fetal heart rate is 148 to 152 with early deceleration down to 142 with contraction and pushing. Her contractions are 4 to 5 minutes apart of good quality. Sandra's mother and sister are present for the birth. Her prenatal record shows no significant pregnancy problems or complications, and her vital signs have been stable within normal limits. Sandra has received two doses of Stadol for a total of 2 mg IV for pain relief during her labor. The last dose was given 2 hours ago. You assist with the vaginal birth of a live baby without an episiotomy. You observe the sex and time as the midwife places the infant girl on the mother's abdomen, suctions out the baby's mouth and nose, and proceeds to clamp the cord. You dry and stimulate the infant to breathe, remove the wet blanket and replace it with a dry one, and place the infant skin to skin on the mother's chest. You assess the need for infant resuscitation. The baby has a lusty cry spontaneously less than 30 seconds after birth. You palpate the cord obtaining a heart rate of 120, and observe that the baby's chest and face are pink, and the legs and arms are flexed with open fist.

1. Explain the changes that must occur in the infant's cardiopulmonary system at birth.	Answer: Pulmonary ventilation is established through lung expansion with the first inspiration in response to mechanical, chemical, thermal, and sensory changes associated with birth. A marked increase in pulmonary circulation occurs as PO_2 rises in the aveoli, relaxing pulmonary arteries and triggering a decrease in pulmonary vascular resistance.
2. What criteria do you look for when you assess the newborn for adequate cardiopulmonary adaptation at birth?	Answer: You determine that the infant's airway is clear. The infant has a good quality cry (has respirations). The infant's color is pink and the muscle tone is good (arms and legs are flexed with fists open or clenched). You use the Apgar score at 1 and 5 minutes to monitor that the infant's condition is stable or improving.
3. What steps do you take to maintain a neutral thermal environment at birth?	Answer: The delivery room should be warm. You would ensure any equipment/ linens to be used on the infant are warmed. Place the infant under a radiant heater or skin to skin on the mother's abdomen or chest. Dry the infant with a warm blanket immediately after birth, remove the wet blanket, and cover the infant with a dry blanket. Place a warm cap on the infant's head.
4. Sandra plans to breastfeed. When would you initiate the first feeding?	Answer: The newborn has the first period of reactivity approximately 30 minutes after birth. During this period the infant is awake and alert. This is a natural time to have the mother and infant together. You assist the mother to bring the infant to the breast. The infant may root and latch on or just root and lick the nipple.
5. Discuss nursing actions that can decrease the probability of high bilirubin levels in the newborn.	Answer: Maintain the infant's skin temperature at 97.8°F or above; monitor for stooling in character and amount; encourage early feeding to promote intestinal elimination and ensure adequate caloric intake.

CHAPTER 29

CRITICAL THINKING IN ACTION: MOTHER LEARNS ABOUT HER NEWBORN

Susan Pine, a 21-year-old G2, now P1011, delivers a 39-week-old female newborn. The vaginal birth is assisted with a vacuum extractor. The prenatal record is significant for an increase of maternal blood pressure to 140/90 on the day of birth. Susan is treated with magnesium sulfate during her labor and has an epidural analgesia for the pain of labor. The baby's Apgar is 8 and 9 at 1 and 5 minutes, and she has been admitted to the newborn nursery. The newborn's admission exam is normal except for a 2-cm round caput. Now, 8 hours later, the baby's condition is stable and she needs to be bottle-fed. You take her to her mother's room where you observe that Susan does not reach out to take her from you. She seems unsure when handling her baby. Susan asks you about the swelling on her baby's head and wonders if it will ever go away.

1. How would you explain the cause of Susan's baby's caput succedaneum?	The swelled area is from the vacuum extraction of the baby's head at birth. The pressure of the vacuum caused compression of blood vessels in the baby's scalp, which caused an increase in tissue fluids and a small amount of bleeding under the skin. The swelled area feels soft and mushy, but this will be absorbed after a few days.
2. Compare the difference between a cephalhematoma and caput succedaneum.	Answer: Cephalhematoma does not cross a suture line, whereas a caput succedaneum does. Caput succedaneum is present at birth; cephalhematomas emerge as defined hematomas between the first and second day.
3. Explore with Susan her baby's reflexes and state of alertness.	Answer: Show the mother the grasping, Moro, rooting, sucking, and stepping reflexes to demonstrate what her baby can do. Point out that in the quiet awake state, her baby is alert and fixates on her face and attends to her voice. Advise that this is the best time to interact with the baby.

4. Susan asks you how she will know what her baby needs. How would you respond?	Answer: Crying is the infant's main method of communicating. Heat, cold, or hunger stimulates the baby to wakefulness. Crying lets you know that she is awake and wants attention. By responding to the baby's cry, the mother will learn what different cries mean such as if the baby is cold, is hungry, or just wants to be held.

CHAPTER 30

CRITICAL THINKING IN ACTION: INSTRUCTING THE MOTHER IN THE CARE OF HER NEWBORN

Alice Fine, age 32, G1, now P1001, spontaneously delivers a 7.25 pound baby girl over a median episiotomy. The baby's Apgars are 7 and 9 at 1 and 5 minutes. The baby is suctioned, stimulated, and given free flow oxygen at birth. As the nurse on duty, you admit baby Fine to the newborn nursery, place her under a radiant heater, and perform a newborn assessment. You obtain the vital signs of temperature 97°F, heart rate 128, respiration 55. A physical exam demonstrates no abnormalities, and you note that there were no significant problems with the pregnancy, the mother's blood type is A+, and she plans to bottle-feed. You monitor the baby until her vital signs are stable and then take her to the mother's room for her first bottle-feeding at 60 minutes old.

1. How would you review measures to promote the safety of the newborn from abduction?	Answer: Inform the mother that the identification bands will be checked each time the baby is brought to her room. She should allow only the people with the proper birthing unit identification to remove the baby from the room. Only the parents or a person with identification bands should bring the baby to the nursery. Advise her not to leave the baby alone in the room.
2. How would you explain the technique to suction the newborn with a bulb syringe?	Answer: Explain to the mother that most newborns are obligatory nose breathers for the first months of life. Newborns can cough or sneeze to clear their airway. However, during the first few days of life, the newborn has increased mucus. Gentle suction with a bulb syringe may be needed. You turn the baby on its side, squeeze the syringe, place the tip in the side (by the cheek) of the mouth, release the bulb, and then squeeze the mucus out onto a tissue. Gently do the same to each nostril. The bulb should be rinsed out after each use.
3. Describe the care of the newborn's cord.	Answer: Instruct the mother to keep the cord clean and dry; fold down the diaper to avoid covering the cord stump which will prevent soiling of the area and promote drying. Contact your physician if you observe signs of infection such as a foul smell, redness and drainage, localized warmth and tenderness, or bleeding.
4. How would you review bottle-feeding with the mother?	Answer: The infant is held for all feedings to provide social and physical contact. Point the nipple directly into the infant's mouth directly on top of the tongue. The nipple should be full of formula at all times to prevent ingestion of extra air. The infant is burped at intervals, preferably at the middle and end of the feeding. Gently pat or stroke the infant's back while holding her upright on the shoulder or in a sitting position on the mother's lap. Advise the mother that newborns frequently regurgitate small amounts of feeding which initially may be due to excessive mucus; keep a "burp cloth" available.

CHAPTER 31

CRITICAL THINKING IN ACTION: BREASTFEEDING TECHNIQUES

Patty Kline, age 28, G1, now P1, delivers a 7.3 pound baby girl by spontaneous vaginal birth over a median episiotomy. The newborn's Apgar scores are 8 and 9 at 1 and 5 minutes. The infant is suctioned in the nose and mouth and given free flow oxygen on the mother's abdomen. Patty received an epidural during labor and birth. Patty initiated breastfeeding within the first hour after the birth, but at that time the newborn did not latch on. The infant was held to the mother's breast, rooted, and licked the nipple. You are the nurse caring for the infant at 2 hours of age. The admission assessment is significant for asymmetric head with a 3-cm caput succedaneum. The infant's temperature is stable. You bring the infant to the mother's room to assist her with breastfeeding.

1. Describe clues that indicate the infant is ready to breastfeed with the mother.	Answer: Early clues that indicate an infant is interested in feeding include hand-to-mouth or hand-passing-mouth motion, whimpering, sucking, and rooting. Advise the mother that crying is a late sign of hunger and may make it more difficult to get the infant latched on if she waits for the infant to cry.
2. How would you explain how to position the infant at the breast?	Answer: The mother should be in a comfortable position with her arms supported. Unwrap the blanket so that the infant is close to the mother's breast. Turn the infant's entire body toward the mother with the infant's mouth adjacent to the mother's nipple. The infant's ear, shoulder, and hip should be in direct alignment. Bring the infant to the mother's breast; tickle the infant's lower lip with her nipple until the infant opens her mouth wide. Direct the nipple straight into the infant's mouth so that during sucking the infant's jaw compresses the ducts directly beneath the areola.

3. Explain what to observe for the infant's proper latch on.	Answer: The infant's nose and chin should touch the breast. If the breast occludes the infant's airway, lifting up the breast will clear the nares. The infant's lips should be relaxed and flanged outward with the tongue over the lower gum.
4. Explain the basics of milk production.	Answer: Breast milk is produced according to demand. The milk is stored in the sinus under the areola. The mother requires adequate fluids to replenish her supply. The milk supply is best established by frequent feedings every $1^1/_2$ to 2 hours. The letdown reflex for the release of milk is initiated by the infant's sucking.
5. Explore helpful measures the mother can attempt in support of breastfeeding.	Answer: Suggest that the infant is awake before attempting to feed; alternate the breast at which the feeding begins; rotate the infant's position at the breast to avoid trauma to the nipples and improve emptying of the ducts. During early feedings, the infant should be offered both breasts at each feeding to stimulate the supply-demand response. Avoid supplementary formula-feeding and pacifiers until lactation is established to prevent nipple confusion in the infant.

CHAPTER 32

CRITICAL THINKING IN ACTION: BIRTH OF AN ILL OR AT-RISK INFANT

As the nurse on duty, you are caring for baby Erin, a 38-week IDM female born by repeat cesarean birth to a 32-year-old G3 now P3 mother. Erin's Apgar scores are 7 and 9 at 1 and 5 minutes. At 2 hours of age, the baby has an elevated respiratory rate of 100 to 110, heart rate of 165 with Grade II/VI intermittent machinery murmur and mild cyanosis. She is now receiving 30% oxygen and has a respiratory rate of 70 to 800. The baby's clinical course, chest x-ray, and lab results are all consistent with transient tachypnea of the newborn and patent ductus arteriosus. The mother calls you to ask about how her baby is doing. She tells you that her last child was born at 30 weeks and had to be hospitalized for 6 weeks. She says, "I really tried to do it right this time," and asks you if this baby will have the same respiratory problem.

1. What should you tell the mother?	Answer: It is important to give the mother clear, factual information regarding the type, cause, and usual course of the infant's respiratory problems. You explain that the infant's laboratory test, chest x-ray, and clinical course are indicative of transient tachypnea of the newborn. Respiratory distress syndrome is probably not the problem since the infant is not premature.
2. What can you do to facilitate mother–infant attachment?	Answer: When transporting the mother from the recovery room, have the mother stop at the nursery so she can see and if possible touch her infant. Give the mother pictures so she can show her baby to visitors and family members. Ask her if she has a name for the infant and call the infant by name.
3. Discuss the emotional response of parents to the birth of an ill or at-risk infant.	Answer: The birth of an ill or at-risk infant is a serious crisis for parents. Each parent experiences an acute grief reaction which follows the loss of the fantasized perfect baby. Parents express grief as shock, disbelief, denial of reality, anger toward self and others, guilt, blame, and concern for the future.
4. Discuss the four psychologic tasks essential for coping with the stress of an at-risk newborn and providing a basis for the maternal-infant relationship (also see discussion in Chapter 31).	Answer: (1) The mother experiences anticipatory grief in preparation for the possible loss of her infant while hoping for her survival. (2) Acknowledgment of the mother's failure to produce a term or perfect newborn expressed as anticipatory grief and depression lasting until the chance of survival is secure. (3) Resumption of the process of relating to the infant. (4) Understanding of the potential special needs and growth pattern of the at-risk infant.
5. Baby Flynn is being discharged tomorrow. Review the elements of discharge and home care instructions.	Answer: Teach the parents routine well-baby care such as bathing, taking a temperature, cord care, preparing formula, and safety for the infant. Arrange for medical follow-up care; make the appointment if possible.

CHAPTER 33

CRITICAL THINKING IN ACTION: PHOTOTHERAPY WITH FIBEROPTIC BLANKET

Rebecca Prince, age 21, G2 now P2, gives birth to a 5-lb baby at 38 weeks' gestation by primary cesarean birth for fetal distress. The infant's Apgars are 7 and 9 at 1 and 5 minutes. The infant is suctioned and given free flow oxygen at birth, then is admitted to the newborn nursery for transitional care and does well. You are the nurse caring for baby Prince at 36 hours old. You review the newborn's record and note that the baby's blood type is A+ and his mother is O+. Rebecca wants to breastfeed. You are performing a shift assessment on Baby Prince when you observe the infant has a unilateral cephalhematoma and is lethargic. You blanch the skin over the sternum and observe a yellow discoloration of the skin. Lab tests reveal a serum bilirubin level of 12 mg/dL, hematocrit 55%, a mildly positive direct Coombs' test, and a positive indirect Coombs' test. Baby Prince is diagnosed with hyperbilirubinemia secondary to ABO incompatibility and cephalhematoma. You provide phototherapy by fiberoptic blanket around the trunk of the infant and take the baby to his mother's room.

1. How would you explain the purpose of phototherapy with the mother?	Answer: Exposure of the newborn to high-intensity light decreases serum bilirubin levels in the skin by facilitating bilary excretion of unconjugated bilirubin. The infant's bilirubin will be lowered by excretion in the stool and urine.
2. Describe the care the mother can give to the newborn.	Answer: Encourage the mother to breastfeed the newborn every 2 to 3 hours to increase the intestinal motility, promote the excretion of unconjugated bilirubin through the clearance of stools, and prevent dehydration. Advise the mother that the infant's stool will change to loose and green color due to the bilirubin. Request that the mother track the number of stools and voids.
3. Discuss the advantage of the fiberoptic blanket phototherapy for the newborn.	Answer: Phototherapy can be provided to the newborn while allowing the newborn to be more accessible to the mother for feedings, holding, and diapering. The blanket eliminates the need for eye patches and allows the newborn to be fully clothed and wrapped, which decreases heat loss. Use of the blanket is less alarming to the parents.
4. Newborns up to 1 month of age are susceptible to organisms that do not cause significant disease in older children. Explore the circumstances that cause susceptibility to infection.	Answer: The newborn's immunologic systems are immature. They lack the complex factors involved in effective phagocytosis and the ability to localize infection or to respond with a well-defined recognizable inflammatory response. All newborns lack IgM immunoglobulin to protect against bacteria because it does not cross the placenta.
5. Describe how to distinguish between oral thrush and milk curds.	Answer: Differentiate white plaque of candidal infection from milk curds by rubbing a cotton tip applicator to the suspect plaque. If it is thrush, removal of the white areas causes raw bleeding areas.

CHAPTER 34

CRITICAL THINKING IN ACTION: POSTPARTAL CARE PROCEDURES FOR THE NEW MOTHER

Janet Burns, a 25-year-old G3 P3, is 2 hours past a low forceps vaginal birth with a right medial lateral episiotomy of a live 8-pound baby boy. You obtain vital signs of BP 118/70, T 98.8°F, P 76, R 14. You observe the fundus is +1 finger above the umbilicus and slightly to the right. Her episiotomy is slightly ecchymotic and well approximated without edema or discharge. Ice has been applied to the episiotomy for the last 20 minutes. Lochia rubra is present and a pad was saturated in 90 minutes. Janet has an intravenous of Ringer's lactate with 10 units of Pitocin infusing at 100 mL/hr in her lower left arm and is complaining of moderate abdominal cramping. She tells you that she is very tired and requests some pain medication so she can sleep for a while.

1. What nursing assessment is of immediate concern?	Answer: A uterus that is above the umbilicus and deviated to the side may indicate that the bladder is full and Janet needs to urinate. Woman often lose their sense of bladder fullness and urge to void after a long second stage with the fetus pressing down on the bladder and meatus. Using nursing interventions, you assist Janet to void. You determine if she has any difficulty urinating or emptying her bladder. After Janet voids, you reassess the uterus for firmness and location. You should not feel the bladder in the lower abdomen.
2. Discuss care of her episiotomy and perineum.	Answer: Demonstrate and describe how to use the perineal rinse bottle to spray warm water from the front (at the symphysis pubis) to the back (around the anus) and pat dry with toilet paper. Encourage the use of witch hazel pads or analgesia ointment over the episiotomy. Apply the pad from front to back. Ice wrapped in gauze can be applied to the episiotomy to decrease edema and discomfort.
3. What other self-care measures could you advise?	Answer: Advise she should call for assistance the first time she gets out of bed as she might experience some dizziness. Encourage the woman to request analgesic medications for discomfort for afterbirth or episiotomy pain. Encourage fluids and snacks. Demonstrate gentle uterine massage and explain changes in lochia. Encourage frequent perineal pad change and use of the perineal rinse bottle, especially after voiding. Keep the perineum clean and dry. Encourage frequent rest periods.
4. Discuss postpartal occurrences that may cause special concern for the mother.	Answer: Explain that a gush of blood that sometimes occurs when she first gets up is due to pooling of blood in the vagina when a woman lies down for a period of time. As the body attempts to eliminate excess fluids that were present during pregnancy, night sweats might occur. Afterbirth pains are more common in multiparas due to uterine contractions.

5. Janet expressed concern about her episiotomy healing. What information can you offer?	Answer: Provide information about the location of the episiotomy. Explain that the sutures will not have to be removed. The sutures will dissolve slowly over the next few weeks as the tissue heals. By the time the sutures are dissolved, the tissues are strong and the incision edges will not separate.

CHAPTER 35

CRITICAL THINKING IN ACTION: POSTPARTUM CONCERNS

Wendy Calahan, a 31-year-old G3, P2, gave birth to an 8.5 pound baby boy by primary cesarean birth for failure to progress. The baby's Apgar score was 9 and 9 at 1 and 5 minutes. The baby was admitted to the newborn nursery for transitional observation. Wendy was transferred to the postpartum unit where you assume her care. You introduce yourself and orient her to the room, call bell, and safety measures. You perform an initial assessment, with all findings within normal limits. Wendy tells you she is very tired and would like to rest while her baby is in the nursery. Her husband and family have left the hospital after spending time with her in the recovery room but will return later. She admits she is disappointed that she could not give birth vaginally even though she pushed for 2 hours. She says, "This baby was just too big."

1. How would you discuss with Wendy the need for frequent assessments after birth?	Answer: Explain that you will assess the mother's fundus, lochia, dressing, vital signs, and comfort level every 30 minutes the next hour, then every hour for 2 hours, and every 4 hours during the rest of her stay to monitor her transition from pregnant to nonpregnant condition.
2. Explain "maternity or baby blues."	Answer: Maternity or baby blues are transient, emotional disturbances commonly occurring around the second or fourth postpartum day, lasting a few hours to 2 weeks. Physiologic factors are rapid hormonal changes, lack of sleep and less effective sleep, and increased energy expenditure.
3. Explore activities to minimize maternity blues.	Answer: Suggest that the mother allow family and friends to help with household tasks and care for older children. She should get plenty of rest, eat a well-balanced diet, drink plenty of fluids but limit caffeine intake, continue taking her prenatal vitamins, perform light exercise daily, ensure some personal time and adult relationships, and avail herself of support groups and other community resources.
4. Discuss concerns of a woman experiencing her second pregnancy.	Answer: Concern for the first child may cause grieving over the dyadic relationship with the first child and her anticipation of the first child's pain. Managing the care of two children may cause a mother to feel overwhelmed. She may have increased expectations of the first child and may doubt her own ability to love two children equally. The second pregnancy may not be as exciting or as desired as the first.
5. Discuss behaviors that inhibit paternal attachment.	Answer: Observe for difficulty adjusting to a new dependent, for failure to relate to the infant, for escape mechanisms such as alcohol and drugs, and for separation from mother and infant because of business or military responsibilities.

CHAPTER 36

CRITICAL THINKING IN ACTION: HOME POSTPARTUM VISIT

Jane Benne, age 23, gravida 1 para 1 gave birth by cesarean for cephalopelvic disproportion to a healthy 7 pound 1 ounce baby boy 5 days ago. You are making a home visit 2 days after Jane was discharged from the hospital to her two-story home. When you arrive the baby is sleeping in a bassinet in Jane's bedroom on the second level. Jane has been trying to breastfeed and complains to you of sore nipples and swollen breasts. She is also having problems getting the baby to latch on and says that she has been supplementing her baby's feedings with a bottle because she is afraid her baby is not getting enough milk from her breasts alone. She also mentions that the baby seems more satisfied after she gives the bottle and seems to sleep longer. You ask her how she has been feeling, and she tells you that she is very tired and upset about her body not making enough milk to feed her child. You assess Jane's breasts and find them to be full and firm, but the nipples are cracked and blistered.

1. What is your focus in the home postpartum visit?	Answer: Home care is focused on assessment, teaching, and counseling the mother and her family rather than on physical care. You assess the mother and infant for signs of complications; the parents' adaptation to the new baby and their skill in bathing, dressing, handling, and comforting the newborn; and the safety of the home environment. You provide answers to questions about infant feedings, provide support and encouragement, and address the need for referrals.

2. What counseling can you give Jane regarding her sore nipples?	Answer: Suggest Jane express some of her milk to soften the breast so the baby can latch on. Observe that the baby is positioned correctly on the breast and alternate positions are used with each feeding. Observe that the nipple and some of the areola is in the baby's mouth. Encourage the mother to hold the baby closely during feedings so the nipple is not constantly being pulled. Assess for breast engorgement and for an inverted nipple. Advise the mother to end the feeding when the baby's sucking slows, before he has a chance to chew on the nipple. Remove the baby from the breast by placing a finger between the baby's gums to ensure the suction is broken. Suggest Jane can apply ice to the nipples and areola for a few minutes before feeding to promote nipple erectness and numb the tissue initially. Air-dry the breasts after feeding to toughen the nipples and promote healing.
3. What suggestion do you give Jane regarding supplemental bottle-feedings?	Answer: Supplemental bottle-feeding for the breastfeeding infant may weaken or confuse the infant's sucking reflex or decrease the infant's interest in breastfeeding. Infants suck differently on a rubber nipple and tend to push the mother's nipple out of their mouth in subsequent breastfeeding attempts. This is frustrating for the mother and baby, so the mother should avoid introducing the bottle until breastfeeding is well established.
4. Explain your assessment of Jane's abdominal incision and provide suggestions for healing.	Answer: Assess the incision for signs of infection such as redness, severe pain, edema, poor tissue approximation, and drainage. Expect some bruising and tenderness. Advise Jane to keep the incision clean and dry. She should allow warm water to flow over the incision in the shower and pat dry the incision. Suggest bringing the baby downstairs during the day to decrease the need to climb stairs frequently. Ask if her husband could carry the bassinet down for the day and up at night. Encourage Jane to rest when the baby sleeps.
5. How would you discuss the baby's voiding patterns to ensure adequate hydration?	Answer: Infants normally void five to eight times a day. Fewer than six to eight wet diapers may indicate the newborn needs more breastfeeding sessions.

CHAPTER 37

CRITICAL THINKING IN ACTION: PERINATAL GRIEF

Marguerite, a 25-year-old, married woman is admitted for delivery of a stillborn baby girl. Through tears, Marguerite shares that she has named the baby, Alicia, after her grandmother. She has already decorated the nursery with the many gifts she received at her baby shower. Marguerite apologizes for "crying so much" and frequently expresses a fear that her husband, John, may blame her for Alicia's death because she worked until the time of the final ultrasound. She wonders aloud if he would be right. She communicates a desire to see and hold Alicia, but is very fearful of how the baby will look and whether people will think that she is morbid for wanting to hold a dead baby. Marguerite apologizes again for crying and shares that she does not know who else to talk to because no one seems to understand what she is going through.

Marguerite is displaying an obvious attachment to her baby and exhibiting very normal grief reactions. How can Marguerite's nurse aid her in normalizing her emotional reactions, viewing and holding her infant, opening dialogue with her husband, and procuring a comprehensive support system?

1. What should the nurse helping families through the crisis of perinatal loss know about grief in general?	Answer: The nurse should know that grief is a natural reaction to loss and encompasses the emotional, cognitive, physical, and spiritual realms. Every grief reaction is as unique as the person experiencing it and no two people will grieve the same way, not even in the same family. There is no right or wrong way to grieve and there is no timetable for completion. There are a variety of factors which will affect a person's response to loss including, but not limited to, age, gender, culture, religion, previous loss history, individual and family personality traits, resilience and hardiness. The safest intervention for responding to grieving individuals will never assume or judge; curiosity is okay, avoidance is not.
2. What should the nurse know about the unique nature of perinatal loss?	Answer: The nurse should know that the grief experienced with perinatal loss is generally more guilt and anger prone, intense and longer lasting. There is more potential for traumatic and complicated grief and finding meaning in the loss is important. The reaction to perinatal loss is based upon the level of attachment, not the length of time the client was pregnant and perinatal loss is often disenfranchised because of this common misconception. Parents having experienced a previous pregnancy loss will generally be more anxious, fearful, and emotional during a subsequent pregnancy.

3. What types of nursing behaviors will facilitate the family's mourning process?	Answer: The nurse should be available and genuine to the grieving family. The nurse should display a nonjudgmental, accepting, and compassionate attitude, treating the family with respect at all times. Care should be taken to avoid the use of unfamiliar medical jargon and clichés when responding to loss. Normalization of the process is crucial and can be facilitated by the reassurance of nonculpability, acceptance of reactions, and affirmation of positive aspects of completed parenting (such as plans made, naming of the baby, planned interactions with other family members).

CHAPTER 38

CRITICAL THINKING IN ACTION: HIV-POSITIVE MOTHER AND INFANT: SUPPORTIVE CARE

Betty Jones, a 32-year-old G4 P2012, is admitted to the postpartum unit after a precipitous birth of a preterm (35 weeks' gestation) 4-lb baby girl followed by a postpartum tubal ligation. Betty's vital signs and postpartum assessment are within normal limits. She has an abdominal dressing which is dry and intact and she is able to void. Her IV with 10 units of Pitocin is infusing well in her lower left arm. She admits to 3 on a pain scale of 10. Betty admits to active use of crack cocaine throughout her pregnancy, and smoked it most recently 5 hours before she gave birth. She is HIV positive with a CD4 count of 726 cells/mm3 and was treated with zidovudine during the pregnancy, labor, and birth. She also has a history of genital herpes and had been treated for chlamydia during the pregnancy. Her infant has been admitted to the special care nursery because of her preterm status. Betty anticipates her baby will be taken into foster care when discharged from the nursery. Wishing to establish as much of a relationship with her infant as possible before that happens, she asks if she can breastfeed the baby while she is in the hospital.

1. What is your response to Betty's request to breastfeed her infant?	Answer: HIV is present in breast milk. Vertical transmission is doubled by breastfeeding. This concern overrides Betty's concern about attachment. You can increase her sense of involvement with her baby with encouraging her to visit her baby and assist with bottle feedings, changing diapers, and touching and holding her baby. Betty's desire to parent her baby would be best supported by seeking drug treatment and carefully following an HIV medical regimen.
2. Over the course of the first postpartum day, Betty appears lethargic and spends most of her time sleeping. After her evening visitors leave, you observe that she is highly energetic and excitable. Would urine testing be useful to help determine if Betty has used cocaine this evening?	Answer: Urine toxicology would not be useful. By her own report, Betty has used cocaine prior to her admission. Other observations may be more useful such as increase in blood pressure and pulse. Your suspicions necessitate further follow-up including social, community, and drug rehabilitation services.
3. Discuss supportive nursing care for infants born of HIV-positive mothers.	Answer: Care involves providing comfort, keeping the newborn well nourished and protected from opportunistic infections, providing good skin care to prevent skin rashes, and facilitating growth, development, and attachment. Caregivers should wear gloves during all diaper changes and examinations. Handwashing is crucial for all newborns at risk for AIDS.
4. Betty wishes for an early discharge from the hospital. What physical criteria must be met before leaving the hospital?	Answer: Betty has to have normal vital signs, appropriate involution of the uterus, and appropriate amount of lochia without evidence of infection. Episiotomy is approximated with a decrease in edema or bruising. She is able to void, pass flatus, and take fluids and food without difficulty. She has received rubella vaccine or RhoGAM if indicated.
5. Discuss when she should contact her physician/CNM after her discharge.	Answer: Betty should notify her caregiver if she experiences a sudden, persistent, or spiking fever; a change in the character of the lochia, such as a foul odor, bright-red bleeding, passage of large clots, or excessive amounts; evidence of increased breast tenderness with reddened areas accompanied by malaise; pain in the calf of her leg with tenderness and redness; urinary frequency or burning with urination; or incapacitating postpartal depression.

© 2008 Pearson Education, Inc.

Olds, London, Ladewig, and Davidson's *Maternal-Newborn Nursing & Women's Health Care* (7th Edition)	Page	Davidson, London, and Ladewig's *Maternal-Newborn Nursing & Women's Health Across the Lifespan* (8th Edition)	Page
Human Papilloma Virus/ Condylomata Acuminata	115	Human Papilloma Virus/ Condylomata Acuminata	117
Pediculosis Pubis (Pubic or Crab Lice)	116	Pediculosis Pubis (Pubic or Crab Lice)	117
Scabies	117	Scabies	118
Viral Hepatitis	117	Viral Hepatitis	118
Acquired Immunodeficiency Syndrome (AIDS)	117	Acquired Immunodeficiency Syndrome (AIDS)	119
Nursing Care Management	118	Nursing Care Management	119
Care of the Woman with Pelvic Inflammatory Disease	119	Care of the Woman with an Upper Genital Tract Infection (Pelvic Inflammatory Disease)	119
Nursing Care Management	120	Nursing Care Management	120
Care of the Woman with a Urinary Tract Infection	120	Care of the Woman with a Urinary Tract Infection	121
Lower Urinary Tract Infection (Cystitis and Urethritis)	121	Lower Urinary Tract Infection (Cystitis and Urethritis)	121
Upper Urinary Tract Infection (Pyelonephritis)	121	Upper Urinary Tract Infection (Pyelonephritis)	122
Nursing Care Management	122	Nursing Care Management	122
Chapter 7: Women's Health Problems	125	Chapter 7: Women's Health Problems	126
Care of the Woman with a Disorder of the Breast	126	Care of the Woman with a Disorder of the Breast	127
Screening Techniques for the Breasts	126	Screening Techniques for the Breasts	127
Benign Breast Conditions	130	Benign Breast Conditions	130
Malignant Breast Disease	131	Malignant Breast Disease	132
Nursing Care Management	134	Nursing Care Management	134
Care of the Woman with Endometriosis	134	Care of the Woman with Endometriosis	145
Nursing Care Management	135	Nursing Care Management	146
Care of the Woman with Toxic Shock Syndrome	135	Care of the Woman with Toxic Shock Syndrome	142
Nursing Care Management	136	Nursing Care Management	143
Care of the Woman During a Pelvic Examination	136	Care of the woman During a Pelvic Examination	135
Vulvar Self-Examination	136	Vulvar Self-Examination	136
Care of the Woman with Vulvitis	138	Care of the Woman with Vulvitis	138
Nursing Care Management	140	Nursing Care Management	138
Care of the Woman with an Abnormal Finding During Pelvic Examination	140	Care of the Woman with an Abnormal Finding During Pelvic Examination	138
Vulvar Lesion	140	Vulvar Lesion	138
Cervicitis	141	Cervicitis	139
Abnormal Pap Smear Results	141	Abnormal Pap Smear Results	139
Abnormal Uterine Bleeding	145	Abnormal Uterine Bleeding	143
Ovarian Masses	145	Ovarian Masses	144
Uterine Masses	146	Uterine Masses	145
Nursing Care Management	147	Nursing Care Management	145
		Care of the Woman with Polycystic Ovarian Syndrome	147
		Nursing Care Management	149
Care of the Woman with Pelvic Relaxation	147	Care of the Woman with Pelvic Relaxation	149
Cystocele	147	Cystocele	149

Olds, London, Ladewig, and Davidson's *Maternal-Newborn Nursing & Women's Health Care* (7th Edition)	Page	Davidson, London, and Ladewig's *Maternal-Newborn Nursing & Women's Health Across the Lifespan* (8th Edition)	Page
Vegetarianism	418	Vegetarianism	431
Factors Influencing Nutrition	419	Factors Influencing Nutrition	431
Eating Disorders	420	Eating Disorders	434
Lactase Deficiency (Lactose Intolerance)	421	Lactase Deficiency (Lactose Intolerance)	432
Pica	421	Pica	435
Common Discomforts of Pregnancy	421	Common Discomforts of Pregnancy	432
		Use of Artificial Sweeteners	432
		Mercury in Fish	433
		Salmonella and Listeria Infection	433
Cultural, Ethnic, and Religious Influences	421	Cultural, Ethnic, and Religious Influences	433
Psychosocial Factors	422	Psychosocial Factors	434
The Pregnant Adolescent	422	Nutritional Care of the Pregnant Adolescent	434
Nutritional Concerns	422	Special Nutrient Concerns	434
		Dietary Patterns	437
Counseling Issues	424	Counseling Issues	437
Postpartum Nutrition	424	Postpartum Nutrition	437
Postpartal Nutritional Status	424	Postpartal Nutritional Status	437
Nutritional Care of Formula-Feeding Mothers	424	Nutritional Care of	437
Nutritional Care of Breastfeeding Mothers	425	Nutritional Care of Breastfeeding Mothers	438
Counseling Issues	425	Counseling Issues	438
Nursing Care Management	425	Nursing Care Management	438
Chapter 19: Pregnancy at Risk: Pregestational Problems	431	Chapter 19: Pregnancy at Risk:	444
Care of the Woman Practicing Substance Abuse	432	Care of the Woman Practicing	445
Substances Commonly Abused During Pregnancy	433	Substances Commonly Abused	446
Clinical Therapy	436	Clinical Therapy	449
Nursing Care Management	436	Nursing Care Management	449
Care of the Women with Diabetes Mellitus	437	Care of the Women with Diabetes Mellitus	450
Normal Glucose Homeostasis	437	Normal Glucose Homeostasis	450
Carbohydrate Metabolism in Normal Pregnancy	437	Carbohydrate Metabolism in	450
Pathophysiology of Diabetes Mellitus	437	Pathophysiology of Diabetes Mellitus	450
Classification of Diabetes Mellitus	438	Classification of Diabetes Mellitus	450
Influence of Pregnancy on Diabetes	438	Influence of Pregnancy on Diabetes	451
Influence of Diabetes on Pregnancy Outcome	439	Influence of Diabetes on Pregnancy	451
Clinical Therapy	440	Clinical Therapy	452
		Antepartal Management of Diabetes	454
		Intrapartal Management of Diabetes Mellitus	455
		Postpartal Management of Diabetes Mellitus	455
Nursing Care Management	443	Nursing Care Management	456
Care of the Woman with Anemia	447	Care of the Woman with Anemia	461
Iron Deficiency Anemia	447	Iron Deficiency Anemia	461
Nursing Care Management	448	Nursing Care Management	462
Folic Acid Deficiency Anemia	448	Folic Acid Deficiency Anemia	462

Olds, London, Ladewig, and Davidson's *Maternal-Newborn Nursing & Women's Health Care* (7th Edition)	Page	Davidson, London, and Ladewig's *Maternal-Newborn Nursing & Women's Health Across the Lifespan* (8th Edition)	Page
Maternal Risks	483	Maternal Risks	496
Fetal-Neonatal Risks	483	Fetal-Neonatal Risks	496
Clinical Therapy	483	Clinical Therapy	496
Nursing Care Management	486	Nursing Care Management	501
Care of the Woman with a Hypertensive Disorder	490	Care of the Woman with a Hypertensive Disorder	504
Preeclampsia and Eclampsia	490	Preeclampsia and Eclampsia	504
Nursing Care Management	498	Nursing Care Management	511
Chronic Hypertension	504	Chronic Hypertension	519
Hypertension with Superimposed Preeclampsia	505	Hypertension with Superimposed Preeclampsia	520
Gestational Hypertension	505	Gestational Hypertension	520
Care of the Woman at Risk for Rh Sensitization	505	Care of the Woman at Risk for Rh Sensitization	520
Fetal-Neonatal Risks	505	Fetal-Neonatal Risks	521
Screening for Rh Imcompatibility and Sensitization	506	Screening for Rh Imcompatibility and Sensitization	521
Clinical Therapy	507	Clinical Therapy	522
Nursing Care Management	508	Nursing Care Management	523
Care of the Woman at Risk Due to ABO Incompatibility	509	Care of the Woman at Risk Due to ABO Incompatibility	524
Care of the Woman Requiring Surgery During Pregnancy	509	Care of the Woman Requiring Surgery During Pregnancy	526
Clinical Therapy	510	Clinical Therapy	526
Nursing Care Management	511	Nursing Care Management	526
Care of the Woman Suffering Trauma from an Accident	512	Care of the Woman Suffering Trauma from an Accident	527
Clinical Therapy	512	Clinical Therapy	527
Nursing Care Management	513	Nursing Care Management	528
Care of the Battered Pregnant Woman	513	Care of the Battered Pregnant Woman	529
Care of the Woman with a Perinatal Infection Affecting the Fetus	514	Care of the Woman with a Perinatal Infection Affecting the Fetus	529
Toxoplasmosis	514	Toxoplasmosis	529
Nursing Care Management	515	Nursing Care Management	530
Rubella	515	Rubella	530
Nursing Care Management	516	Nursing Care Management	531
Cytomegalovirus	516	Cytomegalovirus	531
Herpes Simplex Virus	517	Herpes Simplex Virus	532
Nursing Care Management	517	Nursing Care Management	532
Group B Streptococcal Infection	518	Group B Streptococcal Infection	533
Human B19 Parvovirus	519	Human B19 Parvovirus	534
Other Infections in Pregnancy	519	Other Infections in Pregnancy	534
Chapter 21: Assessment of Fetal Well-Being	525	Chapter 21: Assessment of Fetal Well-Being	541
Psychologic Reactions to Antenatal Testing	526	Psychologic Reactions to Antenatal Testing	542
Nursing Care Management	526	Nursing Care Management	542
Ultrasound	527	Ultrasound	543
Extent of Ultrasound Exams	528	Extent of Ultrasound Exams	544
Methods of Ultrasound Scanning	528	Methods of Ultrasound Scanning	544

© 2008 Pearson Education, Inc.

Olds, London, Ladewig, and Davidson's *Maternal-Newborn Nursing & Women's Health Care* (7th Edition)	Page	Davidson, London, and Ladewig's *Maternal-Newborn Nursing & Women's Health Across the Lifespan* (8th Edition)	Page
Care of the Woman and Fetus at Risk for Precipitous Labor and Birth	699	Care of the Woman and Fetus at Risk for	722
Clinical Therapy	700	Clinical Therapy	722
Nursing Care Management	700	Nursing Care Management	722
Care of the Woman with Postterm Pregnancy	700	Care of the Woman with Postterm Pregnancy	723
Maternal Risks	700	Maternal Risks	723
Fetal-Neonatal Risks	701	Fetal-Neonatal Risks	723
Clinical Therapy	701	Clinical Therapy	723
Nursing Care Management	701	Nursing Care Management	724
Care of the Woman and Fetus at Risk Due to Fetal Malposition	702	Care of the Woman and Fetus at Risk	724
Maternal-Fetal-Neonatal Risks	702	Maternal-Fetal-Neonatal Risks	724
Clinical Therapy	702	Clinical Therapy	724
Nursing Care Management	702	Nursing Care Management	726
Care of the Woman and Fetus at Risk Due to Fetal Malpresentation	704	Care of the Woman and Fetus at Risk	726
Brow Presentation	704	Brow Presentation	726
		Clinical Therapy	726
Nursing Care Management	705	Nursing Care Management	727
Face Presentation	705	Face Presentation	728
Nursing Care Management	706	Nursing Care Management	729
Breech Presentation	706	Breech Presentation	729
Nursing Care Management	708	Nursing Care Management	730
Shoulder Presentation (Transverse Lie) of a Single Fetus	709	Shoulder Presentation (Transverse Lie) of a Single Fetus	731
Nursing Care Management	709	Nursing Care Management	732
Compound Presentation	710	Compound Presentation	732
Care of the Woman and Fetus at Risk Due to Macrosomia	710	Care of the Woman and Fetus at Risk Due to Macrosomia	732
Clinical Therapy	710	Clinical Therapy	733
Nursing Care Management	711	Nursing Care Management	733
Care of the Woman with a Multiple Gestation	712	Care of the Woman with a Multiple Gestation	734
Embryology of Multiple Gestation	712	Embryology of Multiple Gestation	734
Pregnancy Loss in Multiple Gestation	712	Pregnancy Loss in Multiple Gestation	734
Implications	713	Implications	734
Clinical Therapy	714	Clinical Therapy	734
Nursing Care Management	715	Nursing Care Management	737
Care of the Woman and Fetus in the Presence of Nonreassuring Fetal Status	717	Care of the Woman and Fetus in the Presence of Nonreassuring Fetal Status	739
Clinical Therapy	717	Clinical Therapy	740
Nursing Care Management	717	Nursing Care Management	740
Care of the Woman and Fetus at Risk Due to Placental Problems	718	Care of the Woman and Fetus at Risk Due to Placental Problems	741
Abruptio Placentae	719	Abruptio Placentae	741
Nursing Care Management	721	Nursing Care Management	743
Placenta Previa	721	Placenta Previa	743

Olds, London, Ladewig, and Davidson's *Maternal-Newborn Nursing & Women's Health Care* (7th Edition)	Page	Davidson, London, and Ladewig's *Maternal-Newborn Nursing & Women's Health Across the Lifespan* (8th Edition)	Page
Temperature	805	Temperature	830
Skin Characteristics	806	Skin Characteristics	831
Birthmarks	807	Birthmarks	833
Head	808	Head	833
		Hair	835
Face	810	Face	835
		Eyes	836
		Nose	836
		Mouth	838
Neck	813	Neck	838
Chest	813	Chest	838
Cry	813	Cry	838
Respiration	813	Respiration	838
Heart	814	Heart	839
Abdomen	815	Abdomen	840
Umbilical Cord	815	Umbilical Cord	841
Genitals	816	Genitals	841
Anus	816	Anus	842
Extremities	816	Extremities	842
Back	818	Back	843
Assessment of Neurologic Status	818	Assessment of Neurologic Status	843
Newborn Physical Assessment Guide	821	Newborn Physical Assessment Guide	846
Newborn Behavioral Assessment	821	Newborn Behavioral Assessment	846
Chapter 30: The Normal Newborn: Needs and Care	838	Chapter 30: The Normal Newborn: Needs and Care	862
Nursing Care During Admission and the First Four Hours of Life	839	Nursing Care During Admission and the First Four Hours of Life	863
Nursing Assessment and Diagnosis	839	Nursing Assessment and Diagnosis	863
Nursing Plan and Implementation	839	Nursing Plan and Implementation	863
Evaluation	848	Evaluation	872
Nursing Care of Newborn Following Transition	848	Nursing Management of the Newborn Following Transition	872
Nursing Diagnosis	848	Nursing Diagnosis	872
Nursing Plan and Implementation	848	Nursing Plan and Implementation	872
Evaluation	855	Evaluation	878
Nursing Care in Preparation for Discharge	855	Nursing Management in Preparation for Discharge	878
Parent Teaching	855	Parent Teaching	879
Evaluation	862	Evaluation	887
Chapter 31: Newborn Nutrition	865	Chapter 31: Newborn Nutrition	890
Nutritional Needs of the Newborn	866	Nutritional Needs and Milk Composition	891
		Dietary Reference Intakes	891
		Growth	891
		Fluid	892
		Energy	893
		Fats	893
		Carbohydrates	893
		Protein	894
		Vitamins, Minerals, and Trace Elements	894

Olds, London, Ladewig, and Davidson's *Maternal-Newborn Nursing & Women's Health Care* (7th Edition)	Page	Davidson, London, and Ladewig's *Maternal-Newborn Nursing & Women's Health Across the Lifespan* (8th Edition)	Page
Respiratory Distress Syndrome	943	Respiratory Distress Syndrome	988
Nursing Care Management	945	Nursing Care Management	990
Transient Tachypnea of the Newborn	947	Transient Tachypnea of the Newborn	996
Nursing Care Management	951	Nursing Care Management	997
Meconium Aspiration Syndrome	951	Care of the Newborn with Meconium Aspiration Syndrome	997
Nursing Care Management	953	Nursing Care Management	999
Persistent Pulmonary Hypertension of the Newborn	954	Persistent Pulmonary Hypertension of the Newborn	1000
Nursing Care Management	954	Nursing Care Management	1000
Care of the Newborn with Complications Due to Respiratory Therapy	955	Care of the Newborn with Complications Due to Respiratory Therapy	1001
Pulmonary Interstitial Emphysema	955	Pulmonary Interstitial Emphysema	1001
Pneumothorax	955	Pneumothorax	1001
Bronchopulmonary Dysplasia/ Chronic Lung Disease	956	Bronchopulmonary Dysplasia/ Chronic Lung Disease	1002
Nursing Care Management	956	Nursing Care Management	1002
Care of the Newborn with Cold Stress	958	Care of the Newborn with Cold Stress	1004
Nursing Care Management	959	Nursing Care Management	1004
Care of the Newborn with Hypoglycemia	959	Care of the Newborn with Hypoglycemia	1005
Clinical Therapy	959	Clinical Therapy	1005
Nursing Care Management	960	Nursing Care Management	1006
Care of the Newborn with Jaundice	963	Care of the Newborn with Jaundice	1008
		Physiologic Jaundice	1009
Pathophysiology	963	Pathophysiology of Hyperbilirubinemia	1009
Causes of Hyperbilirubinemia	963	Causes of Hyperbilirubinemia	1009
Clinical Therapy	964	Clinical Therapy	1010
Nursing Care Management	966	Nursing Care Management	1012
Care of the Newborn with Anemia	971	Care of the Newborn with Anemia	1021
Clinical Therapy	971	Clinical Therapy	1021
Nursing Care Management	972	Nursing Care Management	1021
Care of the Newborn with Polycythemia	972	Care of the Newborn with Polycythemia	1021
Clinical Therapy	972	Clinical Therapy	1021
Nursing Care Management	972	Nursing Care Management	1021
Care of the Newborn with Infection	973	Care of the Newborn with Infection	1021
Clinical Therapy	973	Clinical Therapy	1024
Nursing Care Management	975	Nursing Care Management	1026
Care of the Family with Birth of an At-Risk Newborn	977	Care of the Family with Birth of an At-Risk Newborn	1027
Parental Responses	977	Parental Responses	1027
Developmental Consequences	978	Developmental Consequences	1028
Nursing Care Management	978	Nursing Care Management	1028
Considerations for the Nurse Who Works with At-Risk Newborns	986	Considerations for the Nurse Who Works with At-Risk Newborns	1035
Part Seven: Postpartum	989	Unit 7: Postpartum	1039
Chapter 34: Postpartal Adaptation and Nursing Assessment	990	Chapter 34: Postpartal Family Adaptation and Nursing Assessment	1040
Postpartal Physical Adaptations	991	Postpartum Physical Adaptations	1041